General Ophthalmology

fifteenth edition

. . . Now do you not see that the eye embraces the beauty of the whole world? It is the lord of astronomy and the maker of cosmography; it counsels and corrects all the arts of mankind; it leads men to the different parts of the world; it is the prince of mathematics, and the sciences founded on it are absolutely certain. It has measured the distances and sizes of the stars; it has found the elements and their locations; it . . . has given birth to architecture, and to perspective, and to the divine art of painting. Oh excellent thing, superior to all others created by God! . . . What peoples, what tongues will fully describe your true function? The eye is the window of the human body through which it feels its way and enjoys the beauty of the world. Owing to the eye the soul is content to stay in its bodily prison, for without it such bodily prison is torture.

—Leonardo da Vinci (1452–1519)

General Ophthalmology

fifteenth edition

Daniel Vaughan, MD
Clinical Professor of Ophthalmology
University of California, San Francisco
Governor, Francis I. Proctor Foundation for
   Research in Ophthalmology, San Francisco

Taylor Asbury, MD
Professor of Ophthalmology
Interim Director, Department of Ophthalmology
College of Medicine
University of Cincinnati, Ohio

Paul Riordan-Eva, FRCS, FRCOphth
Consultant Ophthalmologist
Bromley Hospitals NHS Trust, Kent, UK
Honorary Consultant Neuro-ophthalmologist
National Hospital for Neurology and Neurosurgery
   and King's College Hospital, London, UK

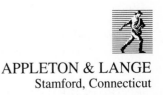

APPLETON & LANGE
Stamford, Connecticut

www.appletonlange.com

99 00 01 02 03 / 10 9 8 7 6 5 4 3 2 1

Prentice Hall International (UK) Limited, *London*
Prentice Hall of Australia Pty. Limited, *Sydney*
Prentice Hall Canada, Inc., *Toronto*
Prentice Hall Hispanoamericana, S.A., *Mexico*
Prentice Hall of India Private Limited, *New Delhi*
Prentice Hall of Japan, Inc., *Tokyo*
Simon & Schuster Asia Pte. Ltd., *Singapore*
Editora Prentice Hall do Brasil Ltda., *Rio de Janeiro*
Prentice Hall, *Upper Saddle River, New Jersey*

ISBN: 0-8385-3137-7
ISBN: 0891-2084

Acquisitions Editor: Shelley Reinhardt
Development Editor: Jim Ransom
Production Editor: Elizabeth Ryan
Associate Art Manager: Maggie Belis Darrow
Cover Designer: Aimee Nordin
Illustrators: Teshin Associates
            Laurel V. Schaubert

ISBN 0-8385-3137-7

90000

9 780838 531372

PRINTED IN THE UNITED STATES OF AMERICA

This edition of
General Ophthalmology
is dedicated to
Dr. Crowell Beard

Contents

Authors

Taylor Asbury, MD
Professor of Ophthalmology, Interim Director, Department of Ophthalmology, College of Medicine, University of Cincinnati, Ohio
Strabismus; Genetic Aspects of Ocular Disorders; Ocular & Orbital Trauma

Roderick Biswell, MD
Associate Clinical Professor of Ophthalmology, University of California, San Francisco
Cornea

David F. Chang, MD
Associate Clinical Professor of Ophthalmology, University of California, San Francisco
Ophthalmologic Examination

J. Brooks Crawford, MD
Clinical Professor of Ophthalmology, University of California, San Francisco
Lids, Lacrimal Apparatus, & Tears; Conjunctiva; Uveal Tract & Sclera; Retina

Emmett T. Cunningham, Jr., MD, PhD, MPH
Assistant Professor and Co-Director, Uveitis Service, Department of Ophthalmology, and Francis I. Proctor Foundation for Research in Ophthalmology, University of California, San Francisco
Internet: emmett@itsa.ucsf.edu
Uveal Tract & Sclera

Philip P. Ellis, MD
Professor, Department of Ophthalmology, University of Colorado Health Sciences Center, Denver
Ophthalmic Therapeutics

Eleanor E. Faye, MD, FACS
Ophthalmologic Consultant, Continuing Education, The Lighthouse, Inc., New York; Attending Ophthalmologist Emeritus, Manhattan Eye and Ear Hospital, New York
Internet: efaye@lighthouse.org
Low Vision; Appendix I. Visual Standards; Appendix II. Practical Factors in Illumination; Appendix III. Resources for Special Services for the Blind & Visually Impaired

Frederick T. Fraunfelder, MD
Professor, Department of Ophthalmology, Casey Eye Institute, Oregon Health Sciences University, Portland
Internet: fraunfel@ohsu.edu
Ophthalmic Therapeutics

Douglas R. Fredrick, MD
Assistant Clinical Professor of Ophthalmology, University of California, San Francisco
Strabismus; Special Subjects of Pediatric Interest

Elizabeth M. Graham, FRCP, FRCOphth
Consultant Medical Ophthalmologist, St. Thomas Hospital and National Hospital for Neurology and Neurosurgery, London, UK
Ocular Disorders Associated With Systemic Diseases

Robert A. Hardy, MD
Associate Clinical Professor of Ophthalmology, University of California School of Medicine, San Francisco; Chief of Ophthalmology, Merrithew Memorial Hospital, Martinez, California
Retina

Richard A. Harper, MD
Assistant Professor of Ophthalmology, University of Arkansas for Medical Sciences, Little Rock
Internet: raharper@acer.uams.edu
Lens

William G. Hodge, MD, MPH, FRCS(C)
Assistant Professor, University of Ottawa Eye Institute, Ottawa, Ontario, Canada
Internet: whodge@ogh.on.ca
Immunologic Diseases of the Eye

William F. Hoyt, MD
Professor of Ophthalmology, Neurology, and Neurosurgery, University of California, San Francisco
Neuro-Ophthalmology

Connor O'Malley, MD
San Jose, California
Internet: ocutom.conor@aol.com
Vitreous

Paul Riordan-Eva, FRCS, FRCOphth
Consultant Ophthalmologist, Bromley Hospitals NHS Trust, Kent, UK; Honorary Consultant Neuro-Ophthalmologist, National Hospital for Neurology and Neurosurgery and King's College Hospital, London, UK
Internet: PaulREva@aol.com
Anatomy & Embryology of the Eye; Glaucoma; Neuro-ophthalmology; Genetic Aspects of Ocular Disorders; Optics & Refraction; Glossary of Terms Relating to the Eye; Abbreviations & Symbols Used in Ophthalmology

Michael D. Sanders, FRCP, FRCS
Consultant Ophthalmologist, National Hospital for Neurology and Neurosurgery, London, UK; Lecturer, University of London
Ocular Disorders Associated With Systemic Diseases

James J. Sanitato, MD
Director of Education, Laser Centers of America, Cincinnati, Ohio
Ocular & Orbital Trauma

Ivan R. Schwab, MD
Professor of Ophthalmology, University of California, Davis
Internet: irschwab@ucdavis.edu
Conjunctiva

John P. Shock, MD
Professor and Chairman, Department of Ophthalmology; Director, Jones Eye Institute, University of Arkansas for Medical Sciences, Little Rock
Internet: jshock@acer.uams.edu
Lens

John H. Sullivan, MD
Clinical Professor of Ophthalmology, University of California, San Francisco
Internet: jsulleye@flash.net
Lids, Lacrimal Apparatus, & Tears; Orbit

Daniel Vaughan, MD
Clinical Professor of Ophthalmology, University of California, San Francisco; Governor, Francis I. Proctor Foundation for Research in Ophthalmology, San Francisco
Glaucoma; Differential Diagnosis of Common Causes of Inflamed Eye

James Berry Wise, MD
Clinical Professor of Ophthalmology, University of Oklahoma, Oklahoma City
Lasers in Ophthalmology

John P. Whitcher, MD, MPH
Professor of Clinical Ophthalmology, University of California, San Francisco; Interim Director, Francis I. Proctor Foundation for Research in Ophthalmology, San Francisco
Lids, Lacrimal Apparatus, & Tears; Preventive Ophthalmology; Blindness

Preface

For four decades, *General Ophthalmology* has served as the most concise, current, and authoritative review of the subject for medical students, ophthalmology residents, practicing ophthalmologists, nurses, optometrists, and colleagues in other fields of medicine and surgery, as well as health related professionals. The fifteenth edition has been revised and updated in keeping with that goal. It contains the following changes from the fourteenth edition:

- Major revisions of the chapters **Uveal Tract & Sclera, Low Vision,** and **Ophthalmic Therapeutics** and **Appendices I–III**
- Significant changes in the chapters **Neuro-ophthalmology, Lasers in Ophthalmology,** and **Ocular Disorders Associated With Systemic Diseases**

As in past revisions, we have relied on the assistance of many authorities in special fields who have given us the benefit of their advice. In particular, we wish to thank our new author, Emmett T. Cunningham, Jr.

Daniel Vaughan, MD
Taylor Asbury, MD
Paul Riordan-Eva, FRCS, FRCOphth

November, 1998

Acknowledgments

Mary Elaine Armacost
Arthur Asbury
Crowell Beard
Laurie Campbell
Patricia Cunnane
William Edward
Hans Gassmann
Margaret Henry
Harry Hind
Geraldine Hruby
Marianne Huslid

Vicente Jocson
Heinrich König
Charles Leiter
Barbara Miller
G. Richard O'Connor
Patricia Pascoe
Kenneth Rogers
Margot Riordan-Eva
Lionel Sorenson
Phillips Thygeson

Anatomy & Embryology of the Eye

1

Paul Riordan-Eva, FRCS, FRCOphth

A thorough understanding of the anatomy of the eye, orbit, visual pathways, upper cranial nerves, and central pathways for the control of eye movements is a prerequisite for proper interpretation of diseases having ocular manifestations. Furthermore, such anatomic knowledge is essential to the proper planning and safe execution of ocular and orbital surgery. Whereas most knowledge of these matters is based on anatomic dissections, either postmortem or during surgery, noninvasive techniques—particularly MRI and ultrasonography—are increasingly providing additional information. Investigating the embryology of the eye is clearly a more difficult area because of the relative scarcity of suitable human material, and thus there is still great reliance on animal studies, with the inherent difficulties in inferring parallels in human development. Nevertheless, a great deal is known about the embryology of the human eye, and—together with the recent expansion in

molecular genetics—this has led to a much deeper understanding of developmental anomalies of the eye.

I. NORMAL ANATOMY

THE ORBIT
(Figures 1–1 and 1–2)

The orbital cavity is schematically represented as a pyramid of four walls that converge posteriorly. The medial walls of the right and left orbit are parallel and are separated by the nose. In each orbit, the lateral and medial walls form an angle of 45 degrees, which re-

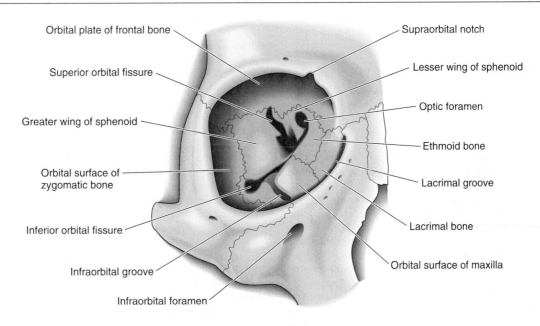

Figure 1–1. Anterior view of bones of right orbit.

1

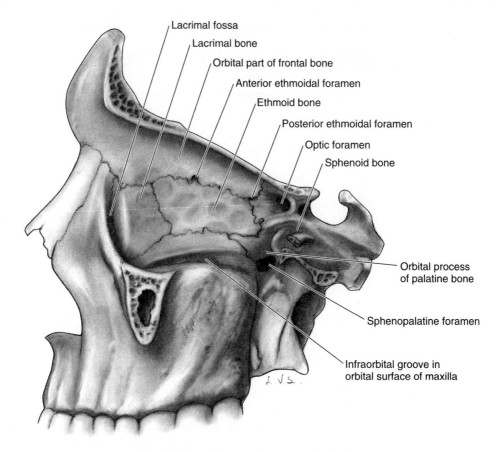

Lacrimal fossa
Lacrimal bone
Orbital part of frontal bone
Anterior ethmoidal foramen
Ethmoid bone
Posterior ethmoidal foramen
Optic foramen
Sphenoid bone

Orbital process
of palatine bone

Sphenopalatine foramen

Infraorbital groove in
orbital surface of maxilla

Figure 1–2. Medial view of bony wall of left orbit.

sults in a right angle between the two lateral walls. The orbit is compared to the shape of a pear, with the optic nerve representing its stem. The anterior circumference is somewhat smaller in diameter than the region just within the rim, which makes a sturdy protective margin.

The volume of the adult orbit is approximately 30 mL, and the eyeball occupies only about one-fifth of the space. Fat and muscle account for the bulk of the remainder.

The anterior limit of the orbital cavity is the **orbital septum,** which acts as a barrier between the eyelids and orbit (see below).

The orbits are related to the frontal sinus above, the maxillary sinus below, and the ethmoid and sphenoid sinuses medially. The thin orbital floor is easily damaged by direct trauma to the globe, resulting in a "blowout" fracture with herniation of orbital contents into the maxillary antrum. Infection within the sphenoid and ethmoid sinuses can erode the paper-thin medial wall (lamina papyracea) and involve the contents of the orbit. Defects in the roof (eg, neurofibromatosis) may result in visible pulsations of the globe transmitted from the brain.

Orbital Walls

The roof of the orbit is composed principally of the orbital plate of the **frontal bone.** The lacrimal gland is located in the lacrimal fossa in the anterior lateral aspect of the roof. Posteriorly, the lesser wing of the **sphenoid bone** containing the optic canal completes the roof.

The lateral wall is separated from the roof by the superior orbital fissure, which divides the lesser from the greater wing of the **sphenoid bone.** The anterior portion of the lateral wall is formed by the orbital surface of the **zygomatic (malar) bone.** This is the strongest part of the bony orbit. Suspensory ligaments, the lateral palpebral tendon, and check ligaments have connective tissue attachments to the lateral orbital tubercle.

The orbital floor is separated from the lateral wall by the inferior orbital fissure. The orbital plate of the **maxilla** forms the large central area of the floor and is the region where blowout fractures most frequently occur. The frontal process of the **maxilla** medially and the **zygomatic bone** laterally complete the inferior orbital rim. The orbital process of the **palatine bone** forms a small triangular area in the posterior floor.

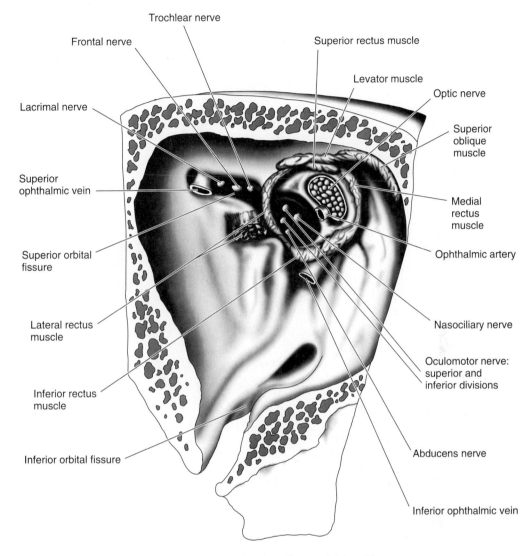

Figure 1–3. Anterior view of apex of right orbit.

The boundaries of the medial wall are less distinct. The **ethmoid bone** is paper-thin but thickens anteriorly as it meets the **lacrimal bone.** The body of the **sphenoid** forms the most posterior aspect of the medial wall, and the angular process of the **frontal bone** forms the upper part of the posterior lacrimal crest. The lower portion of the posterior lacrimal crest is made up of the **lacrimal bone.** The anterior lacrimal crest is easily palpated through the lid and is composed of the frontal process of the **maxilla.** The lacrimal groove lies between the two crests and contains the lacrimal sac.

Orbital Apex
(Figure 1–3)

The apex of the orbit is the entry portal for all nerves and vessels to the eye and the site of origin of all extraocular muscles except the inferior oblique. The **superior orbital fissure** lies between the body and the greater and lesser wings of the sphenoid bone. The superior ophthalmic vein and the lacrimal, frontal, and trochlear nerves pass through the lateral portion of the fissure that lies outside the annulus of Zinn. The superior and inferior divisions of the oculomotor nerve and the abducens and nasociliary nerves pass through the medial portion of the fissure within the annulus of Zinn. The optic nerve and ophthalmic artery pass through the optic canal, which also lies within the annulus of Zinn. The inferior ophthalmic vein may pass through any part of the superior orbital fissure, including the portion adjacent to the body of the sphenoid that lies inferomedial to the annulus of Zinn. The inferior ophthalmic vein frequently joins the superior ophthalmic vein before exiting the orbit.

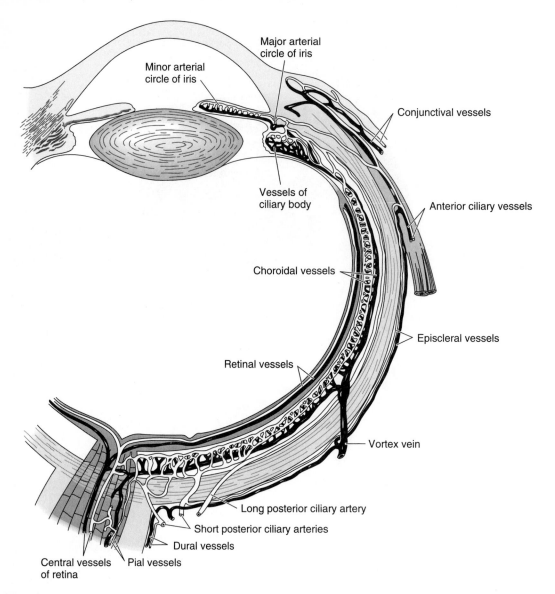

Figure 1–4. Vascular supply to the eye. All arterial branches originate with the ophthalmic artery. Venous drainage is through the cavernous sinus and the pterygoid plexus.

Blood Supply
(Figures 1–4 to 1–6)

The principal arterial supply of the orbit and its structures derives from the ophthalmic artery, the first major branch of the intracranial portion of the internal carotid artery. This branch passes beneath the optic nerve and accompanies it through the optic canal into the orbit. The first intraorbital branch is the central retinal artery, which enters the optic nerve about 8–15 mm behind the globe. Other branches of the ophthalmic artery include the lacrimal artery, supplying the lacrimal gland and upper eyelid; muscular branches to the various muscles of the orbit; long and short posterior ciliary arteries; medial palpebral arteries to both eyelids; and the supraorbital and supratrochlear arteries. The short posterior ciliary arteries supply the choroid and parts of the optic nerve. The two long posterior ciliary arteries supply the ciliary body and anastomose with each other and with the anterior ciliary arteries to form the major arterial circle of the iris. The anterior ciliary arteries are derived from the muscular branches to the rectus muscles. They supply the anterior sclera, episclera, limbus, and conjunctiva as well as contributing to the major arterial circle of the iris. The most anterior branches of the ophthalmic artery contribute to the formation of the

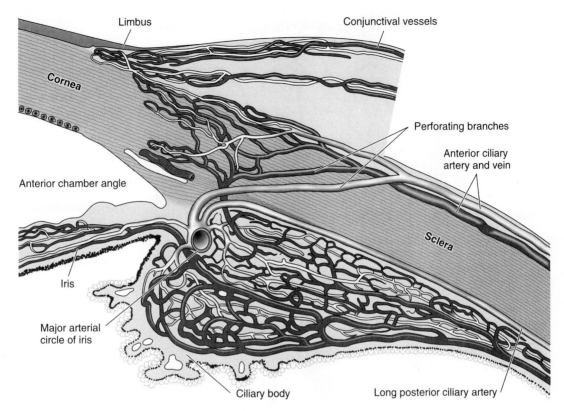

Figure 1–5. Vascular supply of the anterior segment. (Modified, redrawn, and reproduced, with permission, from Wolff E: *Anatomy of the Eye and Orbit,* 4th ed. Blakiston-McGraw, 1954.)

arterial arcades of the eyelids, which make an anastomosis with the external carotid circulation via the facial artery.

The venous drainage of the orbit is primarily through the superior and inferior ophthalmic veins, into which drain the vortex veins, the anterior ciliary veins, and the central retinal vein. The ophthalmic veins communicate with the cavernous sinus via the superior orbital fissure and the pterygoid venous plexus via the inferior orbital fissure. The superior ophthalmic vein is initially formed from the supraorbital and supratrochlear veins and from a branch of the angular vein, all of which drain the skin of the periorbital region. This provides a direct communication between the skin of the face and the cavernous sinus, thus forming the basis of the potentially lethal cavernous sinus thrombosis secondary to superficial infection of the periorbital skin.

THE EYEBALL

The normal adult globe is approximately spherical, with an anteroposterior diameter averaging 24.2 mm.

THE CONJUNCTIVA

The conjunctiva is the thin, transparent mucous membrane that covers the posterior surface of the lids (the palpebral conjunctiva) and the anterior surface of the sclera (the bulbar conjunctiva). It is continuous with the skin at the lid margin (a mucocutaneous junction) and with the corneal epithelium at the limbus.

The **palpebral conjunctiva** lines the posterior surface of the lids and is firmly adherent to the tarsus. At the superior and inferior margins of the tarsus, the conjunctiva is reflected posteriorly (at the superior and inferior fornices) and covers the episcleral tissue to become the bulbar conjunctiva.

The **bulbar conjunctiva** is loosely attached to the orbital septum in the fornices and is folded many times. This allows the eye to move and enlarges the secretory conjunctival surface. (The ducts of the lacrimal gland open into the superior temporal fornix.) Except at the limbus (where Tenon's capsule and the conjunctiva are fused for about 3 mm), the bulbar conjunctiva is loosely attached to Tenon's capsule and the underlying sclera.

A soft, movable, thickened fold of bulbar conjunctiva (the **semilunar fold**) is located at the inner canthus and corresponds to the nictitating membrane of some lower

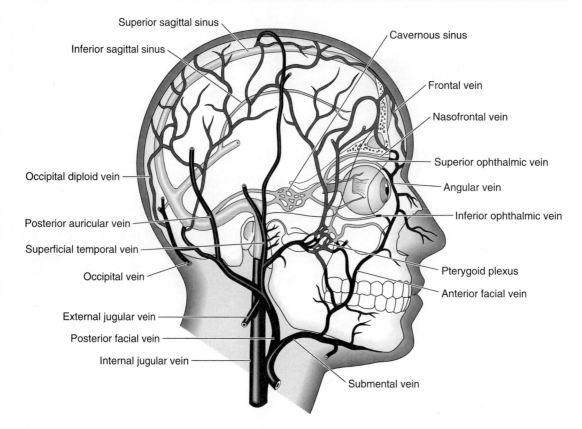

Figure 1–6. Venous drainage system of the eye. (Redrawn and reproduced, with permission, from Wolff E: *Anatomy of the Eye and Orbit,* 4th ed. Blakiston-McGraw, 1954.)

animals. A small, fleshy, epidermoid structure (the **caruncle**) is attached superficially to the inner portion of the semilunar fold and is a transition zone containing both cutaneous and mucous membrane elements.

Histology

The **conjunctival epithelium** consists of two to five layers of stratified columnar epithelial cells, superficial and basal. Conjunctival epithelium near the limbus, over the caruncle, and near the mucocutaneous junctions at the lid margins consists of stratified squamous epithelial cells. The **superficial epithelial cells** contain round or oval mucus-secreting goblet cells. The mucus, as it forms, pushes aside the goblet cell nucleus and is necessary for proper dispersion of the precorneal tear film. The **basal epithelial cells** stain more deeply than the superficial cells and near the limbus may contain pigment.

The **conjunctival stroma** is divided into an adenoid (superficial) layer and a fibrous (deep) layer. The **adenoid layer** contains lymphoid tissue and in some areas may contain "follicle-like" structures without germinal centers. The adenoid layer does not develop until after the first 2 or 3 months of life. This explains why inclusion conjunctivitis of the newborn is papil-

lary in nature rather than follicular and why it later becomes follicular. The **fibrous layer** is composed of connective tissue that attaches to the tarsal plate. This explains the appearance of the papillary reaction in inflammations of the conjunctiva. The fibrous layer is loosely arranged over the globe.

The **accessory lacrimal glands** (glands of Krause and Wolfring), which resemble the lacrimal gland in structure and function, are located in the stroma. Most of the glands of Krause are in the upper fornix, the remaining few in the lower fornix. The glands of Wolfring lie at the superior margin of the upper tarsus.

Blood Supply, Lymphatics, & Nerve Supply

The conjunctival arteries are derived from the anterior ciliary and palpebral arteries. The two arteries anastomose freely and—along with the numerous conjunctival veins that generally follow the arterial pattern—form a considerable conjunctival vascular network. The conjunctival lymphatics are arranged in superficial and deep layers and join with the lymphatics of the eyelids to form a rich lymphatic plexus. The conjunctiva receives its nerve supply from the first (ophthalmic) division of the fifth nerve. It possesses a relatively small number of pain fibers.

TENON'S CAPSULE
(Fascia Bulbi)

Tenon's capsule is a fibrous membrane that envelops the globe from the limbus to the optic nerve. Adjacent to the limbus, the conjunctiva, Tenon's capsule, and the episclera are fused together. More posteriorly, the inner surface of Tenon's capsule lies against the sclera, and its outer aspect is in contact with orbital fat and other structures within the extraocular muscle cone. At the point where Tenon's capsule is pierced by tendons of the extraocular muscles in their passage to their attachments to the globe, it sends a tubular reflection around each of these muscles. These fascial reflections become continuous with the fascia of the muscles, the fused fasciae sending expansions to the surrounding structures and to the orbital bones.

The fascial expansions are quite tough and limit the action of the extraocular muscles and are therefore known as **check ligaments.** The lower segment of Tenon's capsule is thick and fuses with the fascia of the inferior rectus and the inferior oblique muscles to form the suspensory ligament of the eyeball (Lockwood's ligament), upon which the globe rests.

THE SCLERA & EPISCLERA

The **sclera** is the fibrous outer protective coating of the eye consisting almost entirely of collagen (Figure 1–7). It is dense and white and continuous with the cornea anteriorly and the dural sheath of the optic nerve posteriorly. Across the posterior scleral foramen are bands of collagen and elastic tissue, forming the

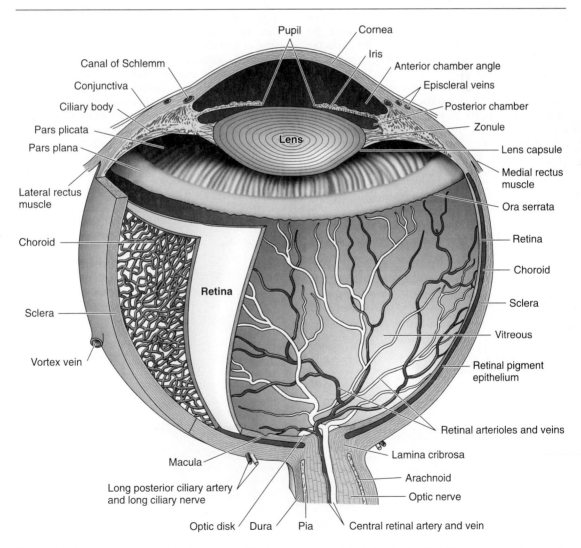

Figure 1–7. Internal structures of the human eye. (Redrawn from an original drawing by Paul Peck and reproduced with permission, from: *The Anatomy of the Eye.* Courtesy of Lederle Laboratories.)

lamina cribrosa, between which pass the axon bundles of the optic nerve. The outer surface of the anterior sclera is covered by a thin layer of fine elastic tissue, the **episclera,** which contains numerous blood vessels that nourish the sclera. The brown pigment layer on the inner surface of the sclera is the lamina fusca, which forms the outer layer of the suprachoroidal space.

At the insertion of the rectus muscles, the sclera is about 0.3 mm thick; elsewhere it is about 0.6 mm thick. Around the optic nerve, the sclera is penetrated by the long and short posterior ciliary arteries and the long and short ciliary nerves (Figure 1–8). The long posterior ciliary arteries and long ciliary nerves pass from the optic nerve to the ciliary body in a shallow groove on the inner surface of the sclera at the 3 and 9 o'clock meridians. Slightly posterior to the equator, the four vortex veins draining the choroid exit through the sclera, usually one in each quadrant. About 4 mm posterior to the limbus, slightly anterior to the insertion of the respective rectus muscle, the four anterior ciliary arteries and veins penetrate the sclera. The nerve supply to the sclera is from the ciliary nerves.

Histologically, the sclera consists of many dense bands of parallel and interlacing collagen bundles, each of which is 10–16 μm thick and 100–140 μm wide. The histologic structure of the sclera is remarkably similar to that of the cornea. The reason for the transparency of the cornea and the opacity of the sclera is the relative deturgescence of the cornea.

THE CORNEA

The cornea is a transparent tissue comparable in size and structure to the crystal of a small wristwatch (Figure 1–9). It is inserted into the sclera at the limbus, the circumferential depression at this junction being known as the scleral sulcus. The average adult cornea is 0.52 mm thick in the center, about 0.65 mm thick at the periphery, and about 11.75 mm in diameter horizontally and 10.6 mm vertically. From anterior to posterior, it has five distinct layers (Figure 1–10): the epithelium (which is continuous with the epithelium of the bulbar conjunctiva), Bowman's layer, the stroma, Descemet's membrane, and the endothelium. The epithelium has five or six layers of cells. Bowman's layer is a clear acellular layer, a modified portion of the stroma. The corneal stroma accounts for about 90% of the corneal thickness. It is composed of intertwining lamellae of collagen fibrils 10–250 μm in width and 1–2 μm in height that run almost the full diameter of the cornea. They run parallel to the surface of the cornea and by virtue of their size and proximity are optically clear. The lamellae lie within a ground substance of hydrated proteoglycans in association with the keratocytes that produce the collagen and ground substance. Descemet's membrane, constituting the basal lamina of the corneal endothelium, has a homogeneous appearance on light microscopy but a laminated appearance on electron microscopy due to structural differences between its pre- and postnatal portions. It is about 3 μm thick at birth but increases in thickness throughout life, reaching 10–12

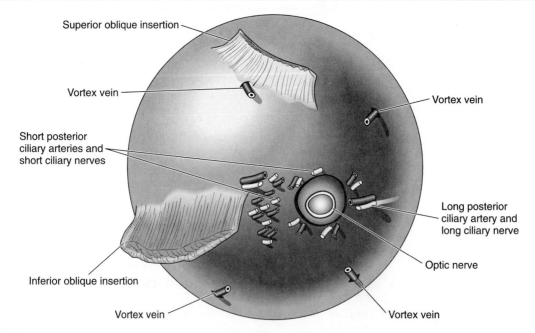

Figure 1–8. Posterior view of left eye. (Redrawn and reproduced, with permission, from Wolff E: *Anatomy of the Eye and Orbit,* 4th ed. Blakiston-McGraw, 1954.)

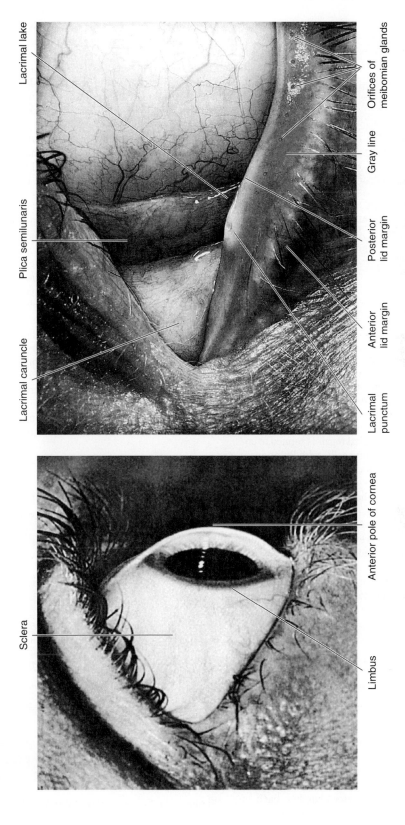

Lacrimal lake

Plica semilunaris

Lacrimal caruncle

Orifices of meibomian glands

Gray line

Posterior lid margin

Anterior lid margin

Lacrimal punctum

Anterior pole of cornea

Sclera

Limbus

Figure 1–9. External landmarks of the eye. The sclera is covered by transparent conjunctiva. (Photo by HL Gibson, from: *Medical Radiography and Photography*. Labeling modified slightly.)

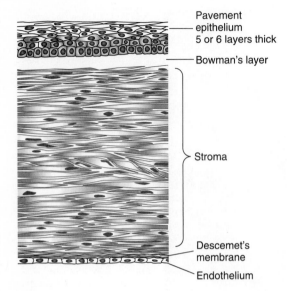

Pavement epithelium 5 or 6 layers thick

Bowman's layer

Stroma

Descemet's membrane

Endothelium

Figure 1–10. Transverse section of cornea. (Reproduced, with permission, from Wolff E: *Anatomy of the Eye and Orbit,* 4th ed. Blakiston-McGraw, 1954.)

μm in adulthood. The endothelium has only one layer of cells, but this is responsible for maintaining the essential deturgescence of the corneal stroma. The endothelium is quite susceptible to injury as well as undergoing loss of cells with age. Endothelial repair is limited to enlargement and sliding of existing cells, with little capacity for cell division. Failure of endothelial function leads to corneal edema.

Sources of nutrition for the cornea are the vessels of the limbus, the aqueous, and the tears. The superficial cornea also gets most of its oxygen from the atmosphere. The sensory nerves of the cornea are supplied by the first (ophthalmic) division of the fifth (trigeminal) cranial nerve.

The transparency of the cornea is due to its uniform structure, avascularity, and deturgescence.

THE UVEAL TRACT

The uveal tract is composed of the iris, the ciliary body, and the choroid (Figure 1–7). It is the middle vascular layer of the eye and is protected by the cornea and sclera. It contributes blood supply to the retina.

Iris

The **iris** is the anterior extension of the ciliary body. It presents as a flat surface with a centrally situated round aperture, the pupil. The iris lies in contiguity with the anterior surface of the lens, dividing the anterior chamber from the posterior chamber, each of which contains aqueous humor. Within the stroma of the iris are the sphincter and dilator muscles. The two heavily pigmented layers on the posterior surface of

the iris represent anterior extensions of the neuroretina and retinal pigment epithelium.

The blood supply to the iris is from the major circle of the iris (Figure 1–4). Iris capillaries have a nonfenestrated endothelium and hence do not normally leak intravenously injected fluorescein. Sensory nerve supply to the iris is via fibers in the ciliary nerves.

The iris controls the amount of light entering the eye. Pupillary size is principally determined by a balance between constriction due to parasympathetic activity transmitted via the third cranial nerve and dilation due to sympathetic activity. (See Chapter 14.)

The Ciliary Body

The **ciliary body,** roughly triangular in cross-section, extends forward from the anterior end of the choroid to the root of the iris (about 6 mm). It consists of a corrugated anterior zone, the pars plicata (2 mm), and a flattened posterior zone, the pars plana (4 mm). The ciliary processes arise from the pars plicata (Figure 1–11). They are composed mainly of capillaries and veins that drain through the vortex veins. The capillaries are large and fenestrated and hence leak intravenously injected fluorescein. There are two layers of ciliary epithelium: an internal nonpigmented layer, representing the anterior extension of the neuroretina; and an external pigmented layer, representing an extension of the retinal pigment epithelium. The ciliary processes and their covering ciliary epithelium are responsible for the formation of aqueous.

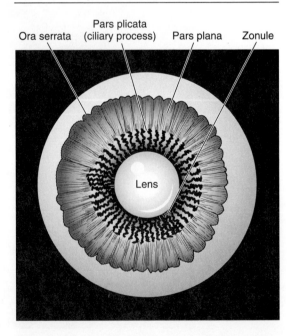

Pars plicata
Ora serrata (ciliary process) Pars plana Zonule

Lens

Figure 1–11. Posterior view of ciliary body, zonule, lens, and ora serrata. (Redrawn and reproduced, with permission, from: Wolff E: *Anatomy of the Eye and Orbit,* 4th ed. Blakiston-McGraw, 1954.)

The **ciliary muscle** is composed of a combination of longitudinal, circular, and radial fibers. The function of the circular fibers is to contract and relax the zonular fibers, which originate in the valleys between the ciliary processes (Figure 1–12). This alters the tension on the capsule of the lens, giving the lens a variable focus for both near and distant objects in the visual field. The longitudinal fibers of the ciliary muscle insert into the trabecular meshwork to influence its pore size.

The blood vessels supplying the ciliary body are derived from the major circle of the iris. The sensory nerve supply of the iris is via the ciliary nerves.

The Choroid

The choroid is the posterior segment of the uveal tract, between the retina and the sclera. It is composed of three layers of choroidal blood vessels: large, medium, and small. The deeper the vessels are placed in the choroid, the wider their lumens (Figure 1–13). The internal portion of the choroid vessels is known as the choriocapillaris. Blood from the choroidal vessels drains via the four vortex veins, one in each of the four posterior quadrants. The choroid is bounded internally by Bruch's membrane and externally by the sclera. The suprachoroidal space lies between the choroid and the sclera. The choroid is firmly attached posteriorly to the margins of the optic nerve. Anteriorly, the choroid joins with the ciliary body.

The aggregate of choroidal blood vessels serves to nourish the outer portion of the underlying retina (Figure 1–4).

THE LENS

The lens is a biconvex, avascular, colorless and almost completely transparent structure, about 4 mm thick and 9 mm in diameter. It is suspended behind the iris by the zonule, which connects it with the ciliary body. Anterior to the lens is the aqueous; posterior to it, the vitreous. The lens capsule (see below) is a semipermeable membrane (slightly more permeable than a capillary wall) that will admit water and electrolytes.

A subcapsular epithelium is present anteriorly (Figure 1–14). The lens nucleus is harder than the cortex. With age, subepithelial lamellar fibers are continuously produced, so that the lens gradually becomes larger and less elastic throughout life. The nucleus and cortex are made up of long concentric lamellae. The suture lines formed by the end-to-end joining of these lamellar fibers are Y-shaped when viewed with the slitlamp (Figure 1–15). The Y is upright anteriorly and inverted posteriorly.

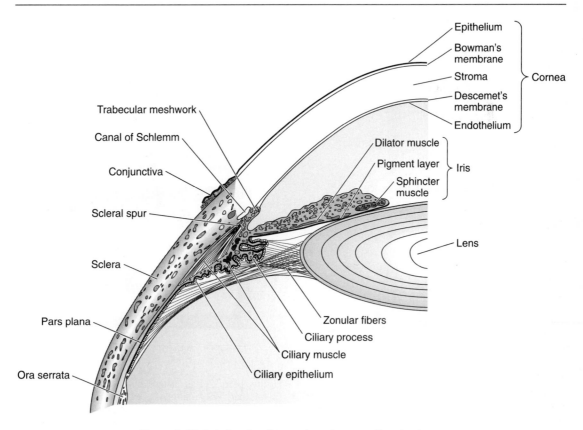

Figure 1–12. Anterior chamber angle and surrounding structures.

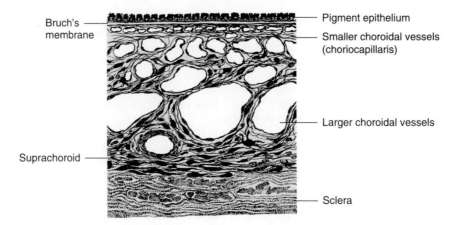

Bruch's membrane — Pigment epithelium

— Smaller choroidal vessels (choriocapillaris)

— Larger choroidal vessels

Suprachoroid —

— Sclera

Figure 1–13. Cross section of choroid. (Redrawn and reproduced, with permission, from Wolff E: *Anatomy of the Eye and Orbit,* 4th ed. Blakiston-McGraw, 1954.)

Each lamellar fiber contains a flattened nucleus. These nuclei are evident microscopically in the peripheral portion of the lens near the equator and are continuous with the subcapsular epithelium.

The lens is held in place by a suspensory ligament known as the zonule (zonule of Zinn), which is composed of numerous fibrils that arise from the surface of the ciliary body and insert into the lens equator.

The lens consists of about 65% water, about 35% protein (the highest protein content of any tissue of the body), and a trace of minerals common to other body tissues. Potassium is more concentrated in the lens than in most tissues. Ascorbic acid and glutathione are present in both oxidized and reduced forms.

There are no pain fibers, blood vessels, or nerves in the lens.

THE AQUEOUS

Aqueous humor is produced by the ciliary body. Entering the posterior chamber, it passes through the pupil into the anterior chamber (Figure 1–7) and then

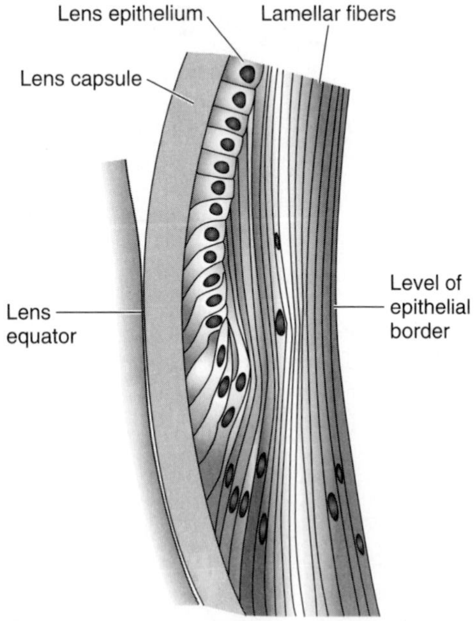

Lens epithelium — Lamellar fibers

Lens capsule —

Lens equator —

— Level of epithelial border

Figure 1–14. Magnified view of lens showing termination of subcapsular epithelium (vertical section). (From Duke-Elder WS: Textbook of Ophthalmology, vol 1. Mosbey, 1942. Drawings first appeared in Salzmann M: Anatomu and History of the Human Eyeball in the Normal State. Univ of Chicago Press, 1912)

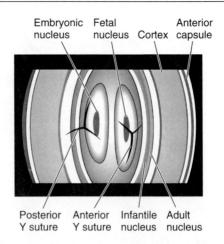

Embryonic nucleus Fetal nucleus Cortex Anterior capsule

Posterior Y suture Anterior Y suture Infantile nucleus Adult nucleus

Figure 1–15. Zones of lens showing Y sutures. (From Duke-Elder WS: *Textbook of Ophthalmology*, vol 1. Mosby, 1942. Drawings first appeared in Salzmann M: *Anatomy and History of the Human Eyeball in the Normal State.* Univ of Chicago Press, 1912.)

peripherally toward the anterior chamber angle. The physiology of the aqueous is discussed in Chapter 11.

THE ANTERIOR CHAMBER ANGLE

The anterior chamber angle lies at the junction of the peripheral cornea and the root of the iris (Figures 1–12, 1–16, and 11–3). Its main anatomic features are Schwalbe's line, the trabecular meshwork (which overlies Schlemm's canal), and the scleral spur.

Schwalbe's line marks the termination of the corneal endothelium. The trabecular meshwork is triangular in cross-section, with its base directed toward the ciliary body. It is composed of perforated sheets of collagen and elastic tissue, forming a filter with decreasing pore size as the canal of Schlemm is approached. The internal portion of the meshwork, facing the anterior chamber, is known as the uveal meshwork; the external portion, adjacent to the canal of Schlemm, is called the corneoscleral meshwork. The longitudinal fibers of the ciliary muscle insert into the trabecular meshwork. The scleral spur is an inward extension of the sclera between the ciliary body and Schlemm's canal, to which the iris and ciliary body are attached. Efferent channels from Schlemm's canal (about 30 collector channels and about 12 aqueous veins) communicate with the episcleral venous system.

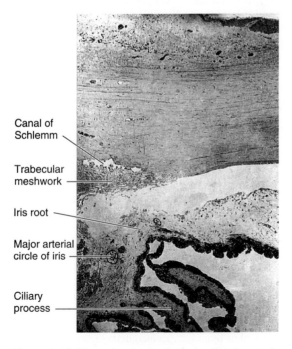

Canal of Schlemm

Trabecular meshwork

Iris root

Major arterial circle of iris

Ciliary process

Figure 1–16. Photomicrograph of anterior chamber angle and related structures. (Courtesy of I Wood and L Garron.)

THE RETINA

The retina is a thin, semitransparent, multilayered sheet of neural tissue that lines the inner aspect of the posterior two-thirds of the wall of the globe. It extends almost as far anteriorly as the ciliary body, ending at that point in a ragged edge, the ora serrata (Figure 1–12). In adults the ora serrata is about 6.5 mm behind Schwalbe's line on the temporal side and 5.7 mm behind it nasally. The outer surface of the sensory retina is apposed to the retinal pigment epithelium and thus related to Bruch's membrane, the choroid, and the sclera. In most areas, the retina and retinal pigment epithelium are easily separated to form the subretinal space, such as occurs in retinal detachment. But at the optic disk and the ora serrata, the retina and retinal pigment epithelium are firmly bound together, thus limiting the spread of subretinal fluid in retinal detachment. This contrasts with the potential suprachoroidal space between the choroid and sclera, which extends to the scleral spur. Choroidal detachments thus extend beyond the ora serrata, under the pars plana and pars plicata. The epithelial layers of the inner surface of the ciliary body and the posterior surface of the iris represent anterior extensions of the retina and retinal pigment epithelium. The inner surface of the retina is apposed to the vitreous.

The layers of the retina, starting from its inner aspect, are as follows: (1) internal limiting membrane; (2) nerve fiber layer, containing the ganglion cell axons passing to the optic nerve; (3) ganglion cell layer; (4) inner plexiform layer, containing the connections of the ganglion cells with the amacrine and bipolar cells; (5) inner nuclear layer of bipolar, amacrine, and horizontal cell bodies; (6) outer plexiform layer, containing the connections of the bipolar and horizontal cells with the photoreceptors; (7) outer nuclear layer of photoreceptor cell nuclei; (8) external limiting membrane; (9) photoreceptor layer of rod and cone inner and outer segments; and (10) retinal pigment epithelium (Figure 1–17). The inner layer of Bruch's membrane is actually the basement membrane of the retinal pigment epithelium.

The retina is 0.1 mm thick at the ora serrata and 0.56 mm thick at the posterior pole. In the center of the posterior retina is the macula. This can be defined clinically as the area of yellowish pigmentation resulting from the presence of luteal pigment (xanthophyll), which is 3 mm in diameter. An alternative histologic definition is that part of the retina in which the ganglion cell layer is more than one cell thick. Clinically, this corresponds to the area bounded by the temporal retinal vascular arcades. In the center of the macula, 4 mm lateral to the optic disk, is the fovea, clinically obvious as a depression that creates a particular reflection when viewed ophthalmoscopically. It corresponds to the retinal avascular zone of fluorescein angiography. Histologically, the fovea is charac-

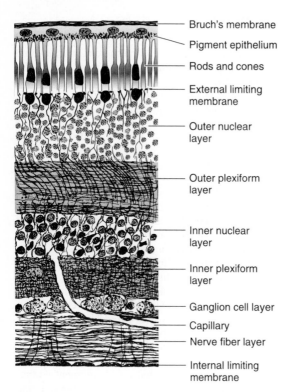

Bruch's membrane

Pigment epithelium

Rods and cones

External limiting membrane

Outer nuclear layer

Outer plexiform layer

Inner nuclear layer

Inner plexiform layer

Ganglion cell layer

Capillary

Nerve fiber layer

Internal limiting membrane

Figure 1–17. Layers of the retina. (Redrawn and reproduced, with permission, from Wolff E: *Anatomy of the Eye and Orbit,* 4th ed. Blakiston-McGraw, 1954.)

terized by thinning of the outer nuclear layer and absence of the other parenchymal layers as a result of the oblique course of the photoreceptor cell axons (Henle fiber layer) and the centrifugal displacement of the retinal layers that are closer to the inner retinal surface. The foveola is the most central portion of the fovea, in which the photoreceptors are all cones, and the thinnest part of the retina (0.25 mm). All these histologic features provide for fine visual discrimination. The normally empty extracellular space of the retina is potentially greatest at the macula, and diseases that lead to accumulation of extracellular material cause considerable thickening of this area.

The retina receives its blood supply from two sources: the choriocapillaris immediately outside Bruch's membrane, which supplies the outer third of the retina, including the outer plexiform and outer nuclear layers, the photoreceptors, and the retinal pigment epithelium; and branches of the central retinal artery, which supply the inner two-thirds (Figure 1–4). The fovea is supplied entirely by the choriocapillaris and is susceptible to irreparable damage when the retina is detached. The retinal blood vessels have a nonfenestrated endothelium, which forms the inner blood-retinal barrier. The endothelium of choroidal vessels is fenestrated. The outer blood-retinal barrier lies at the level of the retinal pigment epithelium.

THE VITREOUS

The vitreous is a clear, avascular, gelatinous body that comprises two-thirds of the volume and weight of the eye. It fills the space bounded by the lens, retina, and optic disk (Figure 1–7). The outer surface of the vitreous—the hyaloid membrane—is normally in contact with the following structures: the posterior lens capsule, the zonular fibers, the pars plana epithelium, the retina, and the optic nerve head. The base of the vitreous maintains a firm attachment throughout life to the pars plana epithelium and the retina immediately behind the ora serrata. The attachment to the lens capsule and the optic nerve head is firm in early life but soon disappears.

The vitreous is about 99% water. The remaining 1% includes two components, collagen and hyaluronic acid, which give the vitreous a gel-like form and consistency because of their ability to bind large volumes of water.

THE EXTERNAL ANATOMIC LANDMARKS

Accurate localization of the position of internal structures with reference to the external surface of the globe is important in many surgical procedures. The distance of structures from the limbus as measured externally is less than their actual length. Externally, the ora serrata is situated approximately 5.5 mm from the limbus on the medial side and 7 mm on the temporal side of the globe. This corresponds to the level of insertion of the rectus muscles. Injections into the vitreous cavity through the pars plana should be given 4–5 mm from the limbus in the phakic eye. In the aphakic eye, it is possible to inject 0.5–1 mm more anteriorly. The pars plicata, which is the target for cyclodestructive procedures in the treatment of intractable glaucoma, occupies the 2–3 mm directly posterior to the limbus.

THE EXTRAOCULAR MUSCLES

Six extraocular muscles control the movement of each eye: four rectus and two oblique muscles.

Rectus Muscles

The four rectus muscles originate at a common ring tendon (annulus of Zinn) surrounding the optic nerve at the posterior apex of the orbit (Figure 1–3). They are named according to their insertion into the sclera on the medial, lateral, inferior, and superior surfaces of the eye. The principal action of the respective muscles is thus to adduct, abduct, depress, and elevate the globe (see Chapter 12). The muscles are about 40 mm long, becoming tendinous 4–9 mm from the point of insertion, where they are about 10 mm wide. The approximate distances of the points of insertion from the corneal limbus are as follows: medial rectus, 5.5 mm: inferior rectus, 6.75 mm; lateral rectus, 7 mm; and superior rectus, 7.5 mm (Figure 1–18). With the eye in the primary position, the vertical rectus muscles make an angle of about 23 degrees with the optic axis.

Oblique Muscles

The two oblique muscles control primarily torsional movement and, to a lesser extent, upward and downward movement of the globe (see Chapter 12).

The **superior oblique** is the longest and thinnest of the ocular muscles. It originates above and medial to the optic foramen and partially overlaps the origin of the levator palpebrae superioris muscle. The superior oblique has a thin, fusiform belly (40 mm long) and passes anteriorly in the form of a tendon to its trochlea, or pulley. It is then reflected backward and downward to attach in a fan shape to the sclera beneath the superior rectus. The trochlea is a cartilaginous structure attached to the frontal bone 3 mm behind the orbital rim. The superior oblique tendon is enclosed in a synovial sheath as it passes through the trochlea.

The **inferior oblique** muscle originates from the nasal side of the orbital wall just behind the inferior orbital rim and lateral to the nasolacrimal duct. It passes beneath the inferior rectus and then under the lateral rectus muscle to insert onto the sclera with a short tendon. The insertion is into the posterotemporal segment of the globe and just over the macular area. The muscle is 37 mm long.

In the primary position, the muscle plane of the su-

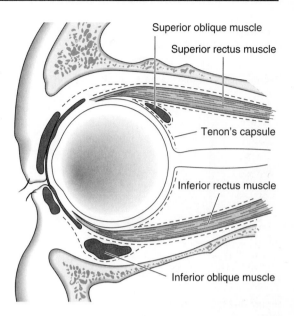

Figure 1–19. Fascia about muscles and eyeball (Tenon's capsule).

perior and inferior oblique muscles forms an angle of 51–54 degrees with the optic axis.

Fascia

All the extraocular muscles are ensheathed by fascia. Near the points of insertion of these muscles the fascia is continuous with Tenon's capsule, and fascial condensations to adjacent orbital structures serve as check ligaments (Figures 1–19 and 1–20).

Nerve Supply

The oculomotor nerve (III) innervates the medial, inferior, and superior rectus muscles and the inferior oblique muscle. The abducens nerve (VI) innervates the lateral rectus muscle; the trochlear nerve (IV) innervates the superior oblique muscle.

Blood Supply

The blood supply to the extraocular muscles is derived from the muscular branches of the ophthalmic artery. The lateral rectus and inferior oblique muscles are also supplied by branches from the lacrimal artery and the infraorbital artery, respectively.

THE OCULAR ADNEXA

1. EYEBROWS

The eyebrows are folds of thickened skin covered with hair. The skin fold is supported by underlying muscle fibers. The glabella is the hairless prominence between the eyebrows.

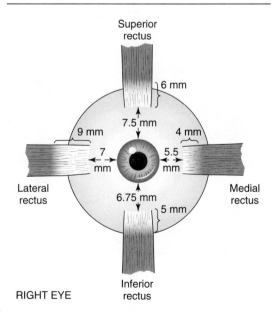

Figure 1–18. Approximate distances of the rectus muscles from the limbus, and the approximate lengths of tendons.

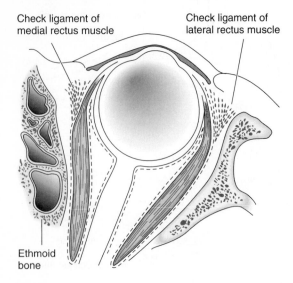

Figure 1–20. Check ligaments of medial and lateral rectus muscles, right eye (diagrammatic).

2. EYELIDS

The upper and lower eyelids (palpebrae) are modified folds of skin that can close to protect the anterior eyeball (Figure 1–21). Blinking helps spread the tear film, which protects the cornea and conjunctiva from dehydration. The upper lid ends at the eyebrows; the lower lid merges into the cheek.

The eyelids consist of five principal planes of tissues. From superficial to deep, they are the skin layer, a layer of striated muscle (orbicularis oculi), areolar tissue, fibrous tissue (tarsal plates), and a layer of mucous membrane (palpebral conjunctiva) (Figure 1–22).

Structures of the Eyelids

A. Skin Layer: The skin of the eyelids differs from skin on most other areas of the body in that it is thin, loose, and elastic and possesses few hair follicles and no subcutaneous fat.

B. Orbicularis Oculi Muscle: The function of the orbicularis oculi muscle is to close the lids. Its muscle fibers surround the palpebral fissure in concentric fashion and spread for a short distance around the orbital margin. Some fibers run onto the cheek and the forehead. The portion of the muscle that is in the lids is known as its pretarsal portion; the portion over the orbital septum is the preseptal portion. The segment outside the lid is called the orbital portion. The orbicularis oculi is supplied by the facial nerve.

C. Areolar Tissue: The submuscular areolar tissue that lies deep to the orbicularis oculi muscle communicates with the subaponeurotic layer of the scalp.

D. Tarsal Plates: The main supporting structure of the eyelids is a dense fibrous tissue layer that—along with a small amount of elastic tissue—is called the

tarsal plate. The lateral and medial angles and extensions of the tarsal plates are attached to the orbital margin by the lateral and medial palpebral ligaments. The upper and lower tarsal plates are also attached by a condensed, thin fascia to the upper and lower orbital margins. This thin fascia forms the orbital septum.

E. Palpebral Conjunctiva: The lids are lined posteriorly by a layer of mucous membrane, the **palpebral conjunctiva,** which adheres firmly to the tarsal plates. A surgical incision through the gray line of the lid margin (see below) splits the lid into an anterior lamella of skin and orbicularis muscle and a posterior lamella of tarsal plate and palpebral conjunctiva.

Lid Margins

The free lid margin is 25–30 mm long and about 2 mm wide. It is divided by the gray line (mucocutaneous junction) into anterior and posterior margins.

A. Anterior Margin:

1. Eyelashes– The eyelashes project from the margins of the eyelids and are arranged irregularly. The upper lashes are longer and more numerous than the lower lashes and turn upward; the lower lashes turn downward.

2. Glands of Zeis– These are small modified sebaceous glands that open into the hair follicles at the base of the eyelashes.

3. Glands of Moll– These are modified sweat glands that open in a row near the base of the eyelashes.

B. Posterior Margin: The posterior lid margin is in close contact with the globe, and along this margin

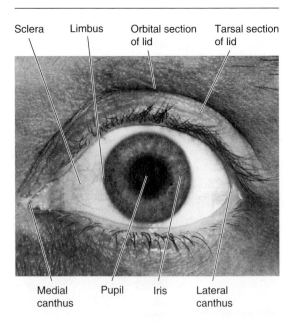

Figure 1–21. External landmarks of the eye. The sclera is covered by transparent conjunctiva. (Photo by HL Gibson, from: *Medical Radiography and Photography.* Labeling modified slightly.)

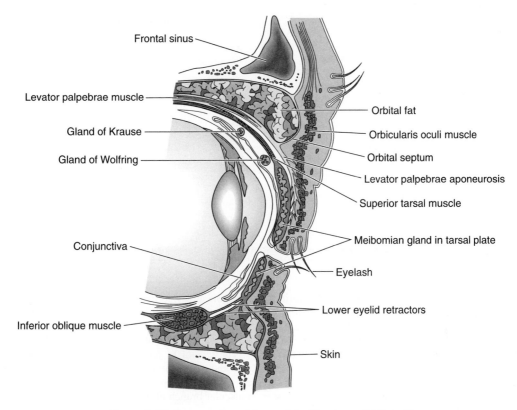

Figure 1–22. Cross section of the eyelids. (Courtesy of C Beard.)

are the small orifices of modified sebaceous glands (meibomian, or tarsal, glands).

C. Lacrimal Punctum: At the medial end of the posterior margin of the lid, a small elevation with a central small opening can be seen on the upper and lower lids. The puncta serve to carry the tears down through the corresponding canaliculus to the lacrimal sac.

Palpebral Fissure

The palpebral fissure is the elliptic space between the two open lids. The fissure terminates at the medial and lateral canthi. The lateral canthus is about 0.5 cm from the lateral orbital rim and forms an acute angle. The medial canthus is more elliptic than the lateral canthus and surrounds the lacrimal lake (Figure 1–21).

Two structures are identified in the lacrimal lake: the **lacrimal caruncle,** a yellowish elevation of modified skin containing large modified sweat glands and sebaceous glands that open into follicles which contain fine hair (Figure 1–9); and the **plica semilunaris,** a vestigial remnant of the third eyelid of lower animal species.

In Orientals, a skin fold known as **epicanthus** passes from the medial termination of the upper lid to the medial termination of the lower lid, hiding the caruncle. Epicanthus may be present normally in young infants of all races and disappears with development of the nasal bridge but persists throughout life in Orientals.

Orbital Septum

The orbital septum is the fascia behind that portion of the orbicularis muscle that lies between the orbital rim and the tarsus and serves as a barrier between the lid and the orbit.

The orbital septum is pierced by the lacrimal vessels and nerves, the supratrochlear artery and nerve, the supraorbital vessels and nerves, the infratrochlear nerve (Figure 1–23), the anastomosis between the angular and ophthalmic veins, and the levator palpebrae superioris muscle.

The **superior orbital septum** blends with the tendon of the levator palpebrae superioris and the superior tarsus; the **inferior orbital septum** blends with the inferior tarsus.

Lid Retractors

The lid retractors are responsible for opening the eyelids. They are formed by a musculofascial complex, with both striated and smooth muscle components, known as the levator complex in the upper lid and the capsulopalpebral fascia in the lower lid.

In the upper lid, the striated muscle portion is the **levator palpebrae superioris,** which arises from the apex of the orbit and passes forward to divide into an aponeurosis and a deeper portion that contains the smooth muscle fibers of **Müller's (superior tarsal) muscle** (Figure 1–22). The aponeurosis elevates the

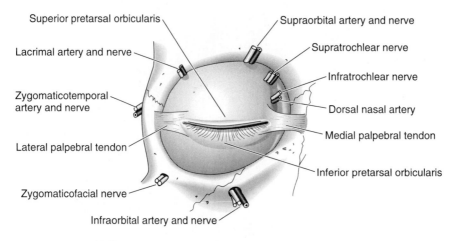

Figure 1–23. Vessels and nerves to extraocular structures.

anterior lamella of the lid, inserting into the posterior surface of the orbicularis oculi and through this into the overlying skin to form the upper lid skin crease. Müller's muscle inserts into the upper border of the tarsal plate and the superior fornix of the conjunctiva, thus elevating the posterior lamella.

In the lower lid, the main retractor is the inferior rectus muscle, from which fibrous tissue extends to enclose the inferior oblique muscle and insert into the lower border of the tarsal plate and the orbicularis oculi. Associated with this aponeurosis are the smooth muscle fibers of the inferior tarsal muscle.

The smooth muscle components of the lid retractors are innervated by sympathetic nerves. The levator and inferior rectus muscles are supplied by the third cranial (oculomotor) nerve. Ptosis is thus a feature of both Horner's syndrome and third nerve palsy.

Levator Palpebrae Superioris Muscle

The levator palpebrae muscle arises with a short tendon from the undersurface of the lesser wing of the sphenoid above and ahead of the optic foramen. The tendon blends with the underlying origin of the superior rectus muscle. The levator belly passes forward, forms an aponeurosis, and spreads like a fan. The muscle, including its smooth muscle component (Müller's muscle), and its aponeurosis form an important part of the upper lid retractor (see above). The palpebral segment of the orbicularis oculi muscle acts as its antagonist.

The two extremities of the levator aponeurosis are called its medial and lateral horns. The medial horn is thin and is attached below the frontolacrimal suture and into the medial palpebral ligament. The lateral horn passes between the orbital and palpebral portions of the lacrimal gland and inserts into the orbital tubercle and the lateral palpebral ligament.

The sheath of the levator palpebrae superioris is attached to the superior rectus muscle inferiorly. The superior surface, at the junction of the muscle belly and

the aponeurosis, forms a thickened band that is attached medially to the trochlea and laterally to the lateral orbital wall, the band forming the check ligaments of the muscle. The band is also known as Whitnall's ligament.

The levator is supplied by the superior branch of the oculomotor nerve (III). Blood supply to the levator palpebrae superioris is derived from the lateral muscular branch of the ophthalmic artery.

Sensory Nerve Supply

The sensory nerve supply to the eyelids is derived from the first and second divisions of the trigeminal nerve (V). The small lacrimal, supraorbital, supratrochlear, infratrochlear, and external nasal nerves are branches of the ophthalmic division of the fifth nerve. The infraorbital, zygomaticofacial, and zygomaticotemporal nerves are branches of the maxillary (second) division of the trigeminal nerve.

Blood Supply & Lymphatics

The blood supply to the lids is derived from the lacrimal and ophthalmic arteries by their lateral and medial palpebral branches. Anastomoses between the lateral and medial palpebral arteries form the tarsal arcades that lie in the submuscular areolar tissue.

Venous drainage from the lids empties into the ophthalmic vein and the veins that drain the forehead and temple. The veins are arranged in pre- and posttarsal plexuses (Figure 1–6).

Lymphatics from the lateral segment of the lids run into the preauricular and parotid nodes. Lymphatics draining the medial side of the lids empty into the submandibular lymph nodes.

3. THE LACRIMAL APPARATUS

The lacrimal complex consists of the lacrimal gland, the accessory lacrimal glands, the canaliculi, the lacrimal sac, and the nasolacrimal duct (Figure 1–24).

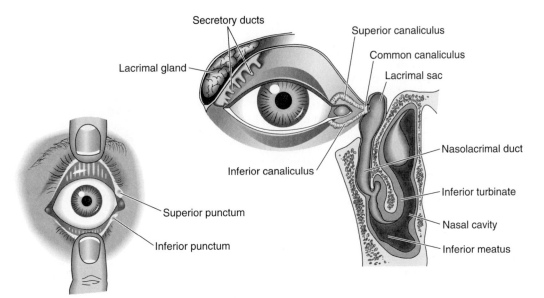

Figure 1–24. The lacrimal drainage system. (Redrawn with modifications and reproduced, with permission, from Thompson J, Elstrom ER: Radiography of the nasolacrimal passageways. Med Radiogr Photogr 1949;25[3]:66.)

The lacrimal gland consists of the following structures:

(1) The almond-shaped **orbital portion,** located in the lacrimal fossa in the anterior upper temporal segment of the orbit, is separated from the palpebral portion by the lateral horn of the levator palpebrae muscle. To reach this portion of the gland surgically, one must incise the skin, the orbicularis oculi muscle, and the orbital septum.

(2) The smaller **palpebral portion** is located just above the temporal segment of the superior conjunctival fornix. Lacrimal secretory ducts, which open by approximately ten fine orifices, connect the orbital and palpebral portions of the lacrimal gland to the superior conjunctival fornix. Removal of the palpebral portion of the gland cuts off all of the connecting ducts and thus prevents secretion by the entire gland.

The accessory lacrimal glands (glands of Krause and Wolfring) are located in the substantia propria of the palpebral conjunctiva.

Tears drain from the lacrimal lake via the upper and lower puncta and canaliculi to the **lacrimal sac,** which lies in the lacrimal fossa. The nasolacrimal duct continues downward from the sac and opens into the inferior meatus of the nasal cavity, lateral to the inferior turbinate. Tears are directed into the puncta by capillary attraction and gravity and by the blinking action of the eyelids. The combined forces of capillary attraction in the canaliculi, gravity, and the pumping action of Horner's muscle, which is an extension of the orbicularis oculi muscle to a point behind the lacrimal sac, all tend to continue the flow of tears down the nasolacrimal duct into the nose.

Blood Supply & Lymphatics

The blood supply of the lacrimal gland is derived from the lacrimal artery. The vein that drains the gland joins the ophthalmic vein. The lymphatic drainage joins with the conjunctival lymphatics to drain into the preauricular lymph nodes.

Nerve Supply

The nerve supply to the lacrimal gland is by (1) the lacrimal nerve (sensory), a branch of the trigeminal first division; (2) the great superficial petrosal nerve (secretory), which comes from the superior salivary nucleus; and (3) sympathetic nerves accompanying the lacrimal artery and the lacrimal nerve.

Related Structures

The **medial palpebral ligament** connects the upper and lower tarsal plates to the frontal process at the inner canthus anterior to the lacrimal sac. The portion of the lacrimal sac below the ligament is covered by a few fibers of the orbicularis oculi muscle. These fibers offer little resistance to swelling and distention of the lacrimal sac. The area below the medial palpebral ligament becomes swollen in acute dacryocystitis, and fistulas commonly open in the area.

The angular vein and artery lie just deep to the skin, 8 mm to the nasal side of the inner canthus. Skin incisions made in surgical procedures on the lacrimal sac should always be placed 2–3 mm to the nasal side of the inner canthus to avoid these vessels.

THE OPTIC NERVE

The trunk of the optic nerve consists of about 1 million axons that arise from the ganglion cells of the retina (nerve fiber layer). The optic nerve emerges from the posterior surface of the globe through the posterior scleral foramen, a short, circular opening in the sclera about 1 mm below and 3 mm nasal to the posterior pole of the eye (Figure 1–8). The nerve fibers become myelinated on leaving the eye, increasing the diameter from 1.5 mm (within the sclera) to 3 mm (within the orbit). The orbital segment of the nerve is 25–30 mm long; it travels within the optic muscle cone, via the bony optic canal, and thus gains access to the cranial cavity. The intracanalicular portion measures 4–9 mm. After a 10 mm intracranial course, the nerve joins the opposite optic nerve to form the optic chiasm.

Eighty percent of the optic nerve consists of visual fibers that synapse in the lateral geniculate body on neurons whose axons terminate in the primary visual cortex of the occipital lobes. Twenty percent of the fibers are pupillary and bypass the geniculate body en route to the pretectal area. Since the ganglion cells of the retina and their axons are part of the central nervous system, they will not regenerate if severed.

Sheaths of the Optic Nerve (Figure 1–25)

The fibrous wrappings that ensheathe the optic nerve are continuous with the meninges. The pia mater

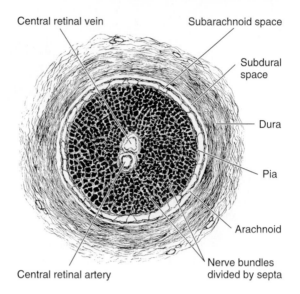

Figure 1–25. Cross section of the optic nerve. (Redrawn and reproduced, with permission, from Wolff E: *Anatomy of the Eye and Orbit,* 6th ed. Blakiston-McGraw, 1968.)

is loosely attached about the nerve near the chiasm and only for a short distance within the cranium, but it is closely attached around most of the intracanalicular and all of the intraorbital portions. The pia consists of some fibrous tissue with numerous small blood vessels (Figure 1–26). It divides the nerve fibers into bundles

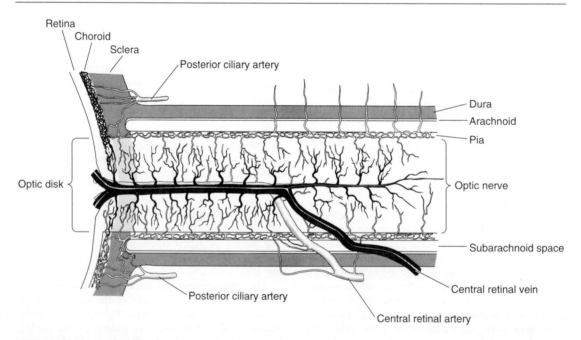

Figure 1–26. Blood supply of the optic nerve. (Redrawn and reproduced, with permission, from: Hayreh SS: Trans Am Acad Ophthalmol Otolaryngol 1974;78:240).

by sending numerous septa into the nerve substance. The pia continues to the sclera, with a few fibers running into the choroid and lamina cribrosa.

The arachnoid comes in contact with the optic nerve at the intracranial end of the optic canal and accompanies the nerve to the globe, where it ends in the sclera and overlying dura. This sheath is a diaphanous connective tissue membrane with many septate connections with the pia mater, which it closely resembles. It is more intimately associated with pia than with dura.

The dura mater lining the inner surface of the cranial vault comes in contact with the optic nerve as it leaves the optic canal. As the nerve enters the orbit from the optic canal, the dura splits, one layer (the periorbita) lining the orbital cavity and the other forming the outer dural covering of the optic nerve. The dura becomes continuous with the outer two-thirds of the sclera. The dura consists of tough, fibrous, relatively avascular tissue lined by endothelium on the inner surface.

The subdural space is between the dura and the arachnoid; the subarachnoid space is between the pia and the arachnoid. Both are more potential than actual spaces under normal conditions but are direct continuations of their corresponding intracranial spaces. Subarachnoid or subdural fluid under sufficient pressure will fill these potential spaces about the optic nerve. The meningeal layers are adherent to each other and to the optic nerve and the surrounding bone within the optic foramen, making the optic nerve resistant to traction from either end.

Blood Supply
(Figure 1–26)

The surface layer of the optic disk receives blood from branches of the retinal arterioles. The rest of the nerve in front of the lamina cribrosa is supplied by branches from the peripapillary choroidal vessels. In the region of the lamina cribrosa, the arterial supply is from the short posterior ciliary arteries. The retrolaminar optic nerve receives some blood from branches of the central retinal artery. The remainder of the intraorbital nerve, as well as the intracanalicular and intracranial portions, are supplied by a pial network of vessels derived from the various branches of the ophthalmic artery and other branches of the internal carotids.

THE OPTIC CHIASM

The optic chiasm is variably situated near the top of the diaphragm of the sella turcica, most often posteriorly, projecting 1 cm above it and at a 45-degree angle upward from the optic nerves as they emerge from the optic canals (Figure 1–27). The lamina terminalis forms the anterior wall of the third ventricle. The internal carotid arteries lie just laterally, adjacent to the cavernous sinuses. The chiasm is made up of the junction of the two optic nerves and provides for crossing of the nasal fibers to the opposite optic tract and passage of temporal fibers to the ipsilateral optic tract. The macular fibers are arranged similarly to the rest of the fibers except that their decussation is farther posteriorly and superiorly. The chiasm receives many small blood vessels from the neighboring circle of Willis.

THE RETROCHIASMATIC VISUAL PATHWAYS

Each optic tract begins at the posterolateral angle of the chiasm and sweeps around the upper part of the cerebral peduncle to end in the lateral geniculate nucleus. Afferent pupillary fibers leave the tract just anterior to the nucleus and pass via the brachium of the superior colliculus to the midbrain. (The pupillary pathway is diagrammed in Figure 14–2.) Afferent visual fibers terminate on cells in the lateral geniculate nucleus that give rise to the geniculocalcarine tract. This tract traverses the posterior limb of the internal capsule and then fans out into a broad bundle called the optic radiation. The fibers in this bundle curve backward around the anterior aspect of the temporal horn of the lateral ventricle and then medially to reach the calcarine cortex of the occipital lobe, where they terminate. The most inferior fibers, which carry projections from the superior aspect of the contralateral half of the visual field, course anteriorly into the temporal lobe in a configuration known as Meyer's loop. Lesions of the temporal lobe that extend 5 cm back from the anterior tip involve these fibers and can produce superior quadrantanopic field defects.

The primary visual cortex (area V1) occupies the upper and lower lips and the depths of the calcarine fissure on the medial aspect of the occipital lobe. Each lobe receives input from the two ipsilateral half-retinas, representing the contralateral half of the binocular visual field. Projection of the visual field onto the visual cortex occurs in a precise and orderly retinotopic pattern. The macula is represented at the medial posterior pole, and the peripheral parts of the retina project to the most anterior part of the calcarine cortex. On either side of area V1 lies area V2, and then area V3. V2 appears to function in a manner very similar to V1. Area V4, situated on the medial surface of the cerebral hemisphere but more anterior and inferior than V1 in the region of the fusiform gyrus, seems to be primarily concerned with color processing. Motion detection localizes to an area at the junction of the occipital and temporal lobes, lateral to area V1 and known as area V5 or MT.

THE OCULOMOTOR NERVE (III)

The oculomotor nerve leaves the brainstem between the cerebral peduncles and passes near the posterior communicating artery of the circle of Willis. Lateral to the pituitary gland, it is closely approximated to the op-

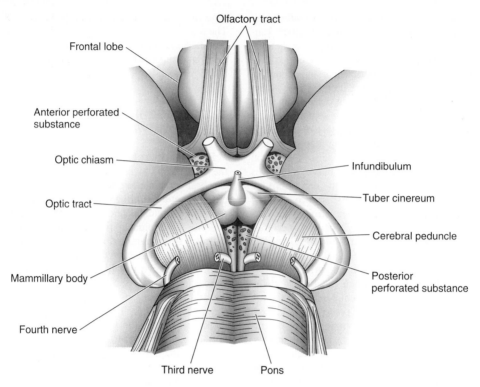

Figure 1–27. Relationship of optic chiasm from inferior aspect. (Redrawn and reproduced, with permission, from Duke-Elder WS: *System of Ophthalmology.* Vol 2. Mosby, 1961.)

tic tract, and here it pierces the dura to course in the lateral wall of the cavernous sinus. As the nerve leaves the cavernous sinus, it divides into superior and inferior divisions. The superior division enters the orbit within the annulus of Zinn at its highest point and adjacent to the trochlear nerve (Figure 1–3). The inferior division enters the annulus of Zinn low and passes below the optic nerve to supply the medial and inferior rectus muscles. A large branch from the inferior division extends forward to supply the inferior oblique. A small twig from the proximal end of the nerve to the inferior oblique carries parasympathetic fibers to the ciliary ganglion.

THE TROCHLEAR NERVE (IV)

Although the thinnest of the cranial nerves, the trochlear nerve (Figure 1–3) has the longest intracranial course, and it is also the only nerve to originate on the dorsal surface of the brain stem. The fibers decussate before they emerge from the brainstem just below the inferior colliculi, where they are subject to injury from the tentorium. The nerve pierces the dura behind the sella turcica and travels within the lateral walls of the cavernous sinus to enter the superior orbital fissure medial to the frontal nerve. From this point it travels within the periorbita of the roof over the levator muscle to the upper surface of the superior oblique muscle.

THE TRIGEMINAL NERVE (V) (FIGURE 1–3)

The trigeminal nerve originates from the pons, and its sensory roots form the trigeminal ganglion. The first (ophthalmic) of the three divisions passes through the lateral wall of the cavernous sinus and divides into the lacrimal, frontal, and nasociliary nerve. The **lacrimal nerve** passes through the upper lateral aspect of the superior orbital fissure, outside the annulus of Zinn, and continuing its lateral course in the orbit to terminate in the lacrimal gland, providing its sensory innervation. Slightly medial to the lacrimal nerve within the superior orbital fissure is the frontal nerve, which is the largest of the first division of branches of the trigeminal nerve. It also crosses over the annulus of Zinn and follows a course over the levator to the medial aspect of the orbit, where it divides into the supraorbital and supratrochlear nerves. These provide sensation to the brow and forehead. The nasociliary nerve is the sensory nerve of the eye. After entering through the medial portion of the annulus of Zinn, it lies between the superior rectus and the optic nerve. Branches to the ciliary ganglion and those forming the ciliary nerves provide sensory supply to the cornea, iris, and ciliary body. The terminal branches are the infratrochlear nerve, which supplies the medial portion of the conjunctiva and eyelids, and the anterior ethmoidal nerve, which provides sensation to the tip of the nose. Thus, the skin on the tip of the nose may be affected with vesicular lesions prior to the onset of herpes zoster ophthalmicus.

The second (maxillary) division of the trigeminal nerve passes through the foramen rotundum and enters the orbit through the inferior orbital fissure. It passes through the infraorbital canal, becoming the **infraorbital nerve,** and exits via the infraorbital foramen, supplying sensation to the lower lid and adjacent cheek. It is frequently damaged in fractures of the orbital floor.

THE ABDUCENS NERVE (VI)

The abducens nerve (Figure 1–3) originates between the pons and medulla and pursues an extended course up the clivus to the posterior clinoid, penetrates the dura, and passes within the cavernous sinus. (All other nerves course through the lateral wall of the cavernous sinus.) After passing through the superior orbital fissure within the annulus of Zinn, the nerve continues laterally to innervate the lateral rectus muscle.

II. EMBRYOLOGY OF THE EYE

The eye is derived from three of the primitive embryonic layers: surface ectoderm, including its derivative the neural crest; neural ectoderm; and mesoderm. Endoderm does not enter into the formation of the eye. Mesenchyme is the term for embryonic connective tissue. Ocular and adnexal connective tissues previously were thought to be derived from mesoderm, but it has now been shown that most of the mesenchyme of all of the head and neck region is derived from the cranial neural crest.

The **surface ectoderm** gives rise to the lens, the lacrimal gland, the epithelium of the cornea, conjunctiva, and adnexal glands, and the epidermis of the eyelids.

The **neural crest,** which arises from the surface ectoderm in the region immediately adjacent to the neural folds of neural ectoderm, is responsible for formation of the corneal keratocytes, the endothelium of the cornea and the trabecular meshwork, the stroma of the iris and choroid, the ciliary muscle, the fibroblasts of the sclera, the vitreous, and the optic nerve meninges. It is also involved in formation of the orbital cartilage and bone, the orbital connective tissues and nerves, the extraocular muscles, and the subepidermal layers of the eyelids.

The **neural ectoderm** gives rise to the optic vesicle and optic cup and is thus responsible for the formation of the retina and retinal pigment epithelium, the pigmented and nonpigmented layers of ciliary epithelium, the posterior epithelium, the dilator and sphincter muscles of the iris, and the optic nerve fibers and glia.

The **mesoderm** is now thought to contribute only to the extraocular muscles and the orbital and ocular vascular endothelium.

Optic Vesicle Stage

The embryonic plate is the earliest stage in fetal development during which ocular structures can be differentiated. At the 2.5 mm (2 week) stage, the edges of the neural groove thicken to form the neural folds (Figure 1–28). The folds then fuse to form the neural tube, which sinks into the underlying mesoderm and detaches itself from the surface epithelium. The site of the optic groove or optic sulcus is in the cephalic neural folds on either side of and parallel to the neural groove. This occurs when neural folds begin to close at 3 weeks.

At the 9 mm (4 week) stage, just before the anterior portion of the neural tube closes completely, neural ectoderm grows outward and toward the surface ectoderm on either side to form the spherical optic vesicles. The optic vesicles are connected to the forebrain by the optic stalks. At this stage also, a thickening of the surface ectoderm (lens plate) begins to form opposite the ends of the optic vesicles.

Optic Cup Stage

As the optic vesicle invaginates to produce the optic cup, the original outer wall of the vesicle approaches its inner wall. The invagination of the ventral surface of the optic stalk and of the optic vesicle occurs simultaneously and creates a groove, the optic (embryonic) fissure. The margins of the optic cup then grow around the optic fissure. At the same time, the lens plate invaginates to form first a cup and then a hollow sphere known as the lens vesicle. By the 9 mm (4 week) stage, the lens vesicle separates from the surface ectoderm and lies free in the rim of the optic cup.

The optic fissure allows the vascular mesoderm to enter the optic stalk and eventually to form the hyaloid system of the vitreous cavity. As invagination is completed, the optic fissure narrows and closes during the 13 mm (6 week) stage, leaving one small permanent opening at the anterior end of the optic stalk through which the hyaloid artery passes. At the 100 mm (4 month) stage, the retinal artery and vein pass through this opening. At this stage also, the ultimate general structure of the eye has been determined.

Further development of the eye consists in differentiation of the individual optic structures. In general, differentiation of the optic structures occurs more rapidly in the posterior than in the anterior segment of the eye during the early stages and more rapidly in the anterior segment during the later stages of gestation.

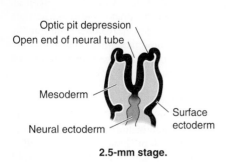

2.5-mm stage.

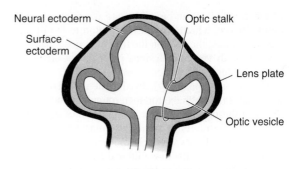

Forebrain of 4-mm embryo, optic vesicle stage.

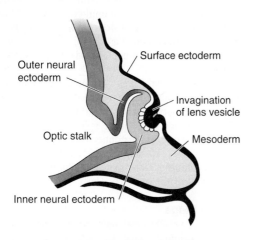

5-mm stage. Beginning formation
of optic cup by invagination.

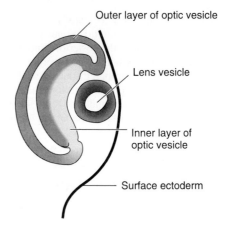

9-mm stage. Lens vesicle has separated from
surface ectoderm and lies free in rim of optic cup.

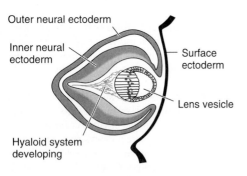

13-mm stage. Choroidal fissure closed.
Posterior lens cells growing forward.

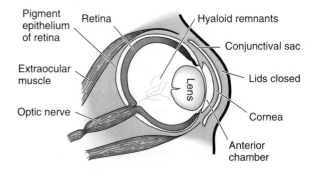

65-mm stage (3 months).

Figure 1–28. Embryologic development of ocular structures. (Redrawn and reproduced, with permission, from Mann IC: *The Development of the Human Eye,* 2nd ed. British Medical Association, 1950).

EMBRYOLOGY OF SPECIFIC STRUCTURES

Lids & Lacrimal Apparatus

The lids develop from mesenchyme except for the epidermis of the skin and the epithelium of the conjunctiva, which are derivatives of surface ectoderm. The lid buds are first seen at 16 mm (6 weeks) growing in front of the eye, where they meet and fuse at the 37 mm (8 week) stage. They separate during the fifth month. The lashes and meibomian and other lid glands develop as downgrowths from the epidermis.

The lacrimal and accessory lacrimal glands develop from the conjunctival epithelium. The lacrimal drainage system (canaliculi, lacrimal sac, and nasolacrimal duct) are also surface ectodermal derivatives, which develop from a solid epithelial cord that becomes buried between the maxillary and nasal processes of the developing facial structures. This cord canalizes just before birth.

Sclera & Extraocular Muscles

The sclera and extraocular muscles are formed from condensations of mesenchyme encircling the optic cup and are first identifiable at the 20 mm (7 week) stage. Development of these structures is well advanced by the fourth month. Tenon's capsule appears about the insertions of the rectus muscles at the 80 mm (12 week) stage and is complete at 5 months.

Anterior Segment

The anterior segment of the globe is formed by invasion of neural crest cells into the space between the surface ectoderm, which develops into the corneal epithelium, and the lens vesicle, which has become separated from it. The invasion of neural crest cells occurs in three stages: The first is responsible for formation of the corneal endothelium, the second for formation of the corneal stroma, and the third for formation of the iris stroma. The anterior chamber angle is formed from a residual condensation of mesenchyme at the anterior rim of the optic cup. The mechanism of formation of the anterior chamber itself—and hence the angle structures—is still debated but certainly seems to involve patterns of migration of neural crest cells and subsequent changes in their structure rather than cleavage of mesodermal tissue as previously thought.

The corneal epithelium and endothelium are first apparent at the 12 mm (5 week) stage. Descemet's membrane is secreted by the flattened endothelial cells by the 75 mm (13 week) stage. The stroma slowly thickens and forms an anterior condensation just under the epithelium that is recognizable at 100 mm (4 months) as Bowman's layer. A definite corneoscleral junction is present at 4 months.

The double row of posterior iris epithelium is a forward extension of the anterior rim of the optic cup. This grows forward during the third month (50 mm stage) to lie posterior to the neural crest cells that form the iris stroma. These two epithelial layers become pigmented in the iris, whereas only the outer layer is pigmented in the ciliary body. By the fifth month (150 mm) stage, the sphincter muscle of the pupil is developing from a bud of nonpigmented epithelium derived from the anterior epithelial layer of the iris near the pupillary margin. Soon after the sixth month, the dilator muscle appears in the anterior epithelial layer near the ciliary body.

The anterior chamber of the eye first appears at 20 mm (7 weeks) and remains very shallow until birth. At 65 mm (9–10 weeks), Schlemm's canal appears as a vascular channel at the level of the recess of the angle and gradually assumes a relatively more anterior location as the angle recess develops. The iris, which in the early stages of development is quite anterior, gradually lies relatively more posteriorly as the chamber angle recess develops, most likely because of the difference in rate of growth of the anterior segment structures. The trabecular meshwork develops from the loose vascular mesenchymal tissue lying originally at the margin of the optic cup. The aqueous drainage system is ready to function before birth.

Lens

Soon after the lens vesicle lies free in the rim of the optic cap (13 mm or 6 week stage), the cells of its posterior wall elongate, encroach on the empty cavity, and finally fill it in (26 mm or 7 week stage). At about this stage (13 mm or 6 week), a hyaline capsule is secreted by the lens cells. Secondary lens fibers elongate from the equatorial region and grow forward under the subcapsular epithelium, which remains as a single layer of cuboidal epithelial cells, and backward under the lens capsule. These fibers meet to form the lens sutures (upright Y anteriorly and inverted Y posteriorly), which are complete by the seventh month. (This growth and proliferation of secondary lens fibers continues at a decreasing rate throughout life; the lens therefore continues to enlarge slowly, causing compression of the lens fibers.)

Ciliary Body & Choroid

The ciliary epithelium is formed from the same anterior extension of the optic cup that is responsible for the posterior iris epithelium. Only the outer layer becomes pigmented. The ciliary muscle and blood vessels are derived from mesenchyme.

At the 6 mm ($3^{1}/_{2}$ week) stage, a network of capillaries encircles the optic cup and develops into the choroid. By the third month, the intermediate and large venous channels of the choroid are developed and drain into the vortex veins to exit from the eye.

Retina

The outer layer of the optic cup remains as a single layer and becomes the pigment epithelium of the retina. Pigmentation begins at the 10 mm (5 week) stage. Secretion of the inner layer of Bruch's membrane occurs by the 13 mm (6 week) stage. The inner layer of the optic cup undergoes a complicated differentiation into the other nine layers of the retina. This occurs slowly throughout gestation. By the seventh month, the outermost cell layer (consisting of the nuclei of the rods and cones) is present as well as the bipolar, amacrine, and ganglion cells and nerve fibers. The macular region is thicker than the rest of the retina until the eighth month, when macular depression begins to develop. Macular development is not complete in anatomic terms until 6 months after birth.

Vitreous

A. First Stage: (Primary vitreous, 4.5 to 13 mm or 3 to 6 week stage.) At about the 4.5 mm stage, mesenchymal cells and fibroblasts derived from mesenchyme at the rim of the optic cup or associated with the hyaloid vascular system, together with minor contributions from the embryonic lens and the inner layer of the optic vesicle, form the vitreous fibrils of the primary vitreous. Ultimately, the primary vitreous comes to lie just behind the posterior pole of the lens in association with remnants of the hyaloid vessels (Cloquet's canal).

B. Second Stage: (Secondary vitreous, 13 to 65 mm or 6 to 10 week stage.) The fibrils and cells (hyalocytes) of the secondary vitreous are thought to originate from the vascular primary vitreous. Anteriorly, the firm attachment of the secondary vitreous to the internal limiting membrane of the retina constitutes the early stages of formation of the vitreous base. The hyaloid system develops a set of vitreous vessels as well as vessels on the lens capsule surface (tunica vasculosa lentis). The hyaloid system is at its height at 40 mm and then atrophies from posterior to anterior.

C. Third Stage: (Tertiary vitreous, 65 mm or 10 weeks on.) During the third month, the marginal bundle of Drualt is forming. This consists of vitreous fibrillar condensations extending from the future ciliary epithelium of the optic cup to the equator of the lens. Condensations then form the suspensory ligament of the lens, which is well developed by the 100 mm or 4 month stage. The hyaloid system atrophies completely during this stage.

Optic Nerve

The axons of the ganglion cells of the retina form the nerve fiber layer. The fibers slowly form the optic stalk and then the optic nerve (26 mm stage). Mesenchymal elements enter the surrounding tissue to form the vascular septa of the nerve. Medullation extends from the brain peripherally down the optic nerve, and at birth has reached the lamina cribrosa. Medullation is completed by age 3 months.

Blood Vessels

Long ciliary arteries bud off from the hyaloid at the 16 mm (6 week) stage and anastomose around the op-

tic cup margin with the major circle of the iris by the 30 mm (7 week) stage.

The hyaloid system (see Vitreous, above) atrophies completely by the eighth month. The hyaloid artery gives rise to the central retinal artery and its branches (100 mm or 4 month stage). Buds begin to grow into the retina and develop the retinal circulation, which reaches the ora serrata at 8 months. The branches of the central retinal vein develop simultaneously.

III. GROWTH & DEVELOPMENT OF THE EYE

Eyeball

At birth, the eye is larger in relation to the rest of the body than is the case in children and adults. In relation to its ultimate size (reached at 7–8 years), it is comparatively short, averaging 16.5 mm in anteroposterior diameter (the only optically significant dimension). This would make the eye quite hyperopic if it were not for the refractive power of the nearly spherical lens.

Cornea

The newborn infant has a relatively large cornea that reaches adult size by the age of 2 years. It is flatter than the adult cornea, and its curvature is greater at the periphery than in the center. (The reverse is true in adults.)

Lens

At birth, the lens is more nearly spherical in shape than later in life, producing a greater refractive power that helps to compensate for the short anteroposterior diameter of the eye. The lens grows throughout life as new fibers are added to the periphery, making it flatter.

The consistency of the lens material changes throughout life. At birth, it may be compared with soft plastic; in old age, the lens is of a glass-like consistency. This accounts for the greater resistance to change of shape in accommodation as one grows older.

Iris

At birth, there is little or no pigment on the anterior surface of the iris; the posterior pigment layer showing through the translucent tissue gives the eyes of most infants a bluish color. As the pigment begins to appear on the anterior surface, the iris assumes its definitive color. If considerable pigment is deposited, the eyes become brown. Less iris stroma pigmentation results in blue, hazel, or green coloration.

Ophthalmologic Examination

2

David F. Chang, MD

Of all the organs of the body, the eye is most accessible to direct examination. Visual function can be quantified by simple subjective testing. The external anatomy of the eye is visible to inspection with the unaided eye and with fairly simple instruments. Even the interior of the eye is visible through the clear cornea. The eye is the only part of the body where blood vessels and central nervous system tissue (retina and optic nerve) can be viewed directly. Important systemic effects of infectious, autoimmune, neoplastic, and vascular diseases may be visible from the internal eye examination.

The purpose of sections I and II of this chapter is to provide an overview of the ocular history and basic complete eye examination as performed by an ophthalmologist. In section III, more specialized examination techniques will be presented.

I. OCULAR HISTORY

The **chief complaint** is characterized according to its duration, frequency, intermittency, and rapidity of onset. The location, the severity, and the circumstances surrounding onset are important as well as any associated symptoms. Current eye medications being used and all other current and past ocular disorders are recorded, and a review of other pertinent ocular symptoms is performed.

The **past medical history** centers on the patient's general state of health and principal systemic illnesses if any. Vascular disorders commonly associated with ocular manifestations—such as diabetes and hypertension—should be asked about specifically. Just as a medical history should include ocular medications being used, the eye history should list the patient's systemic medications. This provides a general indication of health status and may include medications that affect ocular health, such as corticosteroids. Finally, any drug allergies should be recorded.

The **family history** is pertinent for ocular disorders such as strabismus, amblyopia, glaucoma, cataracts,

and retinal problems, such as retinal detachment or macular degeneration. Medical diseases such as diabetes may be relevant as well.

COMMON OCULAR SYMPTOMS

A basic understanding of ocular symptomatology is necessary for performing a proper ophthalmic examination. Ocular symptoms can be divided into three basic categories: abnormalities of vision, abnormalities of ocular appearance, and abnormalities of ocular sensation—pain and discomfort.

Symptoms and complaints should always be fully characterized. Was the **onset** gradual, rapid, or asymptomatic? (For example, was blurred vision in one eye not discovered until the opposite eye was inadvertently covered?) Was the **duration** brief, or has the symptom continued until the present visit? If the symptom was intermittent, what was the frequency? Is the **location** focal or diffuse, and is involvement unilateral or bilateral? Finally, is the **degree** characterized by the patient as mild, moderate, or severe?

One should also determine what therapeutic measures have been tried and to what extent they have helped. Has the patient identified circumstances that trigger or worsen the symptom? Have similar instances occurred before, and are there any other associated symptoms?

The following is a brief overview of ocular complaints. Representative examples of some causes are given here and discussed more fully elsewhere in this book.

ABNORMALITIES OF VISION

Visual Loss

Loss of visual acuity may be due to abnormalities anywhere along the optical and neurologic visual pathway. One must therefore consider refractive (focusing) error, lid ptosis, clouding or interference from the ocular media (eg, corneal edema, cataract, or hemorrhage in the vitreous or aqueous space), and malfunction of the retina (macula), optic nerve, or intracranial visual pathway.

A distinction should be made between decreased central acuity and peripheral vision. The latter may be focal, such as a scotoma, or more expansive as with hemianopia. Abnormalities of the intracranial visual pathway usually disturb the visual field more than central visual acuity.

Transient loss of central or peripheral vision is frequently due to circulatory changes anywhere along the neurologic visual pathway from the retina to the occipital cortex. Examples would be amaurosis fugax or migrainous scotoma.

The degree of visual impairment may vary under different circumstances. For example, uncorrected nearsighted refractive error may seem worse in dark environments. This is because pupillary dilation allows more misfocused rays to reach the retina, increasing the blur. A central focal cataract may seem worse in sunlight. In this case, pupillary constriction prevents more rays from entering and passing around the lens opacity. Blurred vision from corneal edema may improve as the day progresses owing to corneal dehydration from surface evaporation.

Visual Aberrations

Glare or **haloes** may result from uncorrected refractive error, scratches on spectacle lenses, excessive pupillary dilation, and hazy ocular media, such as corneal edema or cataract. **Visual distortion** (apart from blurring) may be manifested as an irregular pattern of dimness, wavy or jagged lines, and image magnification or minification. Causes may include the aura of migraine, optical distortion from strong corrective lenses, or lesions involving the macula and optic nerve. **Flashing** or **flickering** lights may indicate retinal traction (if instantaneous) or migrainous scintillations that last for several seconds or minutes. **Floating spots** may represent normal vitreous strands due to vitreous "syneresis" or separation (see Chapter 9), or the pathologic presence of pigment, blood, or inflammatory cells. **Oscillopsia** is a shaking field of vision due to ocular instability.

It must be determined whether **double vision** is monocular or binocular (ie, disappears if one eye is covered). **Monocular diplopia** is often a split shadow or ghost image. Causes include uncorrected refractive error, such as astigmatism, or focal media abnormalities such as cataracts or corneal irregularities (eg, scars, keratoconus). **Binocular diplopia** (see Chapters 12 and 14) can be vertical, horizontal, diagonal, or torsional. If the deviation occurs or increases in one gaze direction as opposed to others, it is called "incomitant." Neuromuscular dysfunction or mechanical restriction of globe rotation is suspected. "Comitant" deviation is one that remains constant regardless of the direction of gaze. It is usually due to childhood or long-standing strabismus.

ABNORMALITIES OF APPEARANCE

Complaints of "red eye" call for differentiation between redness of the lids and periocular area versus redness of the globe. The latter can be caused by subconjunctival hemorrhage or by vascular congestion of the conjunctiva, sclera, or episclera (connective tissue between the sclera and conjunctiva). Causes of such congestion may be either external surface inflammation, such as conjunctivitis and keratitis, or intraocular inflammation such as iritis and acute glaucoma. Color abnormalities other than redness may include jaundice and hyperpigmented spots on the iris or outer ocular surface.

Other changes in appearance of the **globe** that may be noticeable to the patient include focal lesions of the ocular surface, such as a pterygium, and asymmetry of pupil size, called "anisocoria." The **lids** and **periocular tissues** may be the source of visible signs such as edema, redness, focal growths and lesions, and abnormal position or contour, such as ptosis. Finally, the patient may notice bulging or displacement of the globe, as with exophthalmos.

PAIN & DISCOMFORT

"Eye pain" may be periocular, ocular, retrobulbar (behind the globe), or poorly localized. Examples of **periocular** pain may be tenderness of the lid, tear sac, sinuses, or temporal artery. **Retrobulbar** pain can be due to orbital inflammation of any kind. Certain locations of inflammation, such as optic neuritis or orbital myositis, may produce pain on eye movement. Many **nonspecific** complaints such as "eyestrain," "pulling," "pressure," "fullness," and certain kinds of "headaches" are poorly localized. Causes may include fatigue from ocular accommodation or binocular fusion, or referred discomfort from nonocular muscle tension or fatigue.

Ocular pain itself may seem to emanate from the surface or from deeper within the globe. Corneal epithelial damage typically produces a superficial sharp pain or foreign body sensation exacerbated by blinking. Topical anesthesia will immediately relieve this pain. Deeper internal aching pain occurs with acute glaucoma, iritis, endophthalmitis, and scleritis. The globe is often tender to palpation in these situations. Reflex spasm of the ciliary muscle and iris sphincter can occur with iritis or keratitis, producing brow ache and painful "photophobia" (light sensitivity). This discomfort is markedly improved by instillation of cycloplegic dilating drops (see Chapter 3).

Eye Irritation

Superficial ocular discomfort usually results from surface abnormalities. **Itching,** as a primary symptom, is often a sign of allergic sensitivity. Symptoms of **dryness,** burning, grittiness, and mild foreign body sensation can occur with dry eyes or other types of mild corneal irritation. **Tearing** may be of two general types. Sudden reflex tearing is usually due to irritation of the ocular surface. In contrast, chronic watering and "epiphora" (tears rolling down the cheek) may indicate abnormal lacrimal drainage (see Chapter 4).

Ocular **secretions** are often diagnostically nonspecific. Severe amounts of discharge that cause the lids to be glued shut upon awakening usually indicate viral or bacterial conjunctivitis. More scant amounts of mucoid discharge can also be seen with allergic and noninfectious irritations. Dried matter and crusts on the lashes may occur acutely with conjunctivitis or chronically with blepharitis (lid margin inflammation).

II. BASIC OPHTHALMOLOGIC EXAMINATION

The purpose of the ophthalmologic physical examination is to evaluate both the function and the anatomy of the two eyes. Function includes vision and nonvisual functions, such as eye movements and alignment. Anatomically, ocular problems can be subdivided into three areas: those of the adnexa (lids and periocular tissue), the globe, and the orbit.

VISION

Just as assessment of vital signs is a part of every physical examination, any ocular examination must include assessment of vision, regardless of whether vision is mentioned as part of the chief complaint. Good vision results from a combination of an intact neurologic visual pathway, a structurally healthy eye, and proper focus of the eye. An analogy might be made to a video camera, requiring a functioning cable connection to the monitor, a mechanically intact camera body, and a proper focus setting. In general, measurement of visual acuity is subjective rather than objective, since it requires responses on the part of the patient.

Refraction

The unaided distant focal point of the eye varies among normal individuals depending on the shape of the globe and the cornea (Figure 2–1). An **emmetropic** eye is naturally in optimal focus for distance vision. An **ametropic** eye (ie, one with myopia, hyperopia, or astigmatism) needs corrective lenses to be in proper focus for distance. This optical requirement is called **refractive error. Refraction** is the procedure by which this natural optical error is characterized and quantified (Figure 2–2) (see Chapter 20).

Refraction is often necessary to distinguish between blurred vision caused by refractive (ie, optical) error or by medical abnormalities of the visual system. Thus, in addition to being the basis for prescription of corrective glasses or contact lenses, refraction serves a diagnostic function.

Testing Central Vision

Vision can be divided into central vision and peripheral vision. Central visual acuity is measured with a display of different-sized targets shown at a standard

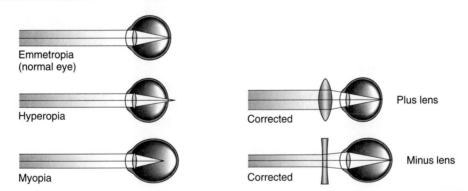

Figure 2–1. Common imperfections of the optical system of the eye **(refractive errors).** Ideally, light rays from a distant target should automatically arrive in focus on the retina if the retina is situated precisely at the eye's natural focal point. Such an eye is called **emmetropic.** In **hyperopia** ("farsightedness"), the light rays from a distant target instead come to a focus behind the retina, causing the retinal image to be blurred. A biconvex (+) lens corrects this by increasing the refractive power of the eye, and shifting the focal point forward. In **myopia** ("nearsightedness"), the light rays come to a focus in front of the retina, as though the eyeball is too long. Placing a biconcave (-) lens in front of the eye diverges the incoming light rays; this effectively weakens the optical power of the eye enough so that the focus is shifted backward and onto the retina. (Modified and reproduced, with permission, from Ganong WF: *Review of Medical Physiology,* 15th ed. Lange, 1991.)

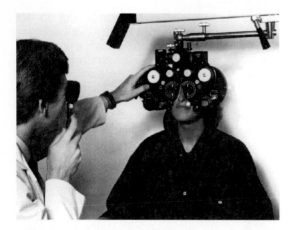

Figure 2–2. Refraction being performed using a "phoropter." This device contains the complete range of corrective lens powers which can quickly be changed back and forth, allowing the patient to subjectively compare various combinations while viewing the eye chart at a distance. (Photo by M Narahara.)

distance from the eye. For example, the familiar "Snellen chart" is composed of a series of progressively smaller rows of random letters used to test distance vision. Each row is designated by a number corresponding to the distance, in feet or meters, from which a normal eye can read all the letters of the row. For example, the letters in the "40" row are large enough for the normal eye to see from 40 feet away.

By convention, vision can be measured either at a distance at 20 feet (6 meters) or at near, 14 inches away. For diagnostic purposes, distance acuity is the standard for comparison and is always tested separately for each eye. Acuity is scored as a set of two numbers (eg, "20/40"). The first number represents the testing distance in feet between the chart and the patient, and the second number represents the smallest row of letters that the patient's eye can read from the testing distance. 20/20 vision is normal; 20/60 vision indicates that the patient's eye can only read from 20 feet letters large enough for a normal eye to read from 60 feet.

Charts containing numerals can be used for patients not familiar with the English alphabet. The "illiterate E" chart is used to test small children or if there is a language barrier. "E" figures are randomly rotated in each of four different orientations throughout the chart. For each target, the patient is asked to point in the same direction as the three "bars" of the E (Figure 2–3). Most children can be tested in this manner beginning at about age 3$\frac{1}{2}$.

Uncorrected visual acuity is measured without glasses or contact lenses. **Corrected** acuity means that these aids were worn. Since poor uncorrected distance acuity may simply be due to refractive (ie, focusing) error, corrected visual acuity is a more relevant assessment of ocular health.

Pinhole Test

If the patient needs glasses or if they are unavailable, the corrected acuity can be estimated by testing vision through a "pinhole." Refractive blur (eg, myopia, hyperopia, astigmatism) is caused by multiple misfocused rays entering through the pupil and reaching the retina. This prevents formation of a sharply focused image.

Viewing the Snellen chart through a placard of multiple tiny pinhole-sized openings prevents most of the misfocused rays from entering the eye. Only a few centrally aligned focused rays will reach the retina, resulting in a sharper image. In this manner, the patient may be able to read within one or two lines of what would be possible if proper corrective glasses were being used.

Testing Poor Vision

The patient unable to read the largest letter on the chart (eg, the "20/200" letter) should be moved closer to the chart until that letter can be read. The distance from the chart is then recorded as the first number. Visual acuity of "5/200" means that the patient can just make out the largest letter from a distance of 5 feet. An eye unable to read any letters is tested by the ability to count fingers. A notation on the chart that reads "CF at 2 ft" indicates that the eye was able to count fingers held 2 feet away but not farther away.

If counting fingers is not possible, the eye may be able to detect a hand moving vertically or horizontally

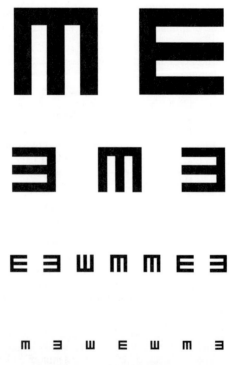

Figure 2–3. "Illiterate E" chart.

("HM," or "hand motions" vision). The next lower level of vision would be the ability to perceive light ("LP," or "light perception"). An eye that cannot perceive light is considered totally blind ("NLP," or "no light perception").

Testing Peripheral Vision

Because it is much grosser than central acuity, side vision is harder to test quantitatively. Specialized tests described in the next section are used when peripheral vision measurements are needed, such as for the diagnosis of early glaucoma.

Gross screening of the peripheral field of vision can be quickly performed using **confrontation testing.** Since the visual fields of the two eyes overlap, each eye must be tested separately. The patient is seated facing the examiner several feet away and begins by covering the left eye while the right eye fixes on the examiner's left eye.

The examiner then briefly shows several fingers of one hand (usually one, two, or four fingers) peripherally in one of the four quadrants. The patient must identify the number of fingers flashed while maintaining straight-ahead fixation. Since patient and examiner are staring eye to eye, any loss of fixation by the patient will be noticed. The upper and lower temporal and the upper and lower nasal quadrants are all tested in this fashion for each eye.

If the examiner closes the right eye while the patient covers the left eye—and if the targets (fingers) are presented at a distance halfway between the patient and the examiner—their respective peripheral fields should be the same. This allows comparison of the patient's field with the examiner's own. Consistent errors indicate gross deficiencies in the quadrant tested, as seen with retinal detachments, optic nerve abnormalities, and ischemic or mass injuries to the intracranial visual pathway. Since dense visual field abnormalities are often asymptomatic, confrontation testing should be included in complete ophthalmologic examinations.

A subtle form of right or left homonymous hemianopia may exist that can only be elicited by simultaneously presenting targets on both sides of the midline—not when targets are presented on one side at a time. To perform **simultaneous confrontation testing,** the examiner holds both hands out peripherally, one on each side. The patient must signify on which side (right, left, or both) the examiner is intermittently wiggling the fingers. Surprisingly, a patient with a mild left hemianopia may still be able to detect one hand wiggling fingers to the left side and may fail to see them (to the left) only when the examiner is simultaneously wiggling the fingers on both hands. This interesting finding indicates partial or relative inattention to the left side as both sides are being equally—and simultaneously—stimulated.

More sophisticated means of visual field testing are discussed later in this chapter.

PUPILS

Basic Examination

The pupils should appear symmetric, and each one should be examined for size, shape (circular or irregular), and reactivity to both light and accommodation. Pupillary abnormalities may be due to (1) neurologic disease, (2) acute intraocular inflammation causing either spasm or atony of the pupillary sphincter, (3) previous inflammation causing adhesions of the iris, (4) prior surgical alteration, (5) the effect of systemic or eye medications, and (6) benign variations of normal.

To avoid accommodation, the patient is asked to stare in the distance as a penlight is directed toward each eye. Dim lighting conditions help to accentuate the pupillary response and may best demonstrate an abnormally small pupil. Likewise, an abnormally large pupil may be more apparent in brighter background illumination. The **direct response** to light refers to constriction of the illuminated pupil. The reaction may be graded as either brisk or sluggish. Normally, a **consensual** constriction will simultaneously occur in the opposite nonilluminated pupil. This is usually a slightly weaker response. The neuroanatomy of the pupillary pathway is discussed in Chapter 14.

Swinging Penlight Test for Marcus Gunn Pupil

As a light is swung back and forth in front of the two pupils, one can compare the direct and consensual reactions of each pupil. Since the direct reaction is usually stronger than the consensual, each pupil as the light falls directly on it should immediately constrict slightly more. Start by shining the light into the right eye, causing consensual constriction of the left pupil. As the light is then swung toward the left eye, the left pupil should constrict slightly more due to the direct light response. The right pupil should behave similarly as the light is swung back toward the right eye.

If the afferent conduction of light in the left optic nerve is impaired as a consequence of disease, the left pupil will have a weak direct response but its consensual efferent response will remain unchanged. As the light is swung from the right to the left eye, the left pupil will then paradoxically *widen* (since its abnormal direct response is weaker than the consensual response initiated by the healthy right optic nerve). This phenomenon is called a Marcus Gunn pupil, or relative afferent pupillary defect, since the paradoxic dilation in response to direct illumination occurs in the eye with the abnormal afferent pathway (ie, optic nerve or retina). Because the Marcus Gunn pupil still reacts and is often of normal size, the swinging flashlight test may be the only means of demonstrating it.

Marcus Gunn pupil is further discussed and illustrated in Chapter 14.

OCULAR MOTILITY

The objective of ocular motility testing is to evaluate the alignment of the eyes and their movements, both individually ("ductions") and in tandem ("versions"). A more complete discussion of motility testing and abnormalities is presented in Chapter 12.

Testing Alignment

Normal patients have binocular vision. Since each eye generates a visual image separate from and independent of that of the other eye, the brain must be able to fuse the two images in order to avoid "double vision." This is achieved by having each eye positioned so that both foveas are simultaneously fixating on the object of regard.

A simple test of binocular alignment is performed by having the patient look toward a penlight held several feet away. A pinpoint light reflection, or "reflex," should appear on each cornea and should be centered over each pupil if the two eyes are straight in their alignment. If the eye positions are convergent, such that one eye points inward ("esotropia"), the light reflex will appear temporal to the pupil in that eye. If the eyes are divergent, such that one eye points outward ("exotropia"), the light reflex will be located more nasally in that eye. This test can be used with infants.

The **cover test** (see Figure 12–3) is a more accurate method of verifying normal ocular alignment. The test requires good vision in both eyes. The patient is asked to gaze at a distant target with both eyes open. If both eyes are fixating together on the target, covering one eye should not affect the position or continued fixation of the other eye.

To perform the test, the examiner suddenly covers one eye and carefully watches to see that the second eye does not move (indicating that it was fixating on the same target already). If the second eye was not identically aligned but was instead turned abnormally inward or outward, it could not have been simultaneously fixating on the target. Thus, it will have to quickly move to find the target once the previously fixating eye is covered. Fixation of each eye is tested in turn.

An abnormal cover test is expected in patients with diplopia. However, diplopia is not always present in many patients with long-standing ocular malalignment. When the test is abnormal, prism lenses of different power can be used to neutralize the refixation movement of the misaligned eye. In this way, the amount of eye deviation can be quantified based on the amount of prism power needed. A more complete discussion of this test and its variations is presented in Chapter 12.

Testing Extraocular Movements

The patient is asked to follow a target with both eyes as it is moved in each of the four cardinal directions of gaze. The examiner notes the speed, smoothness, range, and symmetry of movements and observes for unsteadiness of fixation (eg, nystagmus).

Impairment of eye movements can be due to neurologic problems (eg, cranial nerve palsy), primary extraocular muscular weakness (eg, myasthenia gravis), or mechanical constraints within the orbit limiting rotation of the globe (eg, orbital floor fracture with entrapment of the inferior rectus muscle). If the amount of deviation of ocular alignment is the same in all directions of gaze, is called "comitant." It is "incomitant" if the amount of deviation varies with the direction of gaze.

EXTERNAL EXAMINATION

Before studying the eye under magnification, a general external examination of the ocular adnexa (eyelids and periocular area) is performed. Skin lesions, growths, and inflammatory signs such as swelling, erythema, warmth, and tenderness are evaluated by gross inspection and palpation.

The positions of the eyelids are checked for abnormalities such as ptosis or lid retraction. Asymmetry can be quantified by measuring the central width (in millimeters) of the "palpebral fissure"—the space between the upper and lower lid margins. Abnormal motor function of the lids, such as impairment of upper lid elevation or forceful lid closure, may be due to either neurologic or primary muscular abnormalities.

Gross malposition of the globe, such as proptosis, may be seen with certain orbital diseases. Palpation of the bony orbital rim and periocular soft tissue should always be done in instances of suspected orbital trauma, infection, or neoplasm. The general facial examination may contribute other pertinent information as well. Depending on the circumstances, checking for enlarged preauricular lymph nodes, sinus tenderness, temporal artery prominence, or skin or mucous membrane abnormalities may be diagnostically relevant.

SLITLAMP EXAMINATION

Basic Slitlamp Biomicroscopy

The slitlamp (Figure 2–4) is a table-mounted binocular microscope with a special adjustable illumination source attached. A linear slit beam of incandescent light is projected onto the globe, illuminating an optical cross section of the eye (Figure 2–5). The angle of illumination can be varied along with the width, length, and intensity of the light beam. The magnification can be adjusted as well (normally 10× to 16× power). Since the slitlamp is a binocular microscope, the view is "stereoscopic," or three-dimensional.

The patient is seated while being examined, and the head is stabilized by an adjustable chin rest and fore-

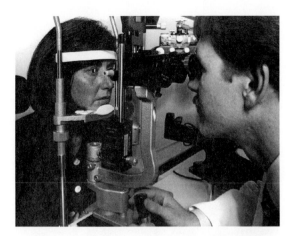

Figure 2–4. Slitlamp examination. (Photo by M Narahara.) (Courtesy of the American Academy of Ophthalmology.)

head strap. Using the slitlamp alone, the anterior half of the globe—the "anterior segment"—can be visualized. Details of the lid margins and lashes, the palpebral and bulbar conjunctival surfaces, the tear film and cornea, the iris, and the aqueous can be studied. Through a dilated pupil, the crystalline lens and the anterior vitreous can be examined as well.

Because the slit beam of light provides an optical cross section of the eye, the precise anteroposterior location of abnormalities can be determined within each of the clear ocular structures (eg, cornea, lens, vitreous body). The highest magnification setting is sufficient to show the abnormal presence of cells within the aqueous, such as red or white blood cells or pigment granules. Aqueous turbidity, called "flare,"

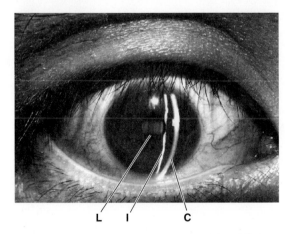

L   I   C

Figure 2–5. Slitlamp photograph of a normal right eye. The curved slit of light to the right is reflected off of the cornea (C), while the slit to the left is reflected off of the iris (I). As the latter slit passes through the pupil, the anterior lens (L) is faintly illuminated in cross section. (Photo by M Narahara.)

resulting from increased protein concentration can be detected in the presence of intraocular inflammation. Normal aqueous is optically clear, without cells or flare.

Adjunctive Slitlamp Techniques

The eye examination with the slitlamp is supplemented by the use of various techniques. Tonometry is discussed separately in a subsequent section.

A. Lid Eversion: Lid eversion to examine the undersurface of the upper lid can be performed either at the slitlamp or without the aid of that instrument. It should always be done if the presence of a foreign body is suspected. A semirigid plate of cartilage called the tarsus gives each lid its contour and shape. In the upper lid, the superior edge of the tarsus lies centrally about 8–9 mm above the lashes. On the undersurface of the lid, it is covered by the tarsal palpebral conjunctiva.

Following topical anesthesia, the patient is positioned at the slitlamp and instructed to look down. The examiner gently grasps the upper lashes with the thumb and index finger of one hand while using the other hand to position an applicator handle just above the superior edge of the tarsus (Figure 2–6). The lid is everted by applying slight downward pressure with the applicator as the lash margin is simultaneously lifted. The patient continues to look down, and the lashes are held pinned to the skin overlying the superior orbital rim, as the applicator is withdrawn. The tarsal conjunctiva is then examined under magnification. To undo eversion the lid margin is gently stroked downward as the patient looks up.

B. Fluorescein Staining: Fluorescein is a specialized dye that stains the cornea and highlights any irregularities of its epithelial surface. Sterile paper strips containing fluorescein are wetted and touched against the inner surface of the lower lid, instilling the yellowish dye into the tear film. The illuminating light of the slitlamp is made blue with a filter, causing the dye to fluoresce.

A uniform film of dye should cover the normal cornea. If the corneal surface is abnormal, excessive amounts of dye will absorb into or collect within the affected area. Abnormalities can range from tiny punctate dots, such as those resulting from excessive dryness or ultraviolet light damage, to large geographic defects in the epithelium such as those seen in corneal abrasions or infectious ulcers.

C. Special Lenses: Special examining lenses can expand and further magnify the slitlamp examination of the eye's interior. A goniolens (Figure 2–7) provides visualization of the anterior chamber "angle" formed by the iridocorneal junction. Other lenses placed on or in front of the dilated eye allow slitlamp evaluation of the posterior half of the globe's interior—the "posterior segment." Since the slitlamp is a binocular microscope, these lenses provide a magnified three-dimensional view of the posterior vitreous,

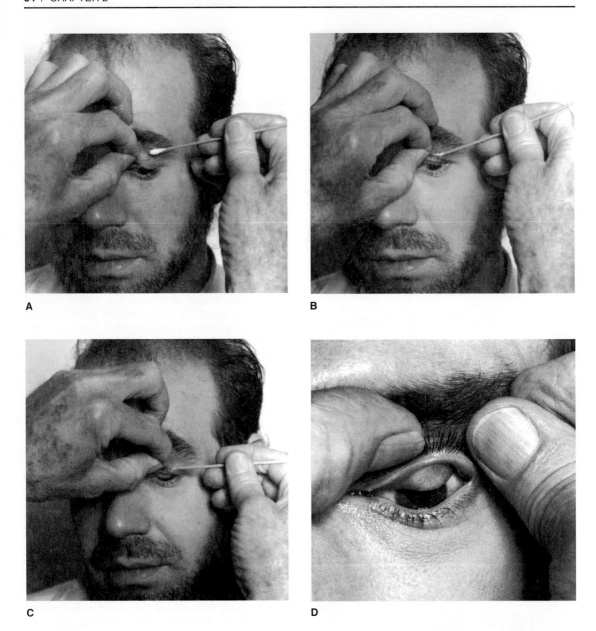

Figure 2–6. Technique of lid eversion. **A:** With the patient looking down, the upper lashes are grasped with one hand as an applicator stick is positioned at the superior edge of the upper tarsus (at the upper lid crease). **B and C:** As the lashes are lifted, slight downward pressure is simultaneously applied with the applicator stick. **D:** The thumb pins the lashes against the superior orbital rim, allowing examination of the undersurface of the tarsus. (Photos by M Narahara.)

the fundus, and the disk. Examples are the Goldmann-style three-mirror lens (Figure 2–7), the Hruby lens, and the Volk-style 90-diopter biconvex lens.

D. Special Attachments: Special attachments to the slitlamp allow it to be used with a number of techniques requiring microscopic visualization. Special camera bodies can be attached for photographic documentation and for special applications such as corneal endothelial cell studies. Special instruments for study of visual potential require attachment to the slitlamp.

Finally, laser sources are attached to a slitlamp to allow microscopic visualization and control of eye treatment.

TONOMETRY

The globe can be thought of as an enclosed compartment through which there is a constant circulation of aqueous humor. This fluid maintains the shape and a relatively uniform pressure within the globe.

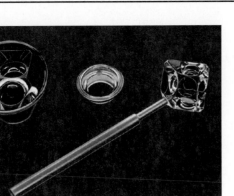

Figure 2–7. Three types of goniolenses. **Left:** Goldmann three-mirror lens. Besides the goniomirror, there are also two peripheral retinal mirrors and a central fourth mirror for examining the central retina. **Center:** Koeppe lens. **Right:** Posner/Zeiss-type lens. (Photo by M Narahara.)

Tonometry is the method of measuring the intraocular fluid pressure using calibrated instruments that indent or flatten the corneal apex. As the eye becomes firmer, a greater force is required to cause the same amount of indentation. Pressures between 10 and 24 mm Hg are considered within the normal range.

Two common types of tonometry are the **Schiotz** and **applanation** methods. The Schiotz tonometer measures the amount of corneal indentation produced by a preset weight or force. The softer the eye, the more a given force will be able to indent the cornea. As the eye becomes firmer, less corneal indentation will result from the same amount of force.

In contrast to the Schiotz tonometer, the applanation tonometer can vary and measure the amount of force applied. The ocular pressure is determined by the force required to flatten the cornea by a predetermined standard amount. At lower intraocular pressures, less tonometer force is needed to achieve the standard degree of corneal flattening than at higher intraocular pressures. Since both methods employ devices that touch the patient's cornea, they require topical anesthetic and disinfection of the instrument tip prior to use. (Tonometer disinfection techniques are discussed in Chapter 21.) While retracting the lids with any method of tonometry, care must be taken to avoid pressing on the globe and artificially increasing its pressure.

Schiotz Tonometry

The advantage of this method is that it is simple, requiring only a portable hand-held instrument—the Schiotz tonometer (Figure 2–8). It can be used in any clinic or emergency room setting, at the hospital bedside, or in the operating room. It is a practical device for the nonophthalmologist, who might use it to screen patients for glaucoma or to diagnose acute angle closure glaucoma in an emergency situation.

The three separate components of the tonometer should be cleaned, assembled, and then disassembled with each use. The tonometer **body** consists of a cylindric hollow plunger barrel fixed to a measuring scale with an indicator needle. The attached handle, which can slide along the outside of the cylindric barrel, supports the weight of the tonometer when it is not resting on the eye. The **plunger** is a slender blunt-tipped rod that is inserted into the barrel shaft, where it can slide back and forth. One end will touch the cornea, while the other end will deflect the needle of the measuring scale. The 5.5 g **weight** screwed onto the upper end of the plunger (farthest from the patient) keeps it from falling out of the shaft.

The patient is placed supine, and topical anesthetic is instilled into each eye. As the patient looks straight ahead, the lids are kept gently opened by lightly retracting the skin against the bony orbital rims. The tonometer is lowered with the other hand until the concave "end" of the barrel balances on the cornea (Figure 2–9). With a force determined by the attached weight, the blunt protruding plunger will press into and slightly indent the central cornea. The corneal resistance, which is proportionate to the intraocular pressure, will displace the plunger upward. As the plunger slides upward within the barrel, it will deflect the needle on the scale. The higher the intraocular pressure, the greater the corneal resistance to indentation, the more the plunger will be displaced upward, and the farther the needle will be deflected along the calibrated scale.

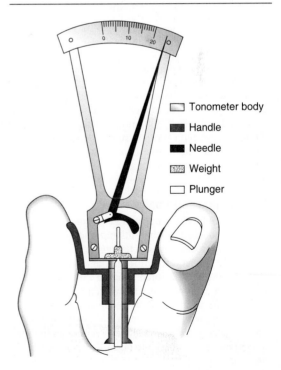

Figure 2–8. Diagram of Schiotz tonometer. The plunger is shown with the 5.5-g weight attached at one end.

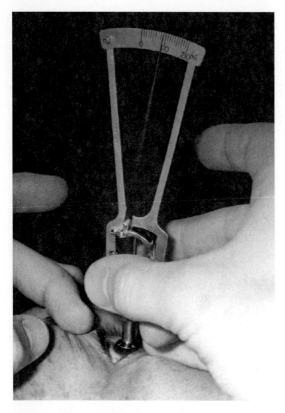

Figure 2–9. Schiotz tonometer placed on cornea. Handle is being held by thumb and third finger of right hand in this photo. (Photo by Diane Beeston.)

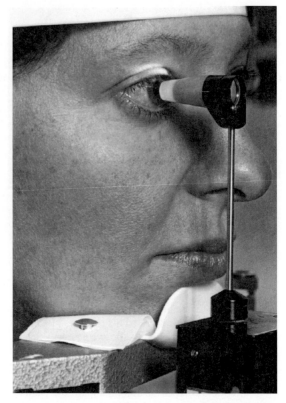

Figure 2–10. Applanation tonometry, using the Goldmann tonometer attached to the slit lamp. (Photo by M Narahara. Courtesy of the American Academy of Ophthalmology.)

A conversion chart is used to translate the reading from the scale into millimeters of mercury. If the eye is firm, additional weights (7.5 g and 10 g) can be added to the plunger to increase the force brought to bear on the cornea. Calibration is checked by placing the tonometer on a "cornea-shaped" metal block that should deflect the needle maximally so that it aligns with the "0" end of the scale.

Applanation Tonometry

The Goldmann applanation tonometer (Figure 2–10) is attached to the slitlamp and measures the amount of force required to flatten the corneal apex by a standard amount. The higher the intraocular pressure, the greater the force required. Since Goldmann applanation tonometer is a more accurate method than Schiotz tonometry, it is preferred by ophthalmologists.

Following topical anesthesia and instillation of fluorescein, the patient is positioned at the slitlamp and the tonometer is swung into place. To visualize the fluorescein, the cobalt blue filter is used with the brightest illumination setting. After grossly aligning the tonometer in front of the cornea, the examiner looks through the slitlamp ocular just as the tip contacts the cornea. A manually controlled counterbalanced spring varies the force applied by the tonometer tip.

Upon contact, the tonometer tip flattens the central cornea and produces a thin circular outline of fluorescein. A prism in the tip visually splits this circle into two semicircles that appear green while viewed through the slitlamp oculars. The tonometer force is adjusted manually until the two semicircles just overlap, as shown in Figure 2–11. This visual end point indicates that the cornea has been flattened by the set standard amount. The amount of force required to do this is translated by the scale into a pressure reading in millimeters of mercury.

A portable electronic applanation tonometer, the **Tono-Pen,** has been developed. Although accurate, it requires daily recalibration. It is more expensive than the Schiotz tonometer and therefore is less often found in clinics and emergency departments. The **Perkins tonometer** is a portable mechanical applanation tonometer with a mechanism similar to the Goldmann tonometer. The **pneumatotonometer** is another applanation tonometer, particularly useful when the cornea has an irregular surface.

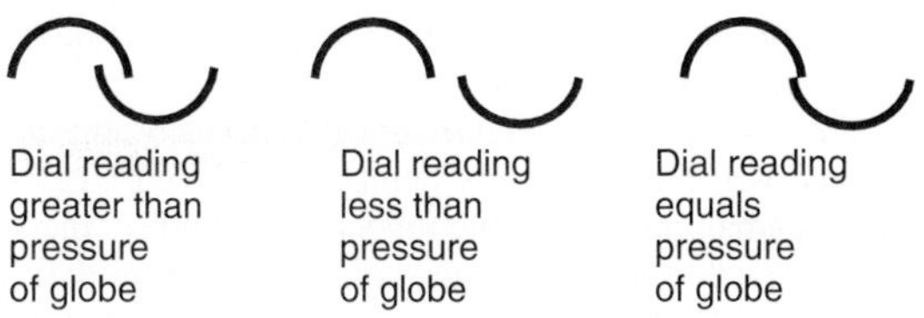

Dial reading
greater than
pressure
of globe

Dial reading
less than
pressure
of globe

Dial reading
equals
pressure
of globe

Figure 2–11. Appearance of fluorescein semicircles, or "mires," through the slit lamp ocular, showing the end point for applanation tonometry.

Noncontact Tonometry

The **noncontact ("air-puff") tonometer** is not as accurate as applanation tonometers. A small puff of air is blown against the cornea. The air rebounding from the corneal surface hits a pressure-sensing membrane in the instrument. This method does not require anesthetic drops, since no instrument touches the eye. Thus, it can be more easily used by technicians and is useful in screening programs.

DIAGNOSTIC MEDICATIONS

Topical Anesthetics

Eye drops such as proparacaine, tetracaine, and benoxinate provide rapid onset, short-acting topical anesthesia of the cornea, and conjunctiva. They are used prior to ocular contact with diagnostic lenses and instruments such as the tonometer. Other diagnostic manipulations utilizing topical anesthetics will be discussed later. These include corneal and conjunctival scrapings, lacrimal canalicular and punctal probing, and scleral depression.

Mydriatic (Dilating) Drops

The pupil can be pharmacologically dilated by either stimulating the iris dilator muscle with a sympathomimetic agent (eg, 2.5% phenylephrine) or by inhibiting the sphincter muscle with an anticholinergic eye drop (eg, 0.5% or 1% tropicamide). Anticholinergic medications also inhibit accommodation, an effect called "cycloplegia." This may aid the process of refraction but causes further inconvenience for the patient. Therefore, drops with the shortest duration of action (usually several hours) are used for diagnostic applications. Combining drops from both pharmacologic classes produces the fastest onset (15–20 minutes) and widest dilation.

Because dilation can cause a small rise in intraocular pressure, tonometry should always be performed before these drops are instilled. There is also a risk of precipitating an attack of acute angle-closure glaucoma if the patient has preexisting narrow anterior chamber angles (between the iris and cornea). Such an eye can be identified using the technique illustrated in Figure 11–4. Finally, excessive instillation of these drops should be avoided because of the systemic ab-

sorption that can occur through the nasopharyngeal mucous membranes following lacrimal drainage.

A more complete discussion of diagnostic drops is found in Chapter 3.

DIRECT OPHTHALMOSCOPY

Instrumentation

The hand-held direct ophthalmoscope provides a magnified (15×) monocular image of the ocular media and fundus. Because of its portability and the detailed view of the disk and retinal vasculature it provides, direct ophthalmoscopy is a standard part of the general medical examination as well as the ophthalmologic examination.

Darkening the room usually causes enough natural pupillary dilation to allow evaluation of the central fundus, including the disk, the macula, and the proximal retinal vasculature. Pharmacologically dilating the pupil greatly enhances the view and permits a more extensive examination of the peripheral retina. The fundus examination is also optimized by holding the ophthalmoscope as close to the patient's pupil as possible (approximately 1–2 inches), just as one can see more through a keyhole by getting as close to it as possible. This requires using the examiner's right eye and hand to examine the patient's right eye and the left eye and hand to examine the patient's left eye (Figure 2–12). If the examiner wears spectacles, they can either be left on or off.

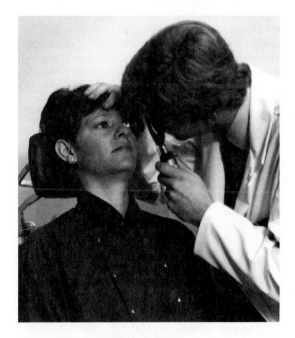

Figure 2–12. Direct ophthalmoscopy. The examiner uses the left eye to evaluate the patient's left eye. (Photo by M Narahara. Courtesy of the American Academy of Ophthalmology.)

The intensity, color, and spot size of the illuminating light can be adjusted as well as the ophthalmoscope's point of focus. The latter is changed using a wheel of progressively higher power lenses that the examiner dials into place. These lenses are sequentially arranged and numbered according to their power in units called "diopters." The descending scale of black numbers designates the (+) converging lenses, whereas the ascending scale of red numbers designates the (−) divergent lenses.

As one dials this focusing wheel counterclockwise from high plus (+) lenses down to zero and on through increasingly minus (−) lenses, the focus is shifted progressively farther away from the ophthalmoscope toward the patient. By starting with a higher (+) lens and dialing in this direction, the examiner will eventually bring the cornea and iris into focus, followed several steps later by the retina. The refractive error (ie, "prescriptions") of the patient's and the examiner's eyes will determine the lens power needed to bring the fundus into optimal focus.

Fundus Examination

The primary value of the direct ophthalmoscope is in examination of the fundus (Figure 2–13). The view may be impaired by cloudy ocular media, such as a cataract, or by insufficient pupillary dilation. As the patient fixates on a distant target with the opposite eye, the examiner first brings retinal details into sharp focus. Since the retinal vessels all arise from the disk, the latter is located by following any major vascular branch back to this common origin. At this point, the ophthalmoscope beam will be aimed slightly nasal to the patient's line of vision, or "visual axis." One should study the shape, size, and color of the disk, the distinctness of its margins, and the size of the pale central "physiologic cup." The ratio of cup size to disk size is of diagnostic importance in glaucoma (Figures 2–14 and 2–15).

The macular area (Figure 2–13) is located approximately two "disk diameters" temporal to the edge of the disk. A small pinpoint white reflection or "reflex" marks the central fovea. This is surrounded by a more darkly pigmented and poorly circumscribed area called the macula. The retinal vascular branches approach from all sides but stop short of the fovea. Thus, its location can be confirmed by the focal absence of retinal vessels or by asking the patient to stare directly into the light.

The major retinal vessels are then examined and followed as far distally as possible in each of the four quadrants (superior, inferior, temporal, and nasal). The veins are darker and wider than their paired arteries. The vessels are examined for color, tortuosity, and caliber as well as for associated abnormalities such as aneurysms, hemorrhages, or exudates. Sizes and distances within the fundus are often measured in "disk diameters (DD)." (The typical optic disk is generally 1.5–2 mm in diameter.) Thus, one might describe a "1 DD area of hemorrhage located 2.5 DD inferotemporal to the fovea."

Dilating the pupil pharmacologically enables more of the periphery to be visualized. The patient is asked to look in the direction of the quadrant one wishes to examine. Thus, the temporal retina of the right eye is seen when the patient looks temporally to the right, while the superior retina is seen when the patient looks up. This principle works because as the globe rotates about a point in the center of the eye, the retina and the cornea move in opposite directions. As the patient looks up, the superior retina rotates downward into the examiner's line of vision.

The spot size and color of the illuminating light can be varied. If the pupil is well dilated, the large spot size of light affords the widest area of illumination.

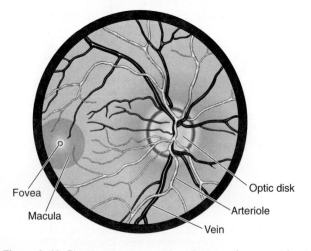
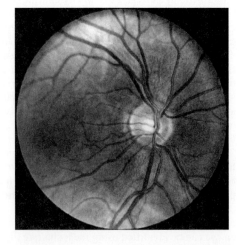

Fovea
Macula
Optic disk
Arteriole
Vein

Figure 2–13. Photo and corresponding diagram of a normal fundus. Note that the retinal vessels all stop short of and do not cross the fovea. (Photo by Diane Beeston.)

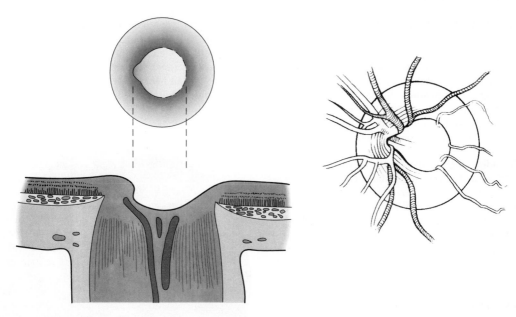

Figure 2–14. Diagram of a moderately cupped disk viewed on end and in profile, with an accompanying sketch for the patient's record. The width of the central cup divided by the width of the disk is the "cup-to-disk ratio." The cup-to-disk ratio of this disk is approximately 0.5.

With a smaller pupil, however, much of this light would be reflected back toward the examiner's eye by the patient's iris, interfering with the view. For this reason, the smaller spot size of light is selected for undilated pupils. The green "red-free" filter assists in the examination of the retinal vasculature and the subtle striations of the nerve fiber layer as they course toward the disk (see Figure 14–6).

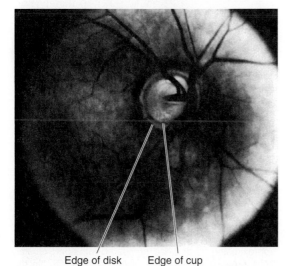

Edge of disk   Edge of cup

Figure 2–15. Cup-to-disk ratio of 0.9 in a patient with end-stage glaucoma. The normal disk tissue is compressed into a peripheral thin rim surrounding a huge pale cup.

Anterior Segment Examination

As discussed earlier, the direct ophthalmoscope can be focused more anteriorly so as to provide a magnified view of the conjunctiva, cornea, and iris. The slit-lamp allows a far superior and more magnified examination of these areas, but it is not portable and may be unavailable.

Red Reflex Examination

If the illuminating light is aligned directly along the visual axis of a dilated pupil, the pupillary space will appear as a homogeneous bright reddish-orange color. This so-called red reflex is a reflection of the fundus color (actually the combined color of the choroidal vasculature and pigmentation) back through clear ocular media—the vitreous, lens, aqueous, and cornea. The red reflex is best observed by holding the ophthalmoscope at arm's length from the patient as he looks toward the illuminating light. By dialing the lens wheel, the bright red reflex will appear when the ophthalmoscope is focused on the plane of the pupil.

Any opacity located along this central optical pathway will block all or part of this bright reflex and appear as a dark spot or shadow. If a small opacity is seen, have the patient look momentarily away and then back toward the light. If the opacity is still moving or floating, it is located within the vitreous (eg, small hemorrhage). If it is stationary, it is probably in the lens (eg, focal cataract) or on the cornea (eg, scar). Less red reflex is visible with a small pupil, limiting the usefulness of this test.

INDIRECT OPHTHALMOSCOPY

Instrumentation

The binocular indirect ophthalmoscope (Figure 2–16) complements and supplements the direct ophthalmoscopic examination. Since it requires wide pupillary dilation and is difficult to learn, this technique is used primarily by ophthalmologists. The patient can be examined while seated, but the supine position is preferable.

The indirect ophthalmoscope is worn on the examiner's head and allows binocular viewing through a set of lenses of fixed power. A bright adjustable light source attached to the headband is directed toward the patient's eye. As with direct ophthalmoscopy, the patient is told to look in the direction of the quadrant being examined. A convex lens is hand-held several inches from the patient's eye in precise orientation so as to simultaneously focus light onto the retina and an image of the retina in midair between the patient and the examiner. Using the preset head-mounted ophthalmoscope lenses, the examiner can then "focus on" and visualize this midair image of the retina.

Comparison of Indirect & Direct Ophthalmoscopy

Indirect ophthalmoscopy is so called because one is viewing an "image" of the retina formed by a hand-held "condensing lens." In contrast, direct ophthalmoscopy allows one to focus on the retina itself.

Compared with the direct ophthalmoscope (15× magnification), indirect ophthalmoscopy provides a much wider field of view (Figure 2–17) with less overall magnification (approximately 3.5× using a standard 20-diopter hand-held condensing lens). Thus, it presents a wide panoramic fundus view from which spe-

A

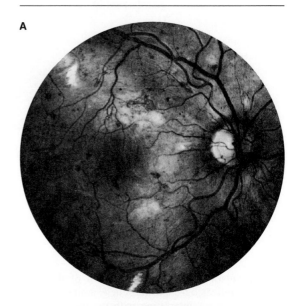

B

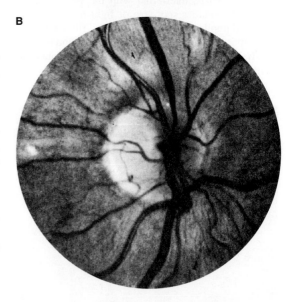

Figure 2–17. Comparison of view within the same fundus using the indirect ophthalmoscope *(A)* and the direct ophthalmoscope *(B).* The field of view with the latter is approximately 10 degrees, compared with approximately 37 degrees using the indirect ophthalmoscope. In this patient with diabetic retinopathy, an important overview is first seen with the indirect ophthalmoscope. The direct ophthalmoscope can then provide magnified details of a specific area. (Photos by M Narahara.)

Figure 2–16. Examination with head-mounted binocular indirect ophthalmoscope. A 20-diopter hand-held condensing lens is used. (Photo by M Narahara.)

cific areas can be selectively studied under higher magnification using either the direct ophthalmoscope or the slitlamp with special auxiliary lenses.

Indirect ophthalmoscopy has three distinct advantages over direct ophthalmoscopy. One is the brighter light source that permits much better visualization through cloudy media. A second advantage is that by using both eyes, the examiner enjoys a stereoscopic view, allowing visualization of elevated masses or retinal detachment in three dimensions. Finally, indirect ophthalmoscopy can be used to examine the entire retina even out to its extreme periphery, the ora serrata. This is possible for two reasons. Optical distortions caused by looking through the peripheral lens and cornea interfere very little with the indirect ophthalmoscopic examination, compared with the direct ophthalmoscope. In addition, the adjunct technique of scleral depression can be used.

Scleral depression (Figure 2–18) is performed as the peripheral retina is being examined with the indirect ophthalmoscope. A smooth, thin metal probe is used to gently indent the globe externally through the lids at a point just behind the corneoscleral junction (limbus). As this is done, the ora serrata and peripheral retina are pushed internally into the examiner's line of view. By depressing around the entire circumference, the peripheral retina can be viewed in its entirety.

Because of all of these advantages, indirect ophthalmoscopy is used preoperatively and intraoperatively in the evaluation and surgical repair of retinal detachments. A minor disadvantage of indirect ophthalmoscopy is that it provides an inverted image of the fundus, which requires a mental adjustment on the examiner's part. Its brighter light source can also be more uncomfortable for the patient.

EYE EXAMINATION BY THE NONOPHTHALMOLOGIST

The preceding sequence of tests would comprise a complete routine or diagnostic ophthalmologic evaluation. A general medical examination would often include many of these same testing techniques.

Assessment of pupils, extraocular movements, and confrontation visual fields is part of any complete neurologic assessment. Direct ophthalmoscopy should always be performed to assess the appearance of the disk and retinal vessels. Separately testing the visual acuity of each eye (particularly with children) may uncover either a refractive or a medical cause of decreased vision. Finally, screening tonometry measurements using the Schiotz tonometer may detect the asymptomatic elevated intraocular pressure of glaucoma, a prevalent condition among the elderly.

The three most common preventable causes of permanent visual loss in developed nations are amblyopia, diabetic retinopathy, and glaucoma. All can

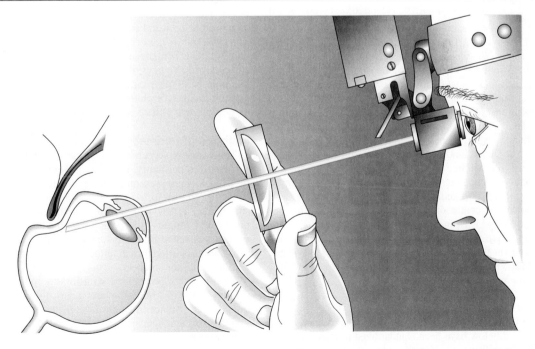

Figure 2–18. Diagrammatic representation of indirect ophthalmoscopy with scleral depression to examine the far peripheral retina. Indentation of the sclera through the lids brings the peripheral edge of the retina into visual alignment with the dilated pupil, the hand-held condensing lens, and the head-mounted ophthalmoscope.

remain asymptomatic while the opportunity for preventive measures is gradually lost. During this time, the pediatrician or general medical practitioner may be the only physician the patient visits.

By testing children for visual acuity in each eye, examining and referring diabetics for regular dilated fundus ophthalmoscopy, and referring patients with suspicious discs or tonometry readings to the ophthalmologist, the nonophthalmologist may indeed be the one who truly "saves" that patient's eyesight. This represents both an important opportunity and responsibility for every primary care physician.

III. SPECIALIZED OPHTHALMOLOGIC EXAMINATIONS

This section will discuss ophthalmologic examination techniques with more specific indications that would not be performed on a routine basis. They will be grouped according to the function or anatomic area of primary interest.

DIAGNOSIS OF VISUAL ABNORMALITIES

1. PERIMETRY

Perimetry is used to examine the central and peripheral visual fields. This technique, which is performed separately for each eye, measures the combined function of the retina, the optic nerve, and the intracranial visual pathway. It is used clinically to detect or monitor field loss due to disease at any of these locations. Damage to specific parts of the neurologic visual pathway may produce characteristic patterns of change on serial field examinations.

The visual field of the eye is measured and plotted in degrees of arc. Measurement of degrees of arc remains constant regardless of the distance from the eye the field is checked. The sensitivity of vision is greatest in the center of the field (corresponding to the fovea) and least in the periphery. Perimetry relies on subjective patient responses, and the results will depend on the patient's psychomotor as well as visual status. Perimetry must always be performed and interpreted with this in mind.

The Principles of Testing

Although perimetry is subjective, the methods discussed below have been standardized to maximize reproducibility and permit subsequent comparison. Perimetry requires (1) steady fixation and attention by the patient; (2) a set distance from the eye to the screen or testing device; (3) a uniform, standard amount of background illumination and contrast; (4) test targets of standard size and brightness; and (5) a universal protocol for administration of the test by examiners.

As the patient's eye fixates on a central target, test objects are randomly presented at different locations throughout the field. If they are seen, the patient responds either verbally or with a hand-held signaling device. Varying the target's size or brightness permits quantification of visual sensitivity of different areas in the field. The smaller or dimmer the target seen, the better the sensitivity of that location.

There are two basic methods of target presentation—static and kinetic—that can be used alone or in combination during an examination. In **static perimetry,** different locations throughout the field are tested one at a time. A difficult test object, such as a dim light, is first presented at a particular location. If it is not seen, the size or intensity of the light is incrementally increased until it is just large enough or bright enough to be detected. This is called the "threshold" sensitivity level of that location. This sequence is repeated at a series of other locations, so that the light sensitivity of multiple points in the field can be evaluated and combined to form a profile of the visual field.

In **kinetic perimetry,** the sensitivity of the entire field to one single test object (of fixed size and brightness) is first tested. The object is slowly moved toward the center from a peripheral area until it is first spotted. By moving the same object inward from multiple different directions, a boundary called an **"isopter"** can be mapped out which is specific for that target. The isopter outlines the area within which the target can be seen and beyond which it cannot be seen. Thus, the larger the isopter, the better the visual field of that eye. The boundaries of the isopter are measured and plotted in degrees of arc. By repeating the test using objects of different size or brightness, multiple isopters can then be plotted for a given eye. The smaller or dimmer test objects will produce smaller isopters.

Methods of Perimetry

The **tangent screen** is the simplest apparatus for standardized perimetry. It utilizes different-sized pins on a black wand presented against a black screen and is used primarily to test the central 30 degrees of visual field. The advantages of this method are its simplicity and rapidity, the possibility of changing the subject's distance from the screen, and the option of using any assortment of fixation and test objects, including different colors.

The more sophisticated **Goldmann perimeter** (Figure 2–19) is a hollow white spherical bowl positioned a set distance in front of the patient. A light of variable size and intensity can be presented by the examiner (seated behind the perimeter) in either static or kinetic fashion. This method can test the full limit of peripheral vision and was for years the primary method for plotting fields in glaucoma patients.

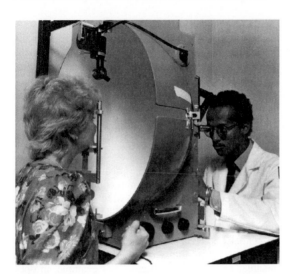

Figure 2–19. Goldmann perimeter. (Photo by M Narahara.)

Computerized automated perimeters (Figure 2–20) now constitute the most sophisticated and sensitive equipment available for visual field testing. Using a bowl similar to the Goldmann perimeter, these instruments display test lights of varying brightness and size but use a quantitative static threshold testing format that is more precise and comprehensive than other methods. Numerical scores (Figure 2–21) corresponding to the threshold sensitivity of each test location can be stored in the computer memory and compared statistically with results from previous examinations or

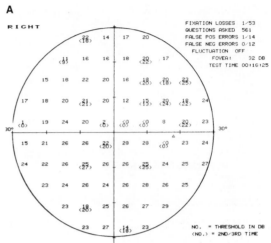

A

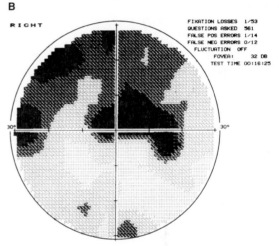

B

Figure 2–21. *A:* Numerical printout of threshold sensitivity scores derived by using the static method of computerized perimetry. This is the 30-degree field of a patient's right eye with glaucoma. The higher the numbers, the better the visual sensitivity. The computer retests many of the points (bracketed numbers) to assess consistency of the patient's responses. ***B:*** Diagrammatic "gray scale" display of these same numerical scores. The darker the area, the poorer the visual sensitivity at that location.

from other normal patients. The higher the numerical score, the better the visual sensitivity of that location in the field. Another important advantage is that the test presentation is programmed and automated, eliminating any variability on the part of the examiner.

2. AMSLER GRID

The Amsler grid is used to test the central 20 degrees of the visual field. The grid (Figure 2–22) is viewed by each eye separately at normal reading distance and with

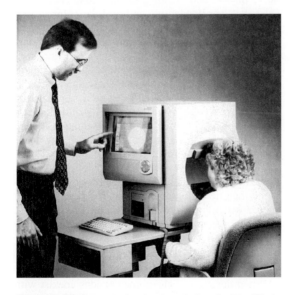

Figure 2–20. Computerized automated perimeter. (Photo Courtesy of Humphrey Instruments.)

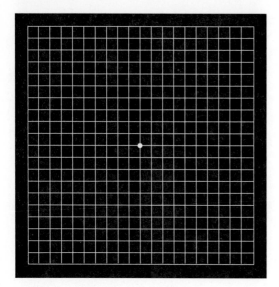

Figure 2–22. Amsler grid.

reading glasses on if the patient uses them. It is most commonly used to test macular function.

While fixating on the central dot, the patient checks to see that the lines are all straight, without distortion, and that no spots or portions of the grid are missing. One eye is compared with the other. A scotoma or blank area—either central or paracentral—can indicate disease of the macula or optic nerve. Wavy distortion of the lines (metamorphopsia) can indicate macular edema or submacular fluid.

The grid can be used by patients at home to test their own central vision. For example, patients with age-related macular degeneration (see Chapter 10) can use the grid to monitor for sudden metamorphopsia. This often is the earliest symptom of acute fluid accumulation beneath the macula arising from leaking subretinal neovascularization. Since these abnormal vessels may be treatable with the laser, early detection is important.

3. BRIGHTNESS ACUITY TESTING

The visual abilities of patients with media opacities may vary depending on conditions of lighting. For example, when dim illumination makes the pupil larger, one may be able to "see around" a central focal cataract, whereas bright illumination causing pupillary constriction would have the contrary effect. Bright lights may also cause disabling glare in patients with corneal edema or diffuse clouding of the crystalline lens due to light scattering.

Because the darkened examining room may not accurately elicit the patient's functional difficulties in real life, instruments have been developed to test the effect of varying levels of brightness or glare on visual acuity. Distance acuity with the Snellen chart is usually tested under standard levels of incrementally increasing illumination, and the information may be helpful in making therapeutic or surgical decisions. Asking cataract patients specific questions about how their vision is affected by various lighting conditions is even more important.

4. COLOR VISION TESTING

Normal color vision requires healthy function of the macula and optic nerve. The most common abnormality is red-green "color blindness," which is present in approximately 8% of the male population. This is due to an X-linked congenital deficiency of one specific type of retinal photoreceptor. Depressed color vision may also be a sensitive indicator of certain kinds of acquired macular or optic nerve disease. For example, in optic neuritis or optic nerve compression (eg, by a mass), abnormal color vision is often an earlier indication of disease than visual acuity, which may still be 20/20.

The most common testing technique utilizes a series of polychromatic plates, such as those of Ishihara or Hardy-Rand-Rittler (Figure 2–23). The plates are made up of dots of the primary colors printed on a background mosaic of similar dots in a confusing variety of secondary colors. The primary dots are arranged in simple patterns (numbers or geometric shapes) that cannot be recognized by patients with deficient color perception.

5. CONTRAST SENSITIVITY TESTING

Contrast sensitivity is the ability of the eye to discern subtle degrees of contrast. Retinal and optic nerve disease and clouding of the ocular media (eg, cataracts) can impair this ability. Like color vision, contrast sensitivity may become depressed before Snellen visual acuity is affected in many situations.

Contrast sensitivity is best tested by using standard preprinted charts with a series of test targets (Figure 2–24). Since illumination greatly affects contrast, it must be standardized and checked with a light meter. Each separate target consists of a series of dark parallel lines in one of three different orientations. They are displayed against a lighter, contrasting gray background. As the contrast between the lines and their background is progressively reduced from one target to the next, it becomes more difficult for the patient to judge the orientation of the lines. The patient can be scored according to the lowest level of contrast at which the pattern of lines can still be discerned.

6. ASSESSING POTENTIAL VISION

When opacities of the cornea or lens coexist with disease of the macula or optic nerve, the visual potential of the eye is often in doubt. The benefit of corneal

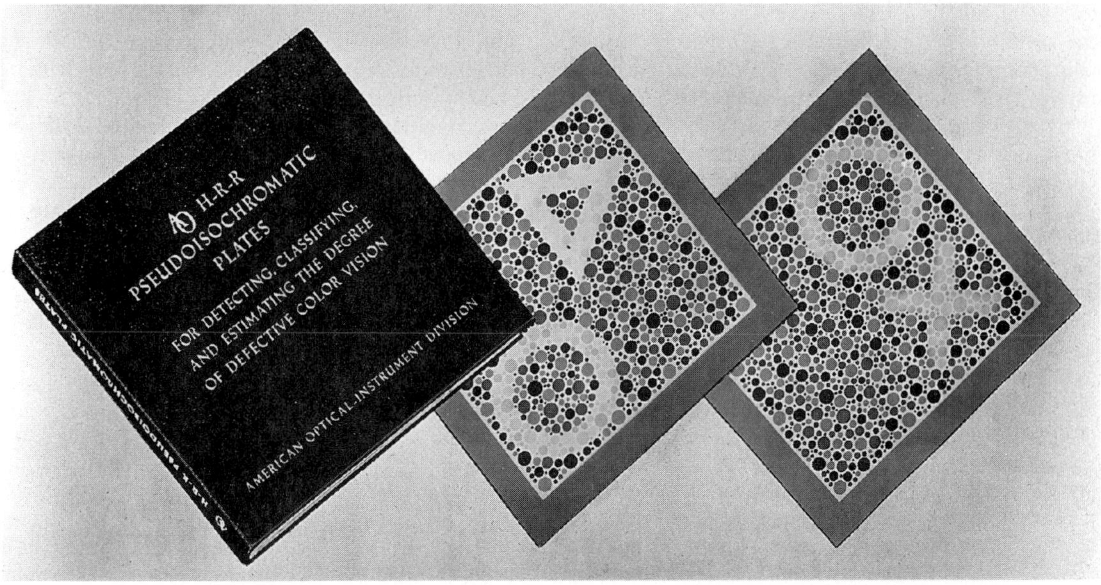

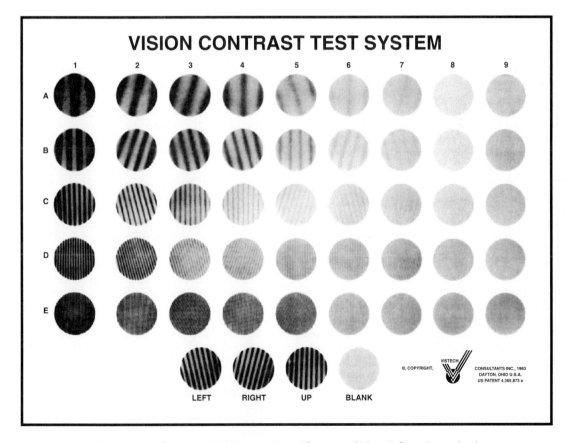

Figure 2–23. Hardy-Rand-Rittler (H-R-R) pseudoisochromatic plates for testing color vision.

Figure 2–24. Contrast sensitivity test chart. (Courtesy of Vistech Consultants, Inc.)

transplantation or cataract extraction will depend on the severity of coexisting retinal or optic nerve impairment. Several methods are available for assessing central visual potential under these circumstances.

Even with a totally opaque cataract that completely prevents a view of the fundus, the patient should still be able to identify the direction of a light directed into the eye from different quadrants. When a red lens is held in front of the light, the patient should be able to differentiate between white and red light. The presence of a Marcus Gunn afferent pupillary defect indicates significant disease of the retina or optic nerve and thus a poor visual prognosis.

A gross test of macular function involves the patient's ability to perceive so-called **entoptic phenomena.** For example, as the eyeball is massaged with a rapidly moving penlight through the closed lids, the patient should be able to visualize an image of the paramacular vascular branches if the macula is healthy. These may be described as looking like "the veins of a leaf." Because this test is highly subjective and subject to interpretation, it is only helpful if the patient is able to recognize the vascular pattern in at least one eye. Absence of the pattern in the opposite eye then suggests macular impairment.

In addition to these gross methods, sophisticated quantitative instruments have been developed for more direct determination of visual potential in eyes with media opacities. These instruments project a narrow beam of light containing a pattern of images through any relatively clear portion of the media (eg, through a less dense region of a cataract) and onto the retina. The patient's vision is then graded according to the size of the smallest patterns that can be seen.

Two different types of patterns are used. **Laser interferometry** employs laser light to generate interference fringes or gratings, which the patient sees as a series of parallel lines. Progressively narrowing the width and spacing of the lines causes an end point to be reached where the patient can no longer discern the orientation of the lines. The narrowest image width the patient can resolve is then correlated with a Snellen acuity measurement to determine the visual potential of that eye. The **potential acuity meter** projects a standard Snellen acuity chart onto the retina. The patient is then graded in the usual fashion, according to the smallest line of letters read.

Although both instruments appear useful in measuring potential visual acuity, false-positive and false-negative results do occur, with a frequency dependent on the type of disease present. Thus, these methods are helpful but not completely reliable in determining the visual prognosis of eyes with cloudy media.

7. TESTS FOR FUNCTIONAL VISUAL LOSS

The measurement of vision is subjective, requiring responses on the part of the patient. The validity of the test may therefore be limited by the alertness or cooperation of the patient. "Functional" visual loss is a subjective complaint of impaired vision without any demonstrated organic or objective basis. Examples include hysterical blindness and malingering.

Recognition of functional visual loss or malingering depends on the use of testing variations in order to elicit inconsistent or contradictory responses. An example would be eliciting "tunnel" visual fields using the tangent screen.

A patient claiming "poor vision" and tested at the standard distance of 1 meter may map out a narrow central zone of intact vision beyond which even large objects—such as a hand—allegedly cannot be seen. The borders ("isopter") of this apparently small area are then marked.

The patient is then moved back to a position 2 meters from the tangent screen. From this position, the field should be twice as large as the area plotted from 1 meter away. If the patient outlines an area of the same size from both testing distances, this raises a strong suspicion of functional visual loss, but a number of conditions such as advanced glaucoma, severe retinitis pigmentosa, and cortical blindness would need to be excluded.

A variety of other different tests can be chosen to assess the validity of different degrees of visual loss that may be in question.

DIAGNOSIS OF OCULAR ABNORMALITIES

1. MICROBIOLOGY & CYTOLOGY

Like any mucous membrane, the conjunctiva can be cultured with swabs for the identification of bacterial infection. Specimens for cytologic examination are obtained by lightly scraping the palpebral conjunctiva (ie, lining the inner aspect of the lid) with a small platinum spatula following topical anesthesia. For the cytologic evaluation of conjunctivitis, Giemsa's stain is used to identify the types of inflammatory cells present, while Gram's stain may demonstrate the presence (and type) of bacteria. These applications are discussed at length in Chapter 5.

The cornea is normally sterile. The base of any suspected infectious corneal ulcer should be scraped with the platinum spatula for Gram staining and culture. This procedure is performed at the slitlamp. Because in many cases only trace quantities of bacteria are recoverable, the spatula should be used to plate the specimen directly onto the culture plate without the intervening use of transport media. Any amount of culture growth, no matter how scant, is considered significant, but many cases of infection may still be "culture-negative."

Culture of intraocular fluids is the only reliable method of diagnosing or ruling out infectious endophthalmitis. Aqueous can be tapped by inserting a short

25-gauge needle on a tuberculin syringe through the limbus parallel to the iris. Care must be taken not to traumatize the lens. The diagnostic yield is better if vitreous is cultured. Vitreous specimens can be obtained by a needle tap through the pars plana or by doing a surgical vitrectomy. In the evaluation of noninfectious intraocular inflammation, cytology specimens are occasionally obtained using similar techniques.

2. TECHNIQUES FOR CORNEAL EXAMINATION

Several additional techniques are available for more specialized evaluation of the cornea. The **keratometer** is a calibrated instrument that measures the radius of curvature of the cornea in two meridians 90 degrees apart. If the cornea is not perfectly spherical, the two radii will be different. This is called **astigmatism** and is quantified by measuring the difference between the two radii of curvature. Keratometer measurements are used in contact lens fitting and for intraocular lens power calculations prior to cataract surgery.

Many corneal diseases result in distortion of the otherwise smooth surface of the cornea, which impairs its optical quality. The **photokeratoscope** is an instrument that assesses the uniformity and evenness of the surface by reflecting a pattern of concentric circles onto it. This pattern, which can be visualized and photographed through the instrument, should normally appear perfectly regular and uniform. Focal corneal irregularities will instead distort the circular patterns reflected from that particular area.

Computerized corneal topography is the most advanced technique of mapping the anterior corneal surface. Whereas keratometry provides only a single corneal curvature measurement and photokeratoscopy provide only qualitative information, these computer systems combine and improve on the features of both. A real time video camera records the concentric keratoscopic rings reflected from the cornea. A personal computer digitizes these data from thousands of locations across the corneal surface and displays these measurements in a color-coded map (Figure 2–25). This enables one to quantify and analyze minute changes in shape and refractive power across the entire cornea induced by disease or surgery.

The endothelium is an irreplaceable monolayer of cells lining the posterior corneal surface. These cells function as fluid pumps and are responsible for keeping the cornea thin and dehydrated, thereby maintaining its optical clarity. If these cells become impaired or depleted, corneal edema and thickening result, ultimately decreasing vision. Central corneal thickness can be accurately measured with a **pachymeter,** a device for quantifying and monitoring these changes. The endothelial cells themselves can be photographed with a special slitlamp camera, enabling one to study cell morphology and perform cell counts.

3. GONIOSCOPY

The anterior chamber—the space between the iris and the cornea—is filled with liquid aqueous humor. The aqueous, which is produced behind the iris by the ciliary body, exits the eye through a tiny sieve-like drainage network called the trabecular meshwork. The meshwork is arranged as a thin circumferential band of tissue just anterior to the base of the iris and within the angle formed by the iridocorneal junction (Figure 11–3). This angle recess can vary in its anatomy, pigmentation, and width of opening—all of which may affect aqueous drainage and be of diagnostic relevance for glaucoma.

Gonioscopy is the method of examination of the anterior chamber angle anatomy using binocular magnification and a special **goniolens.** The Goldmann and Posner/Zeiss types of goniolenses (Figure 2–7) have special mirrors angled so as to provide a line of view parallel with the iris surface and directed peripherally toward the angle recess.

After topical anesthesia, the patient is seated at the slitlamp and the goniolens is placed on the eye (Figure 2–26). Magnified details of the anterior chamber angle are viewed stereoscopically. By rotating the mirror, the entire 360-degree circumference of the angle can be examined. The same lens can be used to direct laser treatment toward the angle as therapy for glaucoma.

A third type of goniolens, the Koeppe lens, requires a special illuminator and a separate handheld binocular microscope. It is used with the patient lying supine and can thus be used either in the office or in the operating room (either diagnostically or for surgery).

4. GOLDMANN THREE-MIRROR LENS

The Goldmann lens is a versatile adjunct to the slitlamp examination (Figure 2–7). Three separate mirrors, all with different angles of orientation, allow the examiner's line of sight to be directed peripherally at three different angles while using the standard slitlamp. The most anterior and acute angle of view is achieved with the goniolens, discussed above.

Through a dilated pupil, the other two mirrored lenses angle the examiner's view toward the retinal mid periphery and far periphery, respectively. As with gonioscopy, each lens can be rotated 360 degrees circumferentially and can be used to aim laser treatment. A fourth central lens (no mirror) is used to examine the posterior vitreous and the centralmost area of the retina. The stereoscopic magnification of this method provides the greatest three-dimensional detail of the macula and disk.

The patient's side of the lens has a concavity designed to fit directly over the topically anesthetized cornea. A clear, viscous solution of methylcellulose is placed in the concavity of the lens prior to insertion onto the patient's eye. This eliminates interference

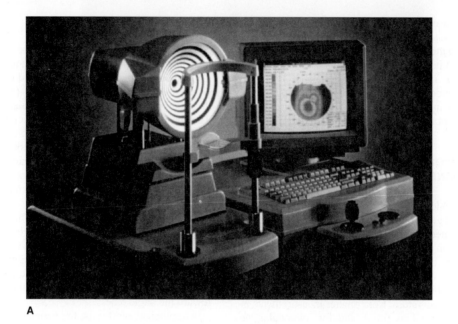

A

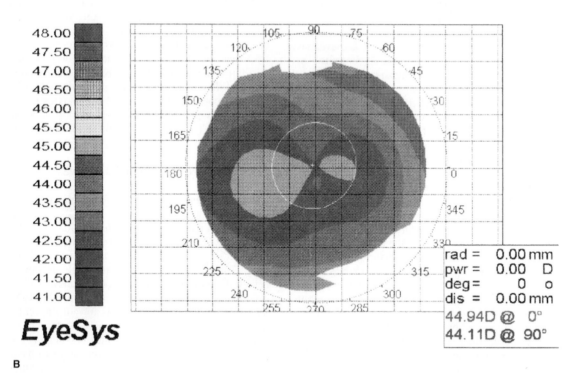

48.00	
47.50	
47.00	
46.50	
46.00	
45.50	
45.00	
44.50	
44.00	
43.50	
43.00	
42.50	
42.00	
41.50	
41.00	

rad = 0.00 mm
pwr = 0.00 D
deg = 0 o
dis = 0.00 mm
44.94D @ 0°
44.11D @ 90°

EyeSys

B

Figure 2–25. A: Computerized corneal topography system utilizing video keratoscope and personal computer. **B:** Color-coded topographic display of curvature and refractive power (in diopters) across the entire corneal surface. (Photos courtesy of EyeSys Technologies, Inc.)

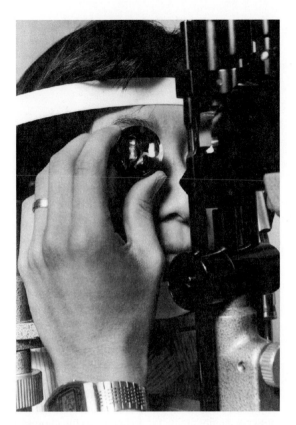

Figure 2–26. Gonioscopy with slitlamp and Goldmann type lens. (Photo by M Narahara.)

from optical interfaces, such as bubbles, and provides mild adhesion of the lens to the eye for stabilization.

5. FUNDUS PHOTOGRAPHY

Special retinal cameras are used to document details of the fundus for study and future comparison. Standard film is used for 35 mm color slides which can be easily stored. As with any form of ophthalmoscopy, a dilated pupil and clear ocular media provide the most optimal view. All of the fundus photographs in this textbook were taken with such a camera.

One of the most common applications is disk photography, used in the evaluation for glaucoma. Since the slow progression of glaucomatous optic nerve damage may be evident only by subtle alteration of the disk's appearance over time (see Chapter 11), precise documentation of its morphology is needed. By slightly shifting the camera angle on two consecutive shots, a "stereo" pair of slides can be produced which will provide a three-dimensional image when studied through a stereoscopic slide viewer. Stereo disk photography thus provides the most sensitive means of detecting increases in glaucomatous cupping.

6. FLUORESCEIN ANGIOGRAPHY

The capabilities of fundus photographic imaging can be tremendously enhanced by fluorescein, a dye whose molecules emit green light when stimulated by blue light. When photographed, the dye highlights vascular and anatomic details of the fundus. Fluorescein angiography has become indispensable in the diagnosis and evaluation of many retinal conditions. Because it can so precisely delineate areas of abnormality, it is an essential guide for planning laser treatment of retinal vascular disease.

Technique

The patient is seated in front of the retinal camera following pupillary dilation. After a small amount of fluorescein is injected into a vein in the arm, it circulates throughout the body before eventually being excreted by the kidneys. As the dye passes through the retinal and choroidal circulation, it can be visualized and photographed because of its properties of fluorescence. Two special filters within the camera produce this effect. A blue **"excitatory"** filter bombards the fluorescein molecules with blue light from the camera flash, causing them to emit a green light. The **"barrier"** filter allows only this emitted green light to reach the photographic film, blocking out all other wavelengths of light. A black and white photograph results in which only the fluorescein image is seen.

Because the fluorescein molecules do not diffuse out of normal retinal vessels, the latter are highlighted photographically by the dye, as seen in Figure 2–27. The diffuse, background "ground glass" appearance

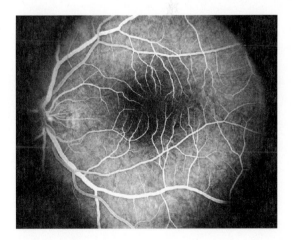

Figure 2–27. Normal angiogram of the central retina. The photo has been taken after the dye (appearing white) has already sequentially filled the choroidal circulation (seen as a diffuse, mottled whitish background), the arterioles and the veins. The macula appears dark due to heavier pigmentation which obscures the underlying choroidal fluorescence that is visible everywhere else. (Photo courtesy of R Griffith and T King.)

results from fluorescein filling of the separate underlying choroidal circulation. The choroidal and retinal circulations are anatomically separated by a thin, homogeneous monolayer of pigmented cells—the "retinal pigment epithelium." Denser pigmentation located in the macula obscures more of this background choroidal fluorescence (Figure 2–27) causing the darker central zone on the photograph. In contrast, focal atrophy of the pigment epithelium causes an abnormal increase in visibility of the background fluorescence (Figure 2–28).

Applications

A high-speed motorized film advance allows for rapid sequence photography of the dye's transit through the retinal and choroidal circulations over time. A fluorescein study or "angiogram" therefore consists of multiple black and white photos of the fundi taken at different times following dye injection (Figure 2–29). Early phase photos document the dye's initial rapid, sequential perfusion of the choroid, the retinal arteries, and the retinal veins. Later phase photos may, for example, demonstrate the gradual, delayed leakage of dye from abnormal vessels. This extravascular dye-stained edema fluid will persist long after the intravascular fluorescein has exited the eye.

Figure 2–29 illustrates several of the retinal vascular abnormalities that are well demonstrated by fluorescein angiography. The dye delineates structural vascular alterations, such as aneurysms or neovascularization. Changes in blood flow such as ischemia and vascular occlusion are seen as an interruption of the normal perfusion pattern. Abnormal vascular permeability is seen as a leaking cloud of dye-stained edema fluid increasing over time. Hemorrhage does not stain with dye but rather appears as a dark, sharply demarcated void. This is due to blockage and obscuration of the underlying background fluorescence.

7. INDOCYANINE GREEN ANGIOGRAPHY

The principal use for fluorescein angiography in age-related macular degeneration (Chapter 10) is in locating subretinal choroidal neovascularization for possible laser photocoagulation. The angiogram may show a well-demarcated neovascular membrane. Frequently, however, the area of choroidal neovascularization is poorly defined ("occult") because of surrounding or overlying blood, exudate, or serous fluid.

Indocyanine green angiography is a separate technique that is superior for imaging the choroidal circulation. Fluorescein diffuses out of the choriocapillaris, creating a diffuse background fluorescence. As opposed to fluorescein, indocyanin green is a larger molecule that binds completely to plasma proteins, causing it to remain in the choroidal vessels. Thus, larger choroidal vessels can be imaged. Unique photochemical properties allow the dye to be transmitted better through melanin (eg, in the retinal pigment epithelium), blood, exudate, and serous fluid. This technique therefore serves as an important adjunct to fluorescein angiography for imaging occult choroidal neovascularization and other choroidal vascular abnormalities.

Following dye injection, angiography is performed using special digital video cameras. The digital images can be further enhanced and analyzed by computer before being printed.

8. ELECTROPHYSIOLOGIC TESTING

Physiologically, "vision" results from a series of electrical signals initiated in the retina and ending in the occipital cortex. Electroretinography, electro-oculography, and visual evoked response testing are methods of evaluating the integrity to the neural circuitry.

Electroretinography (ERG) & Electro-oculography (EOG)

Electroretinography measures the electrical response of the retina to flashes of light, the **flash electroretinogram (ERG),** or to a reversing checkerboard stimulus, the **pattern ERG (PERG).** The recording electrode is placed on the surface of the eye and a reference electrode on the skin of the face. The amplitude of the electrical signal is less than 1 mV, and amplification of the signal and computer averaging of the response to repeated trials are thus necessary to achieve reliable results.

The flash ERG has two major components: the "a

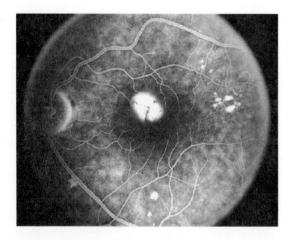

Figure 2–28. Abnormal angiogram in which dye-stained fluid originating from the choroid has pooled beneath the macula. This is one type of abnormality associated with age-related macular degeneration (see Chapter 10). Secondary atrophy of the overlying retinal pigment epithelium in this area causes heightened, unobscured visibility of this increased fluorescence. (Photo courtesy of R Griffith and T King.)

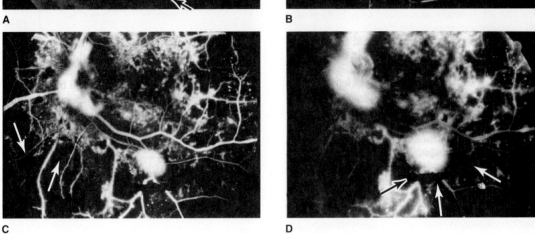

Figure 2–29. Fluorescein angiographic study of an eye with proliferative diabetic retinopathy demonstrating variations in the dye pattern over several minutes' time. **A:** Fundus photograph of left eye (before fluorescein) showing neovascularization (abnormal new vessels) on the disk and inferior to the macula (arrows). This latter area has bled, producing the arcuate preretinal hemorrhage at the bottom of the photo (open arrow). **B:** Early phase angiogram of the same eye, in which fluorescein has initially filled the arterioles and highlighted the area of the disk neovascularization. **C:** Midphase angiogram of the same eye in which dye has begun to leak out of the hyperpermeable areas of neovascularization. In addition to the irregular venous caliber and the microaneurysms (white dots), extensive areas of ischemia are apparent by virtue of the gross absence of vessels (and therefore dye) in many areas (see arrows). **D:** Late-phase photo demonstrating increasing amounts of dye leakage over time. Although the preretinal hemorrhage does not stain with dye, it is detectable as a solid black area since it obscures all underlying fluorescence (arrows). (Photos courtesy of University of California, San Francisco.)

wave" and the "b wave." An early receptor potential (ERP) preceding the "a wave" and oscillatory potentials superimposd on the "b wave" may be recorded under certain circumstances. The early part of the flash ERG reflects photoreceptor function, whereas the later response particularly reflects the function of the Müller cells, which are glial cells within the retina. Varying the intensity, wavelength, and frequency of the light stimulus and recording under conditions of light or dark adaptation modulates the waveform of the flash ERG and allows examination of rod and cone photoreceptor function. The flash ERG is a diffuse response from the whole retina and is thus sensitive only to widespread, generalized diseases of the retina—eg, inherited retinal degenerations (retinitis pigmentosa), in which flash ERG ab-

normalities precede visual loss; congenital retinal dystrophies, in which flash ERG abnormalities may precede ophthalmoscopic abnormalities; and toxic retinopathies from drugs or chemicals (eg, iron intraocular foreign bodies). It is not sensitive to focal retinal disease even when the macula is affected, and is not sensitive to abnormalities of the retinal ganglion cell layer such as in optic nerve disease.

The PERG also has two major components: a positive wave at about 50 ms (P50) and a negative wave at about 95 ms (N95) from the time of the pattern reversal. The P50 seems to reflect macular retinal function, whereas the N95 appears to reflect ganglion cell function. Thus, the PERG is useful in distinguishing retinal and optic nerve dysfunction and in diagnosing macular disease.

Electro-oculography (EOG) measures the standing corneoretinal potential. Electrodes are placed at the medial and lateral canthi to record the changes in electrical potential while the patient performs horizontal eye movements. The amplitude of the corneoretinal potential is least in the dark and maximal in the light. The ratio of the maximum potential in the light to the minimum in the dark is known as the **Arden index.** Abnormalities of the EOG principally occur in diseases diffusely affecting the retinal pigment epithelium and the photoreceptors and often parallel abnormalities of the flash ERG. Certain diseases such as Best's vitelliform dystrophy produce a normal ERG but a characteristically abnormal EOG. EOG is also used to record eye movements.

Visual Evoked Response (VER)

Like electroretinography, the visual evoked response measures the electrical potential resulting from a visual stimulus. However, because it is measured by scalp electrodes placed over the occipital cortex, the entire visual pathway from retina to cortex must be intact in order to produce a normal electrical waveform reading. Like the ERG wave, the VER pattern is plotted on a scale displaying both amplitude and latency (Figure 2–30).

Interruption of neuronal conduction by a lesion will result in reduced amplitude of the VER. Reduced speed of conduction, such as with demyelination, abnormally prolongs the latency of the VER. Unilateral prechiasmatic (retinal or optic nerve) disease can be diagnosed by stimulating each eye separately and comparing the responses. Postchiasmatic disease (eg, homonymous hemianopia) can be identified by comparing the electrode responses measured separately over each hemisphere.

Proportionately, the majority of the occipital lobe area is devoted to the macula. This large cortical area representing the macula is also in close proximity to the scalp electrode, so that the clinically measured VER is primarily a response generated by the macula and optic nerve. An abnormal VER would thus indicate poor central visual acuity, making it a valuable objective test in situations where subjective testing is unreliable. Such patients might include infants, unresponsive individuals, and suspected malingerers.

9. DARK ADAPTATION

In going from conditions of bright light to darkness, a certain period of time must pass before the retina regains its maximal sensitivity to low amounts of light. This phenomenon is called dark adaptation. It can be quantified by measuring the recovery of retinal sensitivity to low light levels over time following a standard period of bright light exposure. Dark adaptation is often abnormal in retinal diseases characterized by rod photoreceptor dysfunction and impaired night vision.

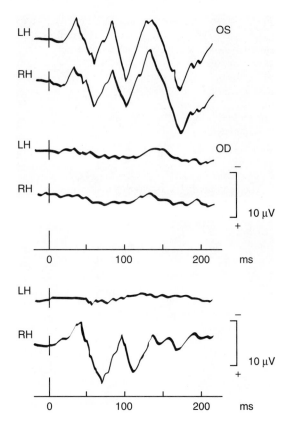

Figure 2–30. Top: Normal VER generated by stimulating the left eye ("OS") is contrasted with the absent response from the right eye ("OD"), which has a severe optic nerve lesion. "LH" and "RH" signify recordings from electrodes over the left and right hemispheres of the occipital lobe. **Bottom:** VER with right homonymous hemianopia. No response is recorded from over the left hemisphere. (Courtesy of M Feinsod.)

DIAGNOSIS OF EXTRAOCULAR ABNORMALITIES

1. LACRIMAL SYSTEM EVALUATION

Evaluation of Tear Production

Tears and their components are produced by the lacrimal gland and accessory glands in the lid and conjunctiva (see Chapter 4). The **Schirmer test** is a simple method for assessing gross tear production. Schirmer strips are disposable dry strips of filter paper in standard 5×35 mm sizes. The tip of one end is folded at the preexisting notch so that it can drape over the lower lid margin just lateral to the cornea.

Tears in the conjunctival sac will cause progressive wetting of the paper strip. The distance between the leading edge of wetness and the initial fold can be measured after 5 minutes, using a millimeter ruler. The ranges of normal measurements vary depending on whether or not topical anesthetic is used. Without anesthesia, irritation from the Schirmer strip itself will cause reflex tearing, thereby increasing the measurement. With anesthesia, less than 5 mm of wetting after 5 minutes is considered abnormal.

Significant degrees of chronic dryness cause surface changes in the exposed areas of the cornea and conjunctiva. **Fluorescein** will stain punctate areas of epithelial loss on the cornea. Another dye, **rose bengal,** is able to stain devitalized cells of the conjunctiva and cornea before they actually degenerate and drop off.

Evaluation of Lacrimal Drainage

The anatomy of the lacrimal drainage system is discussed in Chapters 1 and 4. The pumping action of the lids draws tears nasally into the upper and lower canalicular channels through the medially located "punctal" openings in each lid margin. After collecting in the lacrimal sac, the tears then drain into the nasopharynx via the nasolacrimal duct. Symptoms of watering are frequently due to increased tear production as a reflex response to some type of ocular irritation. However, the patency and function of the lacrimal drainage system must be checked in the evaluation of otherwise unexplained tearing.

The **Jones I** test evaluates whether the entire drainage system as a whole is functioning. Concentrated fluorescein dye is instilled into the conjunctival sac on the side of the suspected obstruction. After 5 minutes, a cotton Calgiswab is used to attempt to recover dye from beneath the inferior nasal turbinate. Alternatively, the patient blows his nose into a tissue which is checked for the presence of dye. Recovery of any dye indicates that the drainage system is functioning.

The **Jones II** test is performed if no dye is recovered, indicating some abnormality of the system. Following topical anesthesia, a smooth-tipped metal probe is used to gently dilate one of the puncta (usually lower). A 3-mL syringe with sterile water or saline is prepared and attached to a special lacrimal irrigating cannula. This blunt-tipped cannula is used to gently intubate the lower canaliculus, and fluid is injected as the patient leans forward. With a patent drainage system, fluid should easily flow into the patient's nasopharynx without resistance.

If fluorescein can now be recovered from the nose following irrigation, a partial obstruction might have been present. Recovery of clear fluid without fluorescein, however, may indicate inability of the lids to initially pump dye into the lacrimal sac with an otherwise patent drainage apparatus. If no fluid can be irrigated through to the nasopharynx using the syringe, total occlusion is present. Finally, some drainage problems may be due to stenosis of the punctal lid opening, in which case the preparatory dilation may be therapeutic.

2. METHODS OF ORBITAL EVALUATION

Exophthalmometry

A method is needed to measure the anteroposterior location of the globe with respect to the bony orbital rim. The lateral orbital rim is a discrete, easily palpable landmark and is used as the reference point.

The exophthalmometer (Figure 2–31) is a hand-held instrument with two identical measuring devices (one for each eye), connected by a horizontal bar. The distance between the two devices can be varied by sliding one toward or away from the other, and each has a notch that fits over the edge of the corresponding lateral orbital rim. When properly aligned, an attached set of mirrors reflects a side image of each eye profiled alongside a measuring scale, calibrated in millimeters.

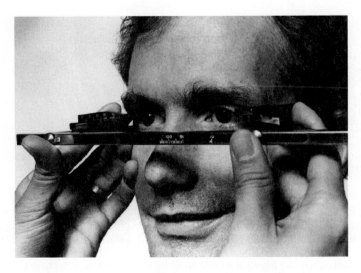

Figure 2–31. Hertel exophthalmometer. (Photo by M Narahara.)

The tip of the corneal image aligns with a scale reading representing its distance from the orbital rim.

The patient is seated facing the examiner. The distance between the two measuring devices is adjusted so that each aligns with and abuts against its corresponding orbital rim. To allow reproducibility for repeat measurements in the future, the distance between the two devices is recorded from an additional scale on the horizontal bar. Using the first mirror scale, the patient's right eye position is measured as it fixates on the examiner's left eye. The patient's left eye is measured while fixating on the examiner's right eye.

The distance from the cornea to the orbital rim typically ranges from 12 to 20 mm, and the two eye measurements are normally within 2 mm of each other. A greater distance is seen in exophthalmos, which can be unilateral or bilateral. This abnormal forward protrusion of the eye can be produced by any significant increase in orbital mass, because of the fixed size of the bony orbital cavity. Causes might include orbital hemorrhage, neoplasm, inflammation, or edema.

Ultrasonography

Ultrasonography utilizes the principle of sonar to study structures that may not be directly visible. It can be used to evaluate either the globe or the orbit. High-frequency sound waves are emitted from a special transmitter toward the target tissue. As the sound waves bounce back off the various tissue components, they are collected by a receiver that amplifies and displays them on an oscilloscope screen.

A single probe that contains both the transmitter and receiver is placed against the eye and used to aim the beam of sound (Figure 2–32). Various structures in its path will reflect separate echoes (which arrive at different times) back toward the probe. Those derived from the most distal structures arrive last, having traveled the farthest.

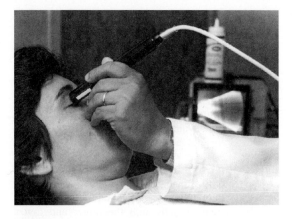

Figure 2–32. Ultrasonography using B-scan probe. The image will appear on the oscilloscope screen, visible in the background. (Photo by M Narahara.)

There are two methods of clinical ultrasonography: A scan and B scan. In **A scan ultrasonography,** the sound beam is aimed in a straight line. Each returning echo is displayed as a spike whose amplitude is dependent on the density of the reflecting tissue. The spikes are arranged in temporal sequence, with the latency of each signal's arrival correlating with that structure's distance from the probe (Figure 2–33). If the same probe is now swept across the eye, a continuous series of individual A scans is obtained. From spatial summation of these multiple linear scans, a two-dimensional image, or **B scan,** can be constructed.

Both A and B scans can be used to image and differentiate orbital disease or intraocular anatomy concealed by opaque media. In addition to defining the size and location of intraocular and orbital masses, A

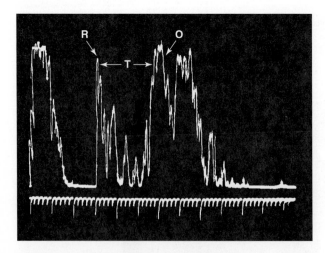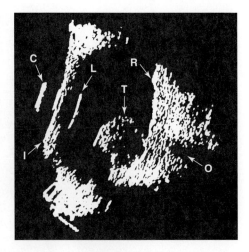

Figure 2–33. A scan *(left)* and B scan *(right)* of an intraocular tumor (melanoma). C = cornea; I = iris; L = posterior lens surface; O = optic nerve; R = retina; T = tumor. (Courtesy of RD Stone.)

and B scans can provide clues to the tissue characteristics of a lesion (eg, solid, cystic, vascular, calcified).

For purposes of measurement, the A scan is the most accurate method. Sound echoes reflected from two separate locations will reach the probe at different times. This temporal separation can be used to calculate the distance between the points, based on the speed of sound in the tissue medium. The most commonly used ocular measurement is the axial length (cornea to retina). This is important in cataract surgery in order to calculate the power for an intraocular lens implant. A scans can also be used to quantify tumor size and monitor growth over time.

The application of pulsed ultrasound and spectral Doppler techniques to orbital ultrasonography provides information on the orbital vasculature. It is certainly possible to determine the direction of flow in the ophthalmic artery and the ophthalmic veins, reversal of flow in these vessels occurring in internal carotid artery occlusion and carotid-cavernous fistula, respectively. As yet, the value of measuring flow velocities in various vessels, including the posterior ciliary arteries, without being able to measure blood vessel diameter is not fully established.

3. OPHTHALMIC RADIOLOGY
(X-Ray, CT Scan)

Plain x-rays and CT scans (Figures 13–1 and 13–2) are useful in the evaluation of **orbital** and **intracranial** conditions. CT scan in particular has become the most widely used method for localizing and characterizing structural disease in the extraocular visual pathway. Common orbital abnormalities demonstrated by CT scan include neoplasms, inflammatory masses, fractures, and extraocular muscle enlargement associated with Graves' disease.

The **intraocular** applications of radiology are primarily in the detection of foreign bodies following trauma and the demonstration of intraocular calcium in tumors such as retinoblastoma. CT scan is useful for foreign body localization because of its multidimensional reformatting capabilities and its ability to image the ocular walls.

4. MAGNETIC RESONANCE IMAGING

The technique of magnetic resonance imaging (MRI) has many applications in orbital and intracranial diagnosis. Improvements such as surface receiver coils and thin section techniques have improved the anatomic resolution in the eye and orbit.

Unlike CT, the MRI technique does not expose the patient to ionizing radiation. Multidimensional views (axial, coronal, and sagittal) are possible without having to reposition the patient. Since MRI might cause movement of metal, it should not be used if a metallic foreign body is suspected.

Because it can better differentiate between tissues of different water content, MRI is superior to CT in its ability to image edema, areas of demyelination, and vascular lesions. Bone generates a weak MRI signal, allowing improved resolution of intraosseous disease and a clearer view of the intracranial posterior fossa. Examples of MRI scans are presented in Chapters 13 and 14.

5. OPHTHALMODYNAMOMETRY

Ophthalmodynamometry gives an approximate measurement of the relative pressures in the central retinal arteries and is an indirect means of assessing carotid artery flow on either side. The test consists of exerting pressure on the sclera with a spring plunger while observing with an ophthalmoscope the vessels emerging from the optic disk. Ophthalmodynamometry is useful in the neurologic evaluation of patients who complain of "blacking out" (amaurosis fugax) in one eye, spells of weakness on one side of the body, or other symptoms of transient cerebral ischemia. A difference of more than 20% in the diastolic pressures between the two eyes suggests insufficiency of the carotid arterial system on the side with the lower reading.

The test is often performed in conjunction with angiography and ultrasonography of the carotid arteries.

REFERENCES

Anderson DR: *Automated Static Perimetry.* Mosby, 1992.

Berkow JW et al: *Fluorescein and Indocyanine Green Angiography: Technique and Interpretation,* 2nd ed. American Academy of Ophthalmology, 1997.

Boothe WA et al: The Tono-Pen: A manometric and clinical study. Arch Ophthalmol 1988;106:1214.

Drake M: *A Primer on Automated Perimetry.* Vol 11, No. 8, in: *Focal Points 1993: Clinical Modules for Ophthalmologists.* American Academy of Ophthalmology, 1993.

Faulkner W: *Macular Function Testing Through Opacities.* Vol 4, Module 2, in: *Focal Points 1986: Clinical Modules for Ophthalmologists.* American Academy of Ophthalmology, 1986.

Fellman RL et al: *Gonioscopy: Key to Successful Management of Glaucoma.* Vol 2, Module 7, in: *Focal Points 1984: Clinical Modules for Ophthalmologists.* American Academy of Ophthalmology, 1984.

Fishman GA, Sokol S: *Electrophysiologic Testing in Disorders of the Retina, Optic Nerve, and Visual Pathway.* American Academy of Ophthalmology, 1990.

Gills JP et al: *Corneal Topography. The State of the Art.* Slack, 1995.

Harrington DO, Drake MV: *The Visual Fields: A Textbook and Atlas of Clinical Perimetry,* 6th ed. Mosby, 1989.

Hirst LW: Clinical evaluation of the corneal endothelium. Vol 4, Module 8, in: *Focal Points 1986: Clinical Modules for Ophthalmologists.* American Academy of Ophthalmology, 1986.

Holder GE: The pattern electroretinogram in anterior visual pathway dysfunction and its relationship to the pattern visual evoked potential: A personal clinical review of 743 eyes. Eye 1997;11:924.

Hoskins HD, Kass M: *Becker-Shaffer's Diagnosis and Therapy of the Glaucomas,* 6th ed. Mosby, 1989.

Hoyt CS et al: Ophthalmological examination of the infant. Surv Ophthalmol 1982;26:177.

Hoyt CS, Paks MM: *How to Examine the Eye of the Neonate.* Vol 7, Module 1, in: *Focal Points 1989: Clinical Modules for Ophthalmologists.* American Academy of Ophthalmology, 1989.

Huber MJE, Reacher MH: *Clinical Tests in Ophthalmology.* Mosby, 1991.

Kline LB: *Computed Tomography in Ophthalmology.* Vol 3, Module 9, in: *Focal Points 1985: Clinical Modules for Ophthalmologists.* American Academy of Ophthalmology, 1985.

Koch DD: *The Role of Glare Testing in Managing the Cataract Patient.* Vol 6, Module 4, in: *Focal Points 1988: Clinical Modules for Ophthalmologists.* American Academy of Ophthalmology, 1988.

Lieberman MF, Drake M: *Computerized Perimetry: A Simplified Guide,* 2nd ed. Slack, 1992.

Maguire LJ: *Computerized Corneal Analysis.* Vol 14, No. 5, in: *Focal Points 1996: Clinical Modules for Ophthalmologists.* American Academy of Ophthalmology, 1996.

Mannis MJ: Making sense of contrast sensitivity testing. Arch Ophthalmol 1987;105:627.

Masters BR: *Noninvasive Diagnostic Techniques in Ophthalmology.* Springer, 1990.

Miller BW: A review of practical tests for ocular malingering and hysteria. Surv Ophthalmol 1973;17:241.

Newman SA: *Automated Perimetry in Neuro-Ophthalmology.* Vol 13, No. 6, in: *Focal Points 1995: Clinical Modules for Ophthalmologists.* American Academy of Ophthalmology, 1995.

Puliafito CA et al: *Optical Coherence Tomography of Ocular Diseases.* Slack, 1996.

Riordan-Eva P et al: Orbital ultrasound in the ocular ischaemic syndrome. Eye 1994;8:93.

Rosenthal ML, Fradin S: The technique of binocular indirect ophthalmoscopy. Highlights Ophthalmol 1966;9:179. (Reprinted as Appendix in: Hilton GF et al: *Retinal Detachment,* 2nd ed. American Academy of Ophthalmology, 1995.

Schuman JS: *Imaging in Glaucoma.* Slack, 1997.

Schwartz B: *Optic Disc Evaluation in Glaucoma.* Vol 8, Module 12, in: *Focal Points 1990: Clinical Modules for Ophthalmologists.* American Academy of Ophthalmology, 1990.

Shaffer RN et al: The use of diagrams to record changes in glaucomatous discs. Am J Ophthalmol 1975;80:460.

Slavin ML: *Functional Visual Loss.* Vol 9, Module 2, in: *Focal Points 1991: Clinical Modules for Ophthalmologists.* American Academy of Ophthalmology, 1991.

Stein HA et al: *The Ophthalmic Assistant: Fundamentals and Clinical Practice,* 6th ed. Mosby, 1994.

Sunness JS: *Clinical Retinal Function Testing.* Vol 9, Module 1, in: *Focal Points 1991: Clinical Modules for Ophthalmologists.* American Academy of Ophthalmology, 1991.

Thompson HS et al: How to measure the relative afferent pupillary defect. Surv Ophthalmol 1981;26:39.

Thompson HS, Kardon RH: *Clinical Importance of Pupillary Inequality.* Vol 10, No. 10, in: *Focal Points 1992: Clinical Modules for Ophthalmologists.* American Academy of Ophthalmology, 1992.

Tomsak RL: *Magnetic Resonance Imaging in Neuro-ophthalmology.* Vol 4, Module 10, in: *Focal Points 1986: Clinical Modules for Ophthalmologists.* American Academy of Ophthalmology, 1986.

von Noorden GK: *Binocular Vision and Ocular Motility,* 5th ed. Mosby, 1996.

Walsh TJ: *Visual Fields: Examination and Interpretation,* 2nd ed. American Academy of Ophthalmology, 1996.

Wilson FM: *Practical Ophthalmology: A Manual for Beginning Residents,* 4th ed. American Academy of Ophthalmology, 1996.

Wirtschafter JD et al: *Magnetic Resonance Imaging and Computed Tomography: Clinical Neuro-orbital Anatomy.* American Academy of Ophthalmology, 1992.

Yannuzzi LA et al: *Indocyanine Green Angiography.* Mosby, 1997.

Ophthalmic Therapeutics

3

Philip P. Ellis, MD, & Frederick T. Fraunfelder, MD

COMMONLY USED EYE MEDICATIONS

Philip P. Ellis, MD

The following is intended to serve as a concise formulary of commonly used ophthalmic drugs. Standard pharmacology and physiology texts should be consulted for more detailed information.

TOPICAL ANESTHETICS

Topical anesthetics are useful for several diagnostic and therapeutic procedures, including tonometry, removal of foreign bodies or sutures, gonioscopy, conjunctival scraping, and minor surgical operations on the cornea and conjunctiva. One or two instillations are usually sufficient, but the dosage may be repeated during the procedure.

Proparacaine, tetracaine, and benoxinate are the most commonly used topical anesthetics. For practical purposes, they can be said to have equivalent anesthetic potency.

Cocaine 1–4% solution is also used for topical anesthesia.

Note: Topical anesthetics should never be prescribed for home use, since prolonged application may cause corneal complications and mask serious ocular disease.

Proparacaine Hydrochloride (Ophthaine, Others)

Preparation: Solution, 0.5%. A combined preparation of proparacaine and fluorescein is available as Fluoracaine.
Dosage: 1 drop and repeat as necessary.
Onset and duration of action: Anesthesia begins within 20 seconds and lasts 10–15 minutes.
Comment: Least irritating of the topical anesthetics.

Tetracaine Hydrochloride (Pontocaine)

Preparations: Solution, 0.5%, and ointment, 0.5%.
Dosage: 1 drop and repeat as necessary.

Onset and duration of action: Anesthesia occurs within 1 minute and lasts for 15–20 minutes.
Comment: Stings considerably on instillation.

Benoxinate Hydrochloride

Preparation (as Fluress): Solution, 0.4%.
Dosage: 1 drop and repeat as necessary.
Onset and duration of action: Anesthesia begins within 1 or 2 minutes and lasts for 10–15 minutes.
Comment: Benoxinate 0.4% and fluorescein 0.25% (Fluress) may be used prior to applanation tonometry.

LOCAL ANESTHETICS FOR INJECTION

Lidocaine, procaine, and mepivacaine are commonly used local anesthetics for eye surgery. Longer-acting agents such as bupivacaine and etidocaine are often mixed with other local anesthetics to prolong the duration of effect. Local anesthetics are extremely safe when used with discretion, but the physician must be aware of the potential systemic toxic action when rapid absorption occurs from the site of the injection, with excessive dosage, or following inadvertent intravascular injection.

The addition of hyaluronidase encourages spreading of the anesthetic and shortens the onset to as little as 1 minute. For these reasons, hyaluronidase is commonly used in retrobulbar and peribulbar injections prior to cataract extraction. Injectable anesthetics are used by ophthalmologists most commonly in older patients, who may be susceptible to cardiac arrhythmias; therefore, *l*-epinephrine should not be used in concentrations greater than 1:200,000.

Lidocaine Hydrochloride (Xylocaine)

Owing to its rapid onset and longer action (1–2 hours), lidocaine has become the most commonly used local anesthetic. It is approximately twice as potent as procaine. Up to 30 mL of 1% solution, without epinephrine, may be used safely. In cataract surgery, 15–20 mL is usually more than adequate. The maximum safe dose is 4.5 mg/kg without epinephrine and 7 mg/kg with epinephrine. Recently, intracameral lidocaine in a 1% solution without preservatives has been employed for anesthesia in cataract surgery.

Procaine Hydrochloride (Novocaine)

Preparations: Solution, 1%, 2%, and 10%.

Dosage: Approximately 50 mL of a 1% solution can be injected without causing systemic effects. The maximum safe dose is 10 mg/kg.

Duration of action: 45–60 minutes.

Mepivacaine Hydrochloride (Carbocaine, Others)

Preparations: Solution, 1%, 1.5%, 2%, and 3%.

Dosage: Infiltration and nerve block, up to 20 mL of 1% or 2% solution.

Duration of action: Approximately 2 hours.

Comment: Carbocaine is similar to lidocaine in potency. It is usually used in patients who are allergic to lidocaine. The maximum safe dose is 7 mg/kg.

Bupivacaine Hydrochloride (Marcaine, Sensorcaine)

Preparations: Solution, 0.25%, 0.5%, and 0.75%.

Dosage: The 0.75% solution has been used most frequently in ophthalmology. The maximum safe dose in an adult is 250 mg with epinephrine and 200 mg without epinephrine. Bupivacaine is frequently mixed with an equal amount of lidocaine.

Onset and duration of action: The onset of action is slower than that of lidocaine, but it persists much longer (up to 6–10 hours).

Etidocaine Hydrochloride (Duranest)

Preparations: Solution, 1% and 1.5%.

Dosage: The maximum safe dose of etidocaine is 4 mg/kg without epinephrine and 5.5 mg/kg with epinephrine. This agent is frequently mixed with lidocaine for local anesthesia in ophthalmic surgery.

Onset and duration of action: The onset of action is slower than that of lidocaine but more rapid than that of bupivacaine. The duration of action is approximately twice as long as that of lidocaine (4–8 hours).

MYDRIATICS & CYCLOPLEGICS

Mydriatics and cycloplegics both dilate the pupil. In addition, cycloplegics cause paralysis of accommodation (patient unable to see near objects, eg, printed words). They are commonly used drugs in ophthalmology, singly and in combination. Their prime uses are (1) for dilating the pupils to facilitate ophthal-

moscopy; (2) for paralyzing the muscles of accommodation, particularly in young patients, as an aid in refraction; and (3) for dilating the pupil and paralyzing the muscles of accommodation in uveitis to prevent synechia formation and relieve pain and photophobia. Since mydriatics and cycloplegics both dilate the pupil, they should be used with extreme caution in eyes with narrow anterior chamber angles since either a mydriatic or a cycloplegic can cause angle-closure glaucoma in such eyes.

1. MYDRIATICS (Sympathomimetics)

Phenylephrine is a mydriatic with no cycloplegic effect.

Phenylephrine Hydrochloride (Neo-Synephrine, Others)

Preparations: Solution, 0.12%, 2.5%, and 10%.

Dosage: 1 drop and repeat in 5–10 minutes.

Onset and duration of action: The effect usually occurs within 30 minutes after instillation and lasts 2–3 hours.

Comment: Phenylephrine is used both singly and with cycloplegics to facilitate ophthalmoscopy, in treatment of uveitis, and to dilate the pupil prior to cataract surgery. It is used almost to the exclusion of all other mydriatics. If a patient is allergic to phenylephrine, hydroxyamphetamine hydrobromide (Paredrine) may be substituted. The 10% solution should not be used in newborn infants, in cardiac patients, or in patients receiving reserpine, guanethidine, or tricyclic antidepressants, because of increased susceptibility to the vasopressor effects.

2. CYCLOPLEGICS (Parasympatholytics)

Atropine Sulfate

Preparations: Solution, 0.5–3%; ointment, 0.5% and 1%.

Dosage: For refraction in children, instill 1 drop of 0.25–0.5% solution in each eye twice a day for 1 or 2 days before the examination and then 1 hour before the examination; ointment, $1/4$-inch ribbon twice a day for 2 days prior to examination.

Onset and duration of action: The onset of action is within 30–40 minutes. A maximum effect is reached in about 2 hours. The effect lasts for up to 2 weeks in a normal eye, but in the presence of acute inflammation the drug must be instilled two or three times daily to maintain its effect.

Toxicity: Atropine drops must be used with caution to avoid toxic reactions resulting from systemic absorption. Restlessness and excited behavior with dryness and flushing of the skin of the face, dry mouth, fever, inhibition of sweating, and tachycardia are prominent toxic symptoms, particularly in young children.

Comment: Atropine is an effective and long-acting cycloplegic. In addition to its use for cycloplegia in children, atropine is applied topically two or three times daily in the treatment of iritis. It is also used to maintain a dilated pupil after intraocular surgical procedures.

Scopolamine Hydrobromide

Preparation: Solution, 0.25%.

Dosage: 1 drop two or three times daily.

Onset and duration of action: Cycloplegia occurs in about 40 minutes and lasts for 3–5 days when scopolamine is used as an aid to refraction in normal eyes. The duration of action is much shorter in inflamed eyes.

Toxicity: Scopolamine occasionally causes dizziness and disorientation, mainly in older people.

Comment: Scopolamine is an effective cycloplegic. It is used in the treatment of uveitis, in refraction of children, and postoperatively.

Homatropine Hydrobromide

Preparations: Solution, 2% and 5%.

Dosage: For refraction, 1 drop in each eye and repeat two or three times at intervals of 10–15 minutes.

Onset and duration of action: Maximal cycloplegic effect lasts for about 3 hours, but complete recovery time is about 36–48 hours. In certain cases, the shorter action is an advantage over scopolamine and atropine.

Toxicity: Sensitivity and side effects associated with the topical instillation of homatropine are rare.

Cyclopentolate Hydrochloride (Cyclogyl, Others)

Preparations: Solution, 0.5%, 1%, and 2%.

Dosage: For refraction, 1 drop in each eye and repeat after 10 minutes.

Onset and duration of action: The onset of dilatation and cycloplegia is within 30–60 minutes. The duration of action is less than 24 hours.

Comment: Cyclopentolate is more popular than homatropine and scopolamine in refraction because of its shorter duration of action. Occasionally, neurotoxicity may occur, manifested by incoherence, visual hallucinations, slurred speech, and ataxia. These reactions are more common in children.

Tropicamide (Mydriacyl, Others)

Preparations: Solution, 0.5% and 1%; 0.25% with 1% hydroxamphetamine hydrobromide (Paremyd).

Dosage: 1 drop of 1% solution two or three times at 5-minute intervals.

Onset and duration of action: The time required to reach the maximum cycloplegic effect is usually 20–25 minutes, and the duration of this effect is only 15–20 minutes; therefore, the timing of the examination after instilling tropicamide is important. Complete recovery requires 5–6 hours.

Comment: Tropicamide is an effective mydriatic with weak cycloplegic action and is therefore most useful for ophthalmoscopy.

Cyclopentolate Hydrochloride-Phenylephrine Hydrochloride (Cyclomydril)

Preparation: Solution, 0.2% cyclopentolate hydrochloride and 1% phenylephrine hydrochloride.

Dosage: 1 drop every 5–10 minutes for two or three doses. Pressure should be applied over the nasolacrimal sac after drop instillation to minimize systemic absorption.

Onset and duration of action: Mydriasis and some cycloplegia occur within the first 3–6 minutes. The duration of action is usually less than 24 hours. This drug combination is of particular value for pupillary dilation in examination of premature and small infants.

DRUGS USED IN THE TREATMENT OF GLAUCOMA

The concentration used and the frequency of instillation should be individualized on the basis of tonometric measurements. Use the smallest dosage that effectively controls the intraocular pressure and prevents optic nerve damage.

1. DIRECT-ACTING CHOLINERGIC (PARASYMPATHOMIMETIC) DRUGS

Pilocarpine Hydrochloride & Nitrate

Preparations: Solution, 0.25%, 0.5–6%, 8%, and 10%; gel, 4%. Also available in a sustained-release system (Ocusert).

Dosage: 1 drop up to six times a day; a $1/2$-inch strip of gel in lower conjunctival cul-de-sac at bedtime.

Comment: Pilocarpine was introduced in 1876 and is still a commonly used antiglaucoma drug.

Carbachol, Topical

Preparations: Solution, 0.75%, 1.5%, 2.25%, and 3%.

Dosage: 1 drop in each eye three or four times a day.

Comment: Carbachol is poorly absorbed through the cornea and usually is used if pilocarpine is ineffective. Its duration of action is 4–6 hours. If benzalkonium chloride is used as the vehicle, the penetration of carbachol is significantly increased.

2. INDIRECT-ACTING REVERSIBLE ANTICHOLINESTERASE DRUGS

Physostigmine Salicylate & Sulfate (Eserine)
Preparations: Solution, 0.25%, and ointment, 0.25%.
Dosage: 1 drop three or four times a day or $1/4$-inch strip of ointment once or twice a day.
Comment: A high incidence of allergic reactions has limited the use of this old and seldom used antiglaucoma drug. It can be combined in the same solution with pilocarpine.

3. INDIRECT-ACTING IRREVERSIBLE ANTICHOLINESTERASE DRUGS

These drugs are strong and long-lasting and are used when other antiglaucoma medications fail to control the intraocular pressure. They are employed less frequently than in the past. The miosis produced is extreme; ciliary spasm and myopia are common. Local irritation is common, and phospholine iodide is believed to be cataractogenic in some patients. Pupillary block may occur. With the development of newer antiglaucoma medications, these agents are used much less commonly than in the past.

Echothiophate Iodide (Phospholine Iodide)
Preparations: Solution, 0.03%, 0.06%, 0.125%, and 0.25%
Dosage: 1 drop once or twice daily or less often, depending upon the response.
Comment: Echothiophate iodide is a long-acting drug similar to isoflurophate that has the advantages of being water-soluble and causing less local irritation. Systemic toxicity may occur in the form of cholinergic stimulation, including salivation, nausea, vomiting, and diarrhea. Ocular side effects include cataract formation, spasm of accommodation, and iris cyst formation.

Demecarium Bromide (Humorsol)
Preparations: Solution, 0.125% and 0.25%.
Dosage: 1 drop once or twice a day.
Comment: Systemic toxicity similar to that associated with echothiophate iodide may occur.

4. ADRENERGIC (SYMPATHOMIMETIC) DRUGS

In the treatment of glaucoma, epinephrine has the advantages of long duration of action (12–72 hours) and no miosis, which is especially important in patients with incipient cataracts (effect on vision not accentuated). At least 25% of patients develop local allergies; others complain of headache and heart palpitation (less common with dipivefrin).

Epinephrine acts by increasing outflow of aqueous humor.

Some of the preparations available for use in open-angle glaucoma are listed below. The dosage is the same for all, ie, 1 drop once or twice daily:

Epinephrine borate (Eppy/N), 0.5%, 1%, and 2%.
Epinephrine hydrochloride (Epifrin, Glaucon), 0.25%, 0.5%, 1%, and 2%.
Dipivefrin hydrochloride (Propine), 0.1%.

5. BETA-ADRENERGIC BLOCKING DRUGS

Timolol Maleate (Timoptic; Timoptic XE, Betimol)
Preparations: Solution, 0.25% and 0.5%; gel, 0.25% and 0.5%.
Dosage: 1 drop of 0.25% or 0.5% in each eye once or twice daily if needed. One drop of gel once daily.
Comment: Timolol maleate is a nonselective beta-adrenergic blocking agent applied topically for treatment of open-angle glaucoma, aphakic glaucoma, and some types of secondary glaucoma. A single application can lower the intraocular pressure for 12–24 hours. Timolol has been found to be effective in some patients with severe glaucoma inadequately controlled by maximum tolerated antiglaucoma therapy with other drugs. The drug does not affect pupillary size or visual acuity. Although timolol is usually well tolerated, it should be prescribed cautiously for patients with known contraindications to systemic use of beta-adrenergic blocking drugs (eg, asthma, heart failure). (See discussion of side effects, below.)

Betaxolol Hydrochloride (Betoptic; Betoptic S)
Preparations: Solution, 0.25% (Betoptic S) and 0.5%.
Dosage: 1 drop once or twice daily.
Comment: Betaxolol has comparable efficacy to timolol in the treatment of glaucoma. Its relative β_1 receptor selectivity reduces the risk of pulmonary side effects, particularly in patients with reactive airway disease.

Levobunolol Hydrochloride
(Betagan)

Preparations: Solution, 0.25% and 0.5%.

Dosage: 1 drop once or twice daily.

Comment: Levobunolol is a nonselective β_1 and β_2 blocker. It has effects comparable to those of timolol in the treatment of glaucoma.

Metipranolol Hydrochloride
(OptiPranolol)

Preparation: Solution, 0.3%.

Dosage: 1 drop once or twice daily.

Comment: Metipranolol is a nonselective β_1 and β_2 blocker with ocular effects similar to those of timolol.

Carteolol Hydrochloride
(Ocupress)

Preparation: Solution, 1%.

Dosage: One drop once or twice daily.

Comment: Carteolol is a nonselective beta-blocker with pharmacologic effects similar to those of other topical beta-blockers used for the treatment of glaucoma.

6. ALPHA-ADRENERGIC AGONISTS

Apraclonidine Hydrochloride
(Iopidine)

Preparation: Solution, 0.5% and 1%.

Dosage: 1 drop of 1% solution before anterior segment laser treatment and a second drop upon completion of the procedure. One drop of 0.5% solution two or three times a day as short-term adjunctive treatment in glaucoma patients receiving other medications.

Comment: Apraclonidine hydrochloride is a selective α-adrenergic agonist that has been applied topically for prevention and management of intraocular pressure elevations after anterior segment laser procedures. It is also used as short-term adjunctive therapy in patients on maximally tolerated medical therapy who need further reduction of intraocular pressure. Apraclonidine lowers intraocular pressure by decreasing aqueous humor formation, the exact mechanism of which is not clearly understood. It may also improve aqueous outflow. Unlike clonidine, apraclonidine does not appear to penetrate blood-tissue barriers easily and produces few side effects. The reported systemic side effects include occasional decreases in diastolic blood pressure, bradycardia, and central nervous system symptoms of insomnia, irritability, and decreased libido. Ocular side effects include conjunctival blanching, upper lid elevation, mydriasis, and burning.

Brimonidine Tartrate
(Alphagan)

Brimonidine is an adrenergic agonist that lowers intraocular pressure by decreasing aqueous production and perhaps also by increasing outflow through the uveoscleral pathway. It has only minimal effect on heart rate and blood pressure.

Preparation: Solution, 0.2%.

Dosage: One drop two or three times daily. May be used as monotherapy or in combination with other glaucoma medications. Frequently used as a replacement drug in patients unable to tolerate beta-blockers.

Toxicity: Dry mouth, stinging, and redness are the most common side reactions.

7. CARBONIC ANHYDRASE INHIBITORS

Inhibition of carbonic anhydrase in the ciliary body reduces the secretion of aqueous. The oral administration of carbonic anhydrase inhibitors is especially useful in reducing the intraocular pressure in selected cases of open-angle glaucoma and can be used with some effect in angle-closure glaucoma.

The carbonic anhydrase inhibitors in use are sulfonamide derivatives. Oral administration produces the maximum effect in approximately 2 hours; intravenous administration, in 20 minutes. The duration of maximal effect is 4–6 hours following oral administration.

The carbonic anhydrase inhibitors are used in patients whose intraocular pressure cannot be controlled with eye drops. They are valuable for this purpose but have many undesirable side effects, including potassium depletion, gastric distress, diarrhea, exfoliative dermatitis, renal stone formation, shortness of breath, fatigue, acidosis, and tingling of the extremities. Since the advent of timolol, topical carbonic anhydrase inhibitors, other newer glaucoma medications, and laser therapy, systemic carbonic anhydrase inhibitors are being used less frequently.

Acetazolamide
(Diamox)

Preparations and dosages:

Oral: Tablets, 125 mg and 250 mg; give 125–250 mg two to four times a day (dosage not to exceed 1 g in 24 hours). Sustained-release capsules, 500 mg; give 1 capsule once or twice a day.

Parenteral: May give 500-mg ampules intramuscularly or intravenously for short periods in patients who cannot tolerate the drug orally.

Methazolamide
(Neptazane)

Preparation: Tablets, 25 and 50 mg.

Dosage: 50–100 mg two or three times daily (total not to exceed 600 mg/d).

Dichlorphenamide
(Daranide)

Preparation: Tablets, 50 mg.

Dosage: Give a priming dose of 100–200 mg followed by 100 mg every 12 hours until the desired response is obtained. The usual maintenance dosage for glaucoma is 25–50 mg three or four times daily. The total daily dosage should not exceed 300 mg daily.

Dorzolamide Hydrochloride
(Trusopt)

Dorzolamide is a topical carbonic anhydrase inhibitor. It is a sulfonamide product with sufficient corneal penetration to reach the secretory epithelium of the ciliary body and reduce intraocular pressure by decreasing aqueous secretion.

Preparation: Solution, 2%.

Dosage: 1 drop two to four times daily. May be used as monotherapy but most frequently used in combination with other glaucoma medications.

Toxicity: Local reactions include burning and stinging, superficial punctate keratopathy, and allergic reactions of the conjunctiva. Bitter after-taste is common. Systemic side reactions associated with oral carbonic anhydrase agents are rare.

8. PROSTAGLANDIN ANALOGS

Latanoprost
(Xalatan)

Latanoprost is a selective prostanoid FP receptor agonist that appears to reduce intraocular pressure by increasing outflow of aqueous humor, mainly via the uveoscleral pathway. This agent may be used alone or in combination with other glaucoma medications.

Preparation: Solution, 0.005%.

Dosage: 1 drop once daily in the evening.

Onset and duration of action: Reduction of intraocular pressure occurs in 3–4 hours, and the maximum effect is reached in 8–12 hours.

Toxicity: Increased brown pigmentation of the iris may occur in some patients. Additionally, conjunctival hyperemia, punctate epithelial keratopathy, and foreign body sensation may occur in a small number of patients.

9. OSMOTIC AGENTS

Hyperosmotic agents such as urea, mannitol, and glycerin are used to reduce intraocular pressure by making the plasma hypertonic to aqueous humor. These agents are generally used in the management of acute (angle-closure) glaucoma and occasionally in pre- or postoperative surgery when reduction of intraocular pressure is indicated. The dosage for all is approximately 1.5 g/kg.

Glycerin
(Osmoglyn)

Preparations and dosage: Glycerin is usually given orally as 50% solution with water, orange juice, or flavored normal saline solution over ice (1 mL of glycerin weighs 1.25 g). Dose is 1–1.5 g/kg.

Onset and duration of action: Maximum hypotensive effect occurs in 1 hour and lasts 4–5 hours.

Toxicity: Nausea, vomiting, and headache occasionally occur.

Comment: Oral administration and the absence of diuretic effect are significant advantages of glycerin over the other hyperosmotic agents.

Isosorbide
(Ismotic)

Preparation: 45% solution.

Dosage: 1.5 g/kg orally.

Onset and duration of action: Similar to glycerin.

Comment: Unlike glycerin, isosorbide does not produce calories or elevated blood sugar. Other side reactions similar to glycerin. Each 220 mL of isosorbide contains 4.6 meq of sodium.

Mannitol
(Osmitrol)

Preparation: 5–25% solution for injection.

Dosage: 1.5–2 g/kg intravenously, usually in 20% concentration.

Onset and duration of action: Maximum hypotensive effect occurs in about 1 hour and lasts 5–6 hours.

Comment: Problems with cardiovascular overload and pulmonary edema are more common with this agent because of the large fluid volumes required.

Urea
(Ureaphil)

Preparation: 30% solution of lyophilized urea in invert sugar.

Dosage: 1–1.5 g/kg intravenously.

Onset and duration of action: Maximum hypotensive effect occurs in about 1 hour and lasts 5–6 hours.

Toxicity: Accidental extravasation at the injection site may cause local reactions ranging from mild irritation to tissue necrosis.

TOPICAL CORTICOSTEROIDS
Indications

Topical corticosteroid therapy is indicated for inflammatory conditions of the anterior segment of the globe. Some examples are allergic conjunctivitis, uveitis, episcleritis, scleritis, phlyctenulosis, superficial punctate keratitis, interstitial keratitis, and vernal conjunctivitis.

Administration & Dosage

The corticosteroids and certain derivatives vary in their anti-inflammatory activity. The relative potency of prednisolone to hydrocortisone is 4 times; of dexamethasone and betamethasone, 25 times. The side effects are not decreased with the higher-potency drugs even though the therapeutic dosage is lower.

The duration of treatment will vary with the type of lesion and may extend from a few days to several months.

Initial therapy for a severely inflamed eye consists of instilling drops every 1 or 2 hours while awake. When a favorable response is observed, gradually reduce the dosage and discontinue as soon as possible. *Caution:* The steroids enhance the activity of the herpes simplex virus, as shown by the fact that perforation of the cornea occasionally occurs when they are used in the eye for treatment of herpes simplex keratitis. Corneal perforation was an extremely rare complication of herpes simplex keratitis before the steroids came into general use. Other side effects of local steroid therapy are fungal overgrowth, cataract formation (unusual), and open-angle glaucoma (common). These effects are produced to a lesser degree with systemic steroid therapy. Any patient receiving local ocular corticosteroid therapy or long-term systemic corticosteroid therapy should be under the care of an ophthalmologist.

The following is a partial list of the available topical corticosteroids for ophthalmologic use:

Hydrocortisone ointment, 0.5%, 0.12%, 0.125%, and 1%.
Prednisolone acetate suspension, 0.125% and 1%.
Prednisolone sodium phosphate solution, 0.125% and 1%.
Dexamethasone sodium phosphate suspension, 0.1%; ointment, 0.05%.
Medrysone suspension, 1%.
Fluorometholone suspension, 0.1% and 0.25%; ointment, 0.1%.
Rimexalone suspension, 1%.

MIXTURES OF CORTICOSTEROIDS & ANTI-INFECTIVE AGENTS

There are numerous commercial products containing fixed-dose combinations of corticosteroids and one or more anti-infective agents. They are used by ophthalmologists chiefly to treat conditions in which both agents may be required, eg, marginal keratitis due to a combined staphylococcal infection and allergic reaction, blepharoconjunctivitis, and phlyctenular keratoconjunctivitis. They are also used postoperatively.

These mixtures should not be used to treat conjunctivitis or blepharitis due to unknown causes. They should not be used as substitutes solely for anti-infec-tive agents but only when a clear indication for corticosteroids exists as well. Mixtures of steroids and anti-infective agents may cause all of the same complications that occur with the topical steroid preparations alone.

NONSTEROIDAL ANTI-INFLAMMATORY AGENTS (NSAIDS)

Oral NSAIDs—indomethacin 75 mg daily or ibuprofen 600 mg daily—are the first-line treatment for scleritis. Gastric irritation and hemorrhage are a risk and may require prophylactic treatment with misoprostol, 100–200 µg orally four times a day, or a proton pump inhibitor. Topical ophthalmic preparations of several NSAIDs have been developed and have become popular in the past few years. They provide ocular bioavailability with little toxicity. These agents act primarily by blocking prostaglandin synthesis through inhibition of cyclooxygenase, the enzyme catalyzing the conversion of arachidonic acid to prostaglandins. Certain NSAIDs also may limit the arachidonic acid available for leukotriene production.

Some ophthalmologists use combinations of topical corticosteroids and NSAIDs to manage ocular inflammation, but the value of adding NSAIDs to adequate steroid therapy is not established. A number of ophthalmologists believe that by using an NSAID, the steroid treatment can be reduced.

Currently, flurbiprofen (Ocufen), 0.03%, and suprofen (Profenal), 1%, have been approved by the Food and Drug Administration for the inhibition of miosis during cataract surgery. Ketorolac (Acular), 0.5%, is approved for use in seasonal allergic conjunctivitis. Diclofenac (Voltaren), 0.1%, is approved for treatment of postoperative inflammation following cataract surgery and for relief of pain and photophobia in patients undergoing laser corneal refractive surgery (PRK). Another preparation, indomethacin suspension (Indocid), 1%, is not available in the USA but is used in some parts of the world to treat cystoid macular edema, to reduce miosis during cataract surgery, and to treat inflammation following trauma, including cataract surgery.

OTHER DRUGS USED IN THE TREATMENT OF ALLERGIC CONJUNCTIVITIS

Cromolyn Sodium (Crolom)

Preparation: Solution, 4%.
Dosage: 1 drop four to six times a day.
Comment: Cromolyn is useful in the treatment of many types of allergic conjunctivitis. Response

to therapy usually occurs within a few days but sometimes not until treatment is continued for several weeks. Cromolyn acts by inhibiting the release of histamine and SRS-A (slow-reacting substance of anaphylaxis) from mast cells. It is not useful in the treatment of acute symptoms.

Lodoxamide Tromethamine (Alomide)

Preparation: Solution, 0.1%.

Dosage: 1 drop four times a day.

Comment: Lodoxamide is a mast cell stabilizer that inhibits type 1 immediate hypersensitivity reactions. It is indicated in the treatment of allergic reactions of the external ocular tissues, including vernal conjunctivitis and vernal keratitis. As with cromolyn, a therapeutic response does not usually occur until after a few days of treatment.

Olapadine Hydrochloride (Patanol)

Preparation: Solution, 0.1%.

Dosage: Twice a day at intervals of 6–8 hours.

Comment: Olapatadine has both antihistamine and mast cell stabilizing actions.

Levocabastine Hydrochloride (Livostin)

Preparation: Suspension, 0.05%.

Dosage: One drop four times a day.

Comment: Levocabastine is a selective, potent histamine H_1-receptor antagonist. It is useful in reducing acute symptoms of allergic conjunctivitis. Relief of symptoms occurs within minutes after application and lasts up to 2 hours.

Vasoconstrictors & Decongestant

These categories of drugs (see below) are also of interest in the treatment of allergic conjunctivitis.

ANTI-INFECTIVE OPHTHALMIC DRUGS

1. TOPICAL ANTIBIOTIC SOLUTIONS & OINTMENTS

Antibiotics are commonly used in the treatment of external ocular infection, including bacterial conjunctivitis, hordeola, marginal blepharitis, and bacterial corneal ulcers. The frequency of use is related to the severity of the condition. Antibiotic treatment of intraocular infection is set forth in Table 3–1.

Bacitracin, neomycin, polymyxin, erythromycin, tetracycline, gentamicin, and tobramycin are the most commonly used topical antibiotics. They are used separately and in combination as solutions and as ointments.

Bacitracin

Preparation: Ointment, 500 units/g. Commercially available in combinations with polymyxin B.

Comment: Most gram-positive organisms are sensitive to bacitracin. It is not used systemically because of its nephrotoxicity.

Erythromycin

Erythromycin ointment, 0.5% is an effective agent, particularly in staphylococcal conjunctivitis. It may be used instead of silver nitrate in prophylaxis of ophthalmia neonatorum.

Neomycin

Preparations: Solution, 2.5 and 5 mg/mL; ointment, 3.5–5 mg/g. Commercially available in combinations with bacitracin and polymyxin B.

Dosage: Apply ointment or drops three or four times daily. Solutions containing 50–100 mg/mL have been used for corneal ulcers.

Comment: Effective against gram-negative and gram-positive organisms. Neomycin is usually combined with some other drug to widen its spectrum of activity. It is best known in ophthalmologic practice as Neosporin, both in ointment and solution form, in which it is combined with polymyxin and bacitracin. Contact skin sensitivity develops in 5% of patients if the drug is continued for longer than a week.

Polymyxin B

Preparations: Ointment, 10,000 units/g; suspension, 10,000 units/mL. Commercially available in combination with bacitracin and neomycin.

Comment: Effective against many gram-negative organisms.

2. TOPICAL PREPARATIONS OF SYSTEMIC ANTIBIOTICS

Topical use of the antibiotics commonly used systemically should be avoided if possible, because sensitization of the patient may interfere with future systemic use. However, in certain instances clinical judgment overrides this principle if the drug is particularly effective locally and the disorder is serious. A prime example of this is tetracycline in the treatment of trachoma, the commonest eye infection in the world.

Fluoroquinolones (ciprofloxacin, norfloxacin) have recently become available for ophthalmic use. These agents are effective against a wide variety of gram-positive and gram-negative ocular pathogens, including *Pseudomonas aeruginosa*. They have been used principally for the treatment of corneal ulcers but have also been administered for the treatment of resistant bacterial conjunctivitis.

Table 3–1. Usual adult dose of selected antimicrobials in endophthalmitis.[1,2]

	Intravitreal Dose (0.1 mL)[3,4]	Subconjunctival Dose (0.5 mL)[3]	Oral or Intravenous Dose[3]
Amikacin (Amikin)	0.4 mg	25 mg	6 mg/kg IV every 12 hours
Amphotericin B (Fungizone)	0.005–0.01 mg	1–2 mg	Varies (determined on case-by-case basis)
Cefamandole (Mandol)	1–2 mg	75 mg	1 g IV every 6–8 hours[5]
Cefazolin (Ancef, Ketzol)	2.25 mg	100 mg	1–1.5 g IV every 6–8 hours
Ceftazidime (Fortraz, others)	2.25 mg	100 mg	1 g IV every 8–12 hours
Ceftriaxone (Rocephin)			1–2 g IV once or twice a day
Ciprofloxacin			750 mg orally twice a day
Clindamycin (Cleocin)	0.5–1 mg	30 mg	600 mg IV every 6 hours
Gentamicin (Garamycin, Jenamycin)	0.1–0.2 mg	20 mg	1 mg/kg IV every 8 hours[5]
Methicillin (Staphcillin)	2 mg	100 mg	1–2 g IV every 6 hours
Miconazole (Monistat)	0.025 mg	5 mg	200–600 mg IV every 8 hours
Tobramycin (Nebcin)	0.5 mg	20 mg	1 mg/kg IV every 8 hours[5]
Vancomycin (Vancocin, others)	1 mg	25 mg	1 g IV every 12 hours

[1] Modified and reproduced, with permission, from Parke DW, Brinton GS: Endophthalmitis. In: *Infections of the Eye,* 2nd ed. Tabbara KF, Hyndiuk RA (editors). Little, Brown, 1996.
[2] Higher doses have been recommended in some cases. The doses listed here are considered appropriate by the present author based on drug toxicity studies.
[3] Principal therapy for microbial endophthalmitis is intravitreal, supplemented by subconjunctival and topical therapy. Systemic therapy does not appear to be of additional advantage in exogenous endophthalmitis following primary intraocular surgery but is indicated in endogenous endophthalmitis and for the treatment and prophylaxis of endophthalmitis complicating ocular trauma.
[4] Intravitreal antibiotic preparations should not contain preservatives.
[5] Nephrotoxic. Dose adjusted based upon creatinine clearance and body weight.

Tetracyclines

Preparations: Suspension, 10 mg/mL; ointment, 10 mg/g.

Comment: Tetracycline, oxytetracycline, and chlortetracycline have limited uses in ophthalmology because their effectiveness is so often impaired by the development of resistant strains. Solutions of these compounds are unstable with the exception of Achromycin in sesame oil, which is widely used in the treatment of trachoma. Ointment may be used for prophylaxis of ophthalmia neonatorum.

Gentamicin (Garamycin, Genoptic, Gentacidin, Gentak)

Preparations: Solution, 3 mg/mL; ointment, 3 mg/g.

Comment: Gentamicin is widely accepted for use in serious ocular infections, especially corneal ulcers caused by gram-negative organisms. It is also effective against many gram-positive staphylococci but is not effective against streptococci. Many strains of bacteria resistant to gentamicin have developed.

Tobramycin (Tobrex, Aktop)

Preparations: Solution, 3 mg/mL; ointment, 3 mg/g.

Comment: Similar antimicrobial activity to gentamicin but more effective against streptococci. Best reserved for treatment of *Pseudomonas* keratitis, for which it is more effective.

Chloramphenicol (Chloromycetin, Chloroptic)

Preparations: Solution, 5 and 10 mg/mL; ointment, 10 mg/g.

Comment: Chloramphenicol is effective against a wide variety of gram-positive and gram-negative organisms. It rarely causes local sensitization, but cases of aplastic anemia have occurred with long-term therapy.

Ciprofloxacin
(Ciloxan)

Preparation: Solution, 3 mg/mL.
Dosage: For treatment of conjunctivitis, 1 drop every 2–4 hours. For treatment of corneal ulcers, 1 drop every 15–30 minutes for the first day, 1 drop every hour the second day, and 1 drop every 4 hours thereafter.

Norfloxacin
(Chibroxin)

Preparation: Solution, 3 mg/mL.
Dosage: For conjunctivitis, same as that of ciprofloxacin.

Ofloxacin
(Ocuflox)

Preparation: Solution, 3 mg/mL.
Dosage: For treatment of bacterial conjunctivitis, 1 drop every 2–4 hours for 2 days, then 1 drop four times a day.

3. COMBINATION ANTIBIOTIC AGENTS

Several ophthalmic preparations are available that contain a mixture of antibiotics and bacteriostatic agents (Table 3–2).

4. SULFONAMIDES

The sulfonamides are the most commonly used drugs in the treatment of bacterial conjunctivitis. Their advantages include (1) activity against both gram-positive and gram-negative organisms, (2) relatively low cost, (3) low allergenicity, and (4) the fact

Table 3–2. Some combination antibiotic preparations.

Generic Name	Trade Name
Bacitracin and polymyxin B	Ak-Poly-Bac, Polycin-B, PolyTracin
Bacitracin (or gramicidin), neomycin, and polymyxin B	Various
Oxytetracycline and polymyxin B	Terramycin w/Polymyxin B, Terak
Polymyxin B and trimethoprim	Polytrim

that their use is not complicated by secondary fungal infections, as sometimes occurs following prolonged use of antibiotics.

The commonest sulfonamides employed are sulfisoxazole and sulfacetamide sodium.

Sulfacetamide Sodium
(Various)

Preparations: Ophthalmic solution, 10%, 15%, and 30%; ointment, 10%.
Dosage: Instill 1 drop frequently, depending upon the severity of the conjunctivitis.

Sulfisoxazole
(Gantrisin)

Preparations: Ophthalmic solution, 4%; ointment, 4%.
Dosage: As for sulfacetamide sodium (above).

5. TOPICAL ANTIFUNGAL AGENTS

Natamycin
(Natacyn)

Preparation: Suspension, 5%.
Dosage: Instill 1 drop every 1–2 hours.
Comment: Effective against filamentary and yeast forms. Initial drug of choice for most mycotic corneal ulcers.

Nystatin
(Mycostatin)

Nystatin is not available in ophthalmic ointment form, but the dermatologic preparation (100,000 units/g) is not irritating to ocular tissues and can be used in the treatment of fungal infection of the eye.

Amphotericin B
(Fungizone)

Amphotericin B is more effective than nystatin but not available in ophthalmic ointment form. The dermatologic preparation is highly irritating. A solution (1.5–8 mg/mL of distilled water in 5% dextrose) must be made up in the pharmacy from the powdered drug. Many patients have extreme ocular discomfort following application of this drug.

Miconazole
(Monistat)

A 1% solution is available in the form of an intravenous preparation that may be applied directly into the eye. The drug is not available in an ophthalmologic form.

Fluconazole
(Diflucan)

An 0.2% parenteral preparation is available and may be applied into the eye. No ophthalmologic product is available.

6. ANTIVIRAL AGENTS

Idoxuridine
(Herplex)

Preparations: Ophthalmic solution, 0.1%; ointment, 0.5%.

Dosage: 1 drop every hour during the day and every 2 hours at night. With improvement (as determined by fluorescein staining), the frequency of instillation is gradually reduced. The ointment may be used four to six times daily, or the solution may be used during the day and the ointment at bedtime.

Comment: Used in the treatment of herpes simplex keratitis. Epithelial infection usually improves within a few days. Therapy should be continued for 3 or 4 days after apparent healing. Many ophthalmologists still prefer to denude the affected corneal epithelium and not use idoxuridine.

Vidarabine
(Vira-A)

Preparation: Ophthalmic ointment, 3%.

Dosage: In herpetic epithelial keratitis, apply four times daily for 7–10 days.

Comment: Vidarabine is effective against herpes simplex virus but not other RNA or DNA viruses. It is effective in some patients unresponsive to idoxuridine. Vidarabine interferes with viral DNA synthesis. The principal metabolite is arabinosylhypoxanthine (Ara-Hx). The drug is effective against herpetic corneal epithelial disease and has limited efficacy in stromal keratitis or uveitis. It may cause cellular toxicity and delay corneal regeneration. The cellular toxicity is less than that of idoxuridine.

Trifluridine
(Viroptic)

Preparation: Solution, 1%.

Dosage: 1 drop every 2 hours (maximum total, 9 drops daily).

Comment: Acts by interfering with viral DNA synthesis. More soluble than either idoxuridine or vidarabine and probably more effective in stromal disease.

Acyclovir
(Zovirax)

Preparation: Capsules, 200 mg.

Comment: Acyclovir is an antiviral agent with inhibitory activity against herpes simplex types 1 and 2, varicella-zoster virus, Epstein-Barr virus, and cytomegalovirus. It is phosphorylated initially by virus-specific thymidine kinase to acyclovir monophosphate and then by cellular kinases to acyclovir triphosphate, which inhibits viral DNA polymerase. Thus, there is a marked selectivity for virus-infected cells. Acyclovir has low toxicity. No commercial ophthalmic preparation is currently available in the USA; a topical product available for treatment of genital herpes should not be used in the eye. An oral preparation is available that may be used for treatment of selected herpes zoster ocular infections.

DIAGNOSTIC DYE SOLUTIONS

Fluorescein Sodium

Preparations: Solution, 2%, in single-use disposable units; as sterile paper strips; as 10% sterile solution for intravenous use in fluorescein angiography.

Dosage: 1 drop.

Comment: Used as a diagnostic agent for detection of corneal epithelial defects, in applanation tonometry, and in fitting contact lenses.

Rose Bengal

Preparation: Solution, 1%, and strips, 1.3 mg.

Dosage: 1 drop.

Comment: Used in diagnosis of keratoconjunctivitis sicca; the mucous shreds and devitalized corneal epithelium stain with rose bengal.

TEAR REPLACEMENT & LUBRICATING AGENTS

Methylcellulose and related chemicals, polyvinyl alcohol and related chemicals, and gelatin are used in the formulation of artificial tears, ophthalmic lubricants, contact lens solutions, and gonioscopic lens solutions. These agents are particularly useful in the treatment of keratoconjunctivitis sicca. (See Chapter 4.)

To increase viscosity and prolong corneal contact time, methylcellulose is sometimes added to eye solutions (eg, pilocarpine). Preservative-free preparations are available for use in patients with sensitivities to these substances.

VASOCONSTRICTORS & DECONGESTANTS

There are many commercially available OTC (over-the-counter) ophthalmic vasoconstrictive agents. The active ingredients in these agents usually are either ephedrine 0.123%, naphazoline 0.012–0.1%, phenylephrine 0.12%, or tetrahydrozoline 0.05–0.15%.

These agents constrict the superficial vessels of the conjunctiva and relieve redness. They also relieve minor surface irritation and itching of the conjunctiva, which can represent a response to noxious or irritating agents such as smog, swimming pool chlorine, etc. Products also are available that contain an antihistamine, antazoline phosphate 0.25–0.5%, or pheniramine maleate 0.3%.

CORNEAL DEHYDRATING AGENTS

Dehydrating solutions and ointments applied topically to the eye reduce corneal edema by creating an osmotic gradient in which the tear film is made hypertonic to the corneal tissues. Temporary clearing of corneal edema results.

Preparations: Anhydrous glycerin solution (Ophthalgan), hypertonic sodium chloride 2% and 5% ointment and solution (Absorbonac, Ak-NaCl, Hypersal, Muro-128).

Dosage: 1 drop of solution or $1/4$-inch strip of ointment to clear cornea. May be repeated every 3–4 hours.

OCULAR & SYSTEMIC SIDE EFFECTS OF DRUGS

F.T. Fraunfelder, MD

Ocular drugs administered both systemically and topically can produce adverse ocular effects, and topical ophthalmic preparations may lead to systemic side effects. Preservatives in topical ocular medications may also be associated with side effects.

Tables 3–3 to 3–5 list possible ocular and systemic side effects of some ocular and systemic medications. This is not a complete listing. Physicians are advised to consult product labels and the references at the end of this chapter.

SYSTEMIC SIDE EFFECTS OF TIMOLOL

One example of a topical ocular drug with serious systemic side effects is timolol. Timolol by topical ocular administration is the most commonly used antiglaucoma medication in the world and has been associated with severe—even fatal—reactions. Plasma drug concentrations sufficient to cause systemic adrenoceptor blocking effects can occasionally result from topical ocular administration. When topical ocular timolol is administered in infants, blood levels are often more than six times what minimum therapeutic levels would be if the drug were given orally. If the lacrimal outflow system is functioning, an estimated 80% of a timolol eye drop is absorbed from the nasal mucosa and passes almost directly into the vascular system. This is called the first-order pass effect and is true for all drugs that can be easily absorbed through mucosal tissue in the head. The venous drainage is to the right atrium (first pass), and this blood containing the drug is pumped back to various target organs before returning to the left atrium (second pass). This blood containing the drug then reaches the liver or kidney, where it is detoxified. Therefore, a small amount applied to the nasal mucosa can result in therapeutic blood levels, whereas if given orally its first pass includes absorption via the gastrointestinal tract and then the liver, where 80–90% is detoxified before reaching the right atrium. In the United States, approximately 8% of the white population, 24% of blacks, and 1% of those of Japanese and Chinese genetic origin lack the cytochrome P450 enzyme (CYP2D6) that metabolizes timolol. Therefore, some groups are at higher risk of developing systemic side effects.

Cardiopulmonary histories should be taken for candidates of beta-blocker glaucoma therapy. Pulmonary function studies should be considered in patients with bronchoconstrictive disease, and electrocardiograms should be ordered on selected patients with cardiac disease. Specifically, the precautions set forth in the package insert should be heeded carefully. Patients with known bronchial asthma, chronic respiratory or cardiovascular disease, or sinus bradycardia may need screening before using timolol. The drug should be used with caution in patients receiving other systemic beta-blocking agents.

WAYS TO DIMINISH SYSTEMIC SIDE EFFECTS

One important principle in avoiding systemic side effects from topical ophthalmic medications is to prevent overdosing. The physician should prescribe the lowest concentration of medication that will be therapeutically effective. Only 1 drop of medication is needed at each dosage, since the volume the conjunctival sac can hold is much less than 1 drop.

The proper method of topical administration of ophthalmic medication is as follows:

(1) Position the patient with head tilted back.

(2) Grasp the lower eyelid below the lashes and gently pull the lid away from the eye (Figure 3–1).

(3) Instill 1 drop of medication into the inferior cul-de-sac nearest the involved area, taking care that the tip of the medication bottle does not touch the lashes or eyelids, thus avoiding contamination (Figure 3–2).

(4) To deepen the inferior cul-de-sac, the lower eyelid should then be gently lifted upward to make contact with the upper lid as the eye looks down (Figure 3–3).

(5) The eyelids should be kept closed for 3 minutes to prevent blinking, which pumps the drug into the nose and increases systemic absorption. The patient may be shown how to obstruct the lacrimal drainage system with firm pressure over the inner corner of the closed eyelids, and this may even be more important than lid closure (Figure 3–4).

(6) Excess medication in the medial canthus should be blotted away before pressure is released or the eyelids opened. The patient receiving multiple topical

Table 3–3. Possible adverse ocular effects secondary to systemic drugs.

Drug	Adverse Effects
Allopurinol	Cataract
Amiodarone	Vortex keratopathy (Figure 15–38), thyroid ophthalmopathy (Figure 15–22)
Amphetamines	Elevation of intraocular pressure
Antibiotics	Conjunctivitis, keratitis
Anticholinergics	Retinal hemorrhage, angle-closure glaucoma, accommodative paresis, nystagmus
Barbiturates	Conjunctivitis, Stevens-Johnson syndrome, ptosis, optic atrophy
Busulfan	Cataract
Cardiac glycosides	Retinal degeneration, changes in color vision
Chloral hydrate	Conjunctivitis
Chlorambucil	Papilledema
Chloramphenicol	Optic neuropathy
Chloroquine	Corneal opacity, retinal degeneration
Chlorpropamide	Stevens-Johnson syndrome, corneal opacity, extraocular muscle paralysis
Clofazimine	Conjunctival deposits, corneal opacity
Corticosteroids	Elevation of intraocular pressure, cataract
Diazepam	Nystagmus
Disulfiram	Optic neuritis
Ethambutol	Optic neuritis
Gold salts	Conjunctival deposits, corneal opacity, nystagmus, pigmentation of lens
Guanethidine	Ptosis
Halogenated hydroxyquinolines	Optic atrophy
Haloperidol	Cataract
Hexamethonium	Retinal vasodilation
Indomethacin	Corneal opacity
Isoniazid	Optic neuritis
Isotretinoin	Conjunctivitis, corneal opacity, papilledema
Ketamine	Nystagmus
Methyldopa	Conjunctivitis
Morphine	Optic neuritis
Nalidixic acid	Papilledema
Naproxen	Corneal opacity
Oral contraceptives	Retinal vascular occlusion, optic neuropathy, papilledema
Penicillamine	Extraocular muscle paralysis, ptosis, optic neuritis
Phenothiazines	Conjunctival deposits, corneal opacity, oculogyric crisis, pigmentation of lens, retinal degeneration
Phenylbutazone	Conjunctivitis, keratitis, retinal hemorrhage
Phenytoin	Nystagmus, extraocular muscle paralysis
Quinacrine	Conjunctival deposits
Quinine	Retinal infarction
Rifampin	Optic neuritis
Salicylates	Nystagmus, retinal hemorrhage
Streptomycin	Conjunctivitis, Stevens-Johnson syndrome, retinal hemorrhage
Tamoxifen	Retinal and corneal deposits, optic neuropathy
Tetracycline	Papilledema
Thioridazine	Corneal and lenticular pigmentation, retinal degeneration, oculogyric crisis
Tricyclic antidepressants	Elevation of intraocular pressure
Vitamin A	Conjunctival deposits, papilledema
Vitamin D	Conjunctival deposits, corneal opacity

medications should wait 10 minutes between doses so that the first drug will not be washed out of the eye by the second.

NATIONAL REGISTRY OF DRUG-INDUCED OCULAR SIDE EFFECTS

The National Registry of Drug-Induced Ocular Side Effects is a clearinghouse of drug information on ocular toxicology. The principle underlying its estab-lishment is the assumption that the suspicions of prac-ticing clinicians regarding possible ocular toxicity of drugs can be pooled to increase the database and de-crease the lag time before recognition of adverse re-sponses. Physicians who wish to report suspected ad-verse drug reactions or would like to receive references pertaining to the data in Tables 3–3 to 3–5 should call or write the Casey Eye Institute, Oregon Health Sciences University, 3375 S.W. Terwilliger Blvd., Portland, OR 97201; phone: 503-494-5686.

Table 3–4. Possible adverse systemic effects of topical ocular medications.

Medication	Adverse Effects
Anesthetics, topical local Benoxinate Proparacaine Tetracaine	Allergic reactions, anaphylactic reactions, convulsions, faintness, hypotension, syncope
Antibiotics Chloramphenicol Sulfacetamide, sulfamethizole, sulfisoxazole Tetracycline, chlortetracycline	Allergic reactions; bone marrow depression, including aplastic anemia; gastrointestinal symptoms Photosensitivity, Stevens-Johnson syndrome Photosensitivity, skin discoloration
Anticholinergics Atropine, homatropine, scopolamine Cyclopentolate, tropicamide	Confusion, dermatitis, dry mouth, excitement, fever, flushed skin, hallucinations, psychosis, tachycardia, thirst Amnesia, ataxia, convulsions, disorientation, dysarthria, fever
Anticholinesterases, long-acting Demecarium, echothiophate, isoflurophate	Abdominal cramps, diarrhea, fatigue, nausea, rhinorrhea, weight loss
Anticholinesterases, short-acting Neostigmine, physostigmine	Abdominal cramps, depigmentation, diarrhea, vomiting
Beta-adrenoceptor blocker Timolol, betaxolol, levobunolol, metipranolol, carteolol	Asthma, bradycardia, cardiac arrhythmia, confusion, depression, dizziness, dyspnea, hallucinations, impotence, myasthenia, psychosis
Parasympathomimetics Carbachol, pilocarpine	Abdominal cramps, diarrhea, hypotension, increased salivation, muscle tremors, nausea, respiratory distress, rhinorrhea, slurred speech, sweating, vomiting, weakness
Sympathomimetics Ephedrine, epinephrine, hydroxyamphetamine, phenylephrine	Cardiac arrhythmias, hypertension, palpitations, subarachnoid hemorrhage, tachycardia

Table 3–5. Possible adverse ocular effects of topical ocular medications.

Medication	Adverse Effects
Anesthetics, local Butacaine, proparacaine, tetracaine	Allergic reactions, corneal opacity, decreased corneal wound healing, iritis
Antibiotics Chlortetracycline, tetracycline Neomycin	Allergic reactions, corneal discoloration Allergic reactions, follicular conjunctivitis, keratitis
Anticholinergics Cyclopentolate, tropicamide	Angle-closure glaucoma, blurred vision, photophobia
Anticholinesterases Demecarium, echothiophate, isoflurophate	Accommodative spasm, cataract, depigmentation of lids, iris cysts, lacrimal outflow obstruction
Anti-inflammatory agents Corticosteroids	Cataracts, corneal thinning, decreased corneal wound healing, glaucoma, infection
Antiglaucoma medications Latanoprost	Increase iris pigment, increase length and darkening of eyelashes, new lashes, anterior uveitis
Antivirals Idoxuridine, trifluridine, vidarabine	Cicatricial pseudopemphigoid, keratitis, lacrimal outflow obstruction
Beta-adrenoceptor blocker Timolol	Blepharoconjunctivitis, corneal anesthesia, diplopia, dry eyes, keratitis, ptosis
Parasympathomimetic Pilocarpine	Accommodative spasm, cicatricial pseudopemphigoid, corneal haze (gel), myopia, retinal detachment
Preservatives Benzalkonium chloride, phenylmercuric nitrate, thimerosal	Allergic reactions, corneal opacity, keratitis
Sympathomimetics Dipivefrin Epinephrine	Allergic reactions, angle-closure glaucoma, follicular conjunctivitis Cicatricial pseudopemphigoid; cystoid macular edema; discoloration of cornea, conjunctiva, and soft contact lens; lacrimal outflow obstruction

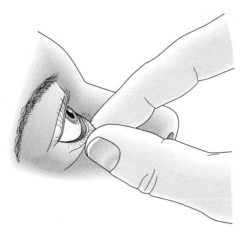

Figure 3–1. With the patient's head tilted back, grasp the lower eyelid below the lashes and gently pull the lid away from the eye.

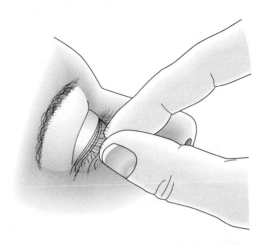

Figure 3–3. While the patient is looking downward, gently lift the lower eyelid to make contact with the upper lid.

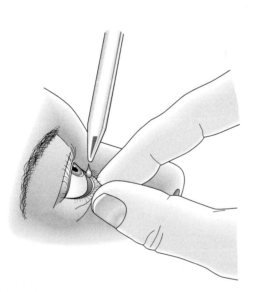

Figure 3–2. The patient should look up to prevent the medication from first "hitting" the cornea, which stimulates tearing and dilutes the medication. One drop of solution or a "match head" amount of ointment should be placed in the inferior cul-de-sac, without touching the bottle to the lashes or eyelids (to prevent contamination).

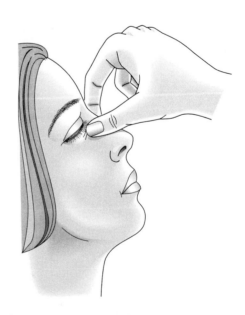

Figure 3–4. For 2 minutes or more, firm pressure is maintained with the forefinger or thumb over the inner corner of the closed eyelids. Lid closure is more important than pressure over the lacrimal sac in decreasing systemic absorption. Any excess medication should be blotted away before pressure is released or the eye is opened.

REFERENCES

Bito LZ (editor): Ocular effects of prostaglandins and other eicosanoids. Surv Ophthalmol 1997;41(Suppl 2). (Entire issue.)

Camras CB: The United States Latanoprost Study Group. Comparison of latanoprost and timolol in patients with ocular hypertension and glaucoma. Ophthalmology 1996;103:138.

Davidson SI et al: Ocular toxicity from systemic drug therapy: An overview of clinically important adverse reactions. Med Toxicol 1986;1:217.

Doft BH et al: Ceftazidime or amikacin: Choice of intravitreal antimicrobials in the treatment of postoperative endophthalmitis. Arch Ophthalmol 1994;112:17.

Edeki TI, Huabing H. Wood AJJ: Pharmacogenetic explanation for excessive β-blockade following timolol eye drops. JAMA 1995;274:20

Endophthalmitis Vitrectomy Study Group: Results of the Endophthalmitis Vitrectomy Study: A randomized trial of immediate vitrectomy and of intravenous antibiotics for the treatment of postoperative bacterial endophthalmitis. Arch Ophthalmol 1995;113:1479.

Fraunfelder FT: *Drug-Induced Ocular Side Effects and Drug Interactions,* 4th ed. Lea & Febiger, 1989.

Fraunfelder FT, Roy FH (editors): *Current Ocular Therapy,* 4th ed. Saunders, 1995.

Grant WM, Schuman JS: *Toxicology of the Eye,* 4th ed. Thomas, 1993.

Lee VH: Review: New directions in the optimization of ocular drug delivery. J Ocul Pharmacol 1990;6:157.

Leibowitz HM: Clinical evaluation of ciprofloxacin 0.3% ophthalmic solution for treatment of bacterial keratitis. Am J Ophthalmol 1991;112:34S.

Mauger TF, Craig EL (editors): *Havener's Ocular Pharmacology,* 6th ed. Mosby, 1994.

Nagasubramanian S et al: Comparisons of apraclonidine and timolol in chronic open-angle glaucoma: A three-month study. Ophthalmology 1993;100:1318.

Neu HC: Microbiologic aspects of fluoroquinolones. Am J Ophthalmol 1991;112:15S.

Ophthalmic Drug Facts. Facts & Comparisons. Lippincott-Raven, 1997.

Palmer EA: How safe are ocular drugs in pediatrics? Ophthalmology 1986;93:1038.

Salminen L: Review: Systemic absorption of topically applied ocular drugs in humans. J Ocul Pharmacol 1990;6:243.

Wilkerson M et al: Four-week safety and efficacy study of dorzolamide, a novel, active topical carbonic anhydrase inhibitor. Arch Ophthalmol 1993;111:1343.

Zimmerman TJ, Kooner KS, Sharir M (editors): *Textbook of Ocular Pharmacology.* Lippincott-Raven, 1997.

Lids, Lacrimal Apparatus, & Tears

John H. Sullivan, MD, J. Brooks Crawford, MD, & John P. Whitcher, MD, MPH

I. LIDS

John H. Sullivan, MD

SURGICAL ANATOMY OF THE LIDS

The eyelids are thin folds of skin, muscle, and fibrous tissue that serve to protect the delicate structures of the eye. The great mobility of the lids is possible because the skin is among the thinnest anywhere on the body. Fine hairs, visible only under magnification, are present on the eyelids. Beneath the skin lies loose areolar tissue which is capable of massive edematous distention. The orbicularis oculi muscle is adherent to the skin. It is innervated on its deep surface by the facial (VII) cranial nerve, and its function is to close the lids. It is divided into orbital, preseptal, and pretarsal divisions. The orbital portion, which functions primarily in forcible closure, is a circular muscle with no temporal insertion. The preseptal and pretarsal muscles have superficial and deep medial heads that participate in the lacrimal pump (see below).

The lid margins are supported by the tarsi, rigid fibrous plates connected to the orbital rim by the medial and lateral canthal tendons. The orbital septum, which originates from the orbital rim, attaches to the levator aponeurosis, which then joins the tarsus. On the lower lid, it joins the inferior border of the tarsus. The septum is an important barrier between the eyelids and the orbit. Behind it lies the preaponeurotic fat pad, a helpful surgical landmark. An additional fat pad lies medially in the upper lid. The lower lid has two anatomically distinct fat pads beneath the orbital septum.

Deep to the fat lies the levator muscle complex—the principal retractor of the upper eyelid—and its equivalent, the capsulopalpebral fascia in the lower lid. The levator muscle originates in the apex of the orbit. As it enters the eyelid, it forms an aponeurosis that attaches to the lower third of the superior tarsus. In the lower lid, the capsulopalpebral fascia originates from the inferior rectus muscle and inserts on the inferior border of the tarsus. It serves to retract the lower lid in downgaze. The superior and inferior tarsal muscles form the next layer, which is adherent to the conjunctiva. These sympathetic muscles are also lid retractors. Conjunctiva lines the inner surface of the lids. It is continuous with that of the eyeball and contains glands essential for lubrication of the cornea.

The upper lid is larger and more mobile than the lower. A deep crease usually present in the mid position of the upper lid in Caucasians represents an attachment of levator muscle fibers. The crease is much lower or is absent in the Asian eyelid. With age, the thin skin of the upper lid tends to hang over the lid crease and may touch the eyelashes. Aging also thins the orbital septum and reveals the underlying fat pads.

The lateral canthus is 1–2 mm higher than the medial. Because of loose tendinous insertion to the orbital rim, the lateral canthus is elevated slightly with upgaze.

INFECTIONS & INFLAMMATIONS OF THE LIDS

HORDEOLUM

Hordeolum is infection of the glands of the eyelid. When the meibomian glands are involved, a large swelling occurs called internal hordeolum (Figure 4–1). The smaller and more superficial external hordeolum (sty) is an infection of Zeis's or Moll's glands.

Pain, redness, and swelling are the principal symptoms. The intensity of the pain is a function of the amount of lid swelling. An internal hordeolum may point to the skin or to the conjunctival surface. An external hordeolum always points to the skin.

Most hordeola are caused by staphylococcal infections, usually *Staphylococcus aureus*. Culture is sel-

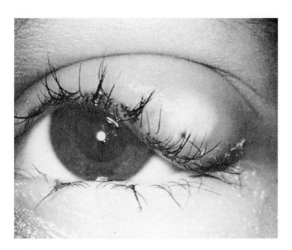

Figure 4–1. Internal hordeolum, left upper eyelid, pointing on skin side. This should be opened by a horizontal skin incision. (Courtesy of A Rosenberg.)

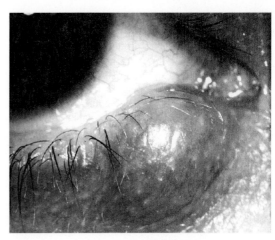

Figure 4–2. Chalazion, right lower eyelid. (Courtesy of K Tabbara.)

dom required. Treatment consists of warm compresses three or four times a day for 10–15 minutes. If the process does not begin to resolve within 48 hours, incision and drainage of the purulent material is indicated. A vertical incision should be made on the conjunctival surface to avoid cutting across the meibomian glands. The incision should not be squeezed to express residual pus. If the hordeolum is pointing externally, a horizontal incision should be made on the skin to minimize scar formation.

Antibiotic ointment applied to the conjunctival sac every 3 hours is beneficial. Systemic antibiotics are indicated if cellulitis develops.

CHALAZION

A chalazion (Figure 4–2) is an idiopathic sterile chronic granulomatous inflammation of a meibomian gland, usually characterized by painless localized swelling that develops over a period of weeks. It may begin with mild inflammation and tenderness resembling hordeolum—differentiated from hordeolum by the absence of acute inflammatory signs. Most chalazia point toward the conjunctival surface, which may be slightly reddened or elevated. If sufficiently large, a chalazion may press on the eyeball and cause astigmatism. If large enough to distort vision or to be a cosmetic blemish, excision is indicated.

Laboratory study is seldom indicated, but on histologic examination there is proliferation of the endothelium of the acinus and a granulomatous inflammatory response that includes Langerhans-type gland cells. Biopsy is indicated for recurrent chalazion, since meibomian gland carcinoma may mimic the appearance of chalazion.

Surgical excision is performed via a vertical inci-

sion into the tarsal gland from the conjunctival surface followed by careful curettement of the gelatinous material and glandular epithelium. Intralesional steroid injections alone may be useful for small lesions, and in combination with surgery in difficult cases.

ANTERIOR BLEPHARITIS

Anterior blepharitis is a common chronic bilateral inflammation of the lid margins. There are two main types: staphylococcal and seborrheic. Staphylococcal blepharitis may be due to infection with *Staphylococcus aureus,* in which case it is often ulcerative, or *Staphylococcus epidermidis* or coagulase-negative staphylococci. Seborrheic blepharitis (nonulcerative) is usually associated with the presence of *Pityrosporum ovale,* although this organism has not been shown to be causative. Often, both types are present (mixed infection). Seborrhea of the scalp, brows, and ears is frequently associated with seborrheic blepharitis.

The chief symptoms are irritation, burning, and itching of the lid margins. The eyes are "red-rimmed." Many scales or "granulations" can be seen clinging to the lashes of both the upper and lower lids. In the staphylococcal type, the scales are dry, the lids are red, tiny ulcerated areas are found along the lid margins, and the lashes tend to fall out. In the seborrheic type, the scales are greasy, ulceration does not occur, and the lid margins are less red. In the more common mixed type, both dry and greasy scales are present and the lid margins are red and may be ulcerated. *S aureus* and *P ovale* can be seen together or singly in stained material scraped from the lid margins.

Staphylococcal blepharitis may be complicated by hordeola, chalazia, epithelial keratitis of the lower third of the cornea, and marginal corneal infiltrates (see Chapter 6). Both forms of anterior blepharitis predispose to recurrent conjunctivitis.

The scalp, eyebrows, and lid margins must be kept clean, particularly in the seborrheic type of blepharitis, by means of soap and water shampoo. Scales must be removed from the lid margins daily with a damp cotton applicator and baby shampoo.

Staphylococcal blepharitis is treated with antistaphylococcal antibiotic or sulfonamide eye ointment applied on a cotton applicator once daily to the lid margins.

The seborrheic and staphylococcal types usually become mixed and may run a chronic course over a period of months or years if not treated adequately; associated staphylococcal conjunctivitis or keratitis usually disappears promptly following local antistaphylococcal medication.

POSTERIOR BLEPHARITIS

Posterior blepharitis is inflammation of the eyelids secondary to dysfunction of the meibomian glands. Like anterior blepharitis, it is a bilateral, chronic condition. Anterior and posterior blepharitis may coexist. Seborrheic dermatitis is commonly associated with meibomian gland dysfunction. Colonization or frank infection with strains of staphylococci is frequently associated with meibomian gland disease and may represent one reason for the disturbance of meibomian gland function. Bacterial lipases may cause inflammation of the meibomian glands and conjunctiva and disruption of the tear film.

Posterior blepharitis is manifested by a broad spectrum of symptoms involving the lids, tears, conjunctiva, and cornea. Meibomian gland changes include inflammation of the meibomian orifices (meibomianitis), plugging of the orifices with inspissated secretions, dilatation of the meibomian glands in the tarsal plates, and production of abnormal soft, cheesy secretion upon pressure over the glands. Hordeola and chalazia may also occur. The lid margin shows hyperemia and telangiectasia. It also becomes rounded and rolled inward as a result of scarring of the tarsal conjunctiva, causing an abnormal relationship between the precorneal tear film and the meibomian gland orifices. The tears may be frothy or abnormally greasy. Hypersensitivity to staphylococci may produce epithelial keratitis. The cornea may also develop peripheral vascularization and thinning, particularly inferiorly, sometimes with frank marginal infiltrates. The gross changes of posterior blepharitis are identical to the ocular findings in acne rosacea (see Chapter 15).

Treatment of posterior blepharitis is determined by the associated conjunctival and corneal changes. Frank inflammation of these structures calls for active treatment, including long-term low-dose systemic antibiotic therapy—usually with tetracycline (250 mg twice daily) or erythromycin (250 mg three times daily), but

guided by results of bacterial cultures from the lid margins—and (preferably short-term) treatment with weak topical steroids, eg, prednisolone, 0.125% twice daily. Topical therapy with antibiotics or tear substitutes is usually unnecessary and may lead to further disruption of the tear film or toxic reactions to their preservatives.

Periodic meibomian gland expression may be helpful, particularly in patients with mild disease that does not warrant long-term therapy with oral antibiotics or topical steroids. Hordeola and chalazia should be treated appropriately.

ANATOMIC DEFORMITIES OF THE LIDS

ENTROPION

Entropion—turning inward of the lid (Figure 4–3)—may be involutional (spastic, senile), cicatricial, or congenital. Involutional entropion is most common and by definition occurs as a result of aging. It always affects the lower lid and is the result of a combination of laxity of the lower lid retractors, upward migration of the preseptal orbicularis muscle, and buckling of the upper tarsal border.

Cicatricial entropion may involve the upper or lower lid and is the result of conjunctival and tarsal scar formation. It is most often found with chronic inflammatory diseases such as trachoma.

Congenital entropion is rare and should not be confused with congenital **epiblepharon,** which usually afflicts Asians. In congenital entropion, the lid margin is rotated toward the cornea, whereas in epiblepharon the pretarsal skin and muscle cause the lashes to rotate around the tarsal border.

Trichiasis is impingement of eyelashes on the cornea and may be due to entropion, epiblepharon, or simply misdirected growth. It causes corneal irritation and encourages ulceration. Chronic inflammatory lid

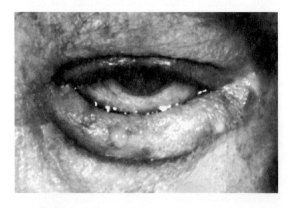

Figure 4–3. Entropion. (Courtesy of M Quickert.)

diseases such as blepharitis may cause scarring of the lash follicles and subsequent misdirected growth.

Distichiasis is a condition manifested by accessory eyelashes, often growing from the orifices of the meibomian glands. It may be congenital or the result of inflammatory metaplastic changes in the glands of the eyelid margin.

Surgery to evert the lid is effective in all kinds of entropion. Useful temporary measures in involutional entropion are to tape the lower lid to the cheek, with tension exerted temporally and inferiorly, or to inject botulinum toxin. Trichiasis without entropion can be temporarily relieved by plucking the offending eyelashes. Permanent relief may be achieved with electrolysis, laser or knife surgery, or cryosurgery.

ECTROPION

Ectropion (sagging and eversion of the lower lid) (Figure 4–4) is usually bilateral and is a frequent finding in older persons. Ectropion may be caused by relaxation of the orbicularis oculi muscle, either as part of the aging process or following seventh nerve palsy. The symptoms are tearing and irritation. Exposure keratitis may occur.

Involutional ectropion is treated surgically by horizontal shortening of the lid. Cicatricial ectropion is caused by contracture of the anterior lamella of the lid. Treatment requires surgical revision of the scar and often skin grafting. Minor degrees of ectropion can be treated by several fairly deep electrocautery penetrations through the conjunctiva 4–5 mm from the lid margins at the inferior aspect of the tarsal plate. The fibrotic reaction that follows will often draw the lid up to its normal position.

COLOBOMA

Congenital coloboma is the result of incomplete fusion of fetal maxillary processes. The consequence is a lid margin cleft of variable size. The medial aspect of the upper lid is most often involved, and there is often an associated dermoid tumor. Surgical reconstruction can usually be delayed for years but should be done immediately if the cornea is at risk. A full-thickness eyelid defect from any cause is sometimes referred to as a coloboma.

EPICANTHUS

Epicanthus (Figure 4–5) is characterized by vertical folds of skin over the medial canthi. It is typical of Asians and is present to some degree in most children of all races. The skinfold is often large enough to cover part of the nasal sclera and cause "pseudo-esotropia." The eye appears to be crossed when the medial aspect of the sclera is not visible. The most frequent type is **epicanthus tarsalis,** in which the superior lid fold is continuous medially with the epicanthal fold. In **epicanthus inversus,** the skinfold blends into the lower lid. Other types are less common. Epicanthal skinfolds may also be acquired after surgery or trauma to the medial eyelid and nose. The cause of epicanthus is vertical shortening of the skin between the canthus and the nose. Surgical correction is directed at vertical lengthening and horizontal shortening. Epicanthal folds in normal children, however, diminish gradually by puberty and seldom require surgery.

TELECANTHUS

The normal distance between the medial canthus of each eye—the intercanthal distance—is equal to the length of each palpebral fissure (approximately 30 mm in adults). A wide intercanthal distance may be the result of traumatic disinsertion or congenital craniofacial dysgenesis. Minor degrees of telecanthus (eg, blepharophimosis syndrome) can be corrected with skin and soft tissue surgery. Major craniofacial reconstruc-

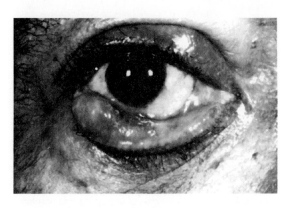

Figure 4–4. Ectropion. (Courtesy of M Quickert.)

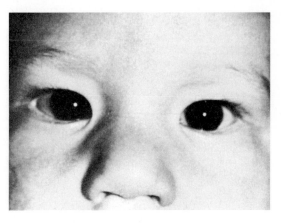

Figure 4–5. Epicanthus tarsalis.

tion, however, is required when the orbits are widely separated, as in Crouzon's disease (see Chapter 17).

BLEPHAROCHALASIS

Blepharochalasis (Figure 4–6) is a rare condition of unknown cause, sometimes familial, which resembles angioneurotic edema. Repeated attacks begin near puberty, diminish during adulthood, and cause atrophy of periorbital structures. Eyelid skin appears thin, wrinkled, and redundant and is described as resembling cigarette paper. A sunken appearance is the result of fat atrophy. Involvement of the levator aponeurosis produces moderate to severe ptosis. Medical management is limited to symptomatic treatment of edema. Surgical repair of levator dehiscence and excision of redundant skin is most likely to be successful after attacks have abated.

DERMATOCHALASIS

Dermatochalasis (Figure 4–7) is eyelid skin redundancy and loss of elasticity, usually as a result of aging. In the upper lid, the preseptal skin and orbicularis muscle, which normally forms a crease near the upper tarsal border in Caucasians, hangs over the pretarsal portion of the lid. When dermatochalasis is severe, the superior visual field is obstructed. Weakness of the orbital septum causes the medial and preaponeurotic fat pads to bulge. "Bags" in the preseptal region of the lower lid represent herniated orbital fat.

Blepharoplasty may be indicated for visual or cosmetic reasons. In the upper lid, superfluous eyelid skin is removed as well as muscle and fat for optimum aesthetics. Lower lid blepharoplasty is considered cosmetic surgery unless extreme redundancy contributes to ectropion of the lid margin. Pulsed CO_2 and erbium lasers have been found effective in tightening periocular skin but must be used with caution on the delicate skin of the lids.

BLEPHAROSPASM

Benign essential blepharospasm is an uncommon type of involuntary muscle contraction characterized by persistent or repetitive spasm of the orbicularis oculi muscle. It is almost always bilateral and is most common in the elderly. The spasms tend to progress in force and frequency, resulting in a grimacing expression and involuntary closure of the eyes. Patients may be incapacitated—able to experience only brief intervals of vision between spasms. When the entire face and neck are involved, the condition is known as Meigs' syndrome.

The cause is not known, but the dysfunction is believed to originate in the basal ganglia. Emotional stress and fatigue sometimes make the condition worse, leading to speculation that this is a psychogenic affliction. Psychotherapy and psychoactive drugs, however, have had very limited success.

It is important to differentiate benign essential blepharospasm from hemifacial spasm. The latter condition tends to be unilateral and to involve the upper and lower face. Hemifacial spasm is thought to be related to compression of the facial nerve by an artery or posterior fossa tumor. Jenetta's neurosurgical decompression is the definitive mode of treatment; however, temporary neuromuscular blockade (see below) is less invasive and more frequently employed.

Other types of involuntary facial movements include **tardive dyskinesia,** which results from prolonged phenothiazine therapy and seldom affects the orbicularis muscle selectively; and **facial tics,** common in children, which are thought to be psychogenic.

Treatment of blepharospasm begins with an attempt to identify the unusual instances of psychoneurotic behavior. Psychotherapy, neuroleptic drug treatment, biofeedback training, and hypnosis can be useful in this subset. Most patients, however, require repeated injections of botulinum toxin type A to produce temporary neuromuscular paralysis. If intolerance or unresponsiveness to the toxin develops, selec-

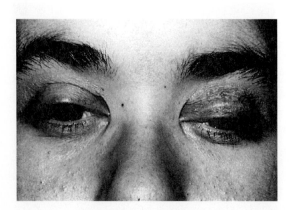

Figure 4–6. Blepharochalasis.

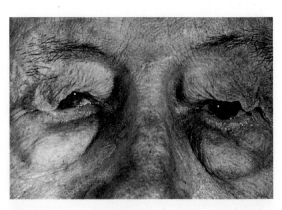

Figure 4–7. Dermatochalasis of upper lids and herniation of orbital fat of lower lids. (Courtesy of M Quickert.)

tive surgical ablation of the facial nerve or selective extirpation of the orbicularis muscles can be performed.

BLEPHAROPTOSIS

The upper lid normally rests approximately midway between the superior limbus and the pupillary margin. Considerable variation may exist as long as symmetry is maintained. Blepharoptosis, or "ptosis" as it is more commonly called, is the condition in which one or both upper eyelids assume an abnormally low position. Blepharoptosis may be congenital or acquired and can be hereditary in either case.

Classification

Classification is important for proper treatment. Beard's revised scheme (Table 4–1) attempts to classify ptosis by etiology.

A. Levator Maldevelopment: Ptosis from levator maldevelopment—formerly classified as true congenital ptosis—is the result of an isolated dystrophy of the levator muscle affecting both contraction and relaxation of the fibers. Ptosis is present in the primary position of gaze, and there is reduced movement of the lid in upgaze and impaired closure on downgaze. Lid lag on downgaze is an important clue to diagnosis of levator maldevelopment. Other ocular abnormali-

Table 4–1. Beard's revised classification of ptosis.

Levator maldevelopment
  Simple
  With superior rectus weakness
Other myogenic ptosis
  Blepharophimosis syndrome
  Chronic progressive external ophthalmoplegia
  Oculopharyngeal syndrome
  Progressive muscular dystrophy
  Myasthenia gravis
  Congenital fibrosis of the extraocular muscles
Aponeurotic ptosis
  Senile ptosis
  Late-developing hereditary ptosis
  Stress or trauma to levator aponeurosis
    Following cataract surgery
    Following other local trauma
    Blepharochalasis
    Associated with pregnancy
    Associated with Graves' disease
Neurogenic ptosis
  Ptosis caused by lesions of the oculomotor nerve
  Posttraumatic ophthalmoplegia
  Misdirected third nerve ptosis
  Marcus Gunn jaw-winking syndrome
  Horner's syndrome
  Ophthalmoplegic migraine
  Multiple sclerosis
Mechanical ptosis
Apparent ptosis
  Due to lack of posterior eyelid support
  Due to hypotropia
  Due to dermatochalasis

ties such as strabismus are sometimes associated with this form of congenital ptosis. In 25% of cases, the superior rectus muscle shares the same dystrophic changes as the levator, resulting in weakness of upgaze. It is important to identify this finding. Successful surgical outcome in the presence of superior rectus weakness requires the resection of an additional length of levator.

The distinction between levator maldevelopment and other forms of ptosis is an important one that cannot always be made by the history. Neurologic and other myogenic ptosis may be present at birth. Application of the surgical principles intended for levator maldevelopment to these types of ptosis patients would result in a gross overcorrection.

B. Other Types of Myogenic Ptosis: Blepharophimosis accounts for 5% of cases of congenital ptosis. Poor levator function and severe ptosis are accompanied by telecanthus, epicanthal folds, and cicatricial ectropion of the lower lids. The condition is familial.

Chronic progressive external ophthalmoplegia is a slowly progressive hereditary neuromuscular disease that begins in mid life. All extraocular muscles including the levator and the muscles of facial expression gradually become affected. Other neurodegenerative disorders may be present. In the form known as oculopharyngeal dystrophy, myopathy of the laryngeal muscles produces dysphagia. In Kearns-Sayre syndrome, ophthalmoplegia is associated with retinitis pigmentosa and heart block.

Ptosis and facial weakness may also be found in **myotonic dystrophy.** Other findings include cataract, pupillary abnormalities, frontal baldness, testicular atrophy, and diabetes.

Ptosis associated with the rare and sometimes familial **congenital fibrosis of the extraocular muscles** may be unilateral.

Ptosis and diplopia are often the initial manifestations of **myasthenia gravis.** The orbicularis oculi muscles are also frequently involved. Cogan's lid twitch is sometimes present—on rapid movements of the eyes from downgaze to the primary position, the upper lid twitches upward. Demonstration of lid fatigue, however, is more consistent. The diagnosis can be confirmed by intravenous administration of edrophonium, which temporarily reverses the weakness. Another useful test is the detection of circulating anti-acetylcholine receptor autoantibodies.

Medical management is usually effective initially, but ptosis surgery often becomes necessary. Thymectomy may be helpful in refractory cases. When lid closure and Bell's phenomenon have been impaired, difficult problems with exposure keratitis may complicate ptosis surgery.

C. Aponeurotic Ptosis: A common form of myogenic ptosis occurs late in life and results from partial disinsertion or dehiscence of the levator aponeurosis from the tarsal plate. Typically, there are sufficient residual attachments to the tarsus to maintain full excursion of the lid with upgaze. Retention of the attachment of the retracted levator aponeurosis to the skin and orbicularis muscle creates an unusually high lid fold. Thinning of the lid may also occur, and on occasion the image of the iris may be seen through the skin of the upper lid. Trauma is often a precipitating cause of disinsertion of the levator. Ptosis following cataract surgery is thought to be due to this mechanism. A hereditary variant is known as "late-developing hereditary ptosis." The mechanism of ptosis associated with ocular surgery, blepharochalasis, pregnancy, and Graves' disease is usually damage to the aponeurosis.

D. Neurogenic Ptosis: In **Marcus Gunn syndrome** (jaw-winking phenomenon), the eye opens when the mandible is opened or is deviated to the opposite side. The ptotic levator muscle is innervated by motor branches of the trigeminal nerve as well as the oculomotor nerve.

Partial or complete oculomotor palsy due to trauma is often complicated by aberrant regeneration, resulting in bizarre movements of the globe, eyelid, and pupil. Congenital oculomotor nerve paralysis, however, is not associated with aberrant regeneration. If the lid is completely closed, deprivational amblyopia will develop unless the ptosis is corrected. Visually immature children with oculomotor nerve paralysis, even after successful ptosis repair, are almost certain to develop strabismic amblyopia without vigorous and early treatment.

Paralysis of Müller's muscle is almost always associated with **Horner's syndrome** and is usually acquired. Rarely is there more than 2 mm of ptosis, and amblyopia is never a threat.

E. Mechanical Ptosis: The upper lid may be prevented from opening completely because of the mass effect of a neoplasm or the tethering effect of scar formation. Excessive horizontal shortening of the upper lid is a common cause of mechanical ptosis. Another form is that seen following enucleation, when absence of support to the levator by the globe permits the lid to drop.

F. Apparent Ptosis: Hypotropia may give the appearance of ptosis. When the eye looks down, the upper lid drops more than the lower lid. The narrowed palpebral fissure and the ptotic upper lid are much more apparent than the hypotropic globe. Occlusion of the opposite eye, however, reveals the true condition. In severe dermatochalasis, a fold of pretarsal orbicularis and skin may conceal the lid margin and give the appearance of blepharoptosis.

Treatment
(Figure 4–8)

With the exception of myasthenia gravis, all types of ptosis are treated surgically. In children, surgery can be performed when accurate evaluation can be obtained and the child is able to cooperate postoperatively. Astigmatism and myopia may be associated with childhood ptosis. Early surgery might be helpful in preventing anisometropic amblyopia, but this has not been proved. Deprivational amblyopia probably occurs only with complete ptosis, as in oculomotor nerve palsy.

Symmetry is the goal of surgery, and symmetry in all positions of gaze is possible only if levator function is unimpaired. In most cases, the best result that can be achieved is to balance the lids in the primary position. With unilateral ptosis, achievement of symmetry in other positions of gaze is proportionate to levator function.

Most ptosis operations involve resection of the levator aponeurosis or superior tarsal muscle (or both). The superior portion of the tarsus is often resected for additional elevation. Many approaches, from both skin and conjunctiva, are currently in use. In recent years, emphasis has been placed on the advantages of confining the operation to advancement and resection of the levator aponeurosis, especially in acquired ptosis.

Patients with little or no levator function require an alternative elevating source. Suspension of the lids to the brow allows the patient to elevate the lids with the natural movement of the frontalis muscle. Autogenous fascia lata is usually considered the best means of suspension.

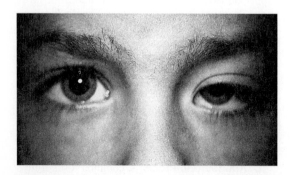 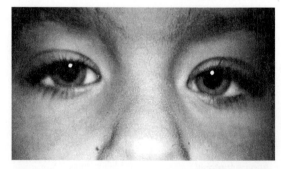

Figure 4–8. Surgical correction of ptosis. **Left:** Before operation, ptosis of the upper lid was present. **Right:** After the operation (levator resection), the ptosis was well corrected and a natural-appearing upper lid fold produced. (Courtesy of C Beard.)

COSMETIC MICROPIGMENTATION OF THE LIDS

Tattooing the lids of women is a controversial procedure whose purpose is to eliminate the need for applying eyeliner. The procedure is also occasionally used to simulate cilia following reconstruction of the lid margin. It is performed under local anesthesia using a power-driven handpiece to implant various pigments adjacent to the eyelashes or eyebrow. Because subcutaneous impregnation of certain mercury-based dyes can cause a local inflammatory reaction, these dyes have been abandoned. Carbon particle tattooing appears to be harmless, but the long-term consequences of dye impregnation at the lid margin are unknown.

As is true also of tattoos elsewhere on the body, the intensity and crispness of the image tends to fade with time. Complete removal of the pigmentation because of misplacement or change in fashion is difficult.

TUMORS OF THE EYELIDS

J. Brooks Crawford, MD

BENIGN LID TUMORS

Benign tumors of the lids are very common and increase in frequency with age. Most are readily distinguished clinically, and excision is done for cosmetic reasons. However, it is often impossible to recognize malignant lesions clinically, and biopsy should always be performed if there is any doubt about the diagnosis.

Nevus

Melanocytic nevi of the eyelids are common benign tumors with the same pathologic structure as nevi found elsewhere. They initially may be relatively unpigmented, enlarging and darkening during adolescence. Many never acquire visible pigment, and many resemble benign papillomas. Nevi rarely become malignant.

Nevi may be removed by shave excision if desired for cosmetic reasons.

Papillomas

Papillomas are the most common benign eyelid tumors. Two types occur: squamous cell papillomas and seborrheic keratoses (basal cell papillomas, senile verrucae). In both, fibrovascular cores permeate thickened (acanthotic and hyperkeratotic) surface epithelium, giving it a papillomatous appearance. Seborrheic keratoses occur in middle-aged and older individuals. They have a friable, verrucous surface and are often pigmented because melanin accumulates in the keratocytes.

Verruca Vulgaris

Another papillomatous, hyperkeratotic nodule that may occur on the skin of the face and eyelids is due to the wart virus, a DNA virus in the papovavirus group.

Molluscum Contagiosum (Figure 4–9)

This tumor, due to a poxvirus, is a small, dome-shaped nodule, often umbilicated centrally. Lid margin lesions may be minute and partially hidden in the cilia but may produce conjunctivitis and even keratitis if the lesion sheds into the conjunctival space.

Cure can usually be achieved by curettement, cautery, or excision.

Keratoacanthoma

Keratoacanthomas are benign inflammatory tumors occurring in sun-exposed skin of adults. Occasionally they are associated with immunodeficiency, xeroderma pigmentosum, or the Muir-Torre syndrome. Many will undergo spontaneous involution, but excisional biopsy is often indicated for cosmetic reasons or to rule out the possibility of squamous cell carcinoma, which they may mimic both clinically and histologically.

Xanthelasma (Figure 4–10)

Xanthelasma is a common disorder that occurs on the anterior surface of the eyelid, usually bilaterally near the inner angle of the eye. The lesions appear as yellow, wrinkled patches on the skin and occur most commonly in elderly people. Xanthelasma represents lipid deposits in histiocytes in the dermis of the lid. They occur in patients with hereditary hyperlipidemia

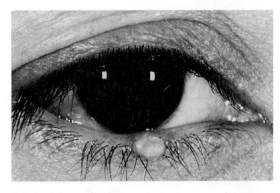

Figure 4–9. Molluscum contagiosum. Note central umbilication.

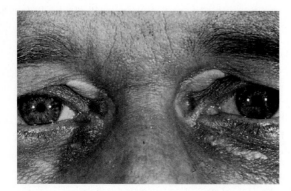

Figure 4–10. Xanthelasma. (Courtesy of M Quickert.)

and in diabetics and other patients with secondary hyperlipidemia, but approximately two-thirds of patients with xanthelasma have normal serum lipids.

Treatment is indicated for cosmetic reasons. Lesions can be excised, cauterized, or treated with laser surgery. Recurrence following removal is not unusual.

Cysts

Cysts in the eyelids are common. Keratinous cysts, lined by epithelium and filled with cheesy-looking keratin and debris, are the result of obstruction of pilosebaceous structures (milia and pilar cysts), or congenital and traumatic subepithelial implantation of surface epithelium (epidermal inclusion cysts).

Dermoid cysts, with adnexal structures such as hair follicles and sebaceous glands in the walls and with hair as well as keratin in the lumen, are congenital but may not become apparent until later in life, when they increase in size or rupture, eliciting a granulomatous inflammatory response. Most are located near the orbital rim superotemporally, and many are associated with a defect in the bone that may communicate with the intracranial cavity.

Hidrocystomas (sudoriferous cysts) arise from the sweat ducts and are filled with a watery material.

Hemangioma
(Figure 4–11)

The most common congenital vascular tumor of the eyelids is the **capillary hemangioma** (strawberry nevus) composed of proliferating capillaries and en-

dothelial cells. They arise at or shortly after birth, often grow rapidly, and usually involute spontaneously by age 7 years. If superficial, they may be bright red (strawberry nevus); deeper lesions may be bluish or violet. Secondary anisometropia, refractive amblyopia, and strabismus are common and must be appropriately treated. Treatment of the tumor is rarely indicated unless it blocks the pupil. If it does, intralesional injection of steroids may produce rapid resolution; if this fails, partial surgical excision is indicated.

Capillary hemangiomas should be differentiated from the much rarer **nevus flammeus (port wine stain),** which is more purple in hue than the bright red of capillary hemangiomas. The nevus flammeus is composed of dilated, cavernous vascular channels. It is always present at birth, does not grow or regress as does a capillary hemangioma, and is often associated with Sturge-Weber syndrome. The cosmetic defect can be treated with laser surgery.

A third type of angioma is the **cavernous hemangioma,** composed of large, endothelium-lined vascular channels with smooth muscle in their walls. They are developmental rather than congenital and tend to arise after the first decade. Unlike capillary hemangiomas, they do not usually regress.

PRIMARY MALIGNANT TUMORS OF THE LIDS

Carcinoma
(Figures 4–12 and 4–13)

Basal cell and squamous cell carcinomas of the lids are the most common malignant ocular tumors. These tumors occur most frequently in fair-complexioned individuals who have had chronic exposure to the sun. Ninety-five percent of lid carcinomas are of the basal cell type. The remaining 5% consist of squamous cell

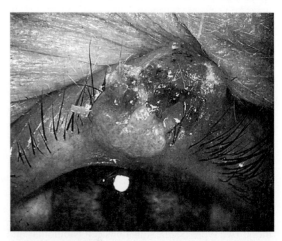

Figure 4–12. Squamous cell carcinoma of upper lid. (Courtesy of A Rosenberg.)

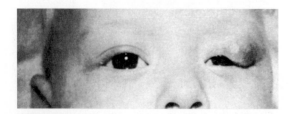

Figure 4–11. Cavernous hemangioma of left upper lid.

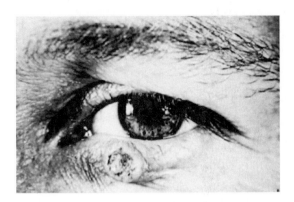

Figure 4–13. Basal cell carcinoma of left lower lid. (Courtesy of S Mettier, Jr.)

carcinomas, meibomian gland carcinomas, and other rare tumors such as Merkel cell carcinomas and carcinomas of the sweat glands.

Treatment of all these carcinomas is by complete excision, which is best achieved by controlling the surgical margins with frozen sections. Many of these malignant tumors and many benign ones as well can have the same appearance; biopsy is usually required to establish the correct diagnosis.

A. Basal Cell Carcinoma: Basal cell carcinoma usually grows slowly and painlessly as a nodule that may or may not become ulcerated. It slowly invades adjacent tissues but rarely metastasizes. A less common type—sclerosing or morphea basal cell carcinoma—tends to extend insidiously and surreptitiously beneath the surface, sometimes producing ectropion, entropion, lid notching or retraction, dimpling of the overlying skin, or loss of eyelashes.

Frozen section study of the surgical margins is particularly important for sclerosing basal cell carcinomas, since the tumor margins are seldom clinically apparent. Microscopically controlled excision (a modified Mohs technique) is used by some dermatologists to achieve complete excision. Selected cases may be treated by other methods such as radiotherapy or cryotherapy with liquid nitrogen.

B. Squamous Cell Carcinoma: Squamous cell carcinomas also grow slowly and painlessly, often starting as a hyperkeratotic nodule that may become ulcerated. Benign inflammatory tumors such as keratoacanthomas may closely resemble carcinomas. The correct diagnosis may depend on biopsy. Like basal cell carcinomas, these tumors can invade and erode through adjacent tissue; they can also spread to regional lymph nodes via the lymphatic system.

C. Sebaceous Gland Carcinoma: Sebaceous gland carcinomas most often arise from the meibomian glands and the glands of Zeis but can also occur in the sebaceous glands of the eyebrow or caruncle. About half resemble benign inflammatory lesions and disorders such as chalazia and chronic blepharitis.

They are more aggressive than squamous cell carcinomas, often extending into the orbit, invading lymphatics, and metastasizing.

Carcinoma Associated With Xeroderma Pigmentosum

This rare disease is characterized by the appearance of a large number of freckles in sun-exposed areas of the skin. These are followed by telangiectases, atrophic patches, and eventually a warty growth that may undergo carcinomatous degeneration. The eyelids are frequently affected and may be the first area to show degenerative changes, causing atrophy and ectropion with secondary inflammatory changes of the conjunctiva, symblepharon, corneal ulceration, and carcinoma of the lids. Malignant tumors include basal cell carcinomas, squamous cell carcinomas, and malignant melanomas. This condition is inherited as an autosomal recessive trait and is due to a defect in the repair of DNA damaged by ultraviolet light. Carriers can often be identified by excessive freckling.

The disease appears early in life and in most cases is fatal by adolescence as a result of metastasis. Life may be prolonged by carefully protecting the skin from actinic rays and treating carcinomatous tumors as rapidly as they appear.

Sarcoma

Soft tissue sarcomas of the lids are rare and usually are anterior extensions of orbital tumors. Rhabdomyosarcomas involving the lids and orbit are the most common primary malignant tumors found in these tissues in the first decade of life. The lid tumor may be the first sign. A combination of radiotherapy and chemotherapy is usually effective in preserving ocular function and preventing death.

Malignant Melanoma

Malignant melanomas of the eyelids are similar to those elsewhere in the skin and include three distinct varieties: superficial spreading melanoma, lentigo maligna melanoma, and nodular melanoma. Not all malignant melanomas are pigmented. Most pigmented lesions on the eyelid skin are not melanomas. Therefore, biopsy should be used to establish the diagnosis. The prognosis for melanomas of the skin depends upon the depth of invasion or the thickness of the lesion. Tumors less than 0.76 mm in thickness rarely metastasize.

METASTATIC TUMORS

Metastatic tumors to eyelids are rare. Because they frequently mimic benign lesions such as chalazions, cysts, and granulomas, the diagnosis is often not suspected. Not infrequently, the lid lesion appears before the primary tumor is discovered.

II. LACRIMAL APPARATUS

John H. Sullivan, MD

The lacrimal system incorporates structures involved in the production and drainage of tears. The secretory component consists of the glands that produce the various ingredients of tear fluid. The nasolacrimal ductules form the excretory element of the system, depositing these secretions into the nose. The tear fluid is distributed over the surface of the eye by the action of blinking.

LACRIMAL SECRETORY SYSTEM

The largest volume of tear fluid is produced by the major lacrimal gland located in the lacrimal fossa in the superior temporal quadrant of the orbit. This almond-shaped gland is divided by the lateral horn of the levator aponeurosis into a larger orbital lobe and a smaller palpebral lobe, each with its own ductule system emptying into the superior temporal fornix (Chapter 1). The palpebral lobe can sometimes be visualized by everting the upper lid. The secretions from the main lacrimal gland are triggered by emotion or physical irritation and cause tears to flow copiously over the lid margin (epiphora). Innervation of the main gland is from the pontine lacrimal nucleus through the nervus intermedius and along an elaborate pathway of the maxillary division of the trigeminal nerve. Denervation is a common consequence of acoustic neuroma and other tumors of the cerebellopontine angle.

The accessory lacrimal glands, although only one-tenth the mass of the major gland, have an essential role. The glands of Krause and Wolfring are identical to the major gland but lack a ductile system. These glands are located in the conjunctiva, mainly in the superior fornix. Unicellular goblet cells, also scattered throughout the conjunctiva, secrete glycoprotein in the form of mucin. Modified sebaceous meibomian and zeisian glands of the lid margin contribute lipid to the tears. The glands of Moll are modified sweat glands that also add to the tear film.

The accessory glands are known as the "basic secretors." Their emissions are sufficient to maintain the cornea without those of the main lacrimal gland. Loss of goblet cells, however, leads to drying of the cornea despite profuse tearing from the lacrimal gland.

DISORDERS OF THE SECRETORY SYSTEM

Alacrima

Congenital absence of tearing occurs in Riley-Day syndrome (familial dysautonomia) and anhidrotic ectodermal dysplasia. Although initially asymptomatic, patients may develop signs typical of keratoconjunctivitis sicca. Absence of tears may also occur after disruption of the lacrimal secretory nerve by acoustic neuroma or following surgery of the cerebellopontine angle. Tumors or inflammation of the lacrimal gland may reduce tear production.

Lacrimal Hypersecretion

Primary hypersecretion is rare and must be distinguished from tearing due to obstruction of the excretory ductules. Secondary hypersecretion may be psychogenic or reflex from irritation of surface epithelium or retina. It is possible to stop hypersecretion by blocking the lacrimal secretory nerve in the sphenopalatine ganglion.

Paradoxic Lacrimation ("Crocodile Tears")

This condition is characterized by tearing while eating. Although it may be congenital, it is usually acquired after Bell's palsy and is the result of aberrant regeneration of the facial nerve.

Bloody Tears

This is a rare clinical entity attributed to a variety of causes. It has been associated with menstruation ("vicarious menses"). Blood-tinged tears may be secondary to conjunctival hemorrhage due to any cause (trauma, blood dyscrasia, etc) or to tumors of the lacrimal sac. They have also been reported in a hypertensive patient suffering from epistaxis with extension through the nasolacrimal duct.

Dacryoadenitis

Acute inflammation of the lacrimal gland is a rare condition most often seen in children as a complication of mumps, measles, or influenza and in adults in association with gonorrhea. Chronic dacryoadenitis may be the result of benign lymphocytic infiltration, lymphoma, leukemia, or tuberculosis. It is occasionally seen bilaterally as a manifestation of sarcoidosis. When combined with parotid gland swelling, it is called Mikulicz's syndrome.

Considerable pain, swelling, and injection occur over the temporal aspect of the upper eyelid, which often imparts to it an S-shaped curve. If bacterial infection is present, systemic antibiotics are given. It is rarely necessary to surgically drain the infection.

LACRIMAL EXCRETORY SYSTEM

The excretory system is composed of the puncta, canaliculi, lacrimal sac, and nasolacrimal duct (see Chapter 1). With each blink, the eyelids close like a zipper—beginning laterally, distributing tears evenly across the cornea, and delivering them to the excretory system on the medial aspect of the lids. Under normal circumstances, tears are produced at about their rate of evaporation, and for that reason few pass through the excretory system. When tears flood the conjunctival sac, they enter the puncta partially by capillary attraction. With lid closure, the specialized portion of pretarsal orbicularis surrounding the ampulla tightens to prevent their escape. Simultaneously, the lid is drawn toward the posterior lacrimal crest, and traction is placed on the fascia surrounding the lacrimal sac, causing the canaliculus to shorten and creating negative pressure within the sac. This dynamic pumping action draws tears into the sac which then pass by gravity and tissue elasticity through the nasolacrimal duct into the inferior meatus of the nose. Valve-like folds of the epithelial lining of the sac tend to resist the retrograde flow of tears and air. The most developed of these flaps is the "valve" of Hasner at the distal end of the nasolacrimal duct. This structure is important because when imperforate in infants it is the cause of congenital obstruction and chronic dacryocystitis.

DISORDERS OF THE EXCRETORY SYSTEM

1. DACRYOCYSTITIS (Figure 4–14)

Infection of the lacrimal sac is a common disease that usually occurs in infants or postmenopausal women. It is most often unilateral and always secondary to obstruction of the nasolacrimal duct. In many adult cases, the cause of obstruction remains unknown. Dacryocystitis is uncommon in the intermediate age groups unless it follows trauma or is caused by a dacryolith. Spontaneous improvement follows passage of a dacryolith, but recurrence is the rule.

In infants, chronic infection accompanies nasolacrimal duct obstruction, but acute dacryocystitis is uncommon. Acute dacryocystitis in children is often a result of *Haemophilus influenzae* infection. Prompt and aggressive treatment should be instituted because of the risk of orbital cellulitis.

Acute dacryocystitis in adults is usually caused by *Staphylococcus aureus* or occasionally β-hemolytic streptococci. In chronic dacryocystitis, *Streptococcus*

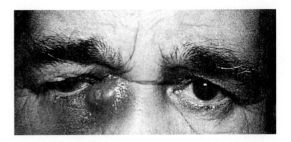

Figure 4–14. Acute dacryocystitis.

pneumoniae or, rarely, *Candida albicans* is the predominant organism—mixed infections do not occur. The infectious agent can be identified microscopically by staining a conjunctival smear taken after expression of the tear sac.

Clinical Findings

The chief symptoms of dacryocystitis are tearing and discharge. In the acute form, inflammation, pain. swelling, and tenderness are present in the tear sac area. Purulent material can be expressed from the sac. In the chronic form, tearing is usually the only sign. Mucoid material can usually be expressed from the sac. It is curious that dacryocystitis is seldom complicated by conjunctivitis even though the conjunctival sac is constantly being bathed with pus exuding through the lacrimal puncta. Corneal ulcer occasionally occurs following minor corneal trauma in the presence of pneumococcal dacryocystitis.

Treatment

Acute dacryocystitis usually responds to appropriate systemic antibiotics, and the chronic form can often be kept latent with antibiotic drops. However, relief of obstruction is the only cure.

In adults, the presence of a mucocele is evidence that the site of obstruction is in the nasolacrimal duct and that **dacryocystorhinostomy** is indicated. The patency of the canalicular system is ensured if mucus or pus is regurgitated through the puncta on compression of the sac. Examination of the nose is important to ensure adequate drainage space between the septum and the lateral nasal wall. Dacryocystorhinostomy consists of forming a permanent anastomosis between the lacrimal sac and the nose. Exposure is gained by an incision over the anterior lacrimal crest. A bony opening is made in the lateral wall of the nose, and the nasal mucosa is sutured to the mucosa of the lacrimal sac. An endoscopic approach through the nose using lasers to help form the opening between the lacrimal sac and the nasal cavity is under investigation. Transluminal balloon dilation of the distal nasolacrimal system may also be useful for patients not suitable for surgery.

Excessive tearing (epiphora) is occasionally due to canalicular stenosis (see below) or obstruction at the junction of the common canaliculus and lacrimal sac. In either case, compression of the sac does not cause regurgitation of fluid, mucus, or pus through the puncta, and no mucocele is present. Intubation and irrigation of the canalicular system with a lacrimal cannula and x-ray studies with contrast media (dacryocystography) will identify the site of obstruction. Common canalicular obstruction may be treated by intubation of the passages with silicone stent for 3–6 months. A thick obstructing scar, however, will necessitate dacryocystorhinostomy and canaliculoplasty with silicone intubation of the canalicular system.

In **infantile dacryocystitis,** the site of stenosis is usually at the valve of Hasner. Failure of canalization is a common occurrence (4–7% of newborns), but normally the duct opens spontaneously within the first month. Forceful compression of the lacrimal sac will sometimes rupture the membrane and establish patency. If stenosis persists more than 6 months or if dacryocystitis develops, probing of the duct is indicated. One probing is effective in 75% of cases. In the remainder, cure can almost always be achieved by repeated probing, by inward fracture of the inferior turbinate, or by a temporary silicone lacrimal splint. Probing should not be attempted in the presence of acute infection.

2. CANALICULAR DISORDERS

Congenital anomalies of the canalicular system include imperforate puncta, accessory puncta, canalicular fistulas, and, rarely, agenesis of the canalicular system. Most cases of canalicular stenosis are acquired, usually the result of viral infections—notably varicella, herpes simplex, and adenovirus infection. Obstruction—even obliteration—may occur with Stevens-Johnson syndrome, pemphigoid, and other conjunctival shrinkage diseases. Systemic chemotherapy with fluorouracil and topical idoxuridine may also cause obstruction. Canaliculitis is an uncommon chronic unilateral infection caused by *Actinomyces israelii* (Figure 4–15), *Candida albicans,* or *Aspergillus* species. It affects the lower canaliculus more often than the upper, occurs exclusively in adults, and causes a secondary purulent conjunctivitis that frequently escapes etiologic diagnosis. Untreated, it will result in canalicular stenosis. The patient complains of a mildly red and irritated eye with a slight discharge. The punctum usually pouts, and material can be expressed from the canaliculus. The organism can be seen microscopically on a direct smear taken from the canaliculus. Curettage of the necrotic material in the involved canaliculus, followed by irrigation, is usually effective in establishing patency. Canaliculotomy is sometimes necessary. Tincture of iodine may be applied to the lining of the canaliculus after canaliculotomy. Recurrence is common.

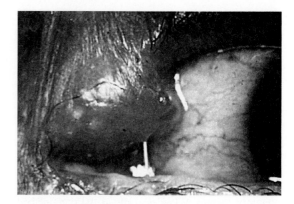

Figure 4–15. *Actinomyces israelii* canaliculitis, left eye. (Courtesy of P Thygeson.)

Total canalicular obstruction necessitates use of an artificial tear duct for relief of epiphora (conjunctivodacryocystorhinostomy). A Pyrex glass tube is placed between the conjunctival sac and the nasal cavity.

Closure of the punctum is sometimes performed in patients with keratitis sicca to allow tears to remain in the conjunctival sac. Temporary closure may be done with silicone or collagen plugs in the canaliculi or by sealing the punctum with a hot cautery. The temporary obstruction will provide an opportunity to evaluate the effect. Permanent closure may be accomplished by deep cautery within the ampulla with thermal, electrocautery, or laser energy or by dividing the canaliculus surgically.

III. TEARS

John P. Whitcher, MD, MPH

Tears form a thin layer approximately 7–10 μm thick that covers the corneal and conjunctival epithelium. The functions of this ultrathin layer are (1) to make the cornea a smooth optical surface by abolishing minute surface epithelial irregularities; (2) to wet and protect the delicate surface of the corneal and conjunctival epithelium; (3) to inhibit the growth of microorganisms by mechanical flushing and antimicrobial action; and (4) to provide the cornea with necessary nutrient substances.

LAYERS OF THE TEAR FILM

The tear film is composed of three layers (Figure 4–16): (1) The superficial layer is a monomolecular

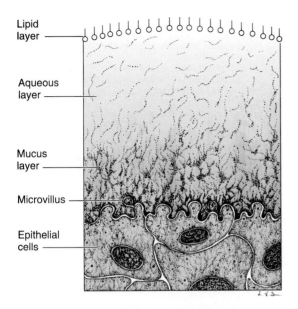

Figure 4–16. The three layers of the tear film covering the superficial epithelial layer of the cornea.

film of lipid derived from meibomian glands. It is thought to retard evaporation and form a watertight seal when the lids are closed. (2) The middle aqueous layer is elaborated by the major and minor lacrimal glands and contains water-soluble substances (salts and proteins). (3) The deep mucinous layer is composed of glycoprotein and overlies the corneal and conjunctival epithelial cells. The epithelial cell membranes are composed of lipoproteins and are therefore relatively hydrophobic. Such a surface cannot be wetted with an aqueous solution alone. Mucin is partly adsorbed onto the corneal epithelial cell membranes and is anchored by the microvilli of the surface epithelial cells. This provides a new hydrophilic surface for the aqueous tears to spread over which is wetted by a lowering of surface tension.

COMPOSITION OF TEARS

The normal tear volume is estimated to be $7 \pm 2 \mu L$ in each eye. Albumin accounts for 60% of the total protein in tear fluid. Globulin and lysozymes are divided equally in the remainder. Immunoglobulins IgA, IgG, and IgE are present. IgA predominates, and differs from serum IgA in that it is not transudated from serum only but is produced by plasma cells located in the lacrimal gland. In certain allergic conditions such as vernal conjunctivitis, the IgE concentration of tear fluid increases. Tear lysozymes form 21–25% of the total protein and—acting synergistically with gamma globulins and other nonlysozyme antibacterial factors—represent an important defense mechanism against infection. Other tear enzymes may

also play a role in diagnosis of certain clinical entities, eg, hexoseaminidase assay for diagnosis of Tay-Sachs disease.

K^+, Na^+, and Cl^- occur in higher concentrations in tears than in plasma. Tears also contain a small amount of glucose (5 mg/dL) and urea (0.04 mg/dL), and changes in blood concentration parallel changes in tear glucose and urea levels. The average pH of tears is 7.35, though a wide normal variation exists (5.20–8.35). Under normal conditions, tear fluid is isotonic. Tear film osmolality ranges from 295 to 309 mosm/L.

DRY EYE SYNDROME (KERATOCONJUNCTIVITIS SICCA)

Dryness of the eye may result from any disease associated with deficiency of the tear film components (aqueous, mucin, or lipid), lid surface abnormalities, or epithelial abnormalities. Although there are many forms of keratoconjunctivitis sicca, those connected with rheumatoid arthritis and other autoimmune diseases are commonly referred to as Sjögren's syndrome.

Etiology

Many of the causes of dry eye syndrome affect more than one component of the tear film or lead to ocular surface alterations that secondarily cause tear film instability. Histopathologic features include the appearance of dry spots on the corneal and conjunctival epithelium, formation of filaments, loss of conjunctival goblet cells, abnormal enlargement of nongoblet epithelial cells, increased cellular stratification, and increased keratinization. The etiology and diagnosis of keratoconjunctivitis sicca are summarized in Table 4–2.

Clinical Findings

Patients with dry eyes complain most frequently of a scratchy or sandy (foreign body) sensation. Other common symptoms are itching, excessive mucus secretion, inability to produce tears, a burning sensation, photosensitivity, redness, pain, and difficulty in moving the lids. In most patients, the most remarkable feature of the eye examination is the grossly normal appearance of the eye. The most characteristic feature on slitlamp examination is the interrupted or absent tear meniscus at the lower lid margin. Tenacious yellowish mucus strands are sometimes seen in the lower conjunctival fornix. The bulbar conjunctiva loses its normal luster and may be thickened, edematous, and hyperemic.

The corneal epithelium shows varying degrees of fine punctate stippling in the interpalpebral fissure. The damaged corneal and conjunctival epithelial cells stain with 1% rose bengal (Figure 4–17), and defects in the corneal epithelium stain with fluorescein. In the

Table 4–2. Etiology and diagnosis of dry eye syndrome.

I. Etiology
  A. Conditions Characterized by Hypofunction of the
     Lacrimal Gland:
     1. Congenital–
        a. Familial dysautonomia (Riley-Day syndrome)
        b. Aplasia of the lacrimal gland (congenital alac-
           rima)
        c. Trigeminal nerve aplasia
        d. Ectodermal dysplasia
     2. Acquired–
        a. Systemic diseases–
           (1) Sjögren's syndrome
           (2) Progressive systemic sclerosis
           (3) Sarcoidosis
           (4) Leukemia, lymphoma
           (5) Amyloidosis
           (6) Hemochromatosis
        b. Infection–
           (1) Mumps
        c. Injury–
           (1) Surgical removal of lacrimal gland
           (2) Irradiation
           (3) Chemical burn
        d. Medications–
           (1) Antihistamines
           (2) Antimuscarinics: atropine, scopolamine
           (3) General anesthetics: halothane, nitrous
               oxide
           (4) Beta-adrenergic blockers: timolol, practolol
        e. Neurogenic Neuroparalytic (facial nerve
           palsy)
  B. Conditions Characterized by Mucin Deficiency:
     1. Avitaminosis A
     2. Stevens-Johnson syndrome
     3. Ocular pemphigoid
     4. Chronic conjunctivitis, eg, trachoma
     5. Chemical burns
     6. Medications–Antihistamines, antimuscarinic

        agents, beta-adrenergic blocking agents
        (eg, practolol)
     7. Folk remedies, eg, kermes
  C. Conditions Characterized by Lipid Deficiency:
     1. Lid margin scarring
     2. Blepharitis
  D. Defective Spreading of Tear Film Caused by the
     Following:
     1. Eyelid abnormalities–
        a. Defects, coloboma
        b. Ectropion or entropion
        c. Keratinization of lid margin
        d. Decreased or absent blinking
           (1) Neurologic disorders
           (2) Hyperthyroidism
           (3) Contact lens
           (4) Drugs
           (5) Herpes simplex keratitis
           (6) Leprosy
        e. Lagophthalmos–
           (1) Nocturnal lagophthalmos
           (2) Hyperthyroidism
           (3) Leprosy
     2. Conjunctival abnormalities–
        a. Pterygium
        b. Symblepharon
     3. Proptosis
II. Diagnostic Tests:
  A. Schirmer test without anesthesia
  B. Tear break-up time
  C. Ocular ferning test
  D. Impression cytology
  E. Fluorescein staining
  F. Rose bengal staining
  G. Tear lysozyme
  H. Tear film osmolality
  I. Tear lactoferrin

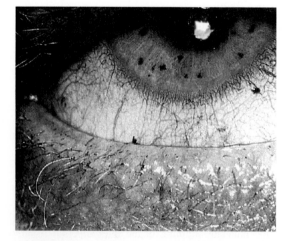

Figure 4–17. Rose bengal staining of corneal and conjunctival cells in a 54-year-old woman with keratoconjunctivitis sicca.

late stages of keratoconjunctivitis sicca, filaments
may be seen—one end of each filament attached to
the corneal epithelium and the other end moving
freely (Figure 4–18).

In patients with Sjögren's syndrome, conjunctival
scrapings may show increased numbers of goblet
cells. Lacrimal gland enlargement occurs uncommonly in patients with Sjögren's syndrome. Diagnosis and grading of the dry eye condition can be
achieved with good accuracy using the following diagnostic methods:

A. Schirmer Test: This test is done by drying the
tear film and inserting Schirmer strips (Whatman filter paper No. 41) into the lower conjunctival cul-de-
sac at the junction of the mid and temporal thirds of
the lower lid. The moistened exposed portion is measured 5 minutes after insertion. Less than 10 mm of
wetting without anesthesia is considered abnormal.

When performed without anesthesia, the test measures the function of the main lacrimal gland, whose
secretory activity is stimulated by the irritating nature
of the filter paper. Schirmer tests performed after topical anesthesia (0.5% tetracaine) measure the function
of the accessory lacrimal glands (the basic secretors).
Less than 5 mm in 5 minutes is abnormal.

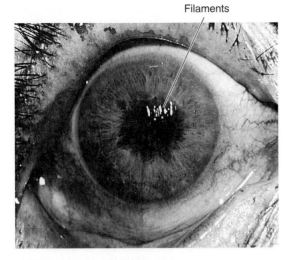

Filaments

Figure 4–18. Corneal filaments in a 56-year-old patient with keratoconjunctivitis sicca.

The Schirmer test is a screening test for assessment of tear production. False-positive and false-negative results occur. Low readings are sporadically found in normals, and normal tests may occur in dry eyes—especially those secondary to mucin deficiency.

B. Tear Film Break-Up Time: Measurement of the tear film break-up time may sometimes be useful to estimate the mucin content of tear fluid. Deficiency in mucin may not affect the Schirmer test but may lead to instability of the tear film. This causes the film's rapid break-up. "Dry spots" (Figure 4–19) are formed in the tear film, and exposure of the corneal or conjunctival epithelium follows. This process ultimately damages the epithelial cells, which can then be stained with rose bengal. Damaged epithelial cells may be shed from the cornea, leaving areas susceptible to punctate staining when the corneal surface is flooded with fluorescein.

The tear film break-up time can be measured by applying a slightly moistened fluorescein strip to the bulbar conjunctiva and asking the patient to blink. The tear film is then scanned with the aid of the cobalt filter on the slitlamp while the patient refrains from blinking. The time that elapses before the first dry spot appears in the corneal fluorescein layer is the tear film break-up time. Normally, the break-up time is over 15 seconds, but it will be reduced appreciably by the use of local anesthetics, by manipulating the eye, or by holding the lids open. The break-up time is shorter in eyes with aqueous tear deficiency and is always shorter than normal in eyes with mucin deficiency.

C. Ocular Ferning Test: A simple and inexpensive qualitative test for the study of conjunctival mucus is performed by drying conjunctival scrapings on a clean glass slide. Microscopic arborization (ferning) is observed in normal eyes. In patients with cicatrizing conjunctivitis (ocular pemphigoid, Stevens-John-son syndrome, diffuse conjunctival cicatrization), ferning of the mucus is reduced or absent.

D. Impression Cytology: Impression cytology is a method by which goblet cell densities on the conjunctival surface can be counted. In normal persons, the goblet cell population is highest in the infranasal quadrant. Loss of goblet cells has been documented in cases of keratoconjunctivitis sicca, trachoma, cicatricial ocular pemphigoid, Stevens-Johnson syndrome, and avitaminosis A.

E. Fluorescein Staining: Touching the conjunctiva with a dry strip of fluorescein is a good indicator of wetness, and the tear meniscus can be seen easily. Fluorescein will stain the eroded and denuded areas as well as microscopic defects of the corneal epithelium.

F. Rose Bengal Staining: Rose bengal is more sensitive than fluorescein. The dye will stain all desiccated nonvital epithelial cells of the cornea as well as conjunctiva.

G. Tear Lysozyme Assay: Reduction in tear lysozyme concentration usually occurs early in the course of Sjögren's syndrome and is helpful in the diagnosis of that disorder. Tears can be collected on Schirmer strips and assayed. The most common method is spectrophotometric assay.

H. Tear Osmolality: Hyperosmolality of tears has been documented in keratoconjunctivitis sicca and in contact lens wearers and is thought to be a consequence of decreased corneal sensitivity. Reports claim that hyperosmolality is the most specific test for keratoconjunctivitis sicca. It can occur even with a normal Schirmer test and normal rose bengal staining.

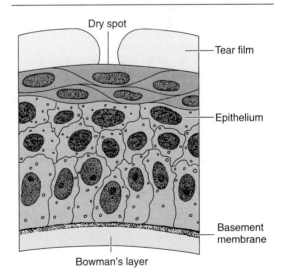

Dry spot

Tear film

Epithelium

Basement membrane

Bowman's layer

Figure 4–19. Baring of the corneal epithelium following formation of a dry spot in the tear film. (Modified and redrawn from Dohlman CH: The function of the corneal epithelium in health and disease. Invest Ophthalmol 1971;10:383.)

I. Lactoferrin: Tear fluid lactoferrin is low in patients with hyposecretion of the lacrimal gland. Testing kits are commercially available.

Complications

Early in the course of keratoconjunctivitis sicca, vision is slightly impaired. As the condition worsens, discomfort can become disabling. In advanced cases, corneal ulceration, corneal thinning, and perforation may develop. Secondary bacterial infection occasionally occurs, and corneal scarring and vascularization may result in marked reduction in vision. Early treatment may prevent these complications.

Treatment

The patient should understand that dry eyes is a chronic condition and complete relief is unlikely except in mild cases when the corneal and conjunctival epithelial changes are reversible. Artificial tears are the mainstay of treatment. Ointment is useful for prolonged lubrication, especially when sleeping. Additional relief can be achieved by using humidifiers, moisture chamber spectacles, or swim goggles.

The primary function of these measures is fluid replacement. Restoration of mucin is a more formidable task. In recent years, high-molecular-weight water-soluble polymers have been added to artificial tears in an attempt to improve and prolong surface wetting.

Other mucomimetic agents include sodium hyaluronate and solutions of the patient's own serum as eye drops. If the mucus is tenacious, as in Sjögren's syndrome, mucolytic agents (eg, acetylcysteine 10%) are helpful.

Patients with excessive tear lipids require specific instructions for removal of lipid from the eyelid margin. Antibiotics topically or systemically may be necessary. Topical vitamin A may be useful in reversing ocular surface metaplasia.

All chemical preservatives in artificial tears induce a certain amount of corneal toxicity. Benzalkonium chloride is the most damaging of the commonly used preparations. Patients who require frequent drops fare better with nonpreserved solutions. Preservatives can also cause idiosyncratic reactions. This is most common with thimerosal.

Patients with dry eyes from any cause are more likely to have concurrent infections. Chronic blepharitis is common and should be treated with hygiene and topical antibiotics. Acne rosacea is associated with keratoconjunctivitis sicca, and treatment with systemic tetracycline may be helpful.

Surgical treatment for dry eyes includes insertion of temporary (collagen) or extended (silicone) punctal plugs to retain lacrimal secretions. Permanent closure of the puncta and canaliculi can be done by thermal, electrocautery, or laser treatment.

REFERENCES

American Academy of Ophthalmology: Botulinum toxin therapy of eye muscle disorders: safety and effectiveness. Ophthalmology 1989;6(Suppl):37.

Beard C: A new classification of blepharoptosis. Int Ophthalmol Clin 1989;29:214.

Becker BB, Berry FD, Koller H: Balloon catheter dilation for treatment of congenital nasolacrimal duct obstruction. Am J Ophthalmol 1996;121:304.

Bron AJ: The Doyne Lecture. Reflections on the tears. Eye 1997;11:583.

Bullock JD, Goldberg SH: Lacrimal sac diverticula. Arch Ophthalmol 1989;107:753.

Callahan MA: Surgically mismanaged ptosis associated with double elevator palsy. Arch Ophthalmol 1981;99:108.

Char DH: *Clinical Ocular Oncology,* 2nd ed. Lippincott-Raven, 1997.

Collin JR: Blepharochalasis: A review of 30 cases. Ophthalmic Plast Reconstr Surg 1991;7:153.

Collin JRO: *A Manual of Systematic Eyelid Surgery,* 2nd ed. Churchill Livingstone, 1989.

Collin JRO, O'Donnell BA: Adjustable sutures in eyelid surgery for ptosis and lid retraction. Br J Ophthalmol 1994;78:167.

Daniels TE, Whitcher JP: Association of labial salivary gland inflammation with keratoconjunctivitis sicca: Analysis of 618 patients with suspected Sjögren's syndrome. Arthritis Rheum 1994;37:869.

Dutton J: Management of periocular basal cell carcinoma: Mohs' micrographic surgery versus radiotherapy. Surv Ophthalmol 1993;38:193.

Fitzpatrick RE: Laser resurfacing of rhytides. Dermatol Clin 1997;15:431.

Fox RI et al: Criteria for diagnosis of Sjögren's syndrome. Rheum Dis Clin North Am 1994;20:391.

Haik BG et al: Capillary hemangioma (infantile periocular hemangioma). Surv Ophthalmol 1994;38:399.

Ilgit ET et al: Transluminal balloon dilatation of the lacrimal drainage system for the treatment of epiphora. AJR Am J Roentgenol 1995;165:1517.

Johnson CC: Developmental abnormalities of the eyelids. Ophthalmic Plast Reconstr Surg 1986;2:2.

Jordan DR et al: Essential blepharospasm and related dystonias. Surv Ophthalmol 1989;34:123.

Kass LG, Hornblass A: Sebaceous carcinoma of the ocular adnexa. Surv Ophthalmol 1989;33:477.

Kersten RC et al: Accuracy of clinical diagnosis of cutaneous eyelid lesions. Ophthalmology 1997;104:479.

Kruize AA et al: Long-term followup of patients with Sjögren's syndrome. Arthritis Rheum 1996;39:297.

Lowery JC, Bartley GB: Complications of blepharoplasty. Surv Ophthalmol 1994;38:327.

Lyons CJ, Rosser PM, Welham RN: The management of punctal agenesis. Ophthalmology 1993;100:1851.

Mansour AM, Hidayat AA: Metastatic eyelid disease. Ophthalmol 1987;94:667.

Noda S, Hayasaka S, Setogawa T: Epiblepharon with inverted eyelashes in Japanese children. Br J Ophthalmol 1989;73:126.

Ratliff CD, Meyer DR: Silicone intubation without intranasal fixation for treatment of congenital nasolacrimal obstruction. Am J Ophthalmol 1994;118:781.

Rodriguez JM, Deutsch GP: The treatment of periocular basal cell carcinomas by radiotherapy. Br J Ophthalmol 1992;76:195.

Schlienger P et al: External radiotherapy for carcinomas of the eyelid: Report of 850 cases treated. Int J Radiat Oncol Biol Phys 1996;34:277.

Shields CL et al: Clinicopathologic review of 142 cases of lacrimal gland lesions. Ophthalmology 1989;96:431.

Shimazaki J, Sakata M, Tsubota K: Ocular surface changes and discomfort in patients with meibomian gland dysfunction. Arch Ophthalmol 1995;113:1266.

Smith RE, Flowers CW: Chronic blepharitis: A review. CLAO J 1995;21:200.

Spencer WH (editor): *Ophthalmic Pathology,* 4th ed. 4 vols. Saunders, 1996.

Steel DHW et al: Botulinum toxin for the temporary treatment of involutional lower lid entropion: A clinical and morphological study. Eye 1997;11:472.

Stewart WB (editor): *Surgery of the Eyelid, Orbit and Lacrimal System.* American Academy of Ophthalmology, Manuals Program, 1993.

Tarbet KJ, Custer PL: External dacryocystorhinostomy: Surgical success, patient satisfaction and economic cost. Ophthalmology 1995;102:1065.

Tucker SM, Linberg JV: Vascular anatomy of the eyelids. Ophthalmology 1994;101:1118.

Tuppurainen K: Cryotherapy for eyelid and periocular basal cell carcinomas: Outcome in 166 cases over an 8-year period. Graefes Arch Clin Exp Ophthalmol 1995;233:205.

Vecsei VP et al: Canaliculitis: Difficulties in diagnosis, differential diagnosis and comparison between conservative and surgical treatment. Ophthalmologica 1994;208:314.

Whitcher JP: Clinical diagnosis of the dry eye. Int Ophthalmol Clin 1987;27:7.

Woog JJ, Metson R, Puliafito CA: Holmium:YAG endonasal laser dacryocystorhinostomy. Am J Ophthalmol 1993;116:1.

Wright M, Dhillon B: Diagnosis and treatment of dry eyes. Practitioner 1997;241:210.

Young JDH, MacEwen CJ: Managing congenital lacrimal obstruction in general practice. BMJ 1997;315:293.

5

Conjunctiva

Ivan R. Schwab, MD, & J. Brooks Crawford, MD

I. CONJUNCTIVITIS

Inflammation of the conjunctiva (conjunctivitis) is the most common eye disease worldwide. It varies in severity from a mild hyperemia with tearing to a severe conjunctivitis with copious purulent discharge. The cause is usually exogenous, but rarely it may be endogenous.

CONJUNCTIVITIS DUE TO INFECTIOUS AGENTS

The types of conjunctivitis and their commonest causes are set forth in Tables 5–1 and 5–2.

Because of its location, the conjunctiva is exposed to many microorganisms and other stressful environmental factors. Several mechanisms protect the surface of the eye from external substances: In the tear film, the aqueous component dilutes infectious material, mucus traps debris, and a pumping action of the lids constantly flushes the tears to the tear duct; the tears contain antimicrobial substances, including lysozyme and antibodies (IgG and IgA).

Common pathogens that can cause conjunctivitis include *Streptococcus pneumoniae, Haemophilus influenzae, Staphylococcus aureus, Neisseria meningitidis,* most human adenovirus strains, herpes simplex virus type 1 and type 2, and two picornaviruses. Two sexually transmitted agents that cause conjunctivitis are *Chlamydia trachomatis* and *Neisseria gonorrhoeae.*

Cytology of Conjunctivitis

Damage to the conjunctival epithelium by a noxious agent may be followed by epithelial edema, cellular death and exfoliation, epithelial hypertrophy, or granuloma formation. There may also be edema of the conjunctival stroma (chemosis) and hypertrophy of the lymphoid layer of the stroma (follicle formation).

Inflammatory cells, including neutrophils, eosinophils, basophils, lymphocytes, and plasma cells, may be seen and often indicate the nature of the damaging agent. The inflammatory cells migrate from the conjunctival stroma through the epithelium to the surface. They then combine with fibrin and mucus from the goblet cells to form the conjunctival exudate, which is responsible for the "mattering" on the lid margins (especially in the morning).

The inflammatory cells appear in the exudate or in scrapings taken with a sterile platinum spatula from the anesthetized conjunctival surface. The material is stained with Gram's stain (to identify the bacterial organisms) and with Giemsa's stain (to identify the cell types and morphology). A predominance of polymorphonuclear leukocytes is characteristic of bacterial conjunctivitis. Generally, a predominance of mononuclear cells—especially lymphocytes—is characteristic of viral conjunctivitis. If a pseudomembrane or true membrane is present (eg, epidemic keratoconjunctivitis or herpes simplex virus conjunctivitis), neutrophils then predominate because of coexistent necrosis. In chlamydial conjunctivitis, neutrophils and lymphocytes are usually present in equal numbers.

In allergic conjunctivitis, eosinophils and basophils are frequently present in conjunctival biopsies, but they are less common on conjunctival smears; eosinophils or eosinophilic granules are commonly found in vernal keratoconjunctivitis. High levels of proteins secreted by eosinophils (eg, eosinophil cationic protein) can be found in the tears of patients with vernal, atopic, or allergic conjunctivitis. Eosinophils and basophils are found in allergic conjunctivitis, and scattered eosinophilic granules and eosinophils are found in vernal keratoconjunctivitis. In all types of conjunctivitis, there are plasma cells in the conjunctival stroma. They do not migrate through the epithelium, however, and are therefore not seen in smears of exudate or of scrapings from the conjunctival surface unless the epithelium has become necrotic, as it may in trachoma; in this event, the rupturing of a follicle allows the plasma cells to reach the epithelial surface. Since the mature follicles of trachoma rupture easily, the finding of large, pale-staining lymphoblastic (germinal center) cells in scrapings strongly suggests trachoma.

Table 5–1. Causes of conjunctivitis.

Bacterial
  Hyperacute (purulent)
    Neisseria gonorrhoeae
    Neisseria meningitidis
    Neisseria gonorrhoeae subsp *kochii*
  Acute (mucopurulent)
    Pneumococcus *(Streptococcus pneumoniae)* (temperate climates)
    Haemophilus aegyptius (Koch-Weeks bacillus) (tropical climates)
  Subacute
    Haemophilus influenzae (temperate climates)
  Chronic, including blepharoconjunctivitis
    Staphylococcus aureus
    Moraxella lacunata (diplobacillus of Morax-Axenfeld)
  Rare types (acute, subacute, chronic)
    Streptococci
    Moraxella catarrhalis
    Coliforms
    Proteus
    Corynebacterium diphtheriae
    Mycobacterium tuberculosis
Chlamydial
  Trachoma *(Chlamydia trachomatis* serotypes A–C)
  Inclusion conjunctivitis *(Chlamydia trachomatis* serotypes D–K)
  Lymphogranuloma venereum (LGV) (*Chlamydia trachomatis* serotypes L1–3)
Viral
  Acute viral follicular conjunctivitis
    Pharyngoconjunctival fever due to adenoviruses types 3 and 7 and other serotypes
    Epidemic keratoconjunctivitis due to adenovirus types 8 and 19
    Herpes simplex virus
    Acute hemorrhagic conjunctivitis due to enterovirus type 70; rarely, coxsackievirus type A24
  Chronic viral follicular conjunctivitis
    Molluscum contagiosum virus
  Viral blepharoconjunctivitis
    Varicella, herpes zoster due to varicella-zoster virus
    Measles virus
Rickettsial (rare)
  Nonpurulent conjunctivitis with hyperemia and minimal infiltration, often a feature of rickettsial diseases
    Typhus
    Murine typhus
    Scrub typhus
    Rocky Mountain spotted fever
    Mediterranean fever
    Q fever
Fungal (rare)
  Chronic exudative
    Candida
  Granulomatous
    Rhinosporidium seeberi
    Coccidioides immitis (San Joaquin Valley fever)
    Sporothrix schenckii
Parasitic (rare but important)
  Chronic conjunctivitis and blepharoconjunctivitis
    Onchocerca volvulus (Central America, Africa)
    Thelazia californiensis
    Loa loa
    Ascaris lumbricoides
    Trichinella spiralis
    Schistosoma haematobium (bladder fluke)
    Taenia solium (cysticercus)
    Pthirus pubis (*Pediculus pubis,* pubic louse)
    Fly larvae (*Oestrus ovis,* etc) (ocular myiasis)
Immunologic (allergic)
  Immediate (humoral) hypersensitivity reactions
    Hay fever conjunctivitis (pollens, grasses, animal danders, etc)
    Vernal keratoconjunctivitis
    Atopic keratoconjunctivitis
    Giant papillary conjunctivitis
  Delayed (cellular) hypersensitivity reactions
    Phlyctenulosis
    Mild conjunctivitis secondary to contact blepharitis

(*continued*)

Table 5–1. Causes of conjunctivitis. (continued)

Immunologic (allergic) (*continued*)
  Autoimmune disease
    Keratoconjunctivitis sicca associated with Sjögen's syndrome
    Cicatricial pemphigoid
Chemical or irritative
  Iatrogenic
    Miotics
    Idoxuridine
    Other topically applied drugs
    Contact lens solutions
  Occupational
    Acids
    Alkalies
    Smoke
    Wind
    Ultraviolet light
  Caterpillar hair
Etiology unknown
  Folliculosis
  Chronic follicular conjunctivitis (orphan's conjunctivitis, Axenfeld's conjunctivitis)
  Ocular rosacea
  Psoriasis
  Erythema multiforme major (Stevens-Johnson syndrome) and minor
  Dermatitis herpetiformis
  Epidermolysis bullosa
  Superior limbic keratoconjunctivitis
  Ligneous conjunctivitis
  Reiter's syndrome
  Mucocutaneous lymph node syndrome (Kawasaki disease)
Associated with systemic disease
  Thyroid disease (exposure, congestive)
  Gouty conjunctivitis
  Carcinoid conjunctivitis
  Sarcoidosis
  Tuberculosis
  Syphilis
Secondary to dacryocystitis or canaliculitis
  Conjunctivitis secondary to dacryocystitis
    Pneumococci or beta-hemolytic streptococci
  Conjunctivitis secondary to canaliculitis
    Actinomyces israelii, Candida spp, *Aspergillus* spp (rarely)

Symptoms of Conjunctivitis

The important symptoms of conjunctivitis are a foreign body sensation, a scratching or burning sensation, a sensation of fullness around the eyes, itching, and photophobia.

Foreign body sensation and a scratching or burning sensation are often associated with the swelling and papillary hypertrophy that normally accompany conjunctival hyperemia. If there is pain, the cornea is probably also affected. Pain of the iris or ciliary body is also suggestive of corneal involvement.

Signs of Conjunctivitis
(Table 5–2)

The important signs of conjunctivitis are hyperemia, tearing, exudation, pseudoptosis, papillary hypertrophy, chemosis, follicles, pseudomembranes and membranes, granulomas, and preauricular adenopathy.

Hyperemia is the most conspicuous clinical sign of acute conjunctivitis. The redness is most marked in the fornix and diminishes toward the limbus by virtue of the dilation of the posterior conjunctival vessels. (A perilimbal dilation or ciliary flush suggests inflammation of the cornea or deeper structures.) A brilliant red suggests bacterial conjunctivitis, and a milky appearance suggests allergic conjunctivitis. Hyperemia without cellular infiltration suggests irritation from physical causes such as wind, sun, smoke, etc, but may occur occasionally with diseases associated with vascular instability (eg, acne rosacea).

Tearing (epiphora) is often prominent in conjunctivitis, the tears resulting from the foreign body sensation, the burning or scratching sensation, or the itching. Mild transudation also arises from the hyperemic vessels and adds to the tearing. An abnormally scant secretion of tears and an increase in mucous threads suggests keratoconjunctivitis sicca.

Exudation is a feature of all types of acute conjunctivitis. The exudate is flaky and amorphous in bacterial conjunctivitis and stringy in allergic conjunctivitis. "Mattering" of the eyelids occurs upon awakening in almost all types of conjunctivitis, and if the exudate is copious and the lids are firmly stuck together, the conjunctivitis is probably bacterial or chlamydial.

Table 5–2. Differentiation of the common types of conjunctivitis.

Clinical Findings and Cytology	Viral	Bacterial	Chlamydial	Allergic
Itching	Minimal	Minimal	Minimal	Severe
Hyperemia	Generalized	Generalized	Generalized	Generalized
Tearing	Profuse	Moderate	Moderate	Moderate
Exudation	Minimal	Profuse	Profuse	Minimal
Preauricular adenopathy	Common	Uncommon	Common only in inclusion conjunctivitis	None
In stained scrapings and exudates	Monocytes	Bacteria, PMNs[1]	PMNs, plasma cells inclusion bodies	Eosinophils
Associated sore throat and fever	Occasionally	Occasionally	Never	Never

[1] Polymorphonuclear cells.

Pseudoptosis is a drooping of the upper lid secondary to infiltration of Müller's muscle. The condition is seen in several types of severe conjunctivitis, eg, trachoma and epidemic keratoconjunctivitis.

Papillary hypertrophy is a nonspecific conjunctival reaction that occurs because the conjunctiva is bound down to the underlying tarsus or limbus by fine fibrils. When the tuft of vessels that forms the substance of the papilla (along with cellular elements and exudates) reaches the basement membrane of the epithelium, it branches over the papilla like the spokes in the frame of an umbrella. An inflammatory exudate accumulates between the fibrils, heaping the conjunctiva into mounds. In necrotizing disease (eg, trachoma), the exudate may be replaced by granulation tissue or connective tissue.

When the papillae are small, the conjunctiva usually has a smooth, velvety appearance. A red papillary conjunctiva suggests bacterial or chlamydial disease (eg, a velvety red tarsal conjunctiva is characteristic of acute trachoma). With marked infiltration of the conjunctiva, giant papillae form which are flat-topped, polygonal, and milky-red in color. On the upper tarsus, they suggest vernal keratoconjunctivitis and giant papillary conjunctivitis with contact lens sensitivities; on the lower tarsus, they suggest atopic keratoconjunctivitis. Giant papillae may also occur at the limbus, especially in the area that is normally exposed when the eyes are open (between 2 and 4 o'clock and between 8 and 10 o'clock). Here they appear as gelatinous mounds that may encroach on the cornea. Limbal papillae are characteristic of vernal keratoconjunctivitis but are rare in atopic keratoconjunctivitis.

Chemosis of the conjunctiva strongly suggests acute allergic conjunctivitis but may also occur in acute gonococcal or meningococcal conjunctivitis and especially in adenoviral conjunctivitis. Chemosis of the bulbar conjunctiva is seen in patients with trichinosis. Occasionally, chemosis may appear before there is any gross cellular infiltration or exudation.

Follicles are seen in most cases of viral conjunctivitis, in all cases of chlamydial conjunctivitis except neonatal inclusion conjunctivitis, in some cases of parasitic conjunctivitis, and in some cases of toxic conjunctivitis induced by topical medications such as idoxuridine, dipivefrin, and miotics. Follicles in the inferior fornix and at the tarsal margins have limited diagnostic value, but when they are located on the tarsi (especially the upper tarsus), chlamydial, viral, or toxic conjunctivitis (following topical medication) should be suspected.

The follicle consists of a focal lymphoid hyperplasia within the lymphoid layer of the conjunctiva and usually contains a germinal center. Clinically, it can be recognized as a rounded, avascular white or gray structure. On slitlamp examination, small vessels can be seen arising at the border of the follicle and encircling it.

Pseudomembranes and **membranes** are the result of an exudative process and differ only in degree. A pseudomembrane is a coagulum on the *surface* of the epithelium, and when it is removed the epithelium remains intact. A membrane is a coagulum involving the *entire* epithelium, and if it is removed a raw, bleeding surface remains. Pseudomembranes or membranes may accompany epidemic keratoconjunctivitis, primary herpes simplex virus conjunctivitis, streptococcal conjunctivitis, diphtheria, cicatricial pemphigoid, and erythema multiforme major. They may also be an aftermath of chemical burns, especially alkali burns.

Ligneous conjunctivitis is a peculiar form of recurring membranous conjunctivitis. It is bilateral, seen mainly in children, predominantly in females, and may be associated with other systemic findings, including nasopharyngitis and vulvovaginitis.

Granulomas of the conjunctiva always affect the stroma and most commonly are chalazia. Other endogenous causes include sarcoid, syphilis, cat-scratch disease, and, rarely, coccidioidomycosis. Parinaud's oculoglandular syndrome includes conjunctival granulomas and a prominent preauricular lymph node, and this group of diseases may require biopsy examination to secure diagnosis.

Phlyctenules represent a delayed hypersensitivity reaction to microbial antigen, eg, staphylococcal or mycobacterial antigens. Phlyctenules of the conjunctiva initially consist of a perivasculitis with lymphocytic cuffing of a vessel. When they progress to ulceration of the conjunctiva, the ulcer bed has many polymorphonuclear leukocytes.

Preauricular lymphadenopathy is an important sign of conjunctivitis. A grossly visible preauricular node is seen in Parinaud's oculoglandular syndrome and, rarely, in epidemic keratoconjunctivitis. A large or small preauricular node, sometimes slightly tender, occurs in primary herpes simplex conjunctivitis, epidemic keratoconjunctivitis, inclusion conjunctivitis, and trachoma. Small but nontender preauricular lymph nodes occur in pharyngoconjunctival fever and acute hemorrhagic conjunctivitis. Occasionally, preauricular lymphadenopathy may be observed in children with infections of the meibomian glands.

BACTERIAL CONJUNCTIVITIS

Two forms of bacterial conjunctivitis are recognized: acute (and subacute) and chronic. Acute bacterial conjunctivitis may be self-limited when caused by certain microorganisms such as *Haemophilus influenzae.* The course may take up to 2 weeks if proper treatment is not given.

Acute bacterial conjunctivitis may become chronic. Treatment with one of the many available antibacterial agents usually cures the condition in a few days.

Purulent conjunctivitis caused by *Neisseria gonorrhoeae* or *Neisseria meningitidis* may lead to serious ocular complications if not treated early.

Clinical Findings

A. Symptoms and Signs: The organisms listed in Table 5–1 account for most cases of bacterial conjunctivitis. They produce bilateral irritation and injection, a purulent exudate with sticky lids on waking, and occasionally lid edema. The infection usually starts in one eye and is spread to the other by the hands. It may be spread from one person to another by fomites.

1. Hyperacute (and subacute) bacterial conjunctivitis–Purulent conjunctivitis (caused by *N gonorrhoeae, Neisseria kochii,* and *N meningitidis*) is marked by a profuse purulent exudate (Figure 5–1). Meningococcal conjunctivitis may occasionally be seen in children. Any severe, profusely exudative conjunctivitis demands immediate laboratory investigation and immediate treatment. If there is any delay, there may be severe corneal damage or loss of the eye, or the conjunctiva could become the portal of entry for either *N gonorrhoeae* or *N meningitidis,* leading to septicemia or meningitis.

Acute mucopurulent (catarrhal) conjunctivitis

often occurs in epidemic form and is called "pinkeye" by most laymen. It is characterized by an acute onset of conjunctival hyperemia and a moderate amount of mucopurulent discharge. The commonest causes are *Streptococcus pneumoniae* in temperate climates and *Haemophilus aegyptius* in warm climates. Less common causes are staphylococci and other streptococci. The conjunctivitis caused by *S pneumoniae* and *H aegyptius* may be accompanied by subconjunctival hemorrhages. *H aegyptius* conjunctivitis in Brazil has been followed by a fatal purpuric fever produced by a plasmid-associated toxin of the bacteria.

Subacute conjunctivitis is caused most often by *H influenzae* and occasionally by *Escherichia coli* and *Proteus* species. *H influenzae* infection is characterized by a thin, watery, or flocculent exudate.

2. Chronic bacterial conjunctivitis–Chronic bacterial conjunctivitis occurs in patients with nasolacrimal duct obstruction and chronic dacryocystitis, which are usually unilateral. It may also be associated with chronic bacterial blepharitis or meibomian gland dysfunction. Patients with floppy lid syndrome or ectropion may develop secondary bacterial conjunctivitis.

Rare bacterial conjunctivitides may be caused by *Corynebacterium diphtheriae* and *Streptococcus pyogenes.* Pseudomembranes or membranes caused by these organisms may form on the palpebral conjunctiva. The rare cases of chronic conjunctivitis produced by *Moraxella catarrhalis,* the coliform bacilli, *Proteus,* etc, are as a rule indistinguishable clinically.

B. Laboratory Findings: In most cases of bacterial conjunctivitis, the organisms can be identified by the microscopic examination of conjunctival scrapings stained with Gram's stain or Giemsa's stain; this reveals numerous polymorphonuclear neutrophils. Conjunctival scrapings for microscopic examination and culture are recommended for all cases and are mandatory if the disease is purulent, membranous, or pseudomembranous. Antibiotic sensitivity studies are also desirable, but empirical antibiotic therapy should be started. When the results of antibiotic sensitivity

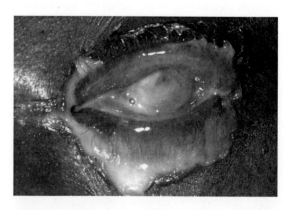

Figure 5–1. Gonococcal conjunctivitis. Profuse purulent exudate. (Courtesy of L Schwab.)

tests become available, specific antibiotic therapy can then be instituted.

Complications & Sequelae

Chronic marginal blepharitis often accompanies staphylococcal conjunctivitis except in very young patients who are not subject to blepharitis. Conjunctival scarring may follow both pseudomembranous and membranous conjunctivitis, and in rare cases corneal ulceration and perforation supervene.

Marginal corneal ulceration may follow infection with *N gonorrhoeae, N kochii, N meningitidis, H aegyptius, S aureus,* and *M catarrhalis*; if the toxic products of *N gonorrhoeae* diffuse through the cornea into the anterior chamber, they may cause toxic iritis.

Treatment

Specific therapy of bacterial conjunctivitis depends on identification of the microbiologic agent. While waiting for laboratory reports, the physician can start topical therapy with an antimicrobial drug. In any purulent conjunctivitis in which Gram's stain shows gram-negative diplococci suggestive of *Neisseria,* both system and topical therapy should be started immediately. If there is no corneal involvement, a single intramuscular dose of ceftriaxone, 1 g, is usually adequate systemic therapy. If there is corneal involvement, a 5-day course of parenteral ceftriaxone, 1–2 g daily, is required.

In acute purulent and mucopurulent conjunctivitis, the conjunctival sac should be irrigated with saline solution as necessary to remove the conjunctival secretions. To prevent spread of the disease, the patient and family should be instructed to give special attention to personal hygiene.

Course & Prognosis

Acute bacterial conjunctivitis is almost always self-limited. Untreated, it may last 10–14 days; if properly treated, 1–3 days. The exceptions are staphylococcal conjunctivitis (which may progress to blepharoconjunctivitis and enter a chronic phase) and gonococcal conjunctivitis (which when untreated can lead to corneal perforation and endophthalmitis). Since the conjunctiva may be the portal of entry for the meningococcus to the bloodstream and meninges, septicemia and meningitis may be the end results of meningococcal conjunctivitis.

Chronic bacterial conjunctivitis may not be self-limited and may become a troublesome therapeutic problem.

CHLAMYDIAL CONJUNCTIVITIS

1. TRACHOMA

Trachoma is one of the most ancient of known diseases. It was recognized as a cause of trichiasis as early as the 27th century BC and affects all races. With 300–600 million of the world's population afflicted, it is one of the most common of all chronic diseases. Its regional variations in prevalence and severity can be explained on the basis of variations in the personal hygiene and standards of living of the world's peoples, the climatic conditions under which they live, the prevailing age at onset, and the frequency and type of the prevailing concomitant bacterial eye infections. Blinding trachoma occurs in many parts of Africa, some parts of Asia, among Australian aborigines, and in northern Brazil. Communities with milder non-blinding trachoma occur in the same regions and in some areas of Latin America and the Pacific Islands.

Trachoma is usually bilateral. It is spread by direct contact or fomites, usually from other family members (siblings, parents), who should also be examined for the disease. Insect vectors, especially flies and gnats, may play a role in transmission. The acute forms of the disease are more infectious than the cicatricial forms, and the larger the inoculum the more severe the disease. Spread is often associated with epidemics of bacterial conjunctivitis and with the dry seasons in tropical and semitropical countries.

Clinical Findings

A. Symptoms and Signs: Trachoma is initially a chronic follicular conjunctivitis of childhood that progresses to conjunctival scarring. In severe cases, inturned eyelashes occur in early adult life as a result of severe conjunctival scarring. The constant abrasion of inturned lashes and a defective tear film lead to corneal scarring, usually after the age of 50 years.

The incubation period of trachoma averages 7 days but varies from 5 to 14 days. In an infant or child, the onset is usually insidious, and the disease may resolve with minimal or no complications. In adults, the onset is often subacute or acute, and complications may develop early. At onset, trachoma often resembles other bacterial conjunctivitis, the signs and symptoms usually consisting of tearing, photophobia, pain, exudation, edema of the eyelids, chemosis of the bulbar conjunctiva, hyperemia, papillary hypertrophy, tarsal and limbal follicles, superior keratitis, pannus formation, and a small, tender preauricular node.

In established trachoma, there may also be superior epithelial keratitis, subepithelial keratitis, pannus, superior limbal follicles, and ultimately the pathognomonic cicatricial remains of these follicles, known as **Herbert's pits**—small depressions in the connective tissue at the limbocorneal junction covered by epithelium. The associated pannus is a fibrovascular membrane arising from the limbus, with vascular loops extending onto the cornea. All of the signs of trachoma are more severe in the upper than in the lower conjunctiva and cornea.

To establish the presence of endemic trachoma in a family or community, a substantial number of children must have at least two of the following signs:

(1) Five or more follicles on the flat tarsal conjunctiva lining the upper eye lid.

(2) Typical conjunctival scarring of the upper tarsal conjunctiva.

(3) Limbal follicles or their sequelae (Herbert's pits).

(4) An even extension of blood vessels onto the cornea, most marked at the upper limbus.

While occasional individuals will meet these criteria, it is the wide distribution of these signs in individual families and in a community that identify the presence of trachoma.

For control purposes, the World Health Organization has developed a simplified method to describe the disease. This includes the following signs:

TF:	Five or more follicles on the upper tarsal conjunctiva.
TI:	Diffuse infiltration and papillary hypertrophy of the upper tarsal conjunctiva obscuring at least 50% of the normal deep vessels.
TS:	Trachomatous conjunctival scarring.
TT:	Trichiasis or entropion (inturned eyelashes).
CO:	Corneal opacity.

The presence of TF and TI indicates active infectious trachoma and a need for treatment. TS is evidence of damage from the disease. TT is potentially blinding and is an indication for corrective lid surgery. CO is the final blinding lesion of trachoma.

B. Laboratory Findings: Chlamydial inclusions can be found in Giemsa-stained conjunctival scrapings, but they are not always present. Inclusions appear in the Giemsa-stained preparations as particulate, dark purple or blue cytoplasmic masses that cap the nucleus of the epithelial cell. Fluorescent antibody stains and enzyme immunoassay tests are available commercially and are widely used in clinical laboratories. These new tests have superseded Giemsa staining of conjunctival smears and isolation of chlamydial agent in cell culture.

The agent of trachoma resembles the agent of inclusion conjunctivitis morphologically, but the two can be differentiated serologically by microimmunofluorescence. Trachoma is caused by *Chlamydia trachomatis* serotypes A, B, Ba, or C.

Differential Diagnosis

Epidemiologic and clinical factors to be considered in differentiating trachoma from other forms of follicular conjunctivitis can be summarized as follows:

(1) No history of exposure to endemic trachoma speaks against the diagnosis.

(2) Viral follicular conjunctivitis (due to infection with adenovirus, herpes simplex virus, picornavirus, and coxsackievirus) usually has an acute onset and is clearly resolving by 2–3 weeks.

(3) Infection with genitally transmitted chlamydial strains usually has an acute onset in sexually active individuals.

(4) Chronic follicular conjunctivitis with exogenous substances (molluscum nodules of the lids, topical eye medications) resolve slowly when the nodules are removed or the drug withdrawn.

(5) Parinaud's oculoglandular syndrome is manifested by massively enlarged preauricular or cervical lymph nodes, though the conjunctival lesion may be follicular.

(6) Young children often have some follicles (like hypertrophied tonsils), a condition known as folliculosis.

(7) The atopic conditions vernal conjunctivitis and atopic keratoconjunctivitis are associated with giant papillae that are elevated and often polygonal, with a milky-red appearance. Eosinophils are present in smears.

(8) Look for a history of contact lens intolerance in patients with conjunctival scarring and pannus; giant papillae in some contact lens wearers can be confused with trachoma follicles.

Complications & Sequelae

Conjunctival scarring is a frequent complication of trachoma and can destroy the ductules of the accessory lacrimal glands and obliterate the orifices of the lacrimal gland. These effects may drastically reduce the aqueous component of the precorneal tear film, and the film's mucous components may be reduced by loss of goblet cells. The scars may also cause distortion of the upper lid with inward deviation of individual lashes (trichiasis) or of the whole lid margin (entropion), so that the lashes constantly abrade the cornea. This often leads to corneal ulceration, bacterial corneal infections, and corneal scarring (Figure 5–2).

Ptosis, nasolacrimal duct obstruction, and dacryocystitis are other common complications of trachoma.

Treatment

Striking clinical improvement can usually be achieved with tetracycline, 1–1.5 g/d orally in four divided doses for 3–4 weeks; doxycycline, 100 mg orally twice daily for 3 weeks; or erythromycin, 1 g/d orally in four divided doses for 3–4 weeks. Several courses are sometimes necessary for actual cure. Systemic tetracyclines should not be given to a child under 7 years of age or to a pregnant woman, since tetracycline binds to calcium in the developing teeth and in the growing bone and may lead to congenital yellowish discoloration of the permanent teeth and skeletal (eg, clavicular) abnormalities.

Topical ointments or drops, including preparations of sulfonamides, tetracyclines, erythromycin, and rifampin, used four times daily for 6 weeks, are equally effective.

From the time therapy is begun, its maximum effect is usually not achieved for 10–12 weeks. The persistence of follicles on the upper tarsus for some weeks

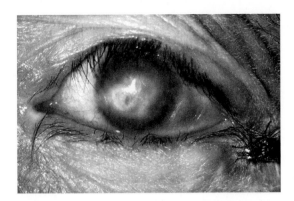

Figure 5–2. Advanced trachoma following corneal ulceration and scarring. Note the fly on the temporal aspect of the lower lid. The fly is a principal vector for trachoma.

after a course of therapy should therefore not be construed as evidence of therapeutic failure.

Surgical correction of inturned eyelashes is essential to prevent scarring from late trachoma in developing countries. Such surgery is sometimes done by nonspecialist physicians or specially trained auxiliary personnel.

Course & Prognosis

Characteristically, trachoma is a chronic disease of long duration. Under good hygienic conditions (specifically, face-washing of young children), the disease resolves or becomes milder so that severe sequelae are avoided. About 6–9 million people in the world today have major visual loss from trachoma.

2. INCLUSION CONJUNCTIVITIS

Inclusion conjunctivitis is often bilateral and usually occurs in sexually active young people. The chlamydial agent infects the urethra of the male and the cervix of the female. Transmission to the eyes of adults is usually by oral-genital sexual practices or hand to eye transmission. About one in 300 persons with genital chlamydial infection develops the eye disease. Indirect transmission has been reported to occur in inadequately chlorinated swimming pools. In newborns, the agent is transmitted during birth by direct contamination of the conjunctiva with cervical secretions. Credé prophylaxis gives only partial protection against inclusion conjunctivitis.

Clinical Findings

A. Symptoms and Signs: Inclusion conjunctivitis may have an acute or a subacute onset. The patient frequently complains of redness of the eyes, pseudoptosis, and discharge, especially in the mornings. Newborns have papillary conjunctivitis and a moderate amount of exudate, and in hyperacute cases

pseudomembranes occasionally form and can lead to scarring. Since the newborn has no adenoid tissue in the stroma of the conjunctiva, there is no follicle formation; but if the conjunctivitis persists for 2–3 months, follicles appear and the conjunctival picture is like that in older children and adults. In the newborn, chlamydial infection may cause pharyngitis, otitis media, and interstitial pneumonitis.

In adults, the conjunctiva of both tarsi—especially the lower tarsus—have papillae and follicles (Figure 5–3). Since pseudomembranes do not usually form in the adult, scarring does not usually occur. Superficial keratitis may be noted superiorly and, less often, a small superior micropannus (< 1–2 mm). Subepithelial opacities, usually marginal, often develop. Otitis media may occur as a result of infection of the auditory tube.

B. Laboratory Findings: The same tests should be performed as for trachoma (above). In neonatal chlamydial ophthalmia, Giemsa-stained smears often have many inclusions. Inclusion conjunctivitis is caused by *C trachomatis* serotypes D–K with occasional isolations of serotype B. Serologic determinations are not useful in the diagnosis of ocular infections, but measurement of IgM antibody levels is extremely valuable in the diagnosis of chlamydial pneumonitis in infants.

Differential Diagnosis

Inclusion conjunctivitis can be clinically differentiated from trachoma on the following grounds:

(1) Active, follicular trachoma occurs commonly in young children or others living in or exposed to a community with endemic trachoma; inclusion conjunctivitis occurs in sexually active adolescents or adults.

(2) Conjunctival scarring is very rare in adult inclusion conjunctivitis.

(3) Herbert's pits are a unique sign that trachoma was present at some time in the past.

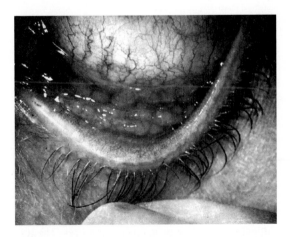

Figure 5–3. Acute follicular conjunctivitis caused by inclusion conjunctivitis in a 22-year-old man with urethritis. (Courtesy of K Tabbara.)

Treatment

A. In Infants: Give oral erythromycin suspension, 40 mg/kg/d in four divided doses for at least 14 days. Oral medication is necessary because chlamydial infection also involves the respiratory and gastrointestinal tracts. Topical antibiotics (tetracyclines, erythromycin, sulfonamides) are not useful in newborns treated with oral erythromycin. Both parents should be treated with oral tetracyclines or erythromycin for their genital tract infection.

B. In Adults: Cure can be achieved with a 3-week course of oral tetracycline, 1–1.5 g/d; doxycycline, 100 mg orally twice daily; or erythromycin, 1 g/d. (Systemic tetracyclines should not be given to a pregnant woman or a child under 7 years of age, since they cause epiphysial problems in the fetus or staining of the young child's teeth.) The patient's sexual partners should be examined and treated.

When one of the standard therapeutic regimens is followed, recurrences are rare. If untreated, inclusion conjunctivitis runs a course of 3–9 months or longer. The average duration is 5 months.

3. CONJUNCTIVITIS CAUSED BY OTHER CHLAMYDIAL AGENTS

Lymphogranuloma venereum conjunctivitis is a rare sexually transmitted disease. Lymphogranuloma venereum causes a dramatic granulomatous conjunctival reaction with greatly enlarged preauricular nodes (Parinaud's syndrome). It is caused by *C trachomatis* serotypes L1, L2 or L3.

Chlamydia psittaci only rarely causes conjunctivitis in humans. Strains from parrots (psittacosis) and cats (feline pneumonitis) have caused follicular conjunctivitis in humans. The prototype strains of *Chlamydia pneumoniae* were isolated from the conjunctiva but have not been identified as a cause of eye disease.

VIRAL CONJUNCTIVITIS

Viral conjunctivitis, a common affliction, can be caused by a wide variety of viruses. Severity ranges from severe, disabling disease to mild, rapidly self-limited infection.

1. ACUTE VIRAL FOLLICULAR CONJUNCTIVITIS

Pharyngoconjunctival Fever

Pharyngoconjunctival fever is characterized by fever of 38.3–40 °C (101–104 °F), sore throat, and a follicular conjunctivitis in one or both eyes. The follicles are often very prominent on both the conjunctiva (Figure 5–4) and the pharyngeal mucosa. The disease can be either bilateral or unilateral. Injection and tearing often occur, and there may be transient superficial epithelial keratitis and occasionally some subepithelial opacities. Preauricular lymphadenopathy (nontender) is characteristic. The syndrome may be incomplete, consisting of only one or two of the cardinal signs (fever, pharyngitis, and conjunctivitis).

Pharyngoconjunctival fever is caused regularly by adenovirus type 3 and occasionally by types 4 and 7. The virus can be grown on HeLa cells and identified by neutralization tests. As the disease progresses, it can also be diagnosed serologically by a rising titer of neutralizing antibody to the virus. Clinical diagnosis is a simple matter, however, and clearly more practical.

Conjunctival scrapings contain predominantly mononuclear cells, and no bacteria grow in cultures. The condition is more common in children than in adults and can be transmitted poorly in chlorinated swimming pools. There is no specific treatment, but the conjunctivitis is self-limited, usually lasting about 10 days.

Epidemic Keratoconjunctivitis

Epidemic keratoconjunctivitis is usually bilateral. The onset is often in one eye only, however, and as a rule the first eye is more severely affected. At onset the patient notes injection, moderate pain, and tearing, followed in 5–14 days by photophobia, epithelial keratitis, and round subepithelial opacities. Corneal sensation is normal. A tender preauricular node is characteristic. Edema of the eyelids, chemosis, and conjunctival hyperemia mark the acute phase, with follicles and subconjunctival hemorrhages often appearing within 48 hours. Pseudomembranes (and occasionally true membranes) may occur and may be followed by flat scars or symblepharon formation (Figure 5–5).

The conjunctivitis lasts for 3–4 weeks at most. The subepithelial opacities are concentrated in the central cornea, usually sparing the periphery, and may persist for months but heal without scars.

Epidemic keratoconjunctivitis is caused by ade-

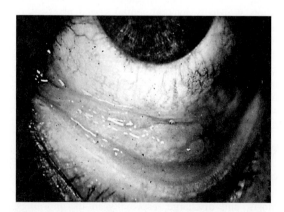

Figure 5–4. Acute follicular conjunctivitis due to adenovirus type 3. (Courtesy of P Thygeson.)

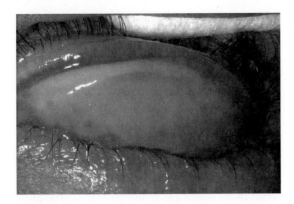

Figure 5–5. Epidemic keratoconjunctivitis. Thick white membrane of upper palpebral conjunctiva.

novirus types 8, 19, 29, and 37 (subgroup D of the human adenoviruses). They can be isolated in cell culture and identified by neutralization tests. Scrapings from the conjunctiva show a primarily mononuclear inflammatory reaction (Figure 5–6); when pseudomembranes occur, neutrophils may also be prominent.

Epidemic keratoconjunctivitis in adults is confined to the external eye, but in children there may be such systemic symptoms of viral infection as fever, sore throat, otitis media, and diarrhea. Nosocomial transmission during eye examinations takes place all too often by way of the physician's fingers, use of improperly sterilized ophthalmic instruments, or use of contaminated solutions. Eye solutions, particularly topical anesthetics, can be contaminated when a dropper tip aspirates infected material from the conjunctiva or cilia. The virus can persist in the solution, which becomes a source of spread.

The danger of contaminated solution bottles can be avoided by the use of individual sterile droppers or unit-dose packages of eye drops. Regular hand washing between examinations and careful cleaning and sterilization of instruments that touch the eyes—especially tonometers—are also mandatory. Applanation tonometers should be cleaned by wiping with alcohol or hypochlorite, then rinsing with sterile water and carefully drying.

There is no specific therapy at present, but cold compresses will relieve some symptoms. Corticosteroids during acute conjunctivitis may prolong the late corneal involvement and so should be avoided. Antibacterial agents should be given if bacterial superinfection occurs.

Herpes Simplex Virus Conjunctivitis

Herpes simplex virus (HSV) conjunctivitis, usually a disease of young children, is an uncommon entity characterized by unilateral injection, irritation, mucoid discharge, pain, and mild photophobia. It occurs during primary infection with HSV or during recurrent episodes of ocular herpes (Figure 5–7). It is

often associated with herpes simplex keratitis, in which the cornea shows discrete epithelial lesions that usually coalesce to form single or multiple branching epithelial (dendritic) ulcers. The conjunctivitis is follicular or, less often, pseudomembranous. (Patients receiving topical antivirals may develop follicular conjunctivitis that can be differentiated because the herpetic follicular conjunctivitis has an acute onset.) Herpetic vesicles may sometimes appear on the eyelids and lid margins, associated with severe edema of the eyelids. Typically, there is a small tender preauricular node.

No bacteria are found in scrapings or recovered in cultures. If the conjunctivitis is follicular, the predominant inflammatory reaction is mononuclear, but if it is pseudomembranous the predominant reaction is polymorphonuclear owing to the chemotaxis of necrosis. Intranuclear inclusions (because of the margination of the chromatin) can be seen in conjunctival and corneal cells if Bouin fixation and the Papanicolaou stain are used but not in Giemsa-stained smears. The finding of multinucleated giant epithelial cells has diagnostic value.

The virus can be readily isolated by gently rubbing

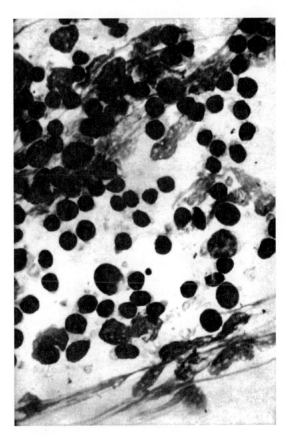

Figure 5–6. Mononuclear cell reaction in conjunctival scrapings of a patient with viral conjunctivitis caused by adenovirus type 8. (Courtesy of M Okumoto.)

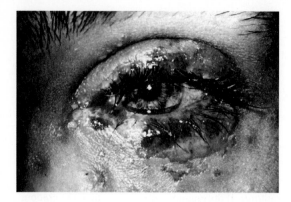

Figure 5–7. Primary ocular herpes. (Courtesy of HB Ostler.)

a dry cotton-tipped applicator over the conjunctiva and transferring the infected cells to a susceptible tissue culture.

HSV conjunctivitis may persist for 2–3 weeks, and if it is pseudomembranous it may leave fine linear or flat scars. Complications consist of corneal involvement (including dendrites) and vesicles on the skin. Although type 1 herpesvirus causes the overwhelming majority of ocular cases, type 2 is the usual cause in newborns and a rare cause in adults. In the newborn, there may be generalized disease with encephalitis, chorioretinitis, hepatitis, etc. Any HSV infection in the newborn must be treated with systemic antiviral therapy (acyclovir) and monitored in a hospital setting.

If the conjunctivitis occurs in a child over 1 year of age or in an adult, it is usually self-limited and may not require therapy. Topical or systemic antivirals should be given, however, to prevent corneal involvement. For corneal ulcers, corneal debridement may be performed by gently wiping the ulcer with a dry cotton swab, applying antiviral drops, and patching the eye for 24 hours. Topical antivirals alone should be applied for 7–10 days: trifluridine every 2 hours while awake, or vidarabine ointment five times a day, or idoxuridine 0.1%, 1 drop every hour while awake and 1 drop every 2 hours during the night. Herpetic keratitis may also be treated with 3% acyclovir ointment (not available in the USA) five times daily for 10 days or with oral acyclovir, 400 mg five times a day for 7 days. The use of steroids is contraindicated, since they may aggravate herpes simplex infections and convert the disease from a short, self-limited process to a severe, greatly prolonged one.

Newcastle Disease Conjunctivitis

Newcastle disease conjunctivitis is a rare disorder characterized by burning, itching, pain, redness, tearing, and (rarely) blurring of vision. It often occurs in small epidemics among poultry workers handling infected birds or among veterinarians or laboratory helpers working with live vaccines or virus.

The conjunctivitis resembles that caused by other viral agents, with chemosis, a small preauricular node, and follicles on the upper and lower tarsus. No treatment is available or necessary for this self-limited disease.

Acute Hemorrhagic Conjunctivitis

All of the continents and most of the islands of the world have had major epidemics of acute hemorrhagic conjunctivitis. It was first recognized in Ghana in 1969. It is caused by enterovirus type 70 and occasionally by coxsackievirus A24.

Characteristically, the disease has a short incubation period (8–48 hours) and course (5–7 days). The usual signs and symptoms are pain, photophobia, foreign body sensation, copious tearing, redness, lid edema, and subconjunctival hemorrhages (Figure 5–8). Chemosis sometimes also occurs. The subconjunctival hemorrhages are usually diffuse but may be punctate at onset, beginning in the upper bulbar conjunctiva and spreading to the lower. Most patients have preauricular lymphadenopathy, conjunctival follicles, and epithelial keratitis. Anterior uveitis has been reported; fever, malaise, and generalized myalgia have been observed in 25% of cases; and motor paralysis of the lower extremities has occurred in rare cases in India and Japan.

The virus is transmitted by close person-to-person contact and by such fomites as common linens, contaminated optical instruments, and water. Recovery occurs within 5–7 days, and there is no known treatment. In the USA, closing of schools has been done to stop epidemics.

2. CHRONIC VIRAL CONJUNCTIVITIS

Molluscum Contagiosum Blepharoconjunctivitis

A molluscum nodule on the lid margins or the skin of the lids or brow may produce unilateral chronic follicular conjunctivitis, superior keratitis, and superior pannus and may resemble trachoma. The inflammatory reaction is predominantly mononuclear (unlike

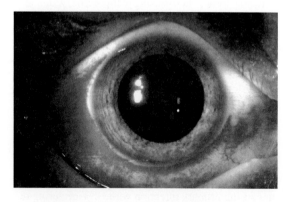

Figure 5–8. Acute hemorrhagic conjunctivitis.

the reaction in trachoma), and the round, waxy, pearly-white, noninflammatory lesion with an umbilicated center is typical of molluscum contagiosum (Figure 5–9). Biopsy shows eosinophilic cytoplasmic inclusions that fill the entire cytoplasm of the enlarged cell, pushing its nucleus to one side.

Excision, simple incision of the nodule to allow peripheral blood to permeate it, or cryotherapy cures the conjunctivitis. On very rare occasions (reports of only two cases have appeared in the literature), molluscum nodules have occurred on the conjunctiva. In these cases, excision of the nodule has also relieved the conjunctivitis. Multiple lid or facial lesions of molluscum contagiosum have been seen in patients with AIDS.

Varicella-Zoster Blepharoconjunctivitis

Hyperemia and an infiltrative conjunctivitis—associated with the typical vesicular eruption along the dermatomal distribution of the ophthalmic branch of the trigeminal nerve—are characteristic of herpes zoster (preferably called simply zoster). The conjunctivitis is usually papillary, but follicles, pseudomembranes, and transitory vesicles that later ulcerate have all been noted. A tender preauricular lymph node occurs early in the disease. Scarring of the lid, entropion, and the misdirection of individual lashes are sequelae.

The lid lesions of varicella, which are like the skin lesions (pox) elsewhere, may appear on both the lid margins and the lids and often leave scars. A mild exudative conjunctivitis often occurs, but discrete conjunctival lesions (except at the limbus) are very rare. Limbal lesions resemble phlyctenules and may go through all the stages of vesicle, papule, and ulcer. The adjacent cornea becomes infiltrated and may vascularize.

In both zoster and varicella, scrapings from lid vesicles contain giant cells and a predominance of polymorphonuclear leukocytes; scrapings from the conjunctiva in varicella and from conjunctival vesicles in zoster may contain giant cells and monocytes. The virus can be recovered in tissue cultures of human embryo cells.

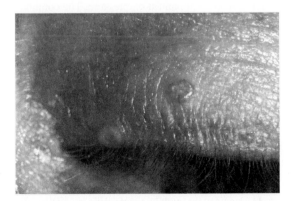

Figure 5–9. Molluscum contagiosum of lid margin. Follicular conjunctivitis was present.

Oral acyclovir in high doses (800 mg orally five times daily for 10 days), if given early in the course of the disease, appears to limit the severity of the illness.

Measles Keratoconjunctivitis

The characteristic enanthem of measles frequently precedes the skin eruption. At this early stage, the conjunctiva may have a peculiar glassy appearance, followed within a few days by swelling of the semilunar fold (Meyer's sign). Several days before the skin eruption, an exudative conjunctivitis with a mucopurulent discharge develops, and at the time of the skin eruption, Koplik's spots appear on the conjunctiva and occasionally on the caruncle. At some time (early in children, late in adults), epithelial keratitis supervenes.

In the immunocompetent patient, measles keratoconjunctivitis has few or no sequelae, but in malnourished or otherwise immunoincompetent patients the ocular disease is frequently associated with a secondary HSV or bacterial infection due to *S pneumoniae, H influenzae,* and other organisms. These agents may lead to purulent conjunctivitis with associated corneal ulceration and severe visual loss. Herpes infection can cause severe corneal ulceration with corneal perforation and loss of vision in poorly nourished children in developing countries.

Conjunctival scrapings show a mononuclear cell reaction unless there are pseudomembranes or secondary infection. Giemsa-stained preparations contain giant cells. Since there is no specific therapy, only supportive measures are indicated unless there is secondary infection.

RICKETTSIAL CONJUNCTIVITIS

All rickettsiae recognized as pathogenic for humans may attack the conjunctiva, and the conjunctiva may be their portal of entry.

Q fever is associated with severe conjunctival hyperemia. Treatment with systemic tetracycline or chloramphenicol is curative.

Marseilles fever (boutonneuse fever) is often associated with ulcerative or granulomatous conjunctivitis and a grossly visible preauricular lymph node.

Endemic (murine) typhus, scrub typhus, Rocky Mountain spotted fever, and **epidemic typhus** have associated, variable, and usually mild conjunctival signs.

FUNGAL CONJUNCTIVITIS

Candidal Conjunctivitis

Conjunctivitis caused by *Candida* species (usually *Candida albicans*) is a rare infection that usually appears as a white plaque. This may occur in diabetics or immunocompromised patients as an ulcerative or granulomatous conjunctivitis.

Scrapings show a polymorphonuclear cell inflammatory reaction. The organism grows readily on blood agar or Sabouraud's medium and can be readily identified as a budding yeast or, rarely, as pseudohyphae.

The infection responds to amphotericin B (3–8 mg/mL) in aqueous (not saline) solution or to applications of nystatin dermatologic cream (100,000 units/g) four to six times daily. The ointment must be applied carefully to be sure that it reaches the conjunctival sac and does not just build up on the lid margins.

Other Fungal Conjunctivitides

Sporothrix schenckii may rarely involve the conjunctiva or the eyelids. It is a granulomatous disease associated with a visible preauricular node. Microscopic examination of a biopsy of the granuloma reveals gram-positive, cigar-shaped conidia (spores).

Rhinosporidium seeberi may rarely affect the conjunctiva, lacrimal sac, lids, canaliculi, and sclera. The typical lesion is a polypoid granuloma that bleeds after minimal trauma. Histologic examination shows a granuloma with enclosed large spherules containing myriads of endospores. Treatment is by simple excision and cauterization of the base.

Coccidioides immitis may rarely cause a granulomatous conjunctivitis associated with a grossly visible preauricular node (Parinaud's oculoglandular syndrome). This is not a primary disease but a manifestation of metastatic infection from a primary pulmonary infection (San Joaquin Valley fever). Disseminated disease suggests a poor prognosis.

PARASITIC CONJUNCTIVITIS*

Thelazia californiensis Infection

The natural habitat of this roundworm is the eye of the dog, but it can also infect the eyes of cats, sheep, black bears, horses, and deer. Accidental infection of the human conjunctival sac has occurred. The disease can be treated effectively by removing the worms from the conjunctival sac with forceps or a cotton-tipped applicator.

Loa loa Infection

L loa is the eye worm of Africa. It lives in the connective tissue of humans and monkeys, and the monkey may be its reservoir. The parasite is transmitted by the bite of the horse or mango fly. The mature worm may then migrate to the lid, the conjunctiva, or the orbit.

Infection with *L loa* is accompanied by a 60–80% eosinophilia, but diagnosis is made by identifying the worm on removal or by finding microfilariae in blood examined at midday.

Diethylcarbamazine is currently the drug of choice. Ivermectin is being evaluated.

---

* Onchocerciasis is discussed in Chapter 7.

Ascaris lumbricoides Infection (Butcher's Conjunctivitis)

Ascaris may cause a rare type of violent conjunctivitis. When butchers or persons performing postmortem examinations cut tissue containing *Ascaris,* the tissue juice of some of the organisms may hit them in the eye. This can be followed by a violent and painful toxic conjunctivitis marked by extreme chemosis and lid edema. Treatment consists of rapid and thorough irrigation of the conjunctival sac.

Trichinella spiralis Infection

This parasite does not cause a true conjunctivitis, but in the course of its general dissemination there may be a doughy edema of the upper and lower eyelids, and over 50% of patients have chemosis—a pale, lemon-yellow swelling most marked over the lateral and medial rectus muscles and fading toward the limbus. The chemosis may last a week or more, and there is often pain on movement of the eyes.

Schistosoma haematobium Infection

Schistosomiasis (bilharziasis) is endemic in Egypt, especially in the region irrigated by the Nile. Granulomatous conjunctival lesions appearing as small, soft, smooth, pinkish-yellow tumors occur, especially in males. The symptoms are minimal. Diagnosis depends on microscopic examination of biopsy material, which shows a granuloma containing lymphocytes, plasma cells, giant cells, and eosinophils surrounding bilharzial ova in various stages of disintegration.

Treatment consists of excision of the conjunctival granuloma and systemic therapy with antimonials such as niridazole.

Taenia solium Infection

This parasite rarely causes conjunctivitis but more often invades the retina, choroid, or vitreous to produce ocular cysticercosis. As a rule, the affected conjunctiva shows a subconjunctival cyst in the form of a localized hemispherical swelling, usually at the inner angle of the lower fornix, which is adherent to the underlying sclera and painful on pressure. The conjunctiva and lid may be inflamed and edematous.

Diagnosis is based on a positive complement fixation or precipitin test or on demonstration of the organism in the gastrointestinal tract. Eosinophilia is a constant feature.

The best treatment is to excise the lesion. The intestinal condition can be treated by niclosamide.

Pthirus pubis Infection (Pubic Louse Infection)

P pubis may infest the cilia and margins of the eyelids. Because of its size, the pubic louse seems to require widely spaced hair. For this reason it has a predilection for the widely spaced cilia as well as for pubic hair. The parasites apparently release an irritating substance (probably feces) that produces a toxic follicular conjunctivitis in children and an irritating papillary conjunctivitis in adults. The lid margin is usually red, and the patient may complain of intense itching.

Finding the adult organism or the ova-shaped nits cemented to the eyelashes is diagnostic.

Lindane (Kwell) 1% or RID (pyrethrins), applied to the pubic area and lash margins after removal of the nits, is usually curative. Application of lindane or RID to the lid margins must be undertaken with great care to avoid contact with the eye. Any ointment applied to the lid margin tends to smother the adult organisms. The patient's family and close contacts should be examined and treated. All clothes and fomites should be washed.

Ophthalmomyiasis

Myiasis is infection with larvae of flies. Many different species of flies may produce myiasis. The ocular tissues may be injured by mechanical transmission of disease-producing organisms and by the parasitic activities of the larvae in the ocular tissues. The larvae are able to invade either necrotic or healthy tissue. Many become infected by accidental ingestion of the eggs or larvae or by contamination of external wounds or skin. Infants and young children, alcoholics, and debilitated unattended patients are common targets for infection with myiasis-producing flies.

These larvae may affect the ocular surface, the intraocular tissues, or the deeper orbital tissues.

Ocular surface involvement may be caused by *Musca domestica,* the housefly, *Fannia,* the latrine fly, and *Oestrus ovis,* the sheep botfly. These flies deposit their eggs at the lower lid margin or inner canthus, and the larvae may remain on the surface of the eye, causing irritation, pain, and conjunctival hyperemia.

Treatment of ocular surface myiasis is by mechanical removal of the larvae after topical anesthesia.

IMMUNOLOGIC (ALLERGIC) CONJUNCTIVITIS

IMMEDIATE HUMORAL HYPERSENSITIVITY REACTIONS

1. HAY FEVER CONJUNCTIVITIS

A mild, nonspecific conjunctival inflammation is commonly associated with hay fever (allergic rhinitis). There is usually a history of allergy to pollens, grasses, animal danders, etc. The patient complains of itching, tearing, and redness of the eyes and often states that the eyes seem to be "sinking into the surrounding tissue." There is mild injection of the palpebral and bulbar conjunctiva, and during acute attacks there is often severe chemosis (which no doubt accounts for the "sinking" description). There may be a small amount of ropy discharge, especially if the patient has been

rubbing the eyes. Eosinophils are difficult to find in conjunctival scrapings. A papillary conjunctivitis can occur if the allergen persists (Figure 5–10).

Treatment consists of the instillation of local vasoconstrictors during the acute phase (epinephrine, 1:1000 solution applied topically, will relieve the chemosis and symptoms within 30 minutes). Cold compresses are helpful to relieve itching, and antihistamines by mouth are of some value. The immediate response to treatment is satisfactory, but recurrences are common unless the antigen is eliminated. Fortunately, the frequency of the attacks and the severity of the symptoms tend to moderate as the patient ages.

2. VERNAL KERATOCONJUNCTIVITIS

This disease, also known as "spring catarrh" and "seasonal conjunctivitis" or "warm weather conjunctivitis," is an uncommon bilateral allergic disease that usually begins in the prepubertal years and lasts for 5–10 years. It occurs much oftener in boys than in girls. The specific allergen or allergens are difficult to identify, but patients with vernal keratoconjunctivitis usually show other manifestations of allergy known to be related to grass pollen sensitivity. The disease is less common in temperate than in warm climates and is almost nonexistent in cold climates. It is almost always more severe during the spring, summer, and fall than in the winter. It is most commonly seen in sub-Saharan Africa and the Middle East.

The patient usually complains of extreme itching and a ropy discharge. There is often a family history of allergy (hay fever, eczema, etc) and sometimes in the young patient as well. The conjunctiva has a milky appearance, and there are many fine papillae in the lower tarsal conjunctiva. The upper palpebral conjunctiva often has giant papillae that give a cobblestone appearance (Figure 5–11). Each giant papilla is polygonal, has a flat top, and contains tufts of capillaries.

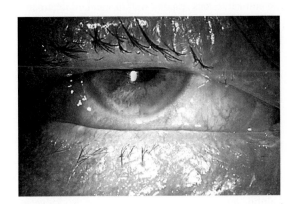

Figure 5–10. Acute hypersensitivity with moderate tylosis, moderate to marked chemosis and mild injection of the conjunctiva. Note that the eye seems to be "sinking" into the surrounding tissue.

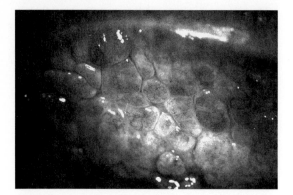

Figure 5–11. Vernal keratoconjunctivitis. "Cobblestone" papillae on superior tarsal conjunctiva.

A stringy conjunctival discharge and a fine, fibrinous pseudomembrane (Maxwell-Lyons sign) may be noted, especially on the upper tarsus on exposure to heat. In some cases, especially in persons of black African ancestry, the most prominent lesions are located at the limbus, where gelatinous swellings (papillae) are noted. A pseudogerontoxon (arcus-like haze) is often noted in the cornea adjacent to the limbal papillae. Trantas' dots are whitish dots seen at the limbus in some patients with vernal keratoconjunctivitis during the active phase of the disease. Many eosinophils and free eosinophilic granules are found in Giemsa-stained smears of the conjunctival exudate and in Trantas' dots.

Micropannus is often seen in both palpebral and limbal vernal keratoconjunctivitis, but gross pannus is unusual. Conjunctival scarring usually does not occur unless the patient has been treated with cryotherapy, surgical removal of the papillae, irradiation, or other damaging procedure. Superficial corneal ("shield") ulcers (oval and located superiorly) may form and may be followed by mild corneal scarring. A characteristic diffuse epithelial keratitis frequently occurs. None of the corneal lesions respond well to standard treatment.

The disease may be associated with keratoconus.

Treatment

Since vernal keratoconjunctivitis is a self-limited disease, it must be recognized that the medication used to treat the symptoms may provide short-term benefit but long-term harm. Topical and systemic steroids, which relieve the itching, affect the corneal disease only minimally, and their side effects (glaucoma, cataract, and other complications) can be severely damaging. Topical cromolyn is a useful prophylactic agent in moderate to severe cases. Vasoconstrictors, cold compresses, and ice packs are helpful, and sleeping (if possible, also working) in cool, air-conditioned rooms can keep the patient reasonably comfortable. Probably the best remedy of all is to move to a cool, moist climate. Patients able to do so are benefited if not completely cured.

The severe symptoms of an extremely photophobic patient who is unable to function can often be relieved by a short course of topical or systemic steroids followed by vasoconstrictors, cold packs, and regular use of histamine-blocking agents as eyedrops. Newer nonsteroidal anti-inflammatory medications, including ketorolac and lodoxamide, may provide significant symptomatic relief. (See discussion in Chapter 3.) As has already been indicated, the prolonged use of steroids must be avoided since it is all too often followed by herpes simplex keratitis, cataract, glaucoma, and fungal and other opportunistic corneal ulcers. Recent clinical studies have shown that topical 2% cyclosporine eye drops are effective in severe unresponsive cases. Supratarsal injection of depot corticosteroids has been demonstrated to be effective for vernal shield ulcers.

Desensitization to grass pollens and other antigens has not been rewarding. Staphylococcal blepharitis and conjunctivitis are frequent complications and should be treated. Recurrences are the rule, particularly in the spring and summer; but after a number of recurrences the papillae disappear completely, leaving no scars.

3. ATOPIC KERATOCONJUNCTIVITIS

Patients with atopic dermatitis (eczema) often also have atopic keratoconjunctivitis. The symptoms and signs are a burning sensation, mucoid discharge, redness, and photophobia. The lid margins are erythematous, and the conjunctiva has a milky appearance. There are fine papillae, but giant papillae are less developed than in vernal keratoconjunctivitis and occur more frequently on the lower tarsus—unlike the giant papillae of vernal keratoconjunctivitis, which are on the upper tarsus (Figure 5–12). Severe corneal signs appear late in the disease after repeated exacerbations of the conjunctivitis. Superficial peripheral keratitis develops and is followed by vascularization. In severe cases, the entire cornea becomes hazy and vascular-

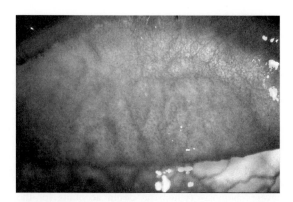

Figure 5–12. Moderate to marked papillary response of upper tarsus seen in atopic keratoconjunctivitis.

ized, and visual acuity is reduced. The disease may be associated with keratoconus.

There is usually a history of allergy (hay fever, asthma, or eczema) in the patient or the patient's family. Most patients have had atopic dermatitis since infancy. Scarring of the flexure creases of the antecubital folds and of the wrists and knees is common. Like the dermatitis with which it is associated, atopic keratoconjunctivitis has a protracted course and is subject to exacerbations and remissions. Like vernal keratoconjunctivitis, it tends to become less active when the patient reaches the fifth decade.

Scrapings of the conjunctiva show eosinophils, though not nearly as many as are seen in vernal keratoconjunctivitis. Scarring of both the conjunctiva and cornea is often seen, and an atopic cataract, a posterior subcapsular plaque, or an anterior shield-like cataract may develop. Keratoconus, retinal detachment, and herpes simplex keratitis are all more than usually frequent in patients with atopic keratoconjunctivitis, and there are many cases of secondary bacterial blepharitis and conjunctivitis, usually staphylococcal.

The management of atopic keratoconjunctivitis is often discouraging. Any secondary infection must be treated. Environmental control should be considered. Oral antihistamines including terfenadine (60–120 mg twice daily), astemizole (10 mg four times daily), or hydroxyzine (50 mg at bedtime, increasing to 200 mg at bedtime) have been shown to be of value. Newer nonsteroidal anti-inflammatory medications, including ketorolac and lodoxamide, show promise for symptomatic relief for these patients (see Chapter 3). A short course of topical steroids may relieve symptoms. In severe cases, plasmapheresis may be an adjunct to therapy. In advanced cases with severe corneal complications, corneal transplantation may be needed to improve the visual acuity.

4. GIANT PAPILLARY CONJUNCTIVITIS

Giant papillary conjunctivitis with signs and symptoms resembling those of vernal conjunctivitis may develop in patients wearing plastic artificial eyes or contact lenses. It is probably a basophil-rich delayed hypersensitivity disorder (Jones-Mote hypersensitivity), perhaps with an IgE humoral component. Use of glass instead of plastic for prostheses and spectacle lenses instead of contact lenses is curative. If the goal is to maintain contact lens wear, additional therapy will be required. Careful contact lens care, including preservative-free agents, is essential. Hydrogen peroxide disinfection and enzymatic cleaning of contact lenses may also help. Changing to a different brand or style of contact lenses may be necessary if other measures fail. If these treatments are unsuccessful, contact lenses should be discontinued.

DELAYED HYPERSENSITIVITY REACTIONS

1. PHLYCTENULOSIS

Phlyctenular keratoconjunctivitis is a delayed hypersensitivity response to microbial proteins, including the proteins of the tubercle bacillus, *Staphylococcus* species, *Candida albicans, Coccidioides immitis, Haemophilus aegyptius,* and *Chlamydia trachomatis* serotypes L1, L2, and L3. Until recently, by far the most frequent cause of phlyctenulosis in the USA was delayed hypersensitivity to the protein of the human tubercle bacillus. This is still the commonest cause in regions where tuberculosis is still prevalent. In the USA, however, most cases are now associated with delayed hypersensitivity to *S aureus.*

The conjunctival phlyctenule begins as a small lesion (usually 1–3 mm in diameter) that is hard, red, elevated, and surrounded by a zone of hyperemia. At the limbus it is often triangular in shape, with its apex toward the cornea. In this location it develops a grayish-white center that soon ulcerates and then subsides within 10–12 days. The patient's first phlyctenule and most of the recurrences develop at the limbus, but there may also be corneal, bulbar, and, very rarely, even tarsal phlyctenules.

Unlike the conjunctival phlyctenule, which leaves no scar, the corneal phlyctenule develops as an amorphous gray infiltrate and always leaves a scar. Consistent with this difference is the fact that scars form on the corneal side of the limbal lesion and not on the conjunctival side. The result is a triangular scar with its base at the limbus—a valuable sign of old phlyctenulosis when the limbus has been involved.

Conjunctival phlyctenules usually produce only irritation and tearing, but corneal and limbal phlyctenules are usually accompanied by intense photophobia (Figure 5–13). Phlyctenulosis is often triggered by active blepharitis, acute bacterial conjunctivitis, and dietary deficiencies. Phlyctenular scarring,

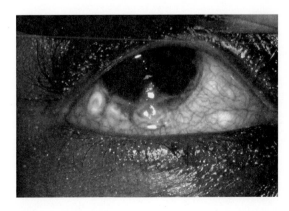

Figure 5–13. Phlyctenulosis. Note three phlyctenules along the inferior limbus, each with an umbilicated center.

which may be minimal or extensive, is often followed by Salzmann's nodular degeneration.

Histologically, the phlyctenule is a focal subepithelial and perivascular infiltration of small round cells, followed by a preponderance of polymorphonuclear cells when the overlying epithelium necrotizes and sloughs—a sequence of events characteristic of the delayed tuberculin type hypersensitivity reaction.

Phlyctenulosis induced by tuberculoprotein and the proteins of other systemic infections responds dramatically to topical corticosteroids. There is a major reduction of symptoms within 24 hours and disappearance of the lesion in another 24 hours. Phlyctenulosis produced by staphylococcal proteins responds somewhat more slowly. Topical antibiotics should be added for active staphylococcal blepharoconjunctivitis. Treatment should be aimed at the underlying disease, and the steroids, when effective, should be used only to control acute symptoms and persistent corneal scarring. Severe corneal scarring may call for corneal transplantation.

2. MILD CONJUNCTIVITIS SECONDARY TO CONTACT BLEPHARITIS

Contact blepharitis caused by atropine, neomycin, broad-spectrum antibiotics, and other topically applied medications is often followed by a mild infiltrative conjunctivitis that produces hyperemia, mild papillary hypertrophy, a mild mucoid discharge, and some irritation (Figure 5–14). Examination of Giemsa-stained scrapings often discloses only a few degenerated epithelial cells, a few polymorphonuclear and mononuclear cells, and no eosinophils.

Treatment should be directed toward finding the offending agent and eliminating it. The contact blepharitis may clear rapidly with topical cortico-steroids, but their use should be limited. Long-term use of steroids on the lids may lead to steroid glaucoma and to skin atrophy with disfiguring telangiectasis.

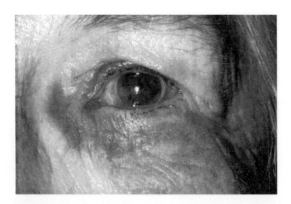

Figure 5–14. Contact dermatitis secondary to neomycin. Note lower lid involvement.

CONJUNCTIVITIS DUE TO AUTOIMMUNE DISEASE

KERATOCONJUNCTIVITIS SICCA (ASSOCIATED WITH SJÖGREN'S SYNDROME)

Sjögren's syndrome is a systemic disease characterized by a triad of disorders: keratoconjunctivitis sicca, xerostomia, and connective tissue dysfunction (arthritis). To establish the diagnosis of Sjögren's syndrome, at least two of the three disorders must be present. The disease is overwhelmingly more common in women at or beyond the menopause than in other groups, though men and younger women can also be affected. The lacrimal gland is infiltrated with lymphocytes and occasionally with plasma cells, and this leads to atrophy and destruction of the glandular structures.

Keratoconjunctivitis sicca is characterized by bulbar conjunctival hyperemia (especially in the palpebral aperture) and symptoms of irritation that are out of proportion to the mild inflammatory signs. It often begins as a mild conjunctivitis with a mucoid discharge. Blotchy epithelial lesions appear on the cornea, more prominently in its lower half, and filaments may be seen. Pain builds up in the afternoon and evening but is absent or only slight in the morning. The tear film is diminished and often contains shreds of mucus. Results of the Schirmer test are abnormal (see Chapter 4). Rose bengal or lissamine green staining of the cornea and conjunctiva in the palpebral aperture is a helpful diagnostic test.

The diagnosis is confirmed by demonstrating lymphocytic and plasma cell infiltration of the accessory salivary glands in a labial biopsy obtained by means of a simple surgical procedure (Figure 5–15).

Treatment should be directed toward preserving and replacing the tear film with artificial tears, with obliteration of the puncta, and with side shields, moisture chambers, and Buller shields. As a rule, the simpler measures should be tried first.

CICATRICIAL PEMPHIGOID

This disease usually begins as a nonspecific chronic conjunctivitis that is resistant to therapy. The conjunctiva may be affected alone or in combination with the mouth, nose, esophagus, vulva, and skin. The conjunctivitis leads to progressive scarring, obliteration of the fornices (especially the lower fornix), and entropion with trichiasis. The patient complains of pain, irritation, and blurring of vision. The cornea is affected only secondarily as a result of trichiasis and lack of the precorneal tear film. The disease is more severe in women than in men. It is typically a disease

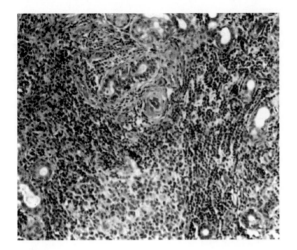

Figure 5–15. Mononuclear infiltration of the accessory salivary glands of a patient with Sjögren's syndrome. (Courtesy of K Tabbara.)

of middle life, occurring very rarely before age 45. In women, it may progress to blindness in a year or less; in men, progress is slower, and spontaneous remission sometimes occurs.

Conjunctival biopsies may contain eosinophils, and the basement membrane will stain positively with certain immunofluorescent stains (IgG, IgM, IgA complement). Oral dapsone and immunosuppressive therapy (eg, sulfapyridine) have been effective in some cases. Treatment must always be instituted at an early stage, prior to the onset of significant scarring. Generally, the course is long and the prognosis poor, with blindness due to complete symblepharon and corneal desiccation the usual outcome.

CHEMICAL OR IRRITATIVE CONJUNCTIVITIS

IATROGENIC CONJUNCTIVITIS FROM TOPICALLY APPLIED DRUGS

A toxic follicular conjunctivitis or an infiltrative, nonspecific conjunctivitis, followed by scarring, is often produced by the prolonged administration of dipivefrin, miotics, idoxuridine, neomycin, and other drugs prepared in toxic or irritating preservatives or vehicles. Silver nitrate instilled into the conjunctival sac at birth (Credé prophylaxis) is a frequent cause of mild chemical conjunctivitis. If tear production is reduced by continual irritation, the conjunctiva can be further damaged by the lack of dilution of the noxious agent as it is instilled into the conjunctival sac.

Conjunctival scrapings often contain keratinized epithelial cells, a few polymorphonuclear neutrophils, and an occasional oddly shaped cell. Treatment consists of stopping the offending agent and using bland drops or none at all. Often the conjunctival reaction persists for weeks or months after its cause has been eliminated.

OCCUPATIONAL CONJUNCTIVITIS FROM CHEMICALS & IRRITANTS

Acids, alkalies, smoke, wind, and almost any irritating substance that enters the conjunctival sac may cause conjunctivitis. Some common irritants are fertilizers, soaps, deodorants, hair sprays, tobacco, makeup preparations (mascara, etc), and various acids and alkalies. In certain areas, smog has become the commonest cause of mild chemical conjunctivitis. The specific irritant in smog has not been positively identified, and treatment is nonspecific. There are no permanent ocular effects, but affected eyes are frequently chronically red and irritated.

In acid burns, the acids denature the tissue proteins and the effect is immediate. Alkalies do not denature the proteins but tend to penetrate the tissues deeply and rapidly and to linger in the conjunctival tissue. Here they continue to inflict damage for hours or days, depending on the molar concentration of the alkali and the amount introduced. Adhesion between the bulbar and palpebral conjunctiva (symblepharon) and corneal leukoma are more likely to occur if the offending agent is an alkali. In either event, pain, injection, photophobia, and blepharospasm are the principal symptoms of caustic burns. A history of the precipitating event can usually be elicited.

Immediate and profuse irrigation of the conjunctival sac with water or saline solution is of importance, and any solid material should be removed mechanically. Do not use chemical antidotes. Further treatment is with intensive topical steroids, ascorbate and citrate eyedrops, cycloplegics, antiglaucoma treatment as necessary, cold compresses, and systemic analgesics (see Chapter 19). Bacterial conjunctivitis may be treated with appropriate antibacterial agents. Corneal scarring may require corneal transplantation, and symblepharon may require a plastic operation on the conjunctiva. Severe conjunctival and corneal burns have a poor prognosis even with surgery, but if proper treatment is started immediately, scarring may be minimized and the prognosis improved.

CATERPILLAR HAIR CONJUNCTIVITIS (OPHTHALMIA NODOSUM)

On rare occasions, caterpillar hairs are introduced into the conjunctival sac, where they produce one or many granulomas (ophthalmia nodosum). Under magnification, each granuloma is seen to contain a small foreign body.

Treatment by removal of each hair individually is effective. If a hair is retained, invasion of the sclera and uveal tract may occur.

CONJUNCTIVITIS OF UNKNOWN CAUSE

FOLLICULOSIS

Folliculosis is a widespread benign, bilateral non-inflammatory conjunctival condition characterized by follicular hypertrophy. It is more common in children than in adults, and the symptoms are minimal. The follicles are more numerous in the lower than in the upper cul-de-sac and tarsal conjunctiva. There is no associated inflammation or papillary hypertrophy, and complications do not occur.

There is no treatment for folliculosis, which disappears spontaneously after a course of 2–3 years. The cause is unknown, but folliculosis may be only a manifestation of a generalized adenoidal hypertrophy.

CHRONIC FOLLICULAR CONJUNCTIVITIS (Axenfeld's Conjunctivitis)

Chronic follicular conjunctivitis is a bilateral transmissible disease of children characterized by numerous follicles in the upper and lower tarsal conjunctiva. There are minimal conjunctival exudates and minimal inflammation but no complications. Treatment is ineffective, but the disease is self-limited within 2 years.

OCULAR ROSACEA

Ocular rosacea is a common complication of acne rosacea and probably occurs more often in light-skinned people, especially of Irish descent, than in dark-skinned people. It is usually a blepharoconjunctivitis, but the cornea is sometimes also affected. The patient complains of mild injection and irritation. There is frequently an accompanying staphylococcal blepharitis. The blood vessels of the lid margins are dilated and the conjunctiva hyperemic, especially in the exposed interpalpebral region. Less often, there may be a nodular conjunctivitis with small gray nodules on the bulbar conjunctiva, especially near the limbus, which may ulcerate superficially. The lesions can be differentiated from phlyctenules by the fact that even after they subside, the large dilated vessels persist.

Microscopic examination of the nodules shows lymphocytes and epithelial cells. The peripheral cornea may ulcerate and vascularize, and the keratitis may have a narrow base at the limbus and a wider infiltrate centrally. The corneal pannus is often segmented or wedge-shaped inferiorly (Figures 5–16 and 5–17).

Treatment of ocular rosacea consists of the elimination of hot, spicy foods and of alcoholic beverages that cause dilation of the facial vessels. Any secondary staphylococcal infection should be treated (Figure 5–18). A course of oral tetracycline or doxycycline is often helpful, and a smaller maintenance dose may be needed to control the disease.

The disease is chronic, recurrences are common, and the response to treatment is usually poor. If the cornea is not affected, the visual prognosis is good; but corneal lesions tend to recur and progress, and the vision grows steadily worse over a period of years.

PSORIASIS

Psoriasis vulgaris usually affects the areas of the skin not exposed to the sun, but in about 10% of cases lesions appear on the skin of the eyelids, and the plaques may extend to the conjunctiva, where they cause irritation, a foreign body sensation, and tearing. Psoriasis can also cause nonspecific chronic conjunctivitis with considerable mucoid discharge. Rarely, the cornea may show marginal ulceration or a deep, vascularized opacity.

The conjunctival and corneal lesions wax and wane with the skin lesions and are not affected by specific treatment. In rare cases, conjunctival scarring (symblepharon, trichiasis), corneal scarring, and occlusion of the nasolacrimal duct have occurred.

ERYTHEMA MULTIFORME MAJOR (STEVENS-JOHNSON SYNDROME)

Erythema multiforme major is a disease of the mucous membranes and skin. The skin lesion is an ery-

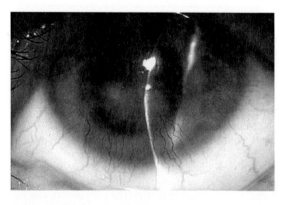

Figure 5–16. Chronic conjunctival injection and inferior keratopathy of rosacea. Note inferior pannus and corneal scarring suggestive of staphylococcal hypersensitivity.

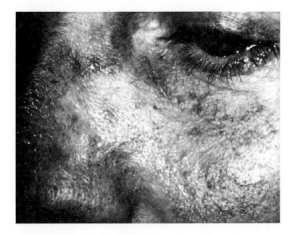

Figure 5–17. Skin lesions in acne rosacea. (Courtesy of HB Ostler.)

thematous, urticarial bullous eruption that appears suddenly and is often distributed symmetrically. Bilateral conjunctivitis, often membranous, is a common manifestation. The patient complains of pain, irritation, discharge, and photophobia. The cornea is affected secondarily, and vascularization and scarring may seriously reduce vision. Stevens-Johnson syndrome is typically a disease of young people, occurring only rarely after age 35.

Cultures are negative for bacteria; conjunctival scrapings show a preponderance of polymorphonuclear cells. Systemic steroids are thought to shorten the course of the systemic disease but have little or no effect on the eye lesions. Careful cleansing of the conjunctiva to remove the accumulated secretion is helpful, however, and tear replacement may be indicated. If trichiasis and entropion supervene, they should be corrected. Topical steroids probably have no beneficial effect, and their protracted use can cause corneal melting and perforation.

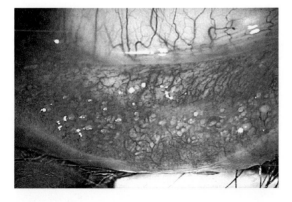

Figure 5–18. Multiple concretions on the inferior tarsus. These are often associated with chronic lid disease caused by staphylococcal species.

The acute episode of Stevens-Johnson syndrome usually lasts about 6 weeks, but the conjunctival scarring, loss of tears, and complications from entropion and trichiasis may result in prolonged morbidity and progressive corneal cicatrization. Recurrences are rare.

DERMATITIS HERPETIFORMIS

This is a rare skin disorder characterized by symmetrically grouped erythematous papulovesicular, vesicular, or bullous lesions. The disease has a predilection for the posterior axillary fold, the sacral region, the buttocks, and the forearms. Itching is often severe. Rarely, a pseudomembranous conjunctivitis occurs and may result in cicatrization resembling that seen in benign mucous membrane pemphigoid. The skin eruption and conjunctivitis usually respond readily to systemic sulfones or sulfapyridine.

EPIDERMOLYSIS BULLOSA

This is a rare hereditary disease characterized by vesicles, bullae, and epidermal cysts. The lesions occur chiefly on the extensor surfaces of the joints and other areas exposed to trauma. The severe dystrophic type that leads to scarring may also produce conjunctival scars similar to those seen in dermatitis herpetiformis and benign mucous membrane pemphigoid. No known treatment is satisfactory.

SUPERIOR LIMBIC KERATOCONJUNCTIVITIS

Superior limbic keratoconjunctivitis is usually bilateral and limited to the upper tarsus and upper limbus. The principal complaints are irritation and hyperemia. The signs are papillary hypertrophy of the upper tarsus, redness of the superior bulbar conjunctiva, thickening and keratinization of the superior limbus, epithelial keratitis, recurrent superior filaments, and superior micropannus (Figure 5–19). Rose bengal staining is a helpful diagnostic test. The keratinized epithelial cells and mucous debris pick up the stain. Scrapings from the upper limbus show keratinizing epithelial cells.

In about 50% of cases, the condition has been associated with abnormal function of the thyroid gland. Applying 0.5% or 1% silver nitrate to the upper palpebral conjunctiva and allowing the tarsus to drop back onto the upper limbus usually result in shedding of the keratinizing cells and relief of symptoms for 4–6 weeks. This treatment can be repeated. There are no complications, and the disease usually runs a course of 2–4 years.

In severe cases, one may consider 5 mm resection of the perilimbal superior conjunctiva.

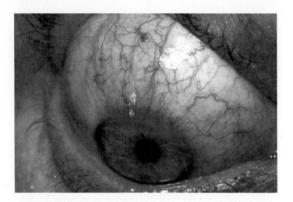

Figure 5–19. Superior limbic keratoconjunctivitis. Note the "corridor" on the bulbar surface.

LIGNEOUS CONJUNCTIVITIS

This is a rare bilateral, chronic or recurrent, pseudomembranous or membranous conjunctivitis that arises early in life, predominantly in young girls, and often persists for many years. Granulomas are often associated with it, and the lids may feel very hard. Cyclosporine may be effective treatment, as suggested by recent reports.

REITER'S SYNDROME

A triad of disease manifestations—nonspecific urethritis, arthritis, and conjunctivitis or iritis—constitutes Reiter's syndrome. The disease occurs much more often in men than in women. The conjunctivitis is papillary in type and usually bilateral. Conjunctival scrapings contain polymorphonuclear cells. No bacteria grow in cultures. The arthritis usually affects the large weight-bearing joints. There is no satisfactory treatment, though nonsteroidal anti-inflammatory agents may be effective. Corticosteroids will help the iridocyclitis. The disease has been found in association with HLA-B27 antigen.

MUCOCUTANEOUS LYMPH NODE SYNDROME (KAWASAKI DISEASE)

This disease of unknown cause was first described in Japan in 1967. Conjunctivitis is one of its six diagnostic features. The others are (1) fever that fails to respond to antibiotics; (2) changes in the lips and oral cavity; (3) such changes in the extremities as erythema of the palms and soles, indurative edema, and membranous desquamation of the fingertips; (4) polymorphous exanthem of the trunk; and (5) acute nonpurulent swelling of the cervical lymph nodes.

The disease occurs almost exclusively in prepubertal children and carries a 1–2% mortality rate from cardiac failure. The conjunctivitis has not been severe, and no corneal lesions have been reported.

Treatment is supportive only.

CONJUNCTIVITIS ASSOCIATED WITH SYSTEMIC DISEASE

CONJUNCTIVITIS IN THYROID DISEASE

In orbital Graves' disease, the conjunctiva may be red and chemotic and the patient may complain of copious tearing. As the disease progresses, the chemosis increases, and in advanced cases the chemotic conjunctiva may extrude between the lids (Figure 5–20).

Treatment is directed toward control of the thyroid disease, and every effort must be made to protect the conjunctiva and cornea by bland ointment, surgical lid adhesions (tarsorrhaphy) if necessary, or even orbital decompression if the lids do not close enough to cover the cornea and conjunctiva.

GOUTY CONJUNCTIVITIS

Patients with gout often complain of a "hot eye" during attacks. On examination, a mild conjunctivitis is found that is less severe than suggested by the symptoms. Gout may also be associated with episcleritis or scleritis, iridocyclitis, keratitis, vitreous opacities, and retinopathy. Treatment is aimed at controlling the gouty attack with colchicine and allopurinol.

CARCINOID CONJUNCTIVITIS

In carcinoid, the conjunctiva is sometimes congested and cyanotic as a result of the secretion of

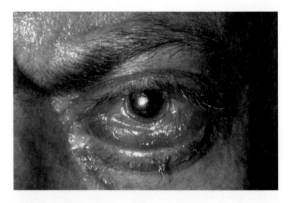

Figure 5–20. Graves' disease. Note conjunctival prolapse, keratinization, and marked chemosis and injection.

serotonin by the chromaffin cells of the gastrointestinal tract. The patient may complain of a "hot eye" during such attacks.

CONJUNCTIVITIS SECONDARY TO DACRYOCYSTITIS OR CANALICULITIS

CONJUNCTIVITIS SECONDARY TO DACRYOCYSTITIS

Both pneumococcal conjunctivitis (often unilateral and unresponsive to treatment) and beta-hemolytic streptococcal conjunctivitis (often hyperacute and purulent) may be secondary to chronic dacryocystitis. The nature and source of the conjunctivitis in both instances are often missed until the lacrimal system is investigated.

CONJUNCTIVITIS SECONDARY TO CANALICULITIS

Canaliculitis due to canalicular infection with *Actinomyces israelii* or *Candida* species (or, very rarely, *Aspergillus* species) may cause unilateral mucopurulent conjunctivitis, often chronic. The source of the condition is often missed unless the characteristic hyperemic, pouting punctum is noted. Expression of the canaliculus (upper or lower, whichever is involved) is curative provided the entire concretion is removed.

Conjunctival scrapings show a predominance of polymorphonuclear cells. Cultures (unless anaerobic) are usually negative. *Candida* grows readily on ordinary culture media, but almost all of the infections are caused by *A israelii,* which requires an anaerobic medium.

II. DEGENERATIVE DISEASES OF THE CONJUNCTIVA

PINGUECULA

Pingueculae are extremely common in adults. They appear as yellow nodules on both sides of the cornea (more commonly on the nasal side) in the area of the palpebral aperture. The nodules, consisting of hyaline and yellow elastic tissue, rarely increase in size, but inflammation is common. In general, no treatment is required, but in certain cases of pingueculitis, weak topical steroids (eg, prednisolone 0.12%) or topical nonsteroidal anti-inflammatory medications may be given (Figure 5–21).

PTERYGIUM

A pterygium is a fleshy, triangular encroachment of a pinguecula onto the cornea, usually on the nasal side bilaterally (Figure 5–22). It is thought to be an irritative phenomenon due to ultraviolet light, drying, and windy environments, since it is common in persons who spend much of their lives out of doors in sunny, dusty, or sandy, windblown surroundings. The pathologic findings in the conjunctiva are the same as those of pinguecula. In the cornea, there is replacement of Bowman's layer by hyaline and elastic tissue.

If the pterygium is enlarging and encroaches on the pupillary area, it should be removed surgically along with a small portion of superficial clear cornea beyond the area of encroachment. Beta-irradiation, topical mitomycin C, and conjunctival autografting have all been used to reduce the risk of recurrent disease.

CLIMATIC DROPLET KERATOPATHY (BIETTI'S BAND-SHAPED NODULAR DYSTROPHY, LABRADOR KERATOPATHY, SPHEROIDAL DEGENERATION)

Climatic droplet keratopathy is an uncommon degenerative disorder of the cornea characterized by aggregates of yellowish-golden spherules that accumulate in the subepithelial layers. The cause is unknown, but certain factors such as exposure to ultraviolet light, aridity, and microtrauma are recognized predisposing factors. The deposits may result in elevation of the epithelium in a band-shaped configuration. The condition is more common in geographic regions with high levels of direct and reflected sunlight.

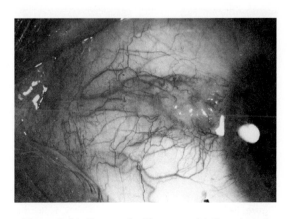

Figure 5–21. Pinguecula. (Courtesy of A Rosenberg.)

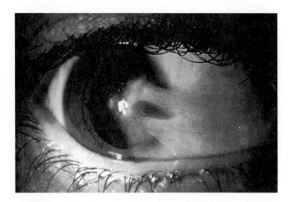

Figure 5–22. Pterygium encroaching on the cornea.

III. MISCELLANEOUS DISORDERS OF THE CONJUNCTIVA

LYMPHANGIECTASIS

Lymphangiectasis is characterized by localized small, clear, tortuous dilations in the conjunctiva. They are merely dilated lymph vessels, and no treatment is indicated unless they are irritating or cosmetically objectionable. They can then be cauterized or excised (Figure 5–23).

CONGENITAL CONJUNCTIVAL LYMPHEDEMA

This is a rare entity, unilateral or bilateral, and characterized by pinkish, fleshy edema of the bulbar conjunctiva. Usually observed as an isolated entity at birth, the condition is thought to be due to a congenital defect in the lymphatic drainage of the conjunctiva. It has been observed in chronic hereditary lymphedema of the lower extremities (Milroy's disease) and is thought to be an ocular manifestation of this disease rather than an associated anomaly.

CYSTINOSIS

Cystinosis is a rare congenital disorder of amino acid metabolism characterized by widespread intracellular deposition of cystine crystals in various body tissues, including the conjunctiva and cornea. Three types are recognized: childhood, adolescent, and adult. Life expectancy is reduced in the first two types.

SUBCONJUNCTIVAL HEMORRHAGE

This common disorder may occur spontaneously, usually in only one eye, in any age group. Its sudden onset and bright red appearance usually alarm the patient. The hemorrhage is caused by rupture of a small conjunctival vessel, sometimes preceded by a bout of severe coughing or sneezing (Figure 5–24).

The best treatment is reassurance. The hemorrhage usually absorbs in 2–3 weeks.

In rare instances the hemorrhages are bilateral or recurrent; the possibility of blood dyscrasias should then be ruled out.

OPHTHALMIA NEONATORUM

Ophthalmia neonatorum in its broad sense refers to any infection of the newborn conjunctiva. In its narrow and commonly used sense, however, it refers to a conjunctival infection, chiefly gonococcal, that follows contamination of the baby's eyes during its passage through the mother's cervix and vagina or during the postpartum period. Because gonococcal conjunctivitis can rapidly cause blindness, the cause of all cases of ophthalmia neonatorum should be verified by examination of smears of exudate, epithelial scrapings, cultures, and rapid tests for gonococci.

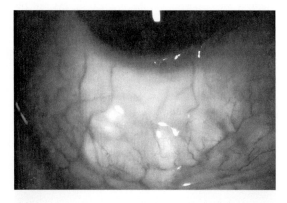

Figure 5–23. Conjunctival lymphangiectasis. Note the clear tortuous dilations in the conjunctiva.

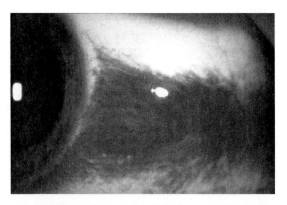

Figure 5–24. Subconjunctival hemorrhage.

Gonococcal neonatal conjunctivitis causes corneal ulceration and blindness if not treated immediately. Chlamydial neonatal conjunctivitis (inclusion blennorrhea) is less destructive but can last months if untreated and may be followed by pneumonia. Other causes include infections with staphylococci, pneumococci, *Haemophilus,* and herpes simplex virus and silver nitrate prophylaxis.

The time of onset is important but not entirely reliable in clinical diagnosis since the two principal types, gonorrheal ophthalmia and inclusion blennorrhea, have widely differing incubation periods: gonococcal disease 2–3 days and chlamydial disease 5–12 days. The third important birth canal infection (HSV-2 keratoconjunctivitis) has a 2- to 3-day incubation period and is potentially quite serious because of the possibility of systemic dissemination.

Treatment for neonatal gonococcal conjunctivitis is with ceftriaxone, 125 mg as a single intramuscular dose; a second choice is kanamycin, 75 mg intramuscularly. To treat chlamydial conjunctivitis in newborns, erythromycin oral suspension is effective at a dosage of 40 mg/kg/d in four divided doses for 2 weeks. In both gonococcal and chlamydial conjunctivitis, the parents need to be treated. Herpes simplex keratoconjunctivitis is treated with acyclovir, 30 mg/kg/d in three divided doses for 14 days. Neonatal disease from HSV requires hospitalization because of the potential neurologic or systemic manifestations. Other types of neonatal conjunctivitis are treated with erythromycin, gentamicin, or tobramycin ophthalmic ointment four times daily.

Credé 1% silver nitrate prophylaxis is effective for the prevention of gonorrheal ophthalmia but not inclusion blennorrhea or herpetic infection. The slight chemical conjunctivitis induced by silver nitrate is minor and of short duration. Accidents with concentrated solutions can be avoided by using wax ampules specially prepared for Credé prophylaxis. Tetracycline and erythromycin ointment are effective substitutes.

OCULOGLANDULAR DISEASE (PARINAUD'S OCULOGLANDULAR SYNDROME)

This is a group of conjunctival diseases, usually unilateral, characterized by low-grade fever, grossly visible preauricular adenopathy, and one or more conjunctival granulomas (Figure 5–25). The commonest cause is cat-scratch disease, but there are many other causes, including *Mycobacterium tuberculosis, Treponema pallidum, Francisella tularensis, Pasteurella (Yersinia) pseudotuberculosis, Chlamydia trachomatis* serotypes L1, L2, and L3, and *Coccidioides immitis.*

Conjunctival Cat-Scratch Disease

This protracted but benign granulomatous conjunctivitis is found most commonly in children who have been in intimate contact with cats. The child often runs

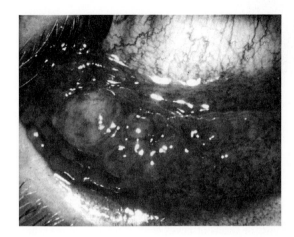

Figure 5–25. Conjunctival granuloma. (Courtesy of P Thygeson.)

a low-grade fever and develops a reasonably enlarged preauricular node and one or more conjunctival granulomas. These may show focal necrosis and may sometimes ulcerate. The regional adenopathy does not suppurate. The clinical diagnosis is supported by serology.

The disease appears to be caused by a slender pleomorphic gram-negative bacillus *(Bartonella* [formerly *Rochalimaea] henselae),* which grows in the walls of blood vessels. With special stains, this organism can be seen in biopsies of conjunctival tissue. The organism closely resembles *Leptotrichia buccalis,* and the disease was previously known as leptotrichosis conjunctivae (Parinaud's conjunctivitis). The organism is commonly found in the mouth in humans and always in the mouth in cats. The eye may be contaminated by saliva on the child's fingers or by cat saliva on the child's pillow. *Afipia felis* has been incriminated also and may still play a role.

The disease is self-limited (without corneal or other complications) and resolves in 2–3 months. The conjunctival nodule can be excised; in the case of a solitary granuloma, this may be curative. Systemic tetracyclines may shorten the course but should not be given to children under 7 years of age.

Conjunctivitis Secondary to Neoplasms (Masquerade Syndrome)

When examined superficially, a neoplasm of the conjunctiva or lid margin is often misdiagnosed as a chronic infectious conjunctivitis or keratoconjunctivitis. Since the underlying lesion is often not recognized, the condition has been referred to as masquerade syndrome. The masquerading neoplasms on record are conjunctival capillary carcinoma, conjunctival carcinoma in situ, infectious papilloma of the conjunctiva, sebaceous gland carcinoma, and verrucae. Verrucae and molluscum tumors of the lid margin may desquamate toxic tumor material that produces a chronic conjunctivitis, keratoconjunctivitis, or (rarely) keratitis alone.

IV. CONJUNCTIVAL TUMORS

J. Brooks Crawford, MD

PRIMARY BENIGN TUMORS OF THE CONJUNCTIVA

Nevus
(Figure 5–26)

One-third of melanocytic nevi of the conjunctiva lack pigment. Over half have cystic epithelial inclusions that can be seen clinically.

Histologically, conjunctival nevi are composed of nests or sheets of nevus cells. Conjunctival nevi, like other nevi, rarely become malignant. Many are excised because they are disfiguring.

Pigmented conjunctival nevi must be distinguished from primary acquired melanosis of the conjunctiva. The latter occurs later in life (after the third decade), is usually unilateral, tends to wax and wane in degree of pigmentation, and, depending on the degree of cellular atypia, has a risk of becoming malignant ranging from nil to 90%.

Papilloma

Conjunctival papillomas occur in two forms: infectious papillomas, associated with a papovavirus, occurs in children and young adults, especially in the inferior fornix and near the medial canthus (Figure 5–27). The other type arises from a broad base, often near the limbus, in older adults and may be indistinguishable from conjunctival intraepithelial neoplasia. A biopsy may be required to establish the diagnosis.

Granulomatous Inflammation

Granulomatous inflammation occurs around foreign bodies, around extravasated sebaceous material in chalazia, and in association with diseases such as coccidioidomycosis and sarcoidosis. These inflamma-

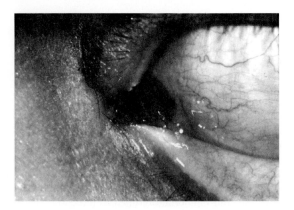

Figure 5–27. Conjunctival papilloma.

tory foci may form elevated plaques or nodules in the skin or the conjunctiva of the eyelids.

Dermoid Tumor
(Figure 5–28)

This congenital tumor appears as a smooth, rounded, yellow elevated mass, frequently with hairs protruding. A dermoid tumor may remain quiescent, though it can increase in size. Removal is indicated only if cosmetic deformity is significant or if vision is impaired or threatened. Limbal dermoids and dermolipomas are most often isolated lesions, but occasionally they may be part of such syndromes as oculoauriculovertebral dysplasia (Goldenhar's syndrome).

Dermolipoma

Dermolipoma is a common congenital tumor that usually appears as a smoothly rounded growth in the upper temporal quadrant of the bulbar conjunctiva near the lateral canthus. Treatment is usually not indicated, but at least partial removal may be indicated if the growth is enlarging or is cosmetically disfiguring. Posterior dissection must be undertaken with extreme care (if at all) since this lesion is frequently continuous with orbital fat; orbital derangement may cause scarring and complications far more serious than the original lesion.

Lymphoma & Lymphoid Hyperplasia

These are conjunctival lesions that may appear in adults without evidence of systemic disease or associated with systemic lymphosarcoma or various blood dyscrasias. The clinical appearance of benign lymphoid hyperplasia and malignant lymphoma can be similar; therefore, biopsy is essential to establish a diagnosis. Since many of these lymphoid tumors may involve the orbit, an MRI or CT scan may be required to determine the true extent of the tumor.

Treatment of both benign and malignant lesions is best accomplished with radiotherapy.

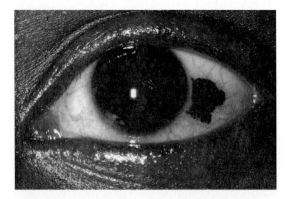

Figure 5–26. Conjunctival nevus. Note sharp borders.

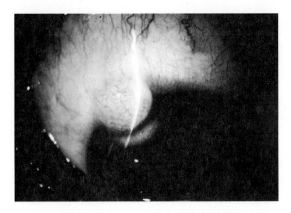

Figure 5–28. Conjunctival dermoid tumor.

Angioma

Conjunctival angiomas may occur as isolated, circumscribed capillary hemangiomas or as more diffuse vascular tumors, often associated with a more extensive lid or orbital capillary or cavernous hemangioma. Hemangiomas should be distinguished from telangiectases involving conjunctival capillaries. Telangiectatic conjunctival vessels may occur as isolated lesions or may be associated with systemic vascular hamartomas in Rendu-Osler-Weber disease or in ataxia-telangiectasia (Louis-Bar syndrome).

Pyogenic granulomas are a variety of capillary hemangiomas. They frequently occur on the palpebral conjunctiva over chalazia or in an area of recent surgery.

In Kaposi's sarcoma associated with AIDS, red-blue vascular nodules may first become apparent in the conjunctiva. They are associated with a herpesvirus. Radiotherapy is the most effective treatment.

Bacillary angiomatosis is another proliferative vascular lesion that may appear similar to Kaposi's sarcoma. It is due to infection with gram-negative bacteria of the genus *Bartonella—B henselae* from cats in patients with AIDS and *B quintana* from body lice in low-income homeless individuals. These tumors respond to antibiotic therapy.

PRIMARY MALIGNANT TUMORS OF THE BULBAR CONJUNCTIVA

Carcinoma

Carcinoma of the conjunctiva arises most frequently at the limbus in the area of the palpebral fissure and less often in nonexposed areas of the conjunctiva. Some of these tumors may resemble pterygia. Most have a gelatinous surface; sometimes, abnormal keratinization of the epithelium produces leukoplakia. Growth is slow, and deep invasion and metastases are extremely rare; therefore, complete excision is effective treatment. Recurrences are common if the lesion is incompletely excised; treatment consists of reexcision. The use of cryotherapy may help to prevent recurrences.

Conjunctival dysplasia, also called atypical epithelial dysplasia, is a benign condition that occurs as an isolated lesion or sometimes over pterygia and pingueculae and can resemble carcinoma in situ clinically and even histologically. The term **conjunctival intraepithelial neoplasia** can be applied to all neoplastic lesions from dysplasia to carcinoma that are confined to the epithelium.

Excisional biopsy will establish a diagnosis and result in cure of most of these lesions.

Malignant Melanoma

Malignant melanomas of the conjunctiva are rare. Most arise from areas of primary acquired melanosis; some arise from conjunctival nevi; a few apparently arise de novo from normal conjunctiva. Some are melanotic; others are heavily pigmented (Figure 5–29).

Many tumors can be locally excised. More radical surgery (eg, exenteration of the orbit) does not usually improve the prognosis. The use of cryotherapy after excision of melanotic tumors may help to prevent recurrences.

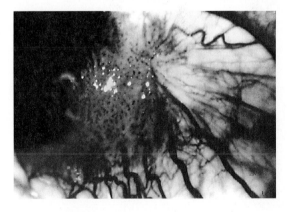

Figure 5–29. Conjunctival malignant melanoma.

REFERENCES

Bernauer W et al: The conjunctiva in acute and chronic mucous membrane pemphigoid: An immunohistochemical analysis. Ophthalmology 1993;100:339.

Buuns DR, Tse DT, Folberg R: Microscopically controlled excision of conjunctival squamous cell carcinoma. Am J Ophthalmol 1994;117:97.

Cameron JA: Shield ulcers and plaques of the cornea in vernal keratoconjunctivitis. Ophthalmology 1995;102:985.

Cano-Parra J et al: Prospective trial of intraoperative mitomycin C in the treatment of primary pterygium. Br J Ophthalmol 1995;79:439.

Char DH: *Clinical Ocular Oncology.* 2nd ed. Lippincott-Raven, 1997.

Dugal PU et al: Ocular adnexal Kaposi's sarcoma in acquired immunodeficiency syndrome. Am J Ophthalmol 1990;110:500.

Elder MJ, Bernauer W: Cryotherapy for trichiasis in ocular cicatricial pemphigoid. Br J Ophthalmol 1994;78:769.

Elder MJ, Leonard J: Sulphapyridine: A new agent for the treatment of ocular cicatricial pemphigoid. Br J Ophthalmol 1996;80:549.

Erie JC, Campbell RJ, Liesegang TJ: Conjunctival and corneal intraepithelial and invasive neoplasia. Ophthalmology 1986;93:176.

Isenberg SJ et al: Povidone-iodine for ophthalmia neonatorum prophylaxis. Am J Ophthalmol 1994;118:701.

Koehler JE et al: Molecular epidemiology of *Bartonella* infections in patients with bacillary angiomatosis-peliosis. N Engl J Med 1997;337:1876.

LeBoit PE et al: Bacillary angiomatosis: The histopathology and differential diagnosis of a pseudoneoplastic infection in patients with human immunodeficiency virus disease. Am J Surg Pathol 1989;13:909.

Lee GA, Hirst LW: Ocular surface squamous neoplasia. Surv Ophthalmol 1995;39:429.

Lee WR, Chawla JC, Reid R: Bacillary angiomatosis of the conjunctiva. Am J Ophthalmol 1994;118:152.

Lin AN et al: Review of ophthalmic findings in 204 patients with epidermolysis bullosa. Am J Ophthalmol 1994;118:384.

Mauriello JA Jr, Napolitano J, McLean I: Actinic keratosis and dysplasia of the conjunctiva: A clinicopathological study of 45 cases. Can J Ophthalmol 1995;30:312.

Montan PG, van Hage-Hamsten M: Eosinophil cationic proteins in tears in allergic conjunctivitis. Br J Ophthalmol 1996;80:556.

O'Leary JJ, Kennedy MM, McGhee JO: Kaposi's sarcoma associated with herpes virus (KSHV/HHV8): Epidemiology, molecular biology and tissue distribution. Mol Pathol 1997;50:40.

Postema EJ, Remeijer L, van der Meijden WI: Epidemiology of genital chlamydial infections in patients with chlamydial conjunctivitis; A retrospective study. Genitourin Med 1996;72:203.

Power WJ et al: Analysis of the acute ophthalmic manifestations of the erythema multiforme/Stevens-Johnson syndrome/toxic epidermal necrolysis disease spectrum. Ophthalmology 1995;102:1669.

Quaterman MJ et al: Ocular rosacea: Signs, symptoms, and tear studies before and after treatment with doxycycline. Arch Dermatol 1997;133:49.

Soparkar CNS et al: Acute and chronic conjunctivitis due to over-the-counter ophthalmic decongestants. Arch Ophthalmol 1997;115:34.

Spencer WH (editor): *Ophthalmic Pathology,* 4th ed. 4 vols. Saunders, 1996.

Tabin G et al: Late recurrences and the need for long-term follow-up in corneal and conjunctival intraepithelial neoplasia. Ophthalmology 1997;104:485.

Uchio E et al: Detection of enterovirus 70 by polymerase chain reaction in acute hemorrhagic conjunctivitis. Am J Ophthalmol 1996;122:273.

Cornea

6

Roderick Biswell, MD

PHYSIOLOGY

The cornea functions as a protective membrane and a "window" through which light rays pass to the retina. Its transparency is due to its uniform structure, avascularity, and deturgescence. Deturgescence, or the state of relative dehydration of the corneal tissue, is maintained by the active bicarbonate "pump" of the endothelium and the barrier function of the epithelium and endothelium. The endothelium is more important than the epithelium in the mechanism of dehydration, and chemical or physical damage to the endothelium is far more serious than damage to the epithelium. Destruction of the endothelial cells causes edema of the cornea and loss of transparency. On the other hand, damage to the epithelium causes only transient, localized edema of the corneal stroma that clears when the epithelial cells regenerate. Evaporation of water from the precorneal tear film produces hypertonicity of the film; that process and direct evaporation are factors that draw water from the superficial corneal stroma in order to maintain the state of dehydration.

Penetration of the intact cornea by drugs is biphasic. Fat-soluble substances can pass through intact epithelium, and water-soluble substances can pass through intact stroma. To pass through the cornea, drugs must therefore have both a lipid-soluble and a water-soluble phase.

CORNEAL RESISTANCE TO INFECTION

The epithelium is an efficient barrier to the entrance of microorganisms into the cornea. Once the epithelium is traumatized, however, the avascular stroma and Bowman's layer become susceptible to infection with a variety of organisms, including bacteria, amebas, and fungi. *Streptococcus pneumoniae* (the pneumococcus) is a true bacterial corneal pathogen; other pathogens require a heavy inoculum or a compromised host (eg, immune deficiency) to produce infection.

Moraxella liquefaciens, which occurs mainly in alcoholics (as a result of pyridoxine depletion), is a classic example of the bacterial opportunist, and in recent years a number of new corneal opportunists have been identified. Among them are *Serratia marcescens, Mycobacterium fortuitum-chelonei* complex, viridans streptococci, *Staphylococcus epidermidis,* and various coliform and *Proteus* organisms, along with viruses and fungi.

Local or systemic corticosteroids modify the host immune reaction in several ways and may allow opportunistic organisms to invade and flourish.

PHYSIOLOGY OF SYMPTOMS

Since the cornea has many pain fibers, most corneal lesions, superficial or deep (corneal foreign body, corneal abrasion, phlyctenule, interstitial keratitis), cause pain and photophobia. The pain is worsened by movement of the lids (particularly the upper lid) over the cornea and usually persists until healing occurs. Since the cornea serves as the window of the eye and refracts light rays, corneal lesions usually blur vision somewhat, especially if centrally located.

Photophobia in corneal disease is the result of painful contraction of an inflamed iris. Dilation of iris vessels is a reflex phenomenon caused by irritation of the corneal nerve endings. Photophobia, severe in most corneal disease, is minimal in herpetic keratitis because of the hypesthesia associated with the disease, which is also a valuable diagnostic sign.

Although tearing and photophobia commonly accompany corneal disease, there is usually no discharge except in purulent bacterial ulcers.

INVESTIGATION OF CORNEAL DISEASE

Symptoms & Signs

The physician examines the cornea by inspecting it under adequate illumination. Examination is often facilitated by instillation of a local anesthetic. Fluorescein staining can outline a superficial epithelial lesion that might otherwise be impossible to see. The biomicroscope (slitlamp) is essential in proper examination of the cornea; in its absence, a loupe and bright illumination can be used. One should follow the course of the light reflection while moving the light carefully over the entire cornea. Rough areas indicative of epithelial defects are demonstrated in this way.

The patient's history is important in corneal disease. A history of trauma can often be elicited—in fact, foreign bodies and abrasions are the two most common corneal lesions. A history of corneal disease may also be of value. The keratitis of herpes simplex infection is often recurrent, but since recurrent erosion is extremely painful and herpetic keratitis is not, these disorders can be differentiated by their symptoms. The patient's use of local medications should be investigated, since corticosteroids may have been used and may have predisposed to bacterial, fungal, or viral disease, especially herpes simplex keratitis. Immunosuppression also occurs with systemic diseases, such as diabetes, AIDS, and malignant disease, as well as with specific immunosuppressive therapy.

Laboratory Studies

To select the proper therapy for corneal infections, especially suppurating ulceration, laboratory aid is essential. Bacterial and fungal ulcers, for example, require completely different medications. Since a delay in identifying the organism may severely compromise the ultimate visual result, scrapings from the ulcer should be stained by both Gram's and Giemsa's stains and the infecting organism identified if possible while the patient waits. Cultures for bacteria and fungi must be done at the same time, since identification of the organism is critical. Appropriate therapy can then be instituted immediately. Therapy should not be withheld if an organism cannot be identified by smear and staining.

Morphologic Diagnosis of Corneal Lesions

A. Epithelial Keratitis: The corneal epithelium is involved in most types of conjunctivitis and keratitis and in rare cases may be the only tissue involved (eg, in superficial punctate keratitis). The epithelial changes vary widely from simple edema and vacuolation to minute erosions, filament formation, partial keratinization, etc. The lesions vary also in their location on the cornea. All of these variations have important diagnostic significance (Table 6–1), and biomicroscopic examination with and without fluorescein staining should be a part of every external eye examination.

B. Subepithelial Keratitis: There are a number of important types of discrete subepithelial lesions. These are often secondary to epithelial keratitis (eg, the subepithelial infiltrates of epidemic keratoconjunctivitis, caused by adenoviruses 8 and 19). They can usually be observed grossly but may also be recognized in the course of biomicroscopic examination of epithelial keratitis.

C. Stromal Keratitis: The responses of the corneal stroma to disease include infiltration, representing accumulation of inflammatory cells; edema manifested as corneal thickening, opacification, or scarring; thinning or melting, which may lead to perforation; and vascularization. The patterns of these responses are less specific for disease entities than those seen in epithelial keratitis, and the clinician often must rely on other clinical information and laboratory studies for clear identification of causes.

D. Endothelial Keratitis: Dysfunction of the corneal endothelium results in corneal edema, initially involving the stroma and later the epithelium. This contrasts with corneal edema due to raised intraocular pressure, in which the epithelium is affected before the stroma. As long as the cornea is not too edematous, it is often possible to visualize morphologic abnormalities of the corneal endothelium with the slitlamp. Inflammatory cells on the endothelium (keratic precipitates, or KPs) are not always an indication of endothelial disease because they are also a manifestation of anterior uveitis, which may or may not accompany stromal keratitis.

CORNEAL ULCERATION

Cicatrization due to corneal ulceration is a major cause of blindness and impaired vision throughout the world. Most of this visual loss is preventable, but only if an etiologic diagnosis is made early and appropriate therapy instituted. Central suppurative ulceration was once caused almost exclusively by *S pneumoniae.* In recent years, however, often as a result of the widespread use of compromising systemic and local medications (at least in the developed countries), opportunistic bacteria, fungi, and viruses have tended to cause more cases of corneal ulcer than *S pneumoniae.*

CENTRAL CORNEAL ULCERS

Central ulcers usually are infectious ulcers that follow epithelial damage. The lesion is situated centrally, away from the vascularized limbus. Hypopyon sometimes accompanies the ulcer. Hypopyon is a collection of inflammatory cells that appears as a pale layer in the inferior anterior chamber and is characteristic of both bacterial and fungal central corneal ulcers. Although hypopyon is sterile in bacterial corneal ulcers unless there has been a rupture of Descemet's membrane, in fungal ulcers it may contain fungal elements.

1. BACTERIAL KERATITIS

Many types of bacterial corneal ulcers look alike and vary only in severity. This is especially true of ulcers caused by opportunistic bacteria (eg, alphahemolytic streptococci, *Staphylococcus aureus, Staphylococcus epidermidis, Nocardia,* and *M fortuitum-chelonei*), which cause indolent corneal ulcers that tend to spread slowly and superficially.

Table 6–1. Principal types of epithelial keratitis (in order of frequency of occurrence).

Minute fluorescein-staining erosions; lower third of cornea affected predominantly. 1. Staphylococcal keratitis	Typically dendritic (occasionally round or oval) with edema and degeneration. 2. Herpetic keratitis (HSK)	More diffuse than lesions of HSK; occasionally linear (pseudodendrites). 3. Varicella-zoster keratitis
Minute fluorescein-staining erosions; diffuse but most conspicuous in pupillary area. 4. Adenovirus keratitis	Minute pleomorphic, fluorescein-staining, damaged epithelium and erosions; epithelial and mucous filaments are typical; lower half of cornea affected predominantly. 5. Keratitis of Sjögren's syndrome	Minute fluorescein-staining, irregular erosions; lower half of cornea affected predominantly. 6. Exposure keratitis—due to lagophthalmos or exophthalmos
Blotchy gray, opaque, syncytiumlike lesions, most conspicuous in upper pupillary area. Sometimes a plaque of opaque epithelium forms.  7. Vernal keratoconjunctivitis	Blotchy epithelial edema; diffuse but predominant in palpebral fissure, 9–3 o'clock.  8. Trophic keratitis—sequela of herpes simplex, herpes zoster, and gasserian ganglion destruction	Minute fluorescein-staining erosions with spotty cellular edema; epithelial whorls. 9. Drug-induced keratitis—especially by many antibiotics and preservatives
Foci of edematous epithelial cells, round or oval; elevated when disease is active.  10. Superficial punctate keratitis (SPK)	Minute fluorescein-staining erosions of upper third of cornea; filaments during exacerbations; bulbar hyperemia, thickened keratinized limbus, micropannus. 11. Superior limbic keratoconjunctivitis	Virus-type lesions like those of SPK; in pupillary area. 12. Rubeola, rubella, and mumps keratitis

Minute fluorescein-staining epithelial erosions affecting upper third of cornea. 13. Trachoma	Spotty gray opacification of individual epithelial cells due to partial keratinization; associated with Bitot's spots. 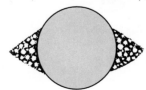 14. Vitamin A deficiency keratitis

Pneumococcal Corneal Ulcer

S pneumoniae is still a common cause of bacterial corneal ulcer in many parts of the world. Before the popularization of dacryocystorhinostomy, pneumococcal ulcers often occurred in patients with obstructed nasolacrimal ducts.

Pneumococcal corneal ulcer usually occurs 24–48 hours after inoculation of an abraded cornea. It typically produces a gray, fairly well circumscribed ulcer that tends to spread erratically from the original site of infection toward the center of the cornea (Figure 6–1). The advancing border shows active ulceration and infiltration as the trailing border begins to heal. (This creeping effect suggested the term "acute serpiginous ulcer.") The superficial corneal layers become involved first and then the deep parenchyma. The cornea surrounding the ulcer is often clear. Hypopyon is common. Scrapings from the leading edge of a pneumococcal corneal ulcer usually contain gram-positive lancet-shaped diplococci. Drugs recommended for use in treatment are listed in Tables 6–2 and 6–3. Concurrent dacryocystitis should also be treated.

Pseudomonas Corneal Ulcer

Pseudomonas corneal ulcer begins as a gray or yellow infiltrate at the site of a break in the corneal epithelium (Figure 6–2). Severe pain usually accompanies it. The lesion tends to spread rapidly in all directions because of the proteolytic enzymes produced by the organisms. Although superficial at first, the ulcer may affect the entire cornea. There is often a large hypopyon that tends to increase in size as the ulcer progresses. The infiltrate and exudate may have a bluish-green color. This is due to a pigment produced by the organism and is pathognomonic of *P aeruginosa* infection.

Pseudomonas is a common cause of bacterial corneal ulcers. Cases of *Pseudomonas* corneal ulcer may follow minor corneal abrasion or the use of soft contact lenses—especially extended wear lenses. Corneal ulcers caused by this organism can vary from

quite benign to devastating. The organism has been shown to adhere to the surface of soft contact lenses. Some cases have been reported following the use of contaminated fluorescein solution or eye drops. It is mandatory that the clinician use sterile medications and sterile technique when caring for patients with corneal injuries.

Scrapings from the ulcer may contain long, thin gram-negative rods that are often few in number. Drugs recommended for use in treatment are listed in Tables 6–2 and 6–3.

Moraxella liquefaciens Corneal Ulcer

M liquefaciens (diplobacillus of Petit) causes an indolent oval ulcer that usually affects the inferior cornea and progresses into the deep stroma over a period of days. There is usually no hypopyon or only a small one, and the surrounding cornea is usually clear. *M liquefaciens* ulcer almost always occurs in a patient with alcoholism, diabetes, or other immunosuppressing disease. Scrapings may contain large, square-ended gram-negative diplobacilli. Drugs recommended for use in treatment are listed in Tables 6–2 and 6–3. Treatment can be difficult and prolonged.

Group A *Streptococcus* Corneal Ulcer

Central corneal ulcers caused by beta-hemolytic streptococci have no identifying features. The surrounding corneal stroma is often infiltrated and edematous, and there is usually a moderately large hypopyon. Scrapings often contain gram-positive cocci in chains. Drugs recommended for use in treatment are listed in Tables 6–2 and 6–3.

Staphylococcus aureus, Staphylococcus epidermidis, & α-Hemolytic *Streptococcus* Corneal Ulcers

Central corneal ulcers caused by these organisms are now being seen more often than formerly, many of them in corneas compromised by topical corticosteroids. The ulcers are often indolent but may be associated with hypopyon and some surrounding corneal infiltration. They are often superficial, and the ulcer bed feels firm when scraped. Scrapings may contain gram-positive cocci—singly, in pairs, or in chains. Infectious crystalline keratopathy (in which the cornea has a crystalline appearance) has been described in patients receiving long-term therapy with topical steroids; the disease is often caused by α-hemolytic streptococci. Tables 6–2 and 6–3 show recommended drug regimens.

Mycobacterium fortuitum-chelonei & *Nocardia* Corneal Ulcers

Ulcers due to *M fortuitum-chelonei* and *Nocardia* are rare. They often follow trauma and are often associated with contact with soil. The ulcers are indolent, and the bed of the ulcer often has radiating lines that make it look like a cracked windshield. Hypopyon may or may

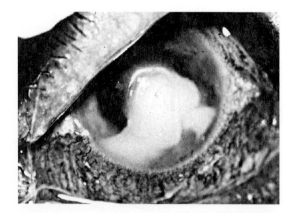

Figure 6–1. Pneumococcal corneal ulcer with hypopyon.

Table 6–2. Treatment of bacterial, fungal, and amebic keratitis.[1]

Organisms	First Choice	Second Choice	Third Choice
Gram-positive cocci: lancet-shaped with capsule = *S pneumoniae* [2]	Cefazolin	Penicillin G	Vancomycin or ceftazidime
Gram-positive rods: slender and varying in length—*Mycobacterium fortuitum, Nocardia* species, *Actinomyces* species	Amikacin	Ciprofloxacin[2]	
Other gram-positive organisms: cocci or rods	Cefazolin	Penicillin G	Vancomycin or ceftazidime
Gram-negative cocci[3]	Ceftriaxone[3]	Penicillin G	Cefazolin or vancomycin
Gram-negative rods: thin = *Pseudomonas*	Tobramycin	Ciprofloxacin	Polymyxin B or carbenicillin
Gram-negative rods: large, square-ended diplobacilli = *Moraxella*	Penicillin G	Gentamicin	Tobramycin
Other gram-negative rods	Tobramycin	Ceftazidime	Gentamicin or carbenicillin
Yeast-like organisms = *Candida* species[4]	Natamycin	Amphotericin B	Nystatin, miconazole, or flucytosine
Hyphae-like organisms = fungal ulcer	Natamycin	Amphotericin B	Miconazole
Cysts, trophozoites = *Acanthamoeba*	Propamidine and polyhexamethylene biguanide	Propamidine and neomycin	Paromomycin or miconazole
No organisms identified; ulcer suggestive of bacterial infection	Tobramycin and cefazolin	Ciprofloxacin	Gentamicin, ceftazidime, or vancomycin
No organisms identified; ulcer suggestive of fungal infection	Natamycin	Amphotericin B	Miconazole

[1] Intensive topical treatment—every hour during the day and every 2 hours during the night for 5 days—is usually sufficient in the first instance. Subconjunctival injections are rarely necessary unless there are concerns about compliance with topical therapy. Systemic therapy is not generally required. It may be used if the corneal ulcer encroaches on the limbus or if there is associated scleritis or endophthalmitis.
[2] Fluoroquinolones are not recommended for streptococcal corneal disease. Norfloxacin and ofloxacin are comparable in efficacy to ciprofloxacin.
[3] Suspected gonococcal keratitis must be treated with systemic therapy (parenteral ceftriaxone, 1–2 g daily for 5 days).
[4] Rarely, *Pityrosporum ovale* or *Pityrosporum orbiculare* may be confused with *Candida* species.

not be present. Scrapings may contain acid-fast slender rods *(M fortuitum-chelonei)* or gram-positive filamentous, often branching organisms *(Nocardia).* See Tables 6–2 and 6–3 for recommended drug regimens.

2. FUNGAL KERATITIS

Fungal corneal ulcers, once seen most commonly in agricultural workers, have become more common in the urban population since the introduction of the corticosteroid drugs for use in ophthalmology. Before the corticosteroid era, fungal corneal ulcers occurred only if an overwhelming inoculum of organisms was introduced into the corneal stroma—an event that can still take place in an agricultural setting. The uncompro-

mised cornea seems to be able to handle the small inocula to which urban residents are ordinarily subjected.

Fungal ulcers are indolent and have a gray infiltrate, often a hypopyon, marked inflammation of the globe, superficial ulceration, and satellite lesions (usually infiltrates at sites distant from the main area of ulceration) (Figure 6–3). The principal lesion—and often the satellite lesions as well—is an endothelial plaque with irregular edges underlying the principal corneal lesions, associated with a severe anterior chamber reaction and a corneal abscess.

Most fungal ulcers are caused by opportunists such as *Candida, Fusarium, Aspergillus, Penicillium, Cephalosporium,* and others. There are no identifying features that help to differentiate one type of fungal ulcer from another.

Table 6–3. Drug concentrations and dosages for treatment of bacterial or fungal keratitis.

Drug	Topical[1]	Subconjunctival[2]	Systemic[3]
Amikacin	50–100 mg/mL	25 mg/0.5 mL/dose	10–15 mg/kg/d in two or three doses
Amphotericin B	1.5–3 mg/mL	0.5–1 mg	...
Carbenicillin	4 mg/mL	125 mg/0.5 mL/dose	100–200 mg/kg/d IV in four doses
Cefazolin	50 mg/mL	100 mg/0.5 mL/dose	15 mg/kg/d IV in four doses
Ceftazidime	50 mg/mL	250 mg (0.5 mL)	1 g IV or IM every 8–12 hours (adult dose)
Ceftriaxone	...	...	1–2 g/d IV or IM
Ciprofloxacin	0.3% solution	...	250–500 mg orally every 4 hours
Flucytosine	1% solution	...	50–150 mg/kg/d orally in four doses
Gentamicin	10–20 mg/mL	20 mg/0.5 mL/dose	...
Miconazole	1% solution or 2% ointment	5–10 mg; 0.5–1 mL/dose	...
Natamycin	5% suspension	...	...
Neomycin	20 mg/mL	...	...
Nystatin	50,000 units/mL or cream (100,000 units/g)	...	...
Paromomyocin	10 mg/mL	...	...
Penicillin G	100,000 units/mL	1 million units/dose (painful)	40,000–50,000 units/kg IV in four doses; or continuously, 2–6 million units IV every 4–6 hours
Polyhexamethylene biguanide	0.01–0.02% solution	...	...
Polymyxin B	1–2 mg/mL	10 mg/0.5 mL/dose	...
Propamidine	0.1 mg/mL solution; 0.15% ointment	...	...
Tobramycin	10–20 mg/mL	20 mg/0.5 mL/dose	...
Vancomycin	50 mg/mL	25 mg/0.5mL/dose	...

[1] Topical: Every hour during the day and every 2 hours during the night for 5 days. The fortified preparations listed must be prepared by pharmacists with special training.
[2] Subconjunctival: One injection daily for 4 days unless otherwise stated; in exceptionally severe cases, initial dose sometimes repeated after 12 hours.
[3] Systemic: Intravenous or oral: One dose daily for 5 days (adult dosage).

Scrapings from fungal corneal ulcers, except those caused by *Candida,* contain hyphal elements; scrapings from *Candida* ulcers usually contain pseudohyphae or yeast forms that show characteristic budding. Tables 6–2 and 6–3 list the drugs recommended for the treatment of fungal ulcers.

3. VIRAL KERATITIS

Herpes Simplex Keratitis

Herpes simplex keratitis occurs in two forms: primary and recurrent. It is the most common cause of corneal ulceration and the most common corneal cause of blindness in the USA. The epithelial form is the ocular counterpart of labial herpes, with which it shares immunologic and pathologic features as well as having a similar time course. The only difference is that the clinical course of the keratitis may be prolonged because of the avascularity of the corneal stroma, which retards the migration of lymphocytes and macrophages to the lesion. HSV ocular infection in the immunocompetent host is usually self-limited, but in the immunologically compromised host, including patients treated with topical corticosteroids, its course can be chronic and damaging. Stromal and endothelial disease has previously been thought to be a purely immunologic response to virus particles or virally in-

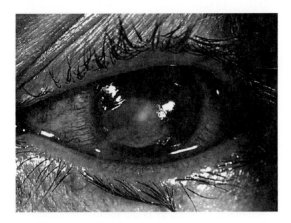

Figure 6–2. *Pseudomonas* ulcer related to 24-hour contact lens wear.

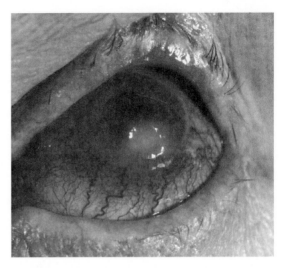

Figure 6–3. Corneal ulcer caused by *Candida albicans.*

duced cellular changes. However, there is increasing evidence that active viral infection can occur within stromal and possibly endothelial cells as well as in other tissues within the anterior segment such as the iris and trabecular endothelium. This highlights the need to assess the relative role of viral replication and host immune responses prior to and during therapy for herpetic disease. Topical corticosteroids may control damaging inflammatory responses but at the expense of facilitation of viral replication. Thus, whenever topical corticosteroids are to be used, antivirals are likely to be necessary. Any patient undergoing topical corticosteroid therapy for herpetic eye disease must be under the supervision of an ophthalmologist.

Serologic studies suggest that almost all adults have been exposed to the virus, though many do not recollect any episodes of clinical disease. Following primary infection, the virus establishes latency in the trigeminal ganglion. The factors influencing the development of recurrent disease, including its site, have yet to be unraveled. There is increasing evidence that the severity of disease is at least partly determined by the strain of virus involved. Most HSV infections of the cornea are still caused by HSV type 1 (the cause of labial herpes), but in both infants and adults a few cases caused by HSV type 2 (the cause of genital herpes) have been reported. The corneal lesions caused by the two types are indistinguishable.

Scrapings of the epithelial lesions of HSV keratitis and fluid from skin lesions contain multinucleated giant cells. The virus can be cultivated on the chorioallantoic membrane of embryonated hens' eggs and in many tissue cell lines—eg, HeLa cells, on which it produces characteristic plaques. In the majority of cases, however, diagnosis can be made clinically on the basis of characteristic dendritic or geographic ulcers and greatly reduced or absent corneal sensation.

A. Clinical Findings: Primary ocular herpes simplex is infrequently seen but is manifested as a vesicular blepharoconjunctivitis, occasionally with corneal involvement, and usually occurs in young children. It is generally self-limited, without causing significant ocular damage. Topical antiviral therapy may be used as prophylaxis against corneal involvement and as therapy for corneal disease.

Attacks of the common recurrent type of herpetic keratitis (Figure 6–4) are triggered by fever, overexposure to ultraviolet light, trauma, psychic stress, the onset of menstruation, or some other local or systemic source of immunosuppression. Unilaterality is the rule, but bilateral lesions develop in 4–6% of cases and are seen most often in atopic patients.

1. Symptoms–The first symptoms are usually irritation, photophobia, and tearing. When the central

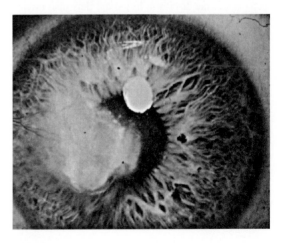

Figure 6–4. Corneal scar caused by recurrent herpes simplex keratitis. (Courtesy of A Rosenberg.)

cornea is affected, there is also some reduction in vision. Since corneal anesthesia usually occurs early in the course of the infection, the symptoms may be minimal and the patient may not seek medical advice. There is often a history of fever blisters or other herpetic infection, but corneal ulceration can occasionally be the only sign of a recurrent herpetic infection.

2. Lesions–The most characteristic lesion is the **dendritic ulcer.** It occurs in the corneal epithelium, has a typical branching, linear pattern with feathery edges, and has terminal bulbs at its ends (Figure 6–5). Fluorescein staining makes the dendrite easy to identify, but unfortunately herpetic keratitis can also simulate many corneal infections and must be considered in the differential diagnosis of many corneal lesions.

Geographic ulceration is a form of chronic dendritic disease in which the delicate dendritic lesion takes a broader form. The edges of the ulcer lose their feathery quality. Corneal sensation, as with dendritic disease, is diminished. The clinician should always test for this sign.

Other corneal epithelial lesions that may be caused by HSV are a blotchy epithelial keratitis, stellate epithelial keratitis, and filamentary keratitis. All of these are usually transitory, however, and often become typical dendrites within a day or two.

Subepithelial opacities can be caused by HSV infection. A ghost-like image, corresponding in shape to the original epithelial defect but slightly larger, can be seen in the area immediately underlying the epithelial lesion. The "ghost" remains superficial but is often enhanced by the use of antiviral drugs, especially idoxuridine. As a rule, these subepithelial lesions do not persist for more than a year.

Disciform keratitis is the most common form of stromal disease in HSV infection. The stroma is edematous in a central, disk-shaped area, without significant infiltration and usually without vascularization. The edema may be sufficient to produce folds in Descemet's membrane. Keratic precipitates may lie directly under the disciform lesion but may also involve the entire endothelium because of the frequently associated anterior uveitis. The pathogenesis of disciform keratitis is generally regarded as an immunologic reaction to viral antigens in the stroma or endothelium, but active viral disease cannot be ruled out. Like most herpetic lesions in immunocompetent individuals, disciform keratitis is normally self-limited, lasting weeks to months. Edema is the most prominent sign, and healing can occur with minimal scarring and vascularization. A similar clinical appearance is seen with primary endothelial keratitis (endothelitis), which can be associated with anterior uveitis together with raised intraocular pressure and a focal inflammation of the iris. This is thought to be due to viral replication within the various anterior chamber structures.

Stromal HSV keratitis in the form of focal areas of infiltration and edema, often accompanied by vascularization, is likely to be predominantly due to viral replication. Corneal thinning and perforation may develop rapidly, particularly if topical corticosteroids are being used. If there is stromal disease in the presence of epithelial ulceration, it may be difficult to differentiate bacterial or fungal superinfection from herpetic disease. The features of the epithelial disease need to be carefully scrutinized for herpetic characteristics, but a bacterial or fungal component may be present and the patient must be managed accordingly. Stromal necrosis also may be caused by an acute immune reaction, again complicating the diagnosis with regard to active viral disease. Hypopyon may be seen with necrosis as well as secondary bacterial or fungal infection.

Peripheral lesions of the cornea can also be caused by HSV. They are usually linear and show a loss of epithelium before the underlying corneal stroma becomes infiltrated. (This is in contrast to the marginal ulcer associated with bacterial hypersensitivity—eg, to *S aureus* in staphylococcal blepharitis, in which the infiltration precedes the loss of the overlying epithelium.) Testing for corneal sensation is unreliable in peripheral herpetic disease. The patient is apt to be far less photophobic than patients with nonherpetic corneal infiltrates and ulceration usually are.

B. Treatment: The treatment of HSV keratitis should be directed at eliminating viral replication within the cornea, while minimizing the damaging effects of the inflammatory response.

1. Debridement–An effective way to treat dendritic keratitis is epithelial debridement, since the virus is located in the epithelium and debridement will also reduce the viral antigenic load to the corneal stroma. Healthy epithelium adheres tightly to the cornea, but infected epithelium is easy to remove. Debridement is accomplished with a tightly wound cotton-tipped applicator. Topical iodine or ether has no value and can cause chemical keratitis. A cycloplegic such as atropine 1% or homatropine 5% is then instilled into the conjunctival sac, and a pressure dressing is applied. The patient should be examined daily and the dressing changed until the corneal defect has healed—usually within 72 hours. Adjunctive therapy with a topical an-

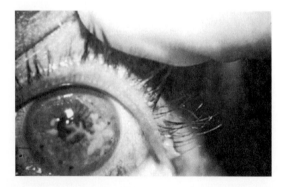

Figure 6–5. Dendritic figures seen in herpes simplex keratitis.

tiviral accelerates epithelial healing. Topical drug therapy without epithelial debridement for epithelial keratitis offers the advantage of not requiring patching but involves a hazard of drug toxicity.

2. Drug therapy–The topical antiviral agents used in herpetic keratitis are idoxuridine, trifluridine, vidarabine, and acyclovir. (Topical acyclovir for ophthalmic use is not available in the USA.) Trifluridine and acyclovir are much more effective in stromal disease than the others. Idoxuridine and trifluridine are frequently associated with toxic reactions. Oral acyclovir may be useful in the treatment of severe herpetic eye disease, particularly in atopic individuals who are susceptible to aggressive ocular and dermal (eczema herpeticum) herpetic disease.

Viral replication in the immunocompetent patient, particularly when confined to the corneal epithelium, usually is self-limited and scarring is minimal. It is then unnecessary and potentially highly damaging to use topical corticosteroids. Regrettably, the clinician sometimes immunosuppresses the patient by using corticosteroids to reduce local inflammation. This is based on the misconception that reducing inflammation reduces the disease. Even when the inflammatory response is thought to be purely immunologically driven, such as in disciform keratitis, topical corticosteroids are often best avoided if the episode is likely to be self-limited. Once topical corticosteroids have been used, this usually commits the patient to requiring the drug to control further episodes of keratitis, with the potential for uncontrolled viral replication and the other steroid-related side effects such as bacterial and fungal superinfection, glaucoma, and cataract. Topical corticosteroids may also accelerate corneal melting, thus increasing the risk of corneal perforation. If it becomes necessary to use topical corticosteroids because of the severity of the inflammatory response, it is absolutely essential that appropriate antiviral therapy be used to control viral replication.

3. Surgical treatment–Penetrating keratoplasty may be indicated for visual rehabilitation in patients with severe corneal scarring, but it should not be undertaken until the herpetic disease has been inactive for many months. Postoperatively, recurrent herpetic infection may occur as a result of the surgical trauma and the topical corticosteroids necessary to prevent corneal graft rejection. It may also be difficult to distinguish corneal graft rejection from recurrent stromal disease. Systemic antiviral agents should be used for several months after keratoplasty to cover the use of topical steroids.

Corneal perforation due to progressive herpetic stromal disease or superinfection with bacteria or fungi may necessitate emergency penetrating keratoplasty. Cyanoacrylate tissue adhesives can be used effectively to seal small perforations, and lamellar "patch" grafts have been successful in selected cases. Lamellar keratoplasty has the advantage over penetrating keratoplasty of reduced potential for corneal graft rejection. A therapeutic soft contact lens or tarsorrhaphy may be required to heal epithelial defects associated with herpes simplex keratitis.

4. Control of trigger mechanisms that reactivate HSV infection–Recurrent HSV infections of the eye are common, occurring in about one-third of cases within 2 years after the first attack. A trigger mechanism can often be discovered by careful questioning of the patient. Once identified, the trigger can often be avoided. Aspirin can be used to avoid fever, excessive exposure to the sun or ultraviolet light can be avoided, situations that might cause psychic stress can be minimized, and aspirin can be taken just prior to the onset of menstruation.

Varicella-Zoster Viral Keratitis

Varicella-zoster virus (VZV) infection occurs in two forms: primary (varicella) and recurrent (herpes zoster). Ocular manifestations are uncommon in varicella but common in ophthalmic zoster. In varicella (chickenpox), the usual eye lesions are pocks on the lids and lid margins. Rarely, keratitis occurs (typically a peripheral stromal lesion with vascularization), and still more rarely epithelial keratitis with or without pseudodendrites. Disciform keratitis, with uveitis of varying duration, has been reported.

In contrast to the rare and benign corneal lesions of varicella, the relatively frequent ophthalmic herpes zoster is often accompanied by keratouveitis that varies in severity according to the immune status of the patient. Thus, although children with zoster keratouveitis usually have benign disease, the aged have severe and sometimes blinding disease. Corneal complications in ophthalmic zoster often occur if there is a skin eruption in areas supplied by the branches of the nasociliary nerve.

Unlike recurrent HSV keratitis that usually affects only the epithelium, VZV keratitis affects the stroma and anterior uvea at onset. The epithelial lesions are blotchy and amorphous except for an occasional linear pseudodendrite that only vaguely resembles the true dendrites of HSV keratitis. Stromal opacities consist of edema and mild cellular infiltration and initially are subepithelial. Deep stromal disease can follow with necrosis and vascularization (Figure 6–6). A disciform keratitis sometimes develops and resembles HSV disciform keratitis. Loss of corneal sensation is always a prominent feature and often persists for months after the corneal lesion appears to have healed. The associated uveitis tends to persist for weeks or months, but with time it eventually heals. Scleritis (sclerokeratitis) can be a serious feature of VZV ocular disease.

Intravenous and oral acyclovir have been used successfully for the treatment of herpes zoster ophthalmicus, particularly in immunocompromised patients. The oral dosage is 800 mg five times daily for 10–14 days. Therapy needs to be started within 72

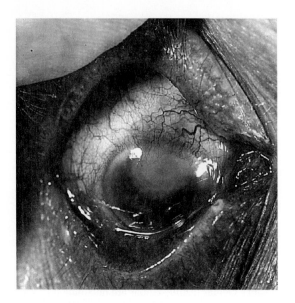

Figure 6–6. Herpes zoster keratitis.

hours after appearance of the rash. The role of topical antivirals is less certain. Topical corticosteroids may be necessary to treat severe keratitis, uveitis, and secondary glaucoma. The use of systemic corticosteroids is controversial. They may be indicated in reducing the incidence and severity of postherpetic neuralgia, but the risk of steroid complications is significant. Unfortunately, systemic acyclovir has little influence on the development of postherpetic neuralgia. However, the condition is self-limited, and reassurance can be helpful as a supplement to analgesics.

4. *ACANTHAMOEBA* KERATITIS

Acanthamoeba is a free-living protozoan that thrives in polluted water containing bacteria and organic material. Corneal infection with *Acanthamoeba* is an increasingly recognized complication of soft contact lens wear, particularly when homemade saline solutions are used. It may also occur in non-contact lens wearers after exposure to contaminated water or soil.

The initial symptoms are pain out of proportion to the clinical findings, redness, and photophobia. The characteristic clinical signs are indolent corneal ulceration, a stromal ring, and perineural infiltrates. The earlier forms of the disease with changes confined to the corneal epithelium are being more frequently recognized. *Acanthamoeba* keratitis is commonly misdiagnosed initially as herpetic keratitis.

The diagnosis is confirmed by scrapings and by culturing on specially prepared media. Corneal biopsy may be required. Histopathologic sections reveal the presence of amebic forms (trophozoites or cysts). Contact lens cases and solutions should be cultured. Often the amebic forms can be identified in the contact lens case fluid.

The differential diagnosis includes fungal keratitis, herpetic keratitis, mycobacterial keratitis, and *Nocardia* infection of the cornea.

In the early stages of the disease, epithelial debridement may be beneficial. Medical treatment is usually started with intensive topical propamidine isethionate (1% solution) and either polyhexamethylene biguanide (0.01–0.02% solution) or fortified neomycin eyedrops (Tables 6–2 and 6–3). *Acanthamoeba* spp may have variable drug sensitivities and may acquire drug resistance. Treatment is also hampered by the organisms' ability to encyst within the corneal stroma, necessitating prolonged treatment. Topical corticosteroids may be required to control the associated inflammatory reaction in the cornea.

Keratoplasty may be necessary in advanced disease to arrest progression of the infection or after resolution and scarring to restore vision. Once the organism has reached the sclera, medical and surgical treatment are usually fruitless.

PERIPHERAL CORNEAL ULCERS

1. MARGINAL INFILTRATES & ULCERS

The majority of marginal corneal ulcers are benign but extremely painful. They are secondary to acute or chronic bacterial conjunctivitis, particularly staphylococcal blepharoconjunctivitis and less often Koch-Weeks *(Haemophilus aegyptius)* conjunctivitis. They are not an infectious process, however, and scrapings do not contain the causal bacteria. They are the result of sensitization to bacterial products, antibody from the limbal vessels reacting with antigen that has diffused through the corneal epithelium.

Marginal infiltrates and ulcers (Figure 6–7) start as oval or linear infiltrates, separated from the limbus by a lucid interval, and only later may ulcerate and vas-

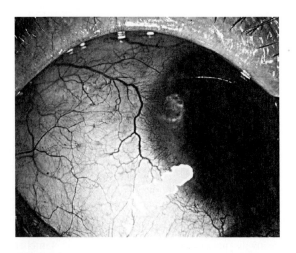

Figure 6–7. Marginal ulcer of temporal cornea, right eye. (Courtesy of P Thygeson.)

cularize. They are self-limited, usually lasting from 7 to 10 days, but those associated with staphylococcal blepharoconjunctivitis usually recur. Treatment for blepharitis (shampoo scrubs, antimicrobials) usually will clear the problem; topical corticosteroids may be needed for severe cases. Topical corticosteroid preparations shorten their course and relieve symptoms, which are often severe, but treatment of the underlying blepharoconjunctivitis is essential if recurrences are to be prevented. Before starting corticosteroid therapy, great care must be taken to distinguish this entity, formerly known as "catarrhal corneal ulceration," from marginal herpetic keratitis. Since marginal herpetic keratitis is usually almost symptomless because of corneal anesthesia, differentiating it from the painful, hypersensitivity-type marginal ulcer is not difficult.

2. MOOREN'S ULCER
(Figure 6–8)

The cause of Mooren's ulcer is still unknown, but an autoimmune origin is suspected. It is a marginal ulcer, unilateral in 60–80% of cases and characterized by painful, progressive excavation of the limbus and peripheral cornea that often leads to loss of the eye. It occurs most commonly in old age but does not seem to be related to any of the systemic diseases that most often afflict the aged. It is unresponsive to both antibiotics and corticosteroids. Surgical excision of the limbal conjunctiva in an effort to remove sensitizing substances has recently been advocated. Lamellar tectonic keratoplasty has been used with success in selected cases. Systemic immunosuppressive therapy may be helpful in advanced disease.

3. PHLYCTENULAR KERATOCONJUNCTIVITIS

This hypersensitivity disease (due to delayed hypersensitivity to bacterial products, eg, the human tubercle bacillus) was formerly a major cause of visual loss in the USA, particularly among the Eskimos and Native Americans. Phlyctenules are localized accumulations of lymphocytes, monocytes, macrophages, and finally neutrophils. They appear first at the limbus, but in recurrent attacks they may involve the bulbar conjunctiva and cornea. Corneal phlyctenules, usually bilateral, cicatrize and vascularize, but conjunctival phlyctenules leave no trace.

Most cases of phlyctenular keratoconjunctivitis in the USA today are caused by delayed hypersensitivity to *S aureus*. The antigen is released locally from staphylococci that proliferate on the lid margin in staphylococcal blepharitis. Rare phlyctenules have occurred in San Joaquin Valley fever, a result of hypersensitivity to a primary infection with *Coccidioides immitis*. In this disease they are not visually important, however.

In the tuberculous type, the attack may be triggered by an acute bacterial conjunctivitis but is associated typically with a transient increase in the activity of a childhood tuberculosis. Untreated phlyctenules run a course to healing in 10–14 days, but topical therapy with corticosteroid preparations dramatically shortens the course to a day or two and often decreases scarring and vascularization. The corticosteroid response in the staphylococcal type is less dramatic, however, and treatment consists essentially of eliminating the causal bacterial infection.

4. MARGINAL KERATITIS IN AUTOIMMUNE DISEASE
(Figure 6–9)

The corneal periphery receives its nourishment from the aqueous humor, the limbal capillaries, and the tear film. It is contiguous with the subconjunctival lym-

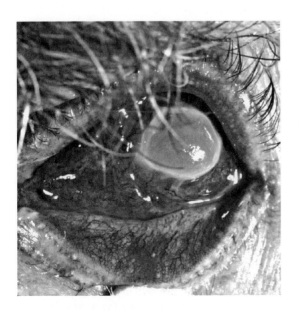

Figure 6–8. Advanced Mooren's ulcer.

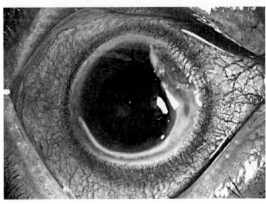

Figure 6–9. Marginal keratitis. (Courtesy of M Hogan.)

phoid tissue and the lymphatic arcades at the limbus. The perilimbal conjunctiva appears to play an important role in the pathogenesis of corneal lesions that arise both from local ocular disease and from systemic disorders, particularly those of autoimmune origin. There is a striking similarity between the limbal capillary network and the renal glomerular capillary network. On the endothelial basement membranes of the capillaries of both networks, immune complexes are deposited and immunologic disease results. Thus, the peripheral cornea often participates in such autoimmune diseases as rheumatoid arthritis, polyarteritis nodosa, systemic lupus erythematosus, scleroderma, midline lethal and Wegener's granulomatosis, ulcerative colitis, Crohn's disease, and relapsing polychondritis. The corneal changes are secondary to scleral inflammation, with or without scleral vascular closure (see Chapter 7). The clinical signs include vascularization, infiltration and opacification, and peripheral guttering that may progress to perforation. Treatment is directed toward control of the associated systemic disease; topical therapy usually is ineffective, and systemic use of potent immunosuppressive drugs often is required. Corneal perforation may require keratoplasty.

5. CORNEAL ULCER DUE TO VITAMIN A DEFICIENCY

The typical corneal ulcer associated with avitaminosis A is centrally located and bilateral, gray and indolent, with a definite lack of corneal luster in the surrounding area (Figure 6–10). The cornea becomes soft and necrotic (hence the term, "keratomalacia"), and perforation is common. The epithelium of the conjunctiva is keratinized, as evidenced by the presence of a Bitot spot. This is a foamy, wedge-shaped area in the conjunctiva, usually on the temporal side,

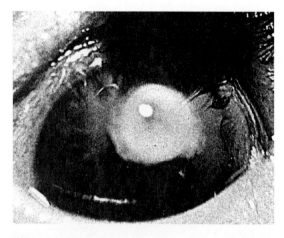

Figure 6–10. Keratomalacia with ulceration associated with xerophthalmia (dietary) in an infant. (Photo by Diane Beeston.)

with the base of the wedge at the limbus and the apex extending toward the lateral canthus. Within the triangle the conjunctiva is furrowed concentrically with the limbus, and dry flaky material can be seen falling from the area into the inferior cul-de-sac. A stained conjunctival scraping from a Bitot spot will show many saprophytic xerosis bacilli (*Corynebacterium xerosis;* small curved rods) and keratinized epithelial cells.

Avitaminosis A corneal ulceration results from dietary lack of vitamin A or impaired absorption from the gastrointestinal tract and impaired utilization by the body. It may develop in an infant who has a feeding problem; in an adult who is on a restricted or generally inadequate diet; or in any person with a biliary obstruction since bile in the gastrointestinal tract is necessary for the absorption of vitamin A. Lack of vitamin A causes a generalized keratinization of the epithelium throughout the body. The conjunctival and corneal changes together are known as **xerophthalmia.** Since the epithelium of the air passages is affected, many patients, if not treated, will die of pneumonia. Avitaminosis A also causes a generalized retardation of osseous growth. This is extremely important in infants; for example, if the skull bones do not grow and the brain continues to grow, increased intracranial pressure and papilledema can result.

Mild vitamin A deficiency should be treatment in adults with a dose of 30,000 units/d for 1 week. Advanced cases will require much higher doses initially (20,000 units/kg/d). Sulfonamide or antibiotic ointment can be used locally in the eye to prevent secondary bacterial infection. The average daily requirement of vitamin A is 1500–5000 IU for children, according to age, and 5000 IU for adults.

6. NEUROTROPHIC KERATITIS

If the trigeminal nerve, which supplies the cornea, is interrupted by trauma, surgery, tumor, inflammation, or in any other way, the cornea loses its sensitivity and one of its best defenses against degeneration, ulceration, and infection—ie, a healthy blink reflex. In the early stages of a typical neurotrophic ulcer, fluorescein solution will produce punctate staining of the superficial epithelium. As this process progresses, patchy areas of denudation appear. Occasionally the epithelium may be absent from a large area of the cornea.

In the absence of corneal sensation, even a severe keratitis may produce little discomfort. Patients must be warned to look out for redness of the eye, reduced vision, or increased conjunctival discharge and to seek ophthalmic care as soon as any of these develop.

Keeping the cornea moist with artificial tears and lubricant ointments may help to protect it. Once a keratitis develops, it must be treated promptly. The most effective management is to keep the eye closed either by careful horizontal taping of the eyelids, by tarsorrhaphy, or by means of ptosis induced with botulinum toxin A. Swim goggles may be useful at night. Secondary corneal infection must be treated appropriately.

7. EXPOSURE KERATITIS

Exposure keratitis may develop in any situation in which the cornea is not properly moistened and covered by the eyelids. Examples include exophthalmos from any cause, ectropion, the floppy lid syndrome, the absence of part of an eyelid as a result of trauma, and inability to close the lids properly, as in Bell's palsy. The two factors at work are the drying of the cornea and its exposure to minor trauma. The uncovered cornea is particularly subject to drying during sleeping hours. If an ulcer develops it usually follows minor trauma and occurs in the inferior third of the cornea.

This type of keratitis will be sterile unless it is secondarily infected, and the therapeutic objective is to provide protection and moisture for the entire corneal surface. The treatment method depends upon the underlying condition: a plastic procedure on the eyelids, correction of exophthalmos, or use of the options mentioned above in the discussion of neurotrophic keratitis.

EPITHELIAL KERATITIS

CHLAMYDIAL KERATITIS

All five principal types of chlamydial conjunctivitis (trachoma, inclusion conjunctivitis, primary ocular lymphogranuloma venereum, parakeet or psittacosis conjunctivitis, and feline pneumonitis conjunctivitis) are accompanied by corneal lesions. Only in trachoma and lymphogranuloma venereum, however, have they been blinding or visually damaging. The corneal lesions of trachoma have been the most studied and are of great diagnostic importance. In order of appearance they consist of (1) epithelial microerosions affecting the upper third of the cornea; (2) micropannus; (3) subepithelial round opacities, commonly called trachoma pustules; (4) limbal follicles and their cicatricial remains, known as Herbert's peripheral pits; (5) gross pannus; and (6) extensive, diffuse, subepithelial cicatrization. Mild cases of trachoma may show only epithelial keratitis and micropannus and may heal without impairing vision.

The rare cases of lymphogranuloma venereum have shown fewer characteristic changes but are known to have caused blindness by diffuse corneal scarring and total pannus. The remaining types of chlamydial infection cause only micropannus, epithelial keratitis, and, rarely, subepithelial opacities which are not visually significant.

Chlamydial keratoconjunctivitis responds to systemic sulfonamides (except for the rare *C psittaci* infections, which are sulfonamide-resistant), tetracyclines, or erythromycin.

DRUG-INDUCED EPITHELIAL KERATITIS

Epithelial keratitis is not uncommonly seen in patients using antiviral medications (idoxuridine and trifluridine) and several of the broad-spectrum and medium-spectrum antibiotics such as neomycin, gentamicin, and tobramycin. It is usually a superficial keratitis affecting predominantly the lower half of the cornea and interpalpebral fissure and may cause permanent scarring. The preservatives in eyedrops, particularly benzalkonium chloride, are a potent cause of toxic keratitis.

KERATOCONJUNCTIVITIS SICCA (SJÖGREN'S SYNDROME)

Epithelial filaments in the lower quadrants of the cornea are the cardinal signs of this autoimmune disease in which secretion of the lacrimal and accessory lacrimal glands is diminished or eliminated. There is also a blotchy epithelial keratitis that affects mainly the lower quadrants. Severe cases show mucous pseudofilaments that stick to the corneal epithelium.

This keratitis of Sjögren's syndrome must be distinguished from the keratitis sicca of such cicatrizing diseases as trachoma and ocular pemphigoid, in which the goblet cells of the conjunctiva have been destroyed. Such cases sometimes still produce tears, but without mucus the corneal epithelium sheds the tears and continues to be dry.

Treatment of keratoconjunctivitis sicca calls for the frequent use of tear substitutes and lubricating ointments, of which there are many commercial preparations. When goblet cells have been destroyed, as in the cicatricial conjunctivitides, mucus substitutes must be used in addition to artificial tears. Topical vitamin A may help to reverse the epithelial keratinization. Moisture chambers or swim goggles may be required. Lacrimal punctal plugs and punctal occlusion are important in the management of advanced cases.

ADENOVIRUS KERATITIS

Keratitis usually accompanies all types of adenoviral conjunctivitis, reaching its peak 5–7 days after onset of the conjunctivitis. It is a fine epithelial keratitis best seen with the slit lamp after instillation of fluorescein. The minute lesions may group together to make up larger ones.

The epithelial keratitis is often followed by subepithelial opacities. In epidemic keratoconjunctivitis (EKC), which is due to adenovirus types 8 and 19, the subepithelial lesions are round and grossly visible. They appear 8–15 days after onset of the conjunctivitis and may persist for months or even (rarely) for several years. Similar lesions occur very exceptionally in other adenoviral infections, eg, those caused by types 3, 4, and 7, but tend to be transitory and mild, lasting a few weeks at most.

Although the corneal opacities of adenoviral keratoconjunctivitis tend to fade temporarily with the use of topical corticosteroids, and although the patient is often made temporarily more comfortable thereby, corticosteroid therapy may prolong the corneal disease and is therefore not recommended. No medication is needed.

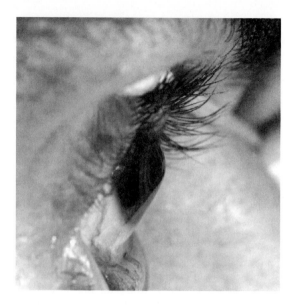

Figure 6–11. Keratoconus.

OTHER VIRAL KERATITIDES

A fine epithelial keratitis may be seen in other viral infections such as measles (in which the central cornea is affected predominantly), rubella, mumps, infectious mononucleosis, acute hemorrhagic conjunctivitis, Newcastle disease conjunctivitis, and verruca of the lid margin. A superior epithelial keratitis and pannus often accompany molluscum contagiosum nodules on the lid margin.

DEGENERATIVE CORNEAL CONDITIONS

KERATOCONUS

Keratoconus is an uncommon degenerative bilateral disease that may be inherited as an autosomal recessive or autosomal dominant trait. Unilateral cases of unknown cause occur rarely. Symptoms appear in the second decade of life. The disease affects all races. Keratoconus has been associated with a number of diseases, including Down's syndrome, atopic dermatitis, retinitis pigmentosa, aniridia, vernal catarrh, Marfan's syndrome, Apert's syndrome, and Ehlers-Danlos syndrome. Pathologically, there are disruptive changes in Bowman's layer with keratocyte degeneration and ruptures in Descemet's membrane.

Blurred vision is the only symptom. Many patients present with rapidly increasing myopic astigmatism. Signs include cone-shaped cornea (Figure 6–11); linear narrow folds centrally in Descemet's membrane (Vogt's lines), which are pathognomonic; an iron ring around the base of the cone (Fleischer's ring); and, in extreme cases, indentation of the lower lid by the cornea when the patient looks down (Munson's sign). There is an irregular or scissor reflex on retinoscopy and a distorted corneal reflection with Placido's disk or the keratoscope—all of which often being more obvious in the early stages than the other corneal signs. Color-coded topography units provide more accurate information on the degree of corneal distortion (Figure 2–26). Generally, the fundi cannot be clearly seen because of corneal astigmatism.

Acute hydrops of the cornea may occur, manifested by sudden diminution of vision associated with central corneal edema. This arises as a consequence of rupture of Descemet's membrane and may be triggered by the patient rubbing the eye. The condition may be mistaken for extreme thinning with impending perforation. Acute hydrops usually clears gradually without treatment but often leaves apical scarring.

Rigid contact lenses will markedly improve vision in the early stages by correcting irregular astigmatism. Keratoconus is one of the most common indications for penetrating keratoplasty. Surgery is indicated when a contact lens can no longer be effectively worn or when peripheral thinning will affect the surgery.

Keratoconus is often slowly progressive between the ages of 20 and 60, although an arrest in progression of the keratoconus may occur at any time. If a corneal transplant is done before extreme corneal thinning occurs, the prognosis is excellent; about 80–95% obtain good best-corrected sight.

CORNEAL DEGENERATION

The corneal degenerations are a rare group of slowly progressive, bilateral, degenerative disorders that usually appear in the second or third decades of life. Some are hereditary. Other cases follow ocular inflammatory disease, and some are of unknown cause.

Marginal Degeneration of the Cornea

A. Terrien's Disease: This is a rare bilateral symmetric degeneration characterized by marginal thinning of the upper nasal quadrants of the cornea. Males are more commonly affected than females, and the condition occurs more frequently in the third and fourth decades. There are no symptoms except for mild irritation during occasional inflammatory episodes, and the condition is slowly progressive. The clinical picture consists of marginal thinning and peripheral vascularization with lipid deposition. Perforation is a known complication, especially from trauma. Tectonic (structural) keratoplasty may be required. Histopathologic studies of affected corneas have revealed vascularized connective tissue with fibrillary degeneration and fatty infiltration of collagen fibers.

Because the course of progression is slow and the central cornea is spared, the prognosis is good.

B. Band (Calcific) Keratopathy: (Figure 6–12.) This disorder is characterized by the deposition of calcium salts in the anterior layers of the cornea. The keratopathy is usually limited to the interpalpebral area and appears as a band. The calcium deposits are noted in the basement membrane, Bowman's layer, and anterior stromal lamellas. A clear margin separates the calcific band from the limbus, and clear holes may be seen in the band, giving the Swiss

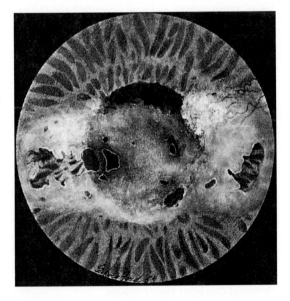

Figure 6–12. Calcific band keratopathy. (Courtesy of M Hogan.)

cheese appearance. Symptoms include irritation, injection, and blurring of vision.

Calcific band keratopathy has been described in a number of inflammatory, metabolic, and degenerative conditions. It is characteristically associated with juvenile rheumatoid arthritis. It has been described in long-standing inflammatory conditions of the eye, glaucoma, and chronic cyclitis. Band keratopathy may also be associated with hyperparathyroidism, vitamin D intoxication, sarcoidosis, and leprosy. Treatment consists of removal of the corneal epithelium by curettage under topical anesthesia followed by irrigation of the cornea with a sterile 0.01-molar solution of ethylenediaminetetraacetic acid (EDTA) or application of EDTA with a cotton applicator. The excimer laser has shown particular value in the treatment of band keratoplasty, or the band can be removed surgically.

Climatic Droplet Keratopathy (Labrador Keratopathy, Spheroid Degeneration of the Cornea) (Figure 6–13)

Climatic droplet keratopathy affects mainly men who work out of doors. The corneal degeneration is thought to be caused by exposure to ultraviolet light and is characterized in the early stages by fine subepithelial yellow droplets in the peripheral cornea. As the disease advances, the droplets become central, with subsequent corneal clouding causing blurred vision. Treatment in advanced cases is by corneal transplantation.

Salzmann's Nodular Degeneration

This disorder is always preceded by corneal inflammation, particularly phlyctenular keratoconjunctivitis or trachoma. Symptoms include redness, irritation, and blurring of vision. There is degeneration of the superficial cornea that involves the stroma, Bowman's layer, and epithelium with superficial whitish-gray elevated nodules sometimes occurring in chains.

Corneal transplantation is rarely required; superficial lamellar keratectomy or phototherapeutic (laser) keratectomy can result in visual improvement.

Rigid contact lenses will significantly improve visual acuity in most cases.

ARCUS SENILIS (CORNEAL ANNULUS, ANTERIOR EMBRYOTOXON)

Arcus senilis is an extremely common, bilateral, benign peripheral corneal degeneration that may occur at any age but is far more common in elderly people as part of the aging process. Arcus senilis in people under age 50 is often associated with hypercholesterolemia; blood lipid studies should be done.

Pathologically, lipid droplets involve the entire

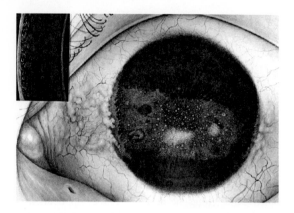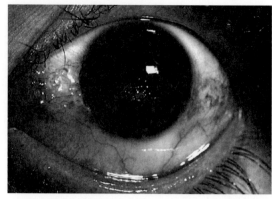

Figure 6–13. Two photos showing climatic droplet (Labrador) keratodystrophy. Inset at left shows slitlamp view. (Photo at left courtesy of A Ahmad.)

corneal thickness but are more concentrated in the superficial and deep layers, being relatively sparse in the corneal stroma.

There are no symptoms. Clinically, arcus senilis appears as a hazy gray ring about 2 mm in width and with a clear space between it and the limbus (Figure 6–14). No treatment is necessary, and there are no complications.

HEREDITARY CORNEAL DYSTROPHIES

This is a group of rare hereditary disorders of the cornea of unknown cause characterized by bilateral abnormal deposition of substances and associated with alteration in the normal corneal architecture that may or may not interfere with vision. These corneal dystrophies usually manifest themselves during the first or second decade but sometimes later. They may be stationary or slowly progressive throughout life.

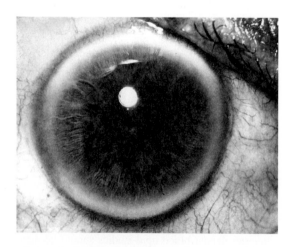

Figure 6–14. Arcus senilis. (Photo by Diane Beeston.)

Corneal transplantation, when indicated, improves vision in most patients with hereditary corneal dystrophy.

Anatomically, corneal dystrophies may be classified as epithelial, stromal, and posterior limiting membrane dystrophies.

Epithelial Corneal Dystrophies

A. Meesman's Dystrophy: This slowly progressive disorder is characterized by microcystic areas in the epithelium. The onset is in early childhood (first 1–2 years of life). The main symptom is slight irritation, and vision is slightly affected. The inheritance is autosomal dominant.

B. Anterior Membrane Dystrophies (Cogan's, Map-Dot-Fingerprint): Map or fingerprint patterns are seen at the level of the epithelial basement membrane. Debris, cysts, and dots also may be noted. Recurrent erosion is common. Vision usually is not significantly affected. In Cogan's dystrophy, intraepithelial opacities are seen in the pupillary area.

C. Others: Reis-Bücklers dystrophy is a dominantly inherited dystrophy affecting primarily Bowman's layer. The disease begins within the first decade of life with symptoms of recurrent erosion. Opacification of Bowman's layer gradually occurs and the epithelium is irregular. No vascularization is usually noted. Vision may be markedly reduced.

Vortex dystrophy, or cornea verticillata, is characterized by pigmented lines occurring in Bowman's layer or the underlying stroma and spreading over the entire corneal surface. Visual acuity is not markedly affected. Such a pattern of radiating pigmented lines may also be seen in patients treated with chlorpromazine, chloroquine, indomethacin, or amiodarone as well as in Fabry's disease.

Stromal Corneal Dystrophies

There are three primary types of stromal corneal dystrophies:

A. Granular Dystrophy: This usually asymptomatic, slowly progressive corneal dystrophy most often begins in early childhood. The lesions consist of central, fine, whitish "granular" lesions in the stroma of the cornea. The epithelium and Bowman's layer may be affected late in the disease. Visual acuity is slightly reduced. Histologically, the cornea shows uniform deposition of hyaline material. Corneal transplant is not needed except in very severe and late cases. The inheritance is autosomal dominant.

B. Macular Dystrophy: This type of stromal corneal dystrophy is manifested by a dense gray central opacity that starts in Bowman's layer. The opacity tends to spread toward the periphery and later involves the deeper stromal layers. Recurrent corneal erosion may occur, and vision is severely impaired. Histologic examination shows deposition of acid mucopolysaccharide in the stroma and degeneration of Bowman's layer. Penetrating keratoplasty is often required.

The inheritance is autosomal recessive.

C. Lattice Dystrophy: Lattice dystrophy starts as fine, branching linear opacities in Bowman's layer in the central area and spreads to the periphery. The deep stroma may become involved, but the process does not reach Descemet's membrane. Recurrent erosion may occur. Histologic examination reveals amyloid deposits in the collagen fibers. Penetrating keratoplasty is common, as is recurrence of the dystrophy in the graft. The hereditary pattern for lattice dystrophy is autosomal dominant.

Posterior Corneal Dystrophies

A. Fuchs' Dystrophy: This disorder begins in the third or fourth decade and is slowly progressive throughout life. Women are more commonly affected than men. There are central wart-like deposits on Descemet's membrane, thickening of Descemet's membrane, and defects of size and shape of the endothelial cells. Decompensation of the endothelium occurs and leads to edema of the corneal stroma and epithelium, causing blurring of vision. Corneal haze is slowly progressive. Histologic examination of the cornea reveals the wart-like excrescences over Descemet's membrane that are secreted by the endothelial cells. Thinning and pigmentation of the endothelium and thickening of Descemet's membrane are characteristics. Penetrating keratoplasty, often combined with extracapsular lens extraction and a posterior lens implant, is often needed. Cataract surgery alone can trigger endothelial decompensation in advanced disease.

B. Posterior Polymorphous Dystrophy: This is a common disorder with onset in early childhood. Polymorphous plaques of calcium crystals are observed in the deep stromal layers. Vesicular lesions may be seen in the endothelium. Edema occurs in the deep stroma. The condition is asymptomatic in most cases, but in severe cases epithelial and total stromal edema may occur. The inheritance is autosomal dominant.

MISCELLANEOUS CORNEAL DISORDERS

THYGESON'S SUPERFICIAL PUNCTATE KERATITIS

Superficial punctate keratitis is an uncommon chronic and recurrent bilateral disorder more common in females. It is characterized by discrete and elevated oval epithelial opacities that show punctate staining with fluorescein, mainly in the pupillary area. The opacities are not visible grossly but can be easily seen with the slit lamp or loupe. Subepithelial opacities underlying the epithelial lesions (ghosts) are often observed as the epithelial disease resolves.

No causative organism has been identified, but a virus is suspected. A varicella-zoster virus has been isolated from the corneal scrapings of one case.

Mild irritation, slight blurring of vision, and photophobia are the only symptoms. The conjunctiva is not involved.

Epithelial keratitis secondary to staphylococcal blepharoconjunctivitis is differentiated from superficial punctate keratitis by its involvement of the lower third of the cornea and lack of subepithelial opacities. Epithelial keratitis in trachoma is ruled out by its location in the upper third of the cornea and the presence of pannus. Many other forms of keratitis involving the superficial cornea are unilateral or are eliminated by their histories.

Short-term instillation of corticosteroid drops will often cause disappearance of the opacities and subjective improvement, but recurrences are the rule. The ultimate prognosis is good since there is no scarring or vascularization of the cornea. Untreated, the disease runs a protracted course of 1–3 years. Long-term treatment with topical corticosteroids may prolong the course of the disease for many years and lead to steroid-induced cataract and glaucoma. Therapeutic soft contact lenses have been used to control symptoms in especially bothersome cases. Cyclosporine topical drops, 1% or 2%, have been effective as a substitute for steroids.

RECURRENT CORNEAL EROSION

This is a fairly common and serious mechanical corneal disorder that presents some classic signs and symptoms but may be easily missed if the physician does not look for it specifically. The patient is usually awakened during the early morning hours by a pain in the affected eye. The pain is continuous, and the eye becomes red, irritated, and photophobic. When the patient attempts to open the eyes in the morning, the lid pulls off the loose epithelium, resulting in pain and redness.

Three types of recurrent corneal erosions can be recognized:

(1) Acquired recurrent erosion (traumatic): The patient usually gives a history of previous corneal injury. It is unilateral, occurs with equal frequency in males and females, and the family history is negative. The recurrent erosion occurs most frequently in the center below the pupil no matter where the site of the previous corneal injury was.

(2) Recurrent erosion associated with corneal disease: After corneal ulceration heals, the epithelium may break down in a recurrent fashion (as in HSV "metaherpetic" ulcer).

(3) Recurrent erosion associated with corneal dystrophies: Recurrent erosions of the cornea may be observed in patients with Cogan's microcystic corneal dystrophy, lattice dystrophy, fingerprint dystrophy, and Reis-Bücklers corneal dystrophy.

Recurrent corneal erosion is due to a defect in the basement membrane of the corneal epithelium. The hemidesmosomes of the basal layer of the corneal epithelium fail to adhere to the basement membrane, and the corneal epithelium remains loose over the basement membrane with very slight subepithelial edema. The loose epithelial layers are vulnerable to separation and erosion.

Instillation of a local anesthetic relieves the symptoms immediately, and fluorescein staining will show the eroded area. This is typically a small area in the lower central cornea.

Treatment consists of a pressure bandage on the eye to promote healing. Mechanical denuding of the loose corneal epithelium may be necessary. The other eye should be kept closed most of the time to minimize movement of the lid over the affected eye. Bed rest is desirable for 24 hours. The cornea usually heals in 2–3 days. To prevent recurrence and to promote continued healing, it is important for these patients to use a bland ointment (eg, boric acid or other ocular lubricant) at bedtime for several months. In more severe cases, artificial tears are instilled during the day. The use of hypertonic ointment (glucose 40%) or 5% saline drops (Adsorbonac 5%) is often of value. Therapeutic soft contact lenses and needle micropuncture of Bowman's layer as well as excimer laser shallow keratectomy have been useful in cases that do not respond to more conservative management.

INTERSTITIAL KERATITIS DUE TO CONGENITAL SYPHILIS

This self-limited inflammatory disease of the cornea is a late manifestation of congenital syphilis. There has been a sharp decrease in the incidence of the disease in recent years—almost to the point of extinction in some parts of the USA. It occasionally starts unilaterally but almost always becomes bilateral weeks to months later. It affects all races and is more common in females than males. Symptoms appear between the ages of 5 and 20. Pathologic findings include edema, lymphocytic infiltration, and vascularization of the corneal stroma.

Interstitial keratitis may be immune in nature since *Treponema pallidum* is not found in the cornea during the acute phase. It has been postulated that these organisms enter the cornea at birth and that later in life there is a violent hypersensitivity to intracorneal viral antigen.

Clinical Findings

A. Symptoms and Signs: Other signs of congenital syphilis may be present, such as saddle nose and Hutchinson's triad (interstitial keratitis, deafness, and notched upper central incisors). The patient complains of pain, photophobia, and blurring of vision. Physical signs include conjunctival injection, corneal edema, vascularization of the deeper corneal layers, and miosis. There is an associated severe anterior granulomatous uveitis and blepharospasm due to photophobia. The grayish-pink appearance of the cornea (due to edema and vascularization) that occurs in the acute phase is sometimes referred to as a "salmon patch."

B. Laboratory Findings: Serologic tests for syphilis are positive.

Complications & Sequelae

Corneal scarring and vascularization occur if the process has been particularly severe and prolonged. Secondary glaucoma may result from the uveitis.

Treatment

There are no specific measures. Treatment is aimed at preventing the development of posterior synechiae, which will occur if the pupil is not dilated.

Both eyes should be dilated with frequent instillation of 2% atropine solution. Corticosteroid drops often relieve the symptoms dramatically but must be continued for long periods to prevent recurrence of symptoms. Dark glasses and a darkened room may be necessary if photophobia is severe. Treatment should be given for systemic syphilis, even though this usually has little effect on the ocular condition.

Corneal scarring may necessitate corneal transplant, and glaucoma, if present, may be difficult to control.

Course & Prognosis

The corneal disease process itself is not affected by treatment, which is aimed at prevention of complications. The inflammatory phase lasts 3 or 4 weeks. The corneas then gradually clear, leaving ghost vessels and scars in the corneal stroma.

INTERSTITIAL KERATITIS DUE TO OTHER CAUSES

Although congenital syphilis is no longer a common cause of interstitial keratitis, the disease still occurs as a complication of other granulomatous diseases, eg, tuberculosis and leprosy. Certain viruses (eg, cytomegalovirus, measles virus, mumps virus) as well as the spirochete of Lyme disease have been described as causing a type of interstitial keratitis. Treatment is usually symptomatic, but it is important to establish the cause.

Cogan's syndrome is a rare disorder generally believed to be a vascular hypersensitivity reaction of unknown origin. It is a disease of young adults and is characterized by nonsyphilitic interstitial keratitis and a vestibuloauditory difficulty. Corticosteroids are reputed to be of value, but some degree of visual impairment and complete nerve deafness usually supervene.

CORNEAL PIGMENTATION

Pigmentation of the cornea may occur with or without ocular or systemic disease. There are several distinct varieties.

Krukenberg's Spindle

In this disorder, brown uveal pigment is deposited bilaterally upon the central endothelial surface in a vertical spindle-shaped fashion. It occurs in a small percentage of people over age 20, usually in myopic women. It can be seen grossly but is best observed with the slitlamp. The visual acuity is only slightly affected, and the progression is extremely slow. Pigmentary glaucoma must be ruled out by yearly intraocular pressure measurements.

Blood Staining

This disorder occurs occasionally as a complication of traumatic hyphema with secondary glaucoma and is due to hemosiderin in the corneal stroma. The cornea is golden brown, and vision is decreased. In most cases the cornea gradually clears in 1–2 years.

Kayser-Fleischer Ring

This is a pigmented ring whose color varies widely from ruby red to bright green, blue, yellow, or brown. The ring is 1–3 mm is diameter and located just inside the limbus posteriorly. In exceptional cases there is a second ring. The pigment is composed of fine granules immediately below the endothelium. It involves Descemet's membrane, rarely the stroma. Electron microscopic studies suggest that the pigment is a copper compound. The intensity of the pigmentation can be reduced markedly by the use of chelating agents.

These rings, which were long considered to be pathognomonic of hepatolenticular degeneration (Wilson's disease), have recently been described in three nonwilsonian patients with chronic hepatobiliary disease and in one patient with chronic cholestatic jaundice. Recognition of the Kayser-Fleischer rings, however, remains important, since such notice calls attention to the possibility that the patient has Wilson's disease. Specific medical treatment with the copper chelating agent penicillamine may dramatically improve a disease that would otherwise inevitably be fatal.

Iron Lines (Hudson-Stähli Line, Fleischer's Ring, Stocker's Line, Ferry's Line)

Localized deposits of iron within the corneal epithelium may occur in sufficient quantity to become visible clinically. The Hudson-Stähli line is a horizontal line at the junction of the middle and lower thirds of the cornea, corresponding to the line of lid closure, in otherwise normal elderly patients. Fleischer's ring surrounds the base of the cone in keratoconus. Stocker's line is a vertical line associated with pterygia, and Ferry's line develops adjacent to limbal filtering blebs. Similar iron deposits are seen at the site of corneal scars.

CONTACT LENSES

Glass contact lenses were first described in 1888 by Adolf Fick and were then used for the treatment of keratoconus by Eugene Kalt. Poor results were achieved until 1945, when Kevin Tuohy of Los Angeles produced a plastic precorneal lens with a diameter of 11 mm. Since that time, advances in contact lens technology have produced several different varieties of lenses, which are broadly divided into two types: rigid and soft lenses. The basic requirement for success of contact lenses is to overcome the effect on oxygen supply to the cornea from wearing an occlusive lens. The optical features of contact lenses are discussed in Chapter 21.

Rigid (Hard) Lenses:

A. Standard Hard Lenses: These direct descendants of Tuohy's lens are made of polymethylmethacrylate (PMMA, Perspex), are impervious to oxygen, and thus rely on pumping of tears into the space between the lens and the cornea during blinking to provide oxygen to the cornea. They are smaller than the corneal diameter. Always for daily wear, these lenses are easy to care for, are relatively inexpensive, and correct vision efficiently, particularly if there is significant astigmatism. Unfortunately, many persons cannot tolerate them. Corneal edema due to corneal hypoxia and spectacle blur (poor vision with spectacle correction after a period of contact lens wear) are common complaints.

B. Gas-Permeable Hard Lenses: These are rigid lenses made from cellulose acetate butyrate, silicone acrylate, or silicone combined with polymethyl-methacrylate. They have the advantage of high oxygen permeability, thus improving corneal metabolism, and greater comfort, while retaining the optical properties of rigid lenses. They are generally used on a daily wear basis but can be used on an extended-wear (24-hour) basis in exceptional circumstances. In keratoconus, the gas-permeable lens has become the lens of first choice.

Soft Lenses

A. Cosmetic Soft Lenses: Hydrogel lenses, based on hydroxymethyl methacrylate (HEMA), are considerably more comfortable than rigid lenses but are flexible and thus conform to the surface of the cornea. Regular astigmatism can be partially corrected by incorporating cylinder into the soft lens; irregular astigmatism is poorly corrected. The oxygen permeability and water content values vary among different types of hydrogel lens. They are more difficult to care for and more expensive than rigid lenses. Complications are also more common and include ulcerative keratitis, (particularly if the lenses are worn overnight), immune corneal reactions to deposits on the lenses, giant papillary conjunctivitis, reactions to lens care solutions (especially those containing the preservative thimerosal), corneal edema, and corneal vascularization.

Cosmetic soft contact lenses are usually worn on a daily wear basis. For aphakic correction, it is occasionally necessary to resort to extended wear because of the patient's inability to insert and remove the lenses themselves. Extended wear increases the risks associated with use of contact lenses.

B. Disposable Soft Lenses: These lenses are designed to be discarded daily or sometimes after extended wear for 1 week. They eliminate the need for contact lens solutions and theoretically reduce the risk of ulcerative keratitis by minimizing bacterial adherence to the lens surface. They do appear to be safe if worn on a daily wear basis, but overnight wear, even for one night, is associated with a significant risk of ulcerative keratitis.

C. Therapeutic Soft Lenses: The use of therapeutic soft contact lenses has become an indispensable part of the ophthalmologist's management of external eye disease. The lenses form a soft barrier between the outside and the cornea, providing protection against trichiasis and exposure. Lenses with high water content can act as a "stent" for epithelial healing, such as in the treatment of recurrent ero-

sions. Patients with pain due to epithelial disease, such as in bullous keratopathy, particularly benefit from therapeutic soft contact lenses. Lenses with low water content can be used to seal small corneal perforations or wound leaks. In all cases of therapeutic contact lens wear, infection can occur. Antimicrobial coverage may be indicated if epithelial defects exist.

Contact Lens Care

It is essential that all contact lens wearers be made aware of the risks associated with contact lens wear—particularly those patients choosing the high-risk varieties such as extended-wear lenses for cosmetic optical correction purely on the grounds of convenience. All wearers must be under the regular care of a contact lens practitioner. Many of the chronic complications of contact lens wear are asymptomatic in their early and easily treated stages. Any contact lens should be removed immediately if the eye becomes uncomfortable or inflamed, and ophthalmic attention must be sought immediately if symptoms do not rapidly resolve.

Contact lenses require regular cleaning and disinfecting, and in the case of soft and gas-permeable lenses removal of protein deposits is required. Disinfection regimens include heat, chemical soaking, and hydrogen peroxide systems. All are effective if used according to the manufacturer's instructions, though heat systems may be preferable for combating resistant organisms such as *Acanthamoeba*. Soft and gas-permeable lenses are much less durable than hard lenses; contact lenses vary in tolerance to disinfection.

There is a significant trend among soft lens wearers toward the use of nonpreserved contact lens care systems because of the development of preservative-related hypersensitivity reactions. It is important that such individuals be aware of the ability of organisms such as *Pseudomonas* and *Acanthamoeba* to survive in nonpreserved saline solutions, such as may be found in their contact lens storage cases. The use of nonpreserved contact lens solutions requires much greater vigilance in the regular disinfection of lenses and lens storage cases.

CORNEAL TRANSPLANTATION

Corneal transplantation (keratoplasty) is indicated for a number of serious corneal conditions, eg, scarring, edema, thinning, and distortion. The term penetrating keratoplasty denotes full-thickness corneal replacement; lamellar keratoplasty denotes a partial-thickness procedure.

Younger donors are preferred for penetrating keratoplasties; there is a direct relationship between age and the health and number of the endothelial cells. Because of the rapid endothelial cell death rate, the eyes should be enucleated soon after death and refrigerated immediately. Whole eyes should be used within 48 hours, preferably within 24 hours. Modern storage media allow for longer storage. Corneoscleral caps stored in nutrient media may be used up to 6 days after donor death, and preservation in tissue culture media allows storage for as long as 6 weeks.

For lamellar keratoplasty, corneas can be frozen, dehydrated, or refrigerated for several weeks; the endothelial cells are not important in this partial-thickness procedure.

Technique

The recipient eye is prepared by a partial-thickness cutting of a circle of diseased cornea with a suction trephine (cookie cutter action) and full-thickness removal with scissors or partial-thickness removal with dissection.

The donor eye is prepared in two ways. For penetrating keratoplasty, the corneoscleral cap is placed endothelium up on a suction Teflon block; the trephine (Figure 6–15) is pressed down into the cornea, and a full-thickness button is punched out. In lamellar keratoplasty, a partial-thickness trephine incision is made in the cornea of a whole globe and the lamellar button is dissected free. Certain refinements in technique, such as free hand grafts, may be necessary.

Refined sutures (Figure 6–16) and instruments and sophisticated operating microscopes and illuminating systems have significantly improved the prognosis in all patients requiring corneal transplants. There is no significant value to blood type matching in corneal transplant surgery.

Corneal graft rejection continues to be a major management problem (see Chapter 16), as does the difficulty in controlling postgraft astigmatism.

REFRACTIVE CORNEAL SURGERY

The inconvenience of spectacles to many wearers and the complications associated with contact lenses have resulted in a search for surgical solutions to the problem of refractive error.

Radial Keratotomy

In the late 1940s, Sato of Japan created anterior and posterior corneal incisions to alter the curvature of the cornea. Results were poor, and endothelial decompensation with corneal edema occurred frequently. In 1972, Fyodorov of the USSR began to use anterior corneal cuts only. Currently, the operation consists of radial incisions involving 90% of the corneal thickness and extending from a clear optical zone (usually the central 3 mm or more of the cornea) toward but not reaching the limbus. The amount of correction achieved is modified by the size of the optical zone and the number and depth of the incisions. Various formulas and computer programs are used to determine the value of these parameters in each case.

There is general agreement that radial keratotomy does reduce the degree of myopia and is most effective for myopia in the lower range (–2 to –4 diopters). There is a significant degree of unpredictability in the final result, with under- or overcorrection or even progressive hyperopia. Glare and fluctuations of vision during the day are commonly reported side effects. Delayed healing of corneal incisions, with corneal infections occurring up to 2 years after the procedure, have been reported. Endophthalmitis, traumatic cataract, and endothelial cell loss are rare but have been reported.

Keratomileusis

In 1961, Barraquer of Colombia reported on the technique of myopic keratomileusis for the correction

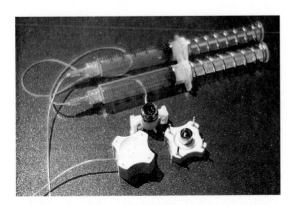

Figure 6–15. A popular vacuum corneal punch and trephine. (Barron-Katena.)

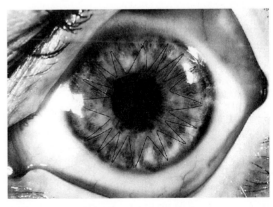

Figure 6–16. Penetrating keratoplasty with 10-0 nylon running suture, 3 months after operation.

of high degrees of myopia. The procedure has been performed in other countries but by relatively few surgeons. A deep lamellar corneal autograft is cut; the tissue is frozen and then reshaped with a cryolathe to obtain a flatter curvature after thawing; and the autograft is then sutured back into position. Expensive cryolathe and microkeratome equipment is required. The procedure has also been used for hyperopia. Automated lamellar keratoplasty (ALK) is a new form of this procedure.

Complications of keratomileusis include improper depth of the lamellar bed, delayed epithelialization over the resutured tissue, interface epithelial growth and opacity, and irregular astigmatism.

Procedures to Correct Astigmatism

Various patterns of keratotomy have been described to correct corneal astigmatism. Irregular astigmatism continues to be a serious problem following most corneal operations, including radial keratotomy and penetrating keratoplasty, and after cataract surgery. Troutman and others have described relaxing incisions, compression sutures, and wedge resections for postkeratoplasty astigmatism, utilizing a surgical keratometer. Various techniques for cataract incision, such as scleral tunnel incisions and clear corneal incisions as well as altering incision location, have been reported as useful in preventing postoperative astigmatism after cataract surgery.

Alloplastic Corneal Implants

Disks of many different materials have been inserted into corneal stromal pockets, initially to control corneal edema but more recently to correct refractive errors. In most cases, the corneal tissue anterior to the implant undergoes necrosis. Hydrogel and polysulfone lenses have been more successful than other types of lenses tried so far. Use of alloplastic corneal implants would remove the need to rely on autologous or homologous material in refractive surgery. A plastic ring meant to be implanted intrastromally is under investigation and shows promise as a refractive surgery procedure.

Clear Lens Removal & Phakic Lens Implants

A few surgeons around the world have advocated the removal of clear lenses in high degrees of myopia, suggesting that the risk of doing so is minimal owing to the safety of extracapsular lens extraction. The procedure is controversial because of a significant risk of retinal detachment in high myopes. Phakic lens implants are under investigation for treatment of high refractive errors.

Lasers

A further approach to refractive corneal surgery involves the use of lasers (see Chapter 24). The excimer laser has received the most publicity, but other machines such as the solid-state neodymium:YAG laser and "minilasers" have been shown to be effective also. Laser photorefractive keratectomy (PRK) produces precisely controlled flattening of the anterior cornea to reduce myopia. The procedure also is done for astigmatism and hyperopia. Anterior stromal haze, irregular astigmatism, and regression have been observed after PRK. In the United States, the FDA has given approval for PRK to two laser companies; the procedure has been done in many other countries for years.

Laser in situ keratomileusis (LASIK) is a procedure that utilizes a motorized microkeratome to cut a shallow lamellar corneal disk which is folded back to allow excimer laser photoablation to the stromal bed. The flap is then folded back into position. The patient is more comfortable immediately after surgery than with PRK, and best vision is restored earlier. Irregular astigmatism and interface problems are among the complications of this procedure.

Controversy exists over the choice between surface ablation (PRK) and LASIK. In general, PRK is used for lower (−6.00 D or less) and LASIK for higher levels of myopia. Improved methods of surface ablation or other techniques may eliminate the need for LASIK in the future. Generally, LASIK is not approved by the FDA.

REFERENCES

Adar MJ et al: Possible consequences of shaking hands with your patients with epidemic keratoconjunctivitis. Am J Ophthalmol 1996;121:711.

Allan BDS, Dart JKG: Strategies for the management of microbial keratitis. Br J Ophthalmol 1995;79:777.

Bacon AS et al: Acanthamoeba keratitis: The value of early diagnosis. Ophthalmology 1993;100:1238.

Bourque LB et al: Spectacle and contact lens wearing six years after radial keratotomy in the Prospective Evaluation of Radial Keratotomy Study. Ophthalmology 1994;100:421.

Bower KS, Kawalski RP, Gordon YJ: Fluoroquinolones in the treatment of bacterial keratitis. Am J Ophthalmol 1996;121:712.

Chatterjee A et al: Results of Excimer Laser Retreatment of Residual Myopia after Previous Photorefractive Keratotomy. Ophthalmol 1997;104:1321-1326.

Clinch TE et al: Microbial Keratitis in children. Am J Ophthalmol 1994; 117:65

Flowers CW et al: Changing indications for penetrating keratoplasty, 1989–1993. Cornea 1995;14:583.

Hersh PS et al: Excimer laser phototherapeutic keratectomy. Ophthalmology 1996;103:1210.

Hope-Ross MW et al: Recurrent corneal erosions: Clinical features. Eye 1994;8:373.

Hyndiuk RA et al: Comparison of ciprofloxacin ophthalmic solution 0.3% to fortified tobramycin-cefazolin in treating bacterial corneal ulcers. Ophthalmology 1996;103:1854.

Jones DB: Emerging antibiotic resistance: Real and relative. Arch Ophthalmol 1996;114:91.

Kawal VO et al: Use of routine antibiotic sensitivity testing for the management of corneal ulcers. Arch Ophthalmol 1997;115:462.

Kershner RM: Clear corneal cataract surgery and the correction of myopia, hyperopia, and astigmatism. Ophthalmology 1997;104:381.

Laibson PR, Rapuano CJ: 100-Year Review of the cornea. Ophthalmology 1996;103(Suppl):517.

Larkin DFP: Corneal allograft rejection. Br J Ophthalmol 1994;78:649.

Luchs JI et al: Ulcerative keratitis in bullous keratopathy. Ophthalmology 1997;104:816.

Lyons CJ et al: Granular corneal dystrophy: Visual results and pattern of recurrence after lamellar or penetrating keratoplasty. Ophthalmology 1994;101:1812.

Maguen E et al: Results of excimer laser photorefractive keratectomy for the correction of myopia. Ophthalmology 1994;101:1548.

Maguire MG et al: Risk factors for corneal graft failure and rejection in the Collaborative Corneal Transplantation Studies. Ophthalmology 1994;101:1536.

Manning CA et al: Intraoperative mitomycin in primary pterygium excision. Ophthalmology 1997;104:844.

McLeod SD et al: The role of smears, cultures, and antibiotic sensitivity testing in the management of suspected infectious keratitis. Ophthalmology 1996;103:23.

O'Brart DPS et al: The effects of ablation diameter on the outcome of excimer laser photorefractive keratectomy: A prospective, randomized, double-blind study. Arch Ophthalmol 1995;113:438.

Ogawa TSH, Hyndiuk RA: Bacterial keratitis and conjunctivitis. In: The Cornea, 3rd ed. Smolin G, Thoft RA (editors). Little, Brown, 1994.

Peacock LW et al: Ocular integrity after refractive procedures. Ophthalmology 1997;104:1079.

Pruett RC: A controlled trial of oral acyclovir for the prevention of stromal keratitis or iritis in patients with herpes simplex virus epithelial keratitis: The epithelial trial. Arch Ophthalmol 1997;115:703.

Pruett RC: Commentary on a case of excessive myopia treated by extraction of the transparent lens. Ophthalmology 1997;115:258.

Remeijer L et al: Newly acquired herpes simplex virus keratitis after penetrating keratoplasty. Ophthalmology 1997;104:648.

Rosa RH, Miller D, Alfonso EC: The changing spectrum of fungal keratitis in south Florida. Ophthalmology 1994;101:1005.

Salah T et al: Excimer laser in situ keratomileusis under a corneal flap for myopia of 2 to 20 diopters. Am J Ophthalmol 1996;121:143.

Schein OD et al: The impact of overnight wear on the risk of contact lens-associated ulcerative keratitis. Arch Ophthalmol 1994;112:186.

Seiler GT, McDonnel PJ: Excimer laser photorefractive keratectomy. Surv Ophthalmol 1995;40:89.

Spencer WH (editor): Ophthalmic Pathology, 4th ed. 4 vols. Saunders, 1996.

Tuft SJ et al: Prognostic factors for the progression of keratoconus. Ophthalmology 1994;101:439.

Vail A et al: Clinical and surgical factors influencing corneal graft survival, visual acuity, and astigmatism. Ophthalmology 1996;103:41.

Wagoner MD: Chemical injuries of the eye. Current concepts in pathophysiology and therapy. Surv Ophthalmol 1997;41:275.

Waring GO III et al: Results of the Prospective Evaluation of Radial Keratotomy (PERK) Study 10 years after surgery. Arch Ophthalmol 1994;112:1298.

Watson PG: Management of Mooren's ulceration. Eye 1997;11:349.

Wilhelmus KR for the Herpetic Eye Disease Study Group: Herpetic Eye Disease Study: A controlled trial of topical corticosteroids for herpes simplex stromal keratitis. Ophthalmology 1994;101:1883.

Wilmer WH: A case of excessive myopia treated by extraction of the transparent lens. Arch Ophthalmol 1898;27:65. (Reprinted in Arch Ophthalmol 1997;115:251.)

7

Uveal Tract & Sclera

Emmett T. Cunningham, Jr., MD, PhD, MPH, & J. Brooks Crawford, MD

I. UVEAL TRACT

Emmett T. Cunningham, Jr., MD, PhD, MPH

The uveal tract consists of the choroid, ciliary body, and iris (Figure 7–1). Uveal tumors and inflammations (uveitis) together comprise the vast majority of diseases affecting these structures. Many neoplastic and inflammatory disorders of the uveal tract are associated with systemic diseases, some of which can be life-threatening if unrecognized. The anterior uveal tract is best examined with a slitlamp, though gross inspection can be performed with a flashlight and loupe. Examination of the posterior uveal tract requires the use of either a direct or indirect ophthalmoscope or a slitlamp.

UVEITIS

The term "uveitis" denotes inflammation of the choroid (choroiditis), ciliary body (intermediate uveitis, cyclitis, peripheral uveitis, or pars planitis), or iris (iritis). However, common usage includes inflammation of the retina (retinitis), retinal vasculature (retinal vasculitis), and optic nerve (optic neuritis). Uveitis may also occur secondary to inflammation of the cornea (keratitis), sclera (scleritis), or both (sclerokeratitis). Uveitis usually affects people 20–50 years of age and accounts for 10–15% of cases of legal blindness in developed countries.

Clinical Findings
A. Symptoms and Signs (Table 7–1) Inflammation of the uveal tract has many causes and may involve one or more regions of the eye simultaneously.

Anterior uveitis is most common and is usually unilateral and acute in onset. Typical symptoms include pain, photophobia, and blurred vision. Examination usually reveals circumcorneal redness with

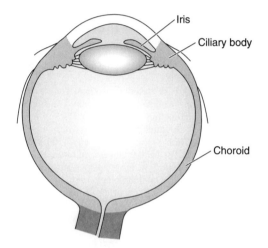

Figure 7–1. The uveal tract consists of the iris, the ciliary body, and the choroid.

minimal palpebral conjunctival injection or discharge. The pupil may be small (miosis) or irregular due to the formation of posterior synechiae. Inflammation limited to the anterior chamber is called "iritis"; inflammation involving both the anterior chamber and the anterior vitreous is called "iridocyclitis." Corneal sensation and intraocular pressure should be checked in every patient with uveitis. Decreased sensation can suggest herpes simplex or herpes zoster infection, whereas increased intraocular pressure can occur with herpes simplex, herpes zoster, or toxoplasmosis, with sarcoidosis, or with an uncommon form of iridocyclitis called glaucomatocyclitic crisis, or Posner-Schlossman syndrome. Clumps of white cells and inflammatory debris—keratic precipitates—are usually evident on the corneal endothelium. Keratic precipitates may be large ("mutton fat," or granulomatous), small (nongranulomatous), or stellate. Granulomatous or nongranulomatous keratic precipitates are usually located inferiorly, particularly in a wedge-shaped region known as Arlt's triangle. Stellate keratic precipitates are usually distributed evenly over the entire corneal endothelium. They are seen in uveitis due to herpes simplex virus, herpes zoster virus, toxoplasmosis, Fuchs' heterochromic iridocyclitis, and sar-

142

Table 7–1. Differentiation of granulomatous and nongranulomatous uveitis.

	Nongranulomatous	Granulomatous
Onset	Acute	Insidious
Pain	Marked	None or minimal
Photophobia	Marked	Slight
Blurred vision	Moderate	Marked
Circumcorneal flush	Marked	Slight
Keratic precipitates	Fine white	Large gray ("mutton fat")
Pupil	Small and irregular	Small and irregular (variable)
Posterior synechiae	Sometimes	Sometimes
Iris nodules	None	Sometimes
Site	Anterior	Anterior, posterior, or diffuse
Course	Acute	Chronic
Recurrence	Common	Sometimes

coidosis. Iris nodules may be present at the iris margin (Koeppe nodules), within the iris stroma (Busacca nodules), or in the anterior chamber angle (Berlin's nodules). Evidence for granulomatous disease, such as mutton fat keratic precipitates or iris nodules, may indicate sarcoidosis or an infectious cause of uveitis. Particularly severe anterior chamber inflammation may result in layering of inflammatory cells in the inferior angle (hypopyon). The iris should be examined carefully for evidence of atrophy or transillumination, which can occur in the setting of herpes simplex or herpes zoster virus infection, or with Fuchs' heterochromic iridocyclitis. The presence of anterior or posterior synechiae (Figures 7–2 to 7–4) should also be noted, as this can predispose the patient to glaucoma.

Intermediate uveitis, also called cyclitis, peripheral uveitis, or pars planitis, is the second most common type of intraocular inflammation, the hallmark of which is vitreous inflammation. Intermediate uveitis is typically bilateral and tends to affect patients in their late teens or early adult years. Men are affected more commonly than women. Typical symptoms include floaters and blurred vision. Pain, photophobia, and redness are usually absent or minimal. The most striking finding on examination is vitritis, often accompanied by vitreous condensates, either free-floating as "snowballs" or layered over the pars plana and ciliary body as "snowbanking." Mild anterior chamber inflammation may be present, but if significant, the uveitis is more appropriately termed diffuse (see below). The cause is unknown in over half of patients, though syphilis, tuberculosis, and sarcoidosis should always be considered. The most common complications include cystoid macular edema, retinal vasculitis, and optic nerve head neovascularization.

Posterior uveitis includes retinitis, choroiditis, retinal vasculitis, and optic neuritis, which may occur alone or in combination. Symptoms typically include floaters, loss of visual field or scotomas, or decreased vision, which can be severe. Retinal detachment, though infrequent, occurs most commonly in posterior uveitis and may be tractional, rhegmatogenous, or exudative in nature.

B. Laboratory Testing: Laboratory testing is usually not required for patients with mild uveitis and a recent history of trauma or surgery—or with clear evidence of herpes simplex or herpes zoster virus infection, such as a concurrent vesicular dermatitis, dendritic or disciform keratitis, or sectoral iris atrophy. Laboratory testing can also be deferred for otherwise healthy and asymptomatic young to middle-aged patients with a first episode of mild to moderately severe acute, unilateral, nongranulomatous iritis or iridocyclitis that responds promptly to treatment with topical corticosteroids and cycloplegics. However, patients with recurrent, severe, bi-

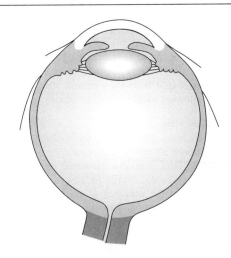

Figure 7–2. Anterior synechiae (adhesions). The peripheral iris adheres to the cornea. Glaucoma may result.

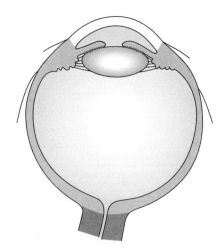

Figure 7–3. Posterior synechiae. The iris adheres to the lens. Iris seclusion, iris bombé, and glaucoma may result.

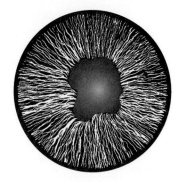

Figure 7–4. Posterior synechiae (anterior view). The iris is adherent to the lens in several places as a result of previous inflammation, causing an irregular, fixed pupil. Appropriate treatment with corticosteroids and cycloplegic agents can often prevent such synechiae.

lateral, granulomatous, intermediate, posterior, or diffuse uveitis should be tested, as should any patient whose uveitis fails to respond promptly to standard therapy. Testing for syphilis should include both a Venereal Disease Research Laboratory (VDRL) or rapid plasma reagin (RPR) test and a more specific test for anti-Treponema pallidum antibodies, such as the FTA-ABS or MHA-TP assays. Tuberculosis and sarcoidosis should be excluded by chest x-ray and skin testing using both purified protein derivative (PPD) and controls, such as mumps and candida. A remote history of having received BCG vaccination should not preclude PPD testing, since a reaction of greater than 5 mm is still considered abnormal. Testing other than for syphilis, tuberculosis, and sarcoidosis should be tailored to findings elicited on history or identified on physical examination. Examples might include an antinuclear antibody (ANA) titer for a young child with chronic iridocyclitis and arthritis suspected of having juvenile rheumatoid arthritis; an HLA-B27 histocompatibility antigen test for patients with arthritis, psoriasis, urethritis, or symptoms consistent with inflammatory bowel disease; or toxoplasmosis IgG and IgM titers for a patient with unilateral diffuse uveitis and focal retinochoroiditis.

Differential Diagnosis

The differential diagnosis for eye redness and decreased vision is extensive and somewhat beyond the scope of this brief overview. However, entities commonly confused with uveitis include conjunctivitis, distinguished by the presence of discharge and redness involving both the palpebral and bulbar conjunctiva; keratitis, distinguished by the presence of epithelial staining or defects or by stromal thickening or infiltrate; and acute angle closure glaucoma, associated with markedly elevated intraocular pressure, corneal haziness and edema, and a narrow anterior chamber angle, often best visualized in the uninvolved eye. (See Inside Front Cover.)

Complications & Sequelae

Anterior uveitis can produce both anterior and posterior synechiae (Figures 7–2 to 7–4). Anterior synechiae can impede aqueous outflow at the chamber angle and cause glaucoma. Posterior synechiae, when extensive, can also cause secondary angle closure glaucoma, usually by producing pupillary seclusion and forward bulging of the iris (iris bombé). Early and aggressive use of corticosteroids and cycloplegics lessens the likelihood of these complications.

Both anterior and posterior chamber inflammation promote lens thickening and opacification. Early, this can cause a simple shift in refractive error, usually toward myopia. With time, however, cataract progresses and often limits best-corrected vision. Treatment involves removal of the cataract but should be done only when the intraocular inflammation is well controlled, since the risk of intraoperative and postoperative complications is greater in patients with active uveitis. Aggressive use of local and systemic corticosteroids is usually necessary before, during, and after cataract surgery in these patients.

Cystoid macular edema is a common cause of visual loss in patients with uveitis, typically observed in the setting of severe anterior or intermediate uveitis. Long-standing or recurrent macular edema can cause permanent loss of vision.

Retinal detachments, including tractional, rhegmatogenous, and exudative forms, occur infrequently in patients with posterior, intermediate, or diffuse uveitis. Exudative retinal detachment suggests significant choroidal inflammation and occurs most commonly in association with Vogt-Koyanagi-Harada syndrome, sympathetic ophthalmia, or posterior scleritis.

Treatment

Corticosteroids and cycloplegics are the mainstays of therapy for uveitis. Care should be taken to rule out an epithelial defect and ruptured globe when a history of trauma is elicited and to check corneal sensation and intraocular pressure to rule out herpes simplex or herpes zoster infection. Aggressive topical therapy with 1% prednisolone acetate, 1 or 2 drops in the affected eye every 1 or 2 hours while awake, usually provides good control of anterior inflammation. Prednisolone acetate is a suspension and needs to be shaken 30 or more times prior to each use. Homatropine, 5%, used two to four times daily, helps prevent synechia formation and reduces discomfort from ciliary spasm.

Intermediate, posterior, and diffuse inflammation responds best to posterior sub-Tenon injection of triamcinolone acetonide, usually 1 mL (40 mg) given superotemporally. Oral prednisone, 0.5–1.5 mg/kg/d, can also be effective. Steroid-sparing agents such as methotrexate, azathioprine, cyclosporine, cyclophosphamide, or chlorambucil are often required to treat severe or chronic cases. Concurrent therapy for specific infectious causes of uveitis is indicated as outlined in Table 7–2.

Complications of Treatment

Cataract and glaucoma are the most common complications of corticosteroid therapy. Cycloplegics weaken accommodation and can be particularly bothersome to patients under 45 years of age. Because oral corticosteroids or steroid-sparing agents can cause numerous systemic complications, dosing and monitoring are best done in close collaboration with an internist, rheumatologist, or oncologist.

Course & Prognosis

The course and prognosis of uveitis depends to a large extent on the severity, location, and cause of the inflammation. In general, severe inflammation takes longer to treat and is more likely to cause intraocular damage and loss of vision than mild or moderate inflammation; and anterior uveitis responds more promptly than intermediate, posterior, or diffuse uveitis. Retinal, choroidal, or optic nerve involvement tends to be associated with a poorer prognosis.

ANTERIOR UVEITIS (TABLE 7–3)

1. UVEITIS ASSOCIATED WITH JOINT DISEASE

About 20% of children with the pauciarticular form of **juvenile rheumatoid arthritis** (JRA) develop a chronic, bilateral, nongranulomatous iridocyclitis. Girls are affected four to five times more commonly than boys. JRA-associated uveitis is usually detected

Table 7–2. Treatment of granulomatous uveitis.

	Anti-Infective Chemotherapy	Use of Corticosteroids
Toxoplasmosis	If central vision is threatened, give pyrimethamine, 75 mg orally as a loading dose for 2 days followed by 25 mg once daily for 4 weeks, in combination with trisulfapyrimidines (sulfadiazine, sulfamerazine, and sulfamethazine, 0.167 g of each per tablet), 2 g orally as loading dose followed by 0.5 g 4 times daily for 4 weeks. If a fall in the white or platelet count occurs during therapy, give folinic acid (leucovorin), 1 mL IM twice weekly or 3 mg orally 3 times a week. Alternative chemotherapeutic approach for ocular toxoplasmosis: Clindamycin, 300 mg orally 4 times a day with sulfonamides (as above), or minocycline, 100 mg orally daily for 3–4 weeks.	If the response is not favorable after 2 weeks, continue anti-infective therapy and give systemic corticosteroids, eg, prednisone, 0.5 mg/kg/d, with tapering over 3–4 weeks. Corticosteroids may activate the organisms of toxoplasmosis and tuberculosis but are given as a calculated risk to control the inflammatory response when it threatens vision. Never stop antiinfective therapy prior to stopping corticosteroids.
Tuberculosis	Isoniazid, 300 mg orally daily; ethambutol, 400 mg orally twice daily; pyridoxine, 50 mg orally daily. Continue treatment for 6–9 months.	If a favorable response does not occur in 6 weeks, continue antimycobacterial therapy and give systemic corticosteroids, eg, prednisone, 0.5–1 mg/kg/d, with tapering as allowed by response.
Sarcoidosis	Treat with local corticosteroids and mydriatics and, during active stages, with systemic corticosteroids such as prednisone, 0.5–1 mg/kg/d, with tapering as allowed by response. The usual contraindications to systemic corticosteroid therapy apply.	
Sympathetic ophthalmia	Treat with local corticosteroids and cycloplegics and with systemic corticosteroids in high doses, eg, prednisone, 1–1.5 mg/kg/d. The usual contraindications to systemic corticosteroid therapy apply, and the drugs may be needed in higher doses and for a longer time. Therefore, management of the side effects is often more difficult. Azathioprine may be helpful in reducing the required dose of corticosteroids. In severe cases that fail to respond to corticosteroids, treatment with cytotoxic agents such as chlorambucil and cyclophosphamide or other immunosuppressants such as cyclosporine has met with some success. *Caution:* White blood counts and platelets must be monitored very carefully in these patients, and these drugs should not be used without careful consideration.	

Table 7–3. Causes of anterior uveitis.

Autoimmune
  Juvenile rheumatoid arthritis
  Ankylosing spondylitis
  Reiter's syndrome
  Ulcerative colitis
  Lens-induced uveitis
  Sarcoidosis
  Crohn's disease
  Psoriasis
Infections
  Syphilis
  Tuberculosis
  Leprosy (Hansen's disease)
  Herpes zoster
  Herpes simplex
  Onchocerciasis
  Leptospirosis
Malignancy
  Masquerade syndrome
    Retinoblastoma
    Leukemia
    Lymphoma
    Malignant melanoma
Other
  Idiopathic
  Traumatic uveitis, including penetrating injuries
  Retinal detachment
  Fuchs' heterochromic iridocyclitis
  Glaucomatocyclitic crisis (Posner-Schlossman syndrome)

at 5–6 years of age following the insidious onset of a difference in color of the two eyes (heterochromia), a difference in the size or shape of the pupil (anisocoria), or ocular misalignment (strabismus). Often these findings are first noted at a screening vision test performed at school. There is no correlation between the onset of the arthritis and that of the uveitis, which may precede the onset of arthritis by up to 10 years. The knee is the most commonly involved joint. The cardinal signs of the disease are cells and flare in the anterior chamber, small to medium-sized white keratic precipitates with or without flecks of fibrin on the endothelium, posterior synechiae often progressing to seclusion of the pupil, and cataract. Band keratopathy, secondary glaucoma, and cystoid macular edema can also be present and cause loss of vision. Patients suspected of having JRA should be evaluated by a rheumatologist and tested for a positive ANA titer.

Treatment of JRA-associated uveitis is challenging. Topical corticosteroids, nonsteroidal anti-inflammatory agents, and cycloplegics are of value. In resistant cases, systemic immunosuppression with corticosteroids, methotrexate, or both may be required to control the disease. The prognosis for cataract surgery is guarded, and intraocular lens implantation is usually contraindicated.

Up to 50% of patients with **ankylosing spondylitis** develop anterior uveitis. There is a marked preponderance for men. The uveitis can vary in severity from mild to severe and often produces pain, photophobia, and blurred vision. Limbal injection can be present. Keratic precipitates, though usually present, are never

granulomatous, and iris nodules do not occur. Posterior synechiae, peripheral anterior synechiae, cataracts, and glaucoma are common complications following severe, recurrent, or poorly controlled bouts of inflammation. Macular edema is uncommon but can occur. Recurrence is the rule and may involve either eye, though bilateral simultaneous involvement is atypical. The HLA-B27 histocompatibility antigen is present in approximately 50% of patients with acute nongranulomatous iritis or iridocyclitis. Of those patients with anterior uveitis who are HLA-B27-positive, roughly half will experience a nonocular complication of their disease, most commonly ankylosing spondylitis but also psoriatic arthritis, Reiter's disease, and inflammatory bowel disease. Sacroiliac radiographs and colonoscopy can occasionally confirm diagnoses suspected on clinical grounds.

2. FUCHS' HETEROCHROMIC IRIDOCYCLITIS

Fuchs' heterochromic iridocyclitis is uncommon, accounting for less than 5% of all cases of uveitis. The onset is typically insidious during the third or fourth decade of life. Redness, pain, and photophobia are minimal. Patients usually complain of blurred vision, due to cataract. Iris heterochromia, best appreciated with natural lighting, can be subtle. Keratic precipitates are often small and stellate and scattered over the entire endothelium. Telangiectatic blood vessels may be seen in the chamber angle on gonioscopy. Posterior synechiae are uncommon. An anterior vitreous reaction may be present but is usually mild. While loss of stromal pigment tends to make heavily pigmented eyes look hypochromic, stromal atrophy affecting lightly colored irides can actually reveal underlying pigment epithelium on the posterior surface of the iris causing paradoxic hyperchromia. Pathologically, the iris and ciliary body show moderate atrophy with patchy depigmentation and diffuse infiltration of lymphocytes and plasma cells.

Cataract eventually develops in most patients, whereas glaucoma is less common but can occur in 10–15% of cases. The prognosis is excellent; cataract surgery can usually be performed without complication, and most patients with glaucoma can be managed with topical medications.

3. LENS-INDUCED UVEITIS

Lens-induced (phacogenic) uveitis is an autoimmune disease directed against lens antigens. There are no data at present to substantiate the implication that lens material per se is toxic, so the term "phacotoxic uveitis" should be avoided. The classic case occurs when the lens develops a hypermature cataract and the lens capsule leaks lens material into the posterior and anterior chambers. This material elicits an inflammatory reaction characterized by accumulation of plasma cells, mononuclear phagocytes, and a few polymorphonuclear cells. Typical anterior uveitis symptoms of pain, photophobia, and blurred vision are common. Lens-induced uveitis may also occur following lens trauma or cataract surgery with retained lens material. Phacolytic glaucoma is a common complication. Definitive treatment requires removal of the lens material. Concurrent treatment with corticosteroids, cycloplegics, and glaucoma medications is often necessary.

INTERMEDIATE UVEITIS (CYCLITIS, PERIPHERAL UVEITIS, PARS PLANITIS)

Intermediate uveitis affects mainly the intermediate zone of the eye—ciliary body, pars plana, peripheral retina, and vitreous. The cause is unknown in over half of cases, though syphilis, tuberculosis, and sarcoidosis should be ruled out with appropriate laboratory and ancillary testing. Intermediate uveitis is seen mainly among young adults, affects both sexes equally, and is bilateral in up to 80% of cases. Common complaints include floaters and blurred vision. Pain, redness, and photophobia are unusual but can accompany a severe first attack. Adequate examination of the ciliary body, pars plana, and peripheral retina requires use of an indirect ophthalmoscope and scleral depression, which often reveals vitreous condensations in the form of snowballs and snowbanking. Adjacent retinal vasculitis is common. Anterior chamber inflammation is invariably mild, and posterior synechiae are uncommon. Posterior subcapsular cataract and cystoid macular edema are the most common causes of decreased vision. In severe cases, cyclitic membranes and retinal detachments may occur. Secondary glaucoma is rare. Corticosteroids are used mainly to treat cystoid macular edema or retinal neovascularization. Topical corticosteroids should be tried first to identify patients predisposed to develop steroid-induced glaucoma. If no improvement is noted and glaucoma does not occur, a posterior sub-Tenon injection of corticosteroid may be effective. Patients with intermediate uveitis usually do well with cataract surgery.

POSTERIOR UVEITIS (TABLE 7–4)

The retina, choroid, and optic nerve are affected by a variety of infectious and noninfectious disorders, the more common of which are listed in Table 7–4.

Most cases of posterior uveitis are associated with some form of systemic disease. The cause can often be established on the basis of (1) the morphology of the lesions, (2) the mode of onset and course of the

Table 7–4. Causes of posterior uveitis.

Infectious disorders
  Viruses
    CMV, herpes simplex, herpes zoster, rubella, rubeola
  Bacteria
    Agents of tuberculosis, brucellosis, sporadic and endemic syphilis; *Borrelia* (Lyme disease); and various hematogenously spread gram-positive and gram-negative pathogens
  Fungi
    Candida, Histoplasma, Cryptococcus, Aspergillus
  Parasites
    Toxoplasma, Toxocara, Cysticercus, Onchocerca
Noninfectious disorders
  Autoimmune disorders
    Behçet's disease
    Vogt-Koyanagi-Harada syndrome
    Polyarteritis nodosa
    Systemic lupus erythematosus
    Wegener's granulomatosis
    Sympathetic ophthalmia
    Retinal vasculitis
  Malignancies
    Intraocular lymphoma
    Malignant melanoma
    Leukemia
    Metastatic lesions
  Unknown etiology
    Sarcoidosis
    Serpiginous choroiditis
    Acute multifocal placoid pigment epitheliopathy
    Birdshot retinochoroidopathy
    Retinal pigment epitheliopathy
    Multiple evanescent white dot syndrome

disease, or (3) the association with systemic symptoms or signs. Other considerations are the age of the patient and whether involvement is unilateral or bilateral. Laboratory and ancillary tests are often helpful.

Lesions of the posterior segment of the eye can be focal, multifocal, geographic, or diffuse. Those that tend to cause clouding of the overlying vitreous should be differentiated from those that give rise to little or no vitreous cells. The type and distribution of vitreous opacities should be described. Inflammatory lesions of the posterior segment are generally insidious in onset, but some may be accompanied by abrupt and profound visual loss.

Worldwide, the most common causes of retinitis in immunocompetent patients are toxoplasmosis, syphilis, and Behçet's disease, whereas the most common causes of choroiditis are sarcoidosis, tuberculosis, and Vogt-Koyanagi-Harada syndrome. Inflammatory optic neuritis can be caused by any of these diseases, but multiple sclerosis should always be suspected, particularly when associated with eye pain worsened by movement (Chapter 14). Less common causes of posterior uveitis include intraocular lymphoma, acute retinal necrosis syndrome, sympathetic ophthalmia, and the "white dot" syndromes such as multiple evanescent white dot syndrome (MEWDS) or acute multifocal posterior placoid epitheliopathy (AMPPE).

Diagnosis & Clinical Features

Diagnostic clues and clinical features of the more commonly encountered posterior uveitis syndromes are described below.

A. Age of the Patient: Posterior uveitis in patients under 3 years of age can be caused by a "masquerade syndrome" such as retinoblastoma or leukemia. Infectious causes of posterior uveitis in this age group include congenital toxoplasmosis, toxocariasis, and perinatal infections due to syphilis, cytomegalovirus, herpes simplex virus, herpes zoster virus, or rubella.

In the age group from 4 to 15 years, the most common causes of posterior uveitis are toxoplasmosis and toxocariasis. Uncommon causes include syphilis, tuberculosis, sarcoidosis, Behçet's disease, and Vogt-Koyanagi-Harada syndrome.

In the age group from 16 to 50 years, the differential diagnosis for posterior uveitis includes syphilis, tuberculosis, sarcoidosis, toxoplasmosis, Behçet's disease, Vogt-Koyanagi-Harada syndrome, and acute retinal necrosis syndrome.

Patients over age 50 years who present with posterior uveitis may have syphilis, tuberculosis, sarcoidosis, intraocular lymphoma, birdshot retinochoroiditis, acute retinal necrosis syndrome, toxoplasmosis, or endogenous endophthalmitis.

B. Laterality: Unilateral posterior uveitis favors a diagnosis of toxoplasmosis, toxocariasis, acute retinal necrosis syndrome, or endogenous bacterial or fungal infection.

C. Symptoms:

1. Reduced vision–Reduced visual acuity may be present in all types of posterior uveitis but especially in the setting of a macular lesion or retinal detachment. Every patient should be examined for an afferent pupillary defect, which, when present, signifies widespread retinal or optic nerve damage.

2. Ocular injection–Eye redness is uncommon in strictly posterior uveitis but can be seen in diffuse uveitis.

3. Pain–Pain is atypical in posterior uveitis but can occur in endophthalmitis, posterior scleritis, or optic neuritis, particularly when caused by multiple sclerosis.

D. Signs: Signs important in the diagnosis of posterior uveitis include hypopyon formation, granuloma formation, glaucoma, vitritis, morphology of the lesions, vasculitis, retinal hemorrhages, and scar formation.

1. Hypopyon–Disorders of the posterior segment that may be associated with significant anterior inflammation and hypopyon include syphilis, tuberculosis, sarcoidosis, endogenous endophthalmitis, Behçet's disease, and leptospirosis. When this occurs, the uveitis is more appropriately termed diffuse.

2. Type of uveitis–Anterior granulomatous uveitis may be associated with conditions that affect the posterior retina and choroid, including syphilis, tuberculosis, sarcoidosis, toxoplasmosis, Vogt-Koyanagi-Harada syndrome, and sympathetic ophthalmia. On the other hand, nongranulomatous anterior uveitis may be associated with Behçet's disease, acute retinal necrosis syndrome, intraocular lymphoma, or the white dot syndromes.

3. Glaucoma–Acute glaucoma in association with posterior uveitis can occur with toxoplasmosis, acute retinal necrosis syndrome, or sarcoidosis.

4. Vitritis–Posterior uveitis is often associated with vitritis, usually due to leakage from the inflammatory foci, from retinal vessels, or from the optic nerve head. Severe vitritis tends to occur with infections involving the posterior pole, such as toxoplasmic retinochoroiditis or bacterial endophthalmitis, whereas mild to moderate inflammation usually occurs with primary outer retinal and choroidal inflammatory disorders. Serpiginous choroiditis and presumed ocular histoplasmosis are typically accompanied by little if any vitritis.

5. Morphology and location of lesions–

a. Retina–The retina is the primary target of many types of infectious agents. Toxoplasmosis is the most common cause of retinitis in immunocompetent hosts. The active lesion of toxoplasmosis is generally seen in the company of old, healed scars that may be heavily pigmented. The lesions may appear in a juxtapapillary location and often give rise to retinal vasculitis. The vitreous is generally clouded when large lesions are present. In contrast, retinal infection with herpesviruses, such as cytomegalovirus and varicella-zoster virus, is more common in immunocompromised hosts. Rubella and rubeola virus retinal infections occur primarily in young children, where they tend to produce diffuse pigmentary changes involving the outer retina referred to as "salt and pepper" retinopathy (see Chapter 15).

b. Choroid–The choroid is the primary target of granulomatous processes such as tuberculosis and sarcoidosis. Patients with tuberculosis and sarcoidosis may present with a focal, multifocal, or geographic choroiditis. Both multifocal and diffuse infiltration of the choroid occur in Vogt-Koyanagi-Harada syndrome and sympathetic ophthalmia. Birdshot retinochoroidopathy and presumed ocular histoplasmosis syndrome, in contrast, almost always produce multifocal choroiditis.

c. Optic nerve–Primary inflammatory optic neuritis can occur from syphilis, tuberculosis, sarcoidosis, toxoplasmosis, multiple sclerosis, Lyme disease, intraocular lymphoma, or systemic *Bartonella henselae* infection, the causative organism in cat-scratch disease. A macular star is often present.

E. Trauma: A history of trauma is important in patients with uveitis to rule out intraocular foreign body or sympathetic ophthalmia. Surgical trauma, including routine operations for cataract and glaucoma, may introduce microorganisms into the eye and lead to acute or subacute endophthalmitis.

F. Mode of Onset: The onset of posterior uveitis may be acute and sudden or slow and insidious. Diseases of the posterior segment of the eye that tend to present with sudden loss of vision include toxoplasmic retinochoroiditis, acute retinal necrosis syndrome, and bacterial endophthalmitis. Most other causes of posterior uveitis have a more insidious onset.

1. OCULAR TOXOPLASMOSIS

Toxoplasmosis is caused by *Toxoplasma gondii,* an obligate intracellular protozoan (Figure 7–5). The ocular lesions may be acquired in utero or following systemic infection. Constitutional symptoms may be mild and easily missed. The domestic cat and other feline species serve as definitive hosts for the parasite. Susceptible women who acquire the disease during pregnancy may transmit the infection to the fetus, where it can be fatal. Sources of human infection include oocysts in soil or airborne in dust, undercooked meat containing bradyzoites (encysted forms of the parasite), and tachyzoites (proliferative form) transmitted across the placenta.

Clinical Findings
(Figure 7–5)

A. Symptoms and Signs: Patients with toxoplasmic retinochoroiditis present with a history of floaters and blurred vision. In severe cases there may also be pain and photophobia. The ocular lesions consist of fluffy-white areas of focal necrotic retinochoroiditis that may be small or large and single or multiple. Active edematous lesions are often adjacent to healed retinal scars. Retinal vasculitis and hemorrhage can be observed. Cystoid macular edema can accompany lesions in or near the macula. Iridocyclitis is frequently seen in patients with severe infections, and intraocular pressure may be elevated.

B. Laboratory Findings: A positive serologic test for *T gondii* with consistent clinical signs is considered diagnostic. An increase in antibody titer is usually not detected during reactivation, but an elevated IgM titer provides strong evidence for recently acquired infection.

Treatment

Small lesions in the retinal periphery not associated with significant vitritis require no treatment. In contrast, severe or posterior infections are usually treated for 4–6 weeks with pyrimethamine, 25–50 mg daily, and trisulfapyrimidine, 0.5–1 g four times daily. Loading doses of 75 mg of pyrimethamine and 2 g of trisulfapyrimidine should be given at the start of therapy. Patients are usually also given 3 mg of leucovorin calcium twice weekly to prevent bone marrow depression. A complete blood count should be performed weekly during therapy (Table 7–2).

An alternative approach for the treatment of ocular toxoplasmosis consists of administration of clindamycin, 300 mg four times daily, with trisulfapyrimidine, 0.5–1 g four times daily. Clindamycin causes pseudomembranous colitis in 10–15% of patients. Other antibiotics effective in ocular toxoplasmosis include spiramycin and minocycline. Subretinal neovascularization can be treated with argon laser photocoagulation.

Anterior uveitis associated with ocular toxoplasmosis may be treated with topical corticosteroids and cycloplegics. Periocular steroid injections are contraindicated. Topical glaucoma medications are occasionally necessary. Systemic corticosteroids can be used in conjunction with antimicrobial therapy for vision-threatening inflammatory lesions but should never be given alone.

2. HISTOPLASMOSIS

In some areas of the United States where histoplasmosis is endemic (the Ohio and Mississippi River Valley areas), the diagnosis of choroiditis due to presumed ocular histoplasmosis is common. Patients usually have a positive skin test to histoplasmin and demonstrate "punched-out" spots in the posterior or peripheral fundus. These spots are small, irregularly round or oval, and usually depigmented centrally with a finely pigmented border. Peripapillary atrophy and hyperpigmentation occur frequently. Macular lesions may produce subretinal neovascularization, a complication that should be suspected in every patient with presumed ocular histoplasmosis who presents with decreased vision or evidence of subretinal fluid or hemorrhage. Subretinal neovascularization is effectively treated with argon laser photocoagulation.

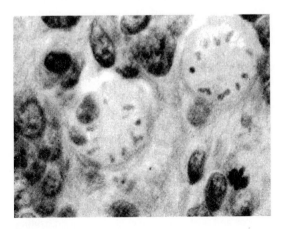

Figure 7–5. *Toxoplasma* cysts in the retina. (Courtesy of K Tabbara.)

3. OCULAR TOXOCARIASIS

Toxocariasis results from infection with *Toxocara cati* (an intestinal parasite of cats) or *Toxocara canis* (of dogs). Visceral larva migrans is a disseminated systemic infection occurring in a young child (Table 7–5). Ocular involvement rarely occurs in visceral larva migrans.

Ocular toxocariasis may occur without systemic manifestations. Children acquire the disease by close association with pets and by eating dirt (pica) contaminated with *Toxocara* ova. The ingested ova form larvae that penetrate the intestinal mucosa and gain access to the systemic circulation and finally to the eye. The parasite does not infect the intestinal tract of humans.

Clinical Findings

A. Symptoms and Signs: The disease is usually unilateral. *Toxocara* larvae lodge in the retina and die, leading to a marked inflammatory reaction and local production of *Toxocara* antibodies. Children are typically brought to the ophthalmologist because of a red eye, blurred vision, or a whitish pupil (leukocoria).

Three clinical presentations are recognized: (1) a localized posterior granuloma, usually near the optic nerve head or fovea; (2) a peripheral granuloma involving the pars plana, often producing an elevated mass that mimics the snowbank of intermediate uveitis; and (3) chronic endophthalmitis.

B. Laboratory Findings: Characteristic clinical findings and a positive enzyme-linked immunosorbent assay (ELISA) for anti-*Toxocara* antibodies, even at low titer, confirm the diagnosis of ocular toxocariasis. Negative ELISAs are common but do not

Table 7–5. Comparison between visceral and ocular larva migrans.

	Visceral Larva Migrans	Ocular Larva Migrans[1]
Average age at onset	2 years	7 years
Fever	+	−
Abdominal symptoms (pain, nausea, diarrhea)	+	−
Nonspecific pulmonary disease	+	−
Hepatosplenomegaly	+	−
Eosinophilia	+	−
Hypergammaglobulinemia	+	−
ELISA (serum anti-*Toxocara* antibodies)	+	±
ELISA (aqueous anti-*Toxocara* antibodies)	−	+
Ocular findings[1]	−	+

[1] Ocular findings of ocular larva migrans: diffuse chronic panuveitis, posterior pole granuloma, or peripheral granuloma.

rule out the possibility of ocular infection. Positive antibody titers of the ocular fluids from patients with suspected ocular toxocariasis have been demonstrated in the setting of a negative serum ELISA, but the test is not routinely available and in any case seldom necessary.

Treatment

Systemic or periocular injections of corticosteroids should be given when there is evidence of significant intraocular inflammation. Vitrectomy may be necessary in patients with marked vitreous opacity or with significant preretinal traction. Systemic anthelmintic therapy is not indicated for limited ocular disease and in fact may worsen the inflammation by producing more rapid killing of the intraocular parasite.

4. ACQUIRED IMMUNODEFICIENCY SYNDROME

Uveitis is common in patients infected with the human immunodeficiency virus (HIV), particularly in advanced stages of the illness when AIDS develops. (See Chapter 15.) CD4 T lymphocyte counts are a good predictor of the risk of opportunistic infections, with the majority occurring at counts of <100 cells/μL. Uveitis occurs most commonly in the setting of posterior segment infection. Cytomegalovirus retinitis, a geographic retinitis often accompanied by hemorrhage, occurs in 30–40% of HIV-positive patients at some point in the course of their illness. Other herpesviruses such as varicella-zoster and herpes simplex can produce a similar retinitis but are usually distinguished by a very rapid progress. Infections caused by other organisms, such as *T gondii*, *Treponema pallidum*, *Cryptococcus neoformans*, *Mycobacterium tuberculosis*, and *Mycobacterium avium-intracellulare* occur in less than 5% of HIV-positive patients but should be considered, particularly when there is a history of infection or exposure, when choroiditis is present, or when the retinitis is atypical in appearance or fails to respond to antiviral therapy. Intraocular lymphoma occurs in less than 1% of HIV-positive patients but should be considered when the retinitis is atypical or is unresponsive to antiviral treatment, especially when neurologic symptoms are present. Diagnosis usually requires vitreous biopsy.

DIFFUSE UVEITIS (TABLE 7–6)

The term "diffuse uveitis" is used to denote a more or less uniform cellular infiltration of both the anterior and posterior segments. Associated findings such as retinitis, vasculitis, or choroiditis can occur and often prompt further diagnostic testing. Tuber-

Table 7–6. Causes of diffuse uveitis.

Sarcoidosis
Tuberculosis
Syphilis
Onchocerciasis
Leptospirosis
Brucellosis
Sympathetic ophthalmia
Behçet's disease
Multiple sclerosis
Cysticercosis
Vogt-Koyanagi-Harada syndrome
Masquerade syndrome: retinoblastoma, leukemia
Retained intraocular foreign body

culosis, sarcoidosis, and syphilis should always be considered in patients with diffuse uveitis. Less common causes include sympathetic ophthalmia, Vogt-Koyanagi-Harada syndrome, Behçet's disease, birdshot retinochoroiditis, and intraocular lymphoma.

1. TUBERCULOUS UVEITIS

Tuberculosis can cause any type of uveitis but deserves special consideration when granulomatous keratic precipitates or iris or choroidal granulomas are present. Such granulomas, or tubercles, consist of giant and epithelioid cells. Caseating necrosis is characteristic on histopathologic examination. Although the infection is said to be transmitted from a primary focus elsewhere in the body, uveal tuberculosis is uncommon in patients with active pulmonary tuberculosis (see Chapter 15). Evaluation should include a chest x-ray and skin testing with both PPD and positive controls such as mumps and candida. Treatment should involve three or more antituberculous medicines for 6–12 months. (See Table 7–2.)

2. SARCOIDOSIS

Sarcoidosis is a chronic granulomatous disease of unknown cause, usually presenting in the fourth or fifth decade of life. Pulmonary involvement occurs in over 90% of patients. Virtually every other organ system can be involved, including the skin, bones, liver, spleen, central nervous system, and eyes. The tissue reaction is much less severe than in tuberculous uveitis, and caseation does not occur. Anergy on skin testing supports the diagnosis. When the parotid glands are involved, the disease is called uveoparotid fever, or Heerfordt's disease. When the lacrimal glands are involved, the disease is called Mikulicz's syndrome.

Uveitis occurs in approximately 25% of patients with systemic sarcoidosis. As with tuberculosis, any form of uveitis can occur, but sarcoid deserves special consideration when the uveitis is granulomatous or

when retinal phlebitis is present, particularly in black patients.

The diagnosis can be supported by an abnormal chest x-ray, especially when hilar adenopathy is present, or by elevated serum angiotensin-converting enzyme, lysozyme, or calcium levels. The strongest evidence comes from histopathologic demonstration of noncaseating granulomas in affected tissues such as lung or conjunctiva. However, biopsies should only be taken when suspicious lesions are clearly evident. A gallium scan of the head, neck, and thorax can provide evidence for subclinical inflammation of the lacrimal, parotid, or salivary glands or of paratracheal or pulmonary lymph nodes.

Corticosteroid therapy given early in the disease may be effective, but recurrences are common. Long-term therapy may require the use of steroid-sparing agents such as methotrexate or azathioprine (Table 7–2).

3. SYPHILIS

Syphilis is an uncommon but treatable cause of uveitis. Intraocular inflammation occurs almost exclusively during the secondary and tertiary stages of infection. All types of uveitis occur. Associated retinitis or optic neuritis is common. Widespread atrophy and hyperplasia of the retinal pigment epithelium can occur late if untreated. Testing should include one of the commonly used (and less expensive) tests for the production of *T pallidum*-induced anticardiolipin antibodies, such as the VDRL or RPR test, as well as a test for the more specific anti-*T pallidum* antibodies such as the FTA-ABS or MH-ATP. While the FTA-ABS and MH-ATP tests display high sensitivity and specificity during both secondary and tertiary stages of infection, the VDRL and RPR can be falsely negative in up to 30% of patients with late or latent disease. Falsely positive results can occur in the setting of other spirochetal infections, biliary cirrhosis, or collagen-vascular disease, whereas falsely negative results can occur in severely immunocompromised patients. Patients with uveitis and a positive serologic test for syphilis should undergo examination of the cerebrospinal fluid to rule out neurosyphilis. Treatment consists of aqueous crystalline penicillin G, 2–4 million units, given intravenously every 4 hours for 10 days.

4. SYMPATHETIC OPHTHALMIA (Figure 7–6)

Sympathetic ophthalmia is a rare but devastating bilateral granulomatous uveitis that comes on 10 days to many years following a perforating eye injury. Ninety percent of cases occur within 1 year after injury. The cause is not known, but the disease is prob-

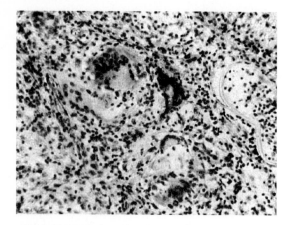

Figure 7–6. Microscopic section of giant cells and lymphocytes in sympathetic ophthalmia involving the choroid. (Courtesy of R Carriker.)

ably related to hypersensitivity to some element of the pigment-bearing cells in the uvea. It very rarely occurs following uncomplicated intraocular surgery for cataract or glaucoma and even less commonly following endophthalmitis.

The injured, or exciting, eye becomes inflamed first and the fellow, or sympathizing, eye secondarily. Patients usually complain of photophobia, redness, and blurred vision though the presence of floaters may be the primary complaint. The uveitis is usually diffuse. Soft yellow-white exudates in the deep layer of the retina (Dalen-Fuchs nodules) are sometimes seen in the posterior segment. Serous retinal detachments also occur.

The recommended treatment of a severely injured sightless eye is enucleation within 10 days after injury. The sympathizing eye should be treated aggressively with local or systemic corticosteroids. Other immunosuppressive agents such as cyclosporine, cyclophosphamide, and chlorambucil may be required as well (see Table 7–2). Without treatment, the disease progresses relentlessly to complete bilateral blindness.

UVEITIS IN DEVELOPING COUNTRIES

All forms of uveitis mentioned above occur in developing countries as well, and some, such as toxoplasmosis and tuberculosis, are relatively common. In addition, more than 95% of all HIV-positive patients live in developing countries, particularly in sub-Saharan Africa and Southeast Asia. In these regions, otherwise opportunistic infections such as cytomegalovirus retinitis are increasing at an alarming rate. A few infectious causes of uveitis deserve special mention, since they occur almost exclusively in patients who either live in or visit developing countries.

1. LEPTOSPIROSIS

Uveitis occurs in up to 10% of patients infected with the spirochete *Leptospira.* Humans are accidental hosts, infected most commonly by contact with or ingestion of infected water supplies. Wild and domestic animals, including rodents, dogs, pigs, and cattle, are the natural hosts and shed large quantities of infectious organisms in their urine. Farmers, veterinarians, and those who work or swim in waters fed by agricultural runoff are at particularly high risk.

Clinical Findings

A. Symptoms and Signs: Fever, malaise, and headache are common constitutional symptoms. Renal failure and death can occur in up to 30% of untreated patients. The uveitis may be of any type but is typically diffuse and often associated with hypopyon and retinal vasculitis.

B. Laboratory Findings: Culture of live organisms is only possible early in the infection. Sensitive and specific anti-*Leptospira* antibody tests are available for use on blood or cerebrospinal fluid. A fourfold rise in antibody titer is strong evidence for recent infection.

Treatment

Treatment of severe infections includes penicillin, 1.5 million units intravenously every 6 hours for 10 days. Less severe infections can be treated with doxycycline, 100 mg given orally twice daily for 7 days. Topical corticosteroids and cycloplegics should be used in conjunction with antibiotic therapy to minimize the complications of anterior uveitis. Posterior sub-Tenon injection of corticosteroids may be necessary for severe intermediate, posterior, or diffuse forms of inflammation.

2. ONCHOCERCIASIS

Onchocerciasis is caused by *Onchocerca volvulus.* The disease afflicts about 30 million people in Africa and Central America and is a major cause of blindness. It is transmitted by *Simulium damnosum,* a black fly that breeds in areas of rapidly flowing streams—thus the term "river blindness." Microfilariae picked up from the skin by the fly mature into larvae that become adult worms in 1 year. The adult parasite produces cutaneous nodules 5–25 mm in diameter on the trunk, thighs, arms, head, and shoulders. Microfilariae cause itching, and healing of skin lesions may lead to loss of skin elasticity and areas of depigmentation.

Clinical Findings

A. Symptoms and Signs: Skin nodules may be seen. The cornea reveals nummular keratitis and sclerosing keratitis. Microfilariae swimming actively in the anterior chamber look like silver threads. Death of the microfilariae causes an intense inflammatory reaction and severe uveitis, vitritis, and retinitis. Focal retinochoroiditis may be seen. Optic atrophy may develop secondary to glaucoma.

B. Laboratory Findings: The diagnosis of onchocerciasis is made by skin biopsy and microscopic examination looking for live microfilariae.

Treatment

The preferred treatment for onchocerciasis is with nodulectomy and ivermectin. Diethylcarbamazine and suramin have significant toxicity and should be used only when ivermectin is not available.

The great advantage of ivermectin over diethylcarbamazine is that a single oral dose of 100 or 200 µg/kg reduces the worm burden in the skin and anterior chamber more slowly and therefore with a significant reduction in systemic and ocular reactions. The reduction also persists longer.

The minimum effective dose remains to be determined. A dose of 100 µg/kg may be as effective as 200 µg/kg and is associated with fewer of the mild and transient side effects: fever, headache, etc. Treatment is repeated at 6 or 12 months.

Topical therapy with corticosteroids and cycloplegics is helpful for uveitis.

3. CYSTICERCOSIS

Cysticercosis is a common cause of serious ocular morbidity. The disease is endemic in Mexico and other Central and South American countries, with ocular involvement occurring in about one-third of patients. It is caused either by the ingestion of eggs of *Taenia solium* or by reverse peristalsis in cases of intestinal obstruction caused by adult tapeworms. Eggs mature and embryos penetrate intestinal mucosa, thus gaining access to the circulation. The larva *(Cysticercus cellulosae)* is the most common tapeworm that invades the human eye.

Clinical Findings

The larvae may reach the subretinal space, producing acute retinitis with retinal edema and subretinal exudates, or the vitreous cavity, where a translucent cyst with a dense white spot formed by the invaginated scolex develops. Larvae may live in the eye for as long as 2 years. Death of the larvae inside the eye leads to a severe inflammatory reaction. Movements of larvae within the ocular tissue may stimulate a chronic inflammatory reaction and fibrosis. In rare instances, the larva may be seen in the anterior chamber. Involvement of the brain can cause seizures. Focal calcification may be seen in the subcutaneous tissues by x-ray.

Treatment

Treatment of cysticercosis is by surgical removal, usually by pars plana vitrectomy.

TUMORS INVOLVING THE UVEAL TRACT

J. Brooks Crawford, MD

Several important tumors that may be first identified during ophthalmoscopic examination are discussed below.

Nevus

Nevi (Figures 7–7 and 7–8) are usually flat lesions with or without pigment lying in the stroma of the tissue. On the anterior surface of the iris, they may be noted as iris "freckles." Posteriorly in the choroid, one may see flat pigmented areas. Large choroidal nevi are difficult to differentiate from malignant melanomas. Their flat appearance and especially their lack of growth on repeat serial examinations are important in the differential diagnosis from malignant melanoma.

Because of the difficulties in differentiation from malignant melanomas, fundus photographs or careful line drawings should be made of all suspicious lesions. The elevation or thickness of these lesions can best be measured and documented by ultrasonography. Observations should be made periodically for changes.

Ocular & Oculodermal Melanocytosis

Hyperpigmentation of tissue due to an abundance of large, pigmented uveal melanocytes and episcleral melanocytes occurs in both ocular and oculodermal melanocytosis. Melanocytes located deep in the dermis give the skin around the eye a bluish or slate-gray color in oculodermal melanocytosis. Eyes with melanosis—particularly ocular melanosis, which is most common in Caucasians—have a slightly in-

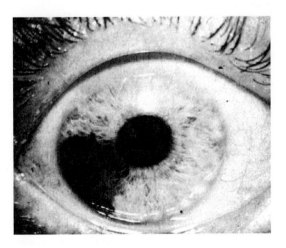

Figure 7–7. Nevus of the iris. (Courtesy of A Rosenberg.)

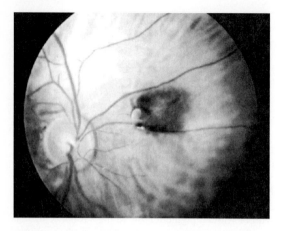

Figure 7–8. Nevus of the choroid. (Photo by Diane Beeston.)

creased risk of developing uveal and orbital melanomas.

Hemangioma of the Choroid

Choroidal hemangiomas occur as isolated localized tumors or as diffuse hamartomas associated with Sturge-Weber syndrome. Ultrasonography can help distinguish these orange-colored tumors from amelanotic choroidal melanomas. Visual loss is the result of secondary retinal detachment, degenerative changes in the retinal pigment epithelium or sensory retina, and secondary glaucoma.

Occasionally, choroidal hemangiomas can be treated with photocoagulation to limit the extent and degree of associated serous detachment of the retina. Those that fail to respond to photocoagulation—and especially the more diffuse tumors—may require radiotherapy. Enucleation may be necessary for tumors associated with intractable, painful glaucoma.

Medulloepitheliomas of the Ciliary Body

Benign and malignant medulloepitheliomas are rare tumors that may arise from the ciliary body epithelium, which is the anterior extension of the retina (see Chapter 10), and are therefore not truly tumors of the uveal tract. Those with one or more heteroplastic elements, such as hyaline cartilage, brain tissue, or rhabdomyoblasts, are called teratoid medulloepitheliomas. Those that arise soon after birth may infiltrate the area around the lens and produce a white pupillary reflex similar to that seen in eyes with retinoblastoma.

Malignant Melanoma

It has been estimated that intraocular malignant melanoma occurs in 0.02–0.06% of the total eye patient population in the USA. It is seen only in the uveal tract and is the most common intraocular malignant tumor in the white population. It is almost always unilateral. Eighty-five percent appear in the choroid (Figure 7–9), 9% in the ciliary body, and 6% in the iris.

This tumor may be seen in its early stages only accidentally during routine ophthalmoscopic examination or because of blurring due to macular invasion. Blood-borne metastases may occur at any time. Glaucoma may be a late manifestation.

Histologically, these tumors are composed of spindle-shaped cells, with or without prominent nucleoli, and large epithelioid tumor cells. Tumors composed of the former have a good prognosis; tumors with the latter a poorer prognosis.

Intraocular malignant melanomas may extend into adjacent intraocular tissues or outside the eye through the scleral canals or by intravascular invasion.

Clinical manifestations are usually absent unless the macula is involved. In the later stages, growth of the tumor may lead to retinal detachment with loss of visual field. A tumor located in the iris may change the color of the iris or deform the pupil. Pain does not occur in the absence of glaucoma or inflammation.

The first step in diagnosis is to suspect the lesion. Most intraocular malignant melanomas can be seen ophthalmoscopically. Always suspect the presence of a tumor in eyes with nonrhegmatogenous retinal detachment. A significant incidence of intraocular melanomas has been found in blind, painful eyes; ultrasonography will help detect these.

Enucleation of an eye with a choroidal melanoma has been the traditional treatment. Recently, other forms of therapy, particularly local resection or radiotherapy with charged particles such as helium ions and protons or with plaques of radioactive isotopes sutured to the sclera, have been used for eyes with all but the largest tumors. Very small melanomas (< 10 mm in diameter) have an excellent prognosis and are often impossible to differentiate from benign nevi;

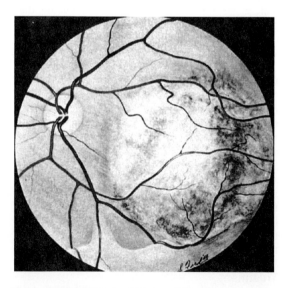

Figure 7–9. Malignant melanoma of the choroid, macular area, left eye (drawing). (Courtesy of F Cordes.)

therefore, most authorities advocate not treating these tumors until unequivocal growth can be documented (usually with serial photographs or ultrasound measurements). In patients with metastatic disease, the median survival time is less than 1 year, the value of chemotherapy is limited, and treatment to the affected eye is for symptomatic relief only.

Small melanomas of the iris that have not invaded the iris root can be safely observed until growth is documented; then they can be removed by iridectomy. Lesions that invade the iris root and ciliary body can be treated with iridocyclectomy unless the tumor has extended around the trabecular meshwork and Schlemm's canal to form a ring melanoma with secondary glaucoma. Iris melanomas have an excellent prognosis; the mortality rate is less than 1%. Many pigmented iris tumors are actually large nevi rather than malignant melanomas. Iris cysts, traumatic foreign bodies, and inflammatory nodules can also mimic melanomas.

Choroidal Metastases

Because of its rich blood supply, the choroid is an important site for blood-borne metastases. In females, carcinoma of the breast is much the most common source. In males, lung, genitourinary, and gastrointestinal malignancies are the usual primaries. Metastasis to the choroid usually becomes apparent within 2 years after diagnosis of the primary malignancy, but occasionally it does not become manifest until many years later. Occasionally—especially for lung carcinomas—the appearance of a choroidal metastasis may precede the diagnosis of the primary neoplasm.

The usual presenting symptoms of choroidal metastasis are decreased vision and photopsia. The tumor appears as a pale, non-pigmented elevation of the choroid, often associated with serous retinal detachment. There may be multiple lesions involving one or both eyes, in which case the diagnosis is relatively easily made. A solitary metastasis may be mistaken for an amelanotic choroidal malignant melanoma. Ultrasonography and fine-needle biopsy may aid in differentiation.

Chemotherapy for concurrent metastatic disease is usually effective against the choroidal component. In the absence of other metastases, local radiotherapy is the treatment of choice.

II. SCLERA

Emmett T. Cunningham, Jr., MD, PhD, MPH

BLUE SCLERAS

The normal sclera is white and opaque, so that the underlying uveal structures are not visible. Structural changes of the scleral collagen fibers and thinning of the sclera may allow the underlying uveal pigment to be seen, giving the sclera a bluish discoloration. Blue scleras also occur in several disorders that lead to disturbances in the connective tissues, such as osteogenesis imperfecta, Ehlers-Danlos syndrome, pseudoxanthoma elasticum, and Marfan's syndrome (Chapter 15). Blue scleras are sometimes noted in normal newborn infants and in patients with keratoconus or keratoglobus.

SCLERAL ECTASIA

Prolonged elevation of intraocular pressure early in infancy, as may occur with congenital glaucoma, can lead to stretching and thinning of the sclera. Scleral ectasia may also occur as a congenital anomaly surrounding the disk or involving the macular area or following inflammation or injury of the sclera.

STAPHYLOMA

Staphyloma results from bulging of the uvea into ectatic sclera. It may be anterior, equatorial, or posterior. Anterior staphylomas are generally located over the ciliary body (ciliary staphyloma) (Figure 7–10) or between the ciliary body and the limbus (intercalary staphyloma). Equatorial staphylomas are located at the equator and posterior staphylomas posterior to the equator. Posterior staphylomas are most commonly seen near the optic nerve head. Patients with posterior staphyloma generally have poor vision and high myopia, though cases of congenital peripapillary staphyloma in patients with normal or nearly normal vision have been reported. Posterior staphyloma usually produces choroidal atrophy and may be associated with subretinal neovascularization. Staphyloma must be differentiated from extreme myopia and central coloboma of the optic nerve head.

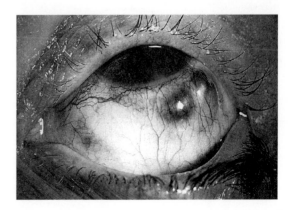

Figure 7–10. Ciliary staphyloma. (Courtesy of P Thygeson.)

INTRASCLERAL NERVE LOOPS OF AXENFELD

The intrascleral nerve loops are sites of branching of the long ciliary nerves. They enter the sclera close to the ciliary body, usually 3–4 mm posterior to the limbus. They are more commonly seen nasally, tend to be pigmented, and are usually accompanied by a small anterior ciliary artery.

INFLAMMATION OF THE EPISCLERA & SCLERA

Inflammation involving the episclera, the thin layer of vascularized connective tissue overlying the sclera, is referred to as episcleritis. Scleritis, in contrast, refers to primary inflammation of the sclera itself. Scleritis tends to be much more painful and is more often associated with an underlying systemic infection or autoimmune disease.

1. EPISCLERITIS

Episcleritis is a relatively common localized inflammation of the vascularized connective tissue overlying the sclera. It tends to affect young people, typically in the third or fourth decade of life; affects women three times as frequently as men; and is unilateral in about two-thirds of cases. Recurrence is the rule. The cause is not known. An associated local or systemic disorder, such as ocular rosacea, atopy, gout, infection, or collagen-vascular disease, is present in up to one-third of patients.

Symptoms of episcleritis include redness and mild irritation or discomfort. Ocular examination reveals episcleral injection, which may be nodular, sectoral, or diffuse (Figure 7–11). There is no inflammation or

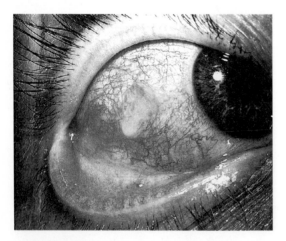

Figure 7–11. Nodular episcleritis, right eye. (Photo by Diane Beeston.)

edema of the underlying sclera, and keratitis and uveitis are uncommon. Conjunctivitis is ruled out by the lack of palpebral conjunctival injection or discharge.

The condition is benign, and the course is generally self-limited in 1–2 weeks. In the absence of a systemic disease, associated treatment should include chilled artificial tears every 4–6 hours until the redness resolves. However, for cases associated with a local or systemic disorder, more specific therapy may be needed—eg, doxycycline, 100 mg twice daily for rosacea; antimicrobial therapy for tuberculosis, syphilis, or herpesvirus infection; or local or systemic nonsteroidal anti-inflammatory agents or corticosteroids for collagen-vascular disease.

2. SCLERITIS

Scleritis is an uncommon disorder characterized by cellular infiltration, destruction of collagen, and vascular remodeling. These changes may be immunologically mediated or, less commonly, the result of infection. Local trauma can precipitate the inflammation (Table 7–7). Laboratory studies are often helpful in identifying associated systemic diseases, which occur in up to two-thirds of patients (Table 7–8).

Scleritis is bilateral in one-third of cases and affects women more commonly than men, typically in the fifth or sixth decades of life. Patients with scleritis almost always complain of pain, which is typically se-

Table 7–7. Causes of scleritis.

Autoimmune diseases
  Ankylosing spondylitis
  Rheumatoid arthritis
  Polyarteritis nodosa
  Relapsing polychondritis
  Wegener's granulomatosis
  Systemic lupus erythematosus
  Pyoderma gangrenosum
  Ulcerative colitis
  IgA nephropathy
  Psoriatic arthritis
Granulomatous and infectious diseases
  Tuberculosis
  Syphilis
  Sarcoidosis
  Toxoplasmosis
  Herpes simplex
  Herpes zoster
  Pseudomonas infection
  Streptococcal infection
  Staphylococcal infection
  Aspergillosis
  Leprosy
Others
  Physical agents (irradiation, thermal burns)
  Chemical agents (alkali or acid burns)
  Mechanical causes (trauma, surgery)
  Lymphoma
  Rosacea
Unknown

Table 7–8. Laboratory workup for scleritis.

Complete blood count and sedimentation rate
Serum rheumatoid factor (RF)
Serum antinuclear antibodies (ANA)
Serum antineutrophil cytoplasmic antibodies (ANCA)
PPD, chest x-ray
Serum FTA-ABS, VDRL
Serum uric acid
Urinalysis

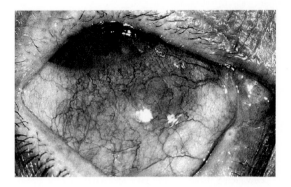

Figure 7–12. Nodular scleritis, left eye, associated with rheumatoid arthritis. (Courtesy of GR O'Connor.)

vere and boring in nature and tends to wake them at night. The globe is frequently tender. Visual acuity is often slightly reduced, and intraocular pressure may be mildly elevated. Concurrent keratitis or uveitis occurs in up to one-third of patients. A key clinical sign is deep violaceous discoloration of the globe due to dilation of the deep vascular plexus of the sclera and episclera, which may be nodular, sectoral, or diffuse (Figure 7–12). Use of the red-free filter of the slitlamp highlights the vascular changes. Areas of avascularity usually result from an occlusive vasculitis and portend a poor prognosis. Scleral thinning often follows bouts of inflammation. Scleral necrosis in the absence of inflammation is referred to as scleromalacia perforans, and is seen almost exclusively in patients with rheumatoid arthritis.

Posterior scleritis usually presents with pain and decreased vision with little or no redness. Mild vitritis, optic nerve head edema, serous retinal detachment, or choroidal folds may be present. Diagnosis is based on detection of thickening of the posterior sclera and choroid on ultrasonography or CT scan. Localized thickening may be mistaken on ultrasonography for a choroidal tumor.

The same disease associations described above for episcleritis also occur with scleritis, though they occur more frequently and tend to be more severe. Failure to control scleral inflammation can, if severe, result in perforation. Initial treatment of scleritis is with systemic nonsteroidal anti-inflammatory agents. Either indomethacin, 75 mg daily, or ibuprofen, 600 mg daily, may be used. In most cases, there is a virtually immediate reduction in pain and subsequent resolution of inflammation. If there is no response in 1–2 weeks, or if vascular closure becomes apparent, oral prednisone, 0.5–1.5 mg/kg/d, should be started. Occasionally, severe disease necessitates intravenous pulse therapy with methylprednisolone, 1 g. Other immunosuppressive agents can also be used. Cyclophosphamide is particularly valuable if perforation is imminent. Topical therapy is not effective on its own but may be useful as an adjunct to systemic therapy, particularly when uveitis is present. Specific antimicrobial therapy should be given if an infectious cause is identified. Surgery may be required to repair scleral or corneal perforations. Scleromalacia perforans is rarely associated with perforation unless trauma or glaucoma occurs.

HYALINE DEGENERATION

Hyaline degeneration is a fairly frequent finding in the scleras of persons over age 60. It is manifested by small, round, translucent gray areas that are usually about 2–3 mm in diameter and located anterior to the insertion of the rectus muscles. These lesions cause no symptoms or complications.

REFERENCES

DISEASES OF THE UVEAL TRACT

Akduman L, Kaplan HJ, Tyschen L: Prevalence of uveitis in an outpatient juvenile arthritis clinic: Onset of uveitis more than a decade after onset of arthritis. J Pediatr Ophthalmol Strabismus 1997;34:101.

Brockhurst RJ, Jakobiec FA (section editors): Uveal tract. In: *Principles and Practice of Ophthalmology. Clinical Practice.* Volume 1. Alberts DM, Jakobiec FA (editors). Saunders, 1994.

Cano MR: Ocular cysticercosis. In: *Retina,* 2nd ed. Ryan SJ (editor). Mosby, 1994.

Chan CC et al: 32 cases of sympathetic ophthalmia: A retrospective study at the National Eye Institute

Bethesda, Md., from 1982–1992. Arch Ophthalmol 1995;113:597.

Ciulla TA, Gragoudas ES: Serpiginous choroiditis. Int Ophthalmol Clin 1996;36:135.

Dana M-R et al: Prognosticators for visual outcome in sarcoid uveitis. Ophthalmology 1996;103:1846.

Golnik KC et al: Ophthalmic manifestations of *Rochalimaea* species. Am J Ophthalmol 1994;118:145.

Hawkins BS, Alexander J, Schachat AP: Ocular histoplasmosis. In: *Retina,* 2nd ed. Ryan SJ (editor). Mosby, 1994.

Helm CJ, Holland GN: Ocular tuberculosis. Surv Ophthalmol 1993;38:229.

Jabs DA: Ocular manifestations of HIV infection. Trans Am Ophthalmol Soc 1995;93:623.

Jabs DA, Bartlett JG: AIDS and ophthalmology: A period of transition. Am J Ophthalmol 1997;124:227.

Jacobson MA: Treatment of cytomegalovirus retinitis in patients with the acquired immunodeficiency syndrome. N Engl J Med 1997;337:105.

Kauffmann DJH, Wornser GP: Ocular Lyme disease: Case report and review of the literature. Br J Ophthalmol 1990;74:325.

La Hey E, de Jong PT, Kijlstra A: Fuchs' heterochromic cyclitis: Review of the literature on the pathogenetic mechanisms. Br J Ophthalmol 1994;78:307.

Lewallen S, Courtright P: HIV and AIDS and the eye in developing countries: A review. Arch Ophthalmol 1997;115:1291.

Linssen A, Meenken C: Outcomes of HLA-B27-positive and HLA-B27-negative acute anterior uveitis. Am J Ophthalmol 1995;120:351.

Margo CE, Hamed LM: Ocular syphilis. Surv Ophthalmol 1992;37:203.

Moorthy RS, Inomata H, Rao NA: Vogt-Koyanagi-Harada syndrome. Surv Ophthalmol 1995;39:265.

Moorthy RS et al: Management of varicella zoster virus retinitis in AIDS. Br J Ophthalmol 1997;81:189.

Nussenblatt RB, Whitcup SM, Palestine AG: *Uveitis: Fundamentals and Clinical Practice,* 3rd ed. Mosby, 1996.

Pavesio CE, Lightman S: *Toxoplasma gondii* and ocular toxoplasmosis: Pathogenesis. Br J Ophthalmol 1996;80:1099.

Pepose JS, Holland GN, Wilhelmus KR: *Ocular Infection and Immunity.* Mosby, 1996.

Rathinam SR et al: Uveitis associated with an epidemic outbreak of leptospirosis. Am J Ophthalmol 1997;124:71.

Rodriguez A et al: Referral patterns of uveitis in a tertiary eye care center. Arch Ophthalmol 1996;114:593.

Rose DN, Schechter CB, Adler JJ: Interpretation of the tuberculin skin test. J Gen Intern Med 1995;10:635.

Rosenbaum JT, Wernick R: Selection and interpretation of laboratory tests for patients with uveitis. Int Ophthalmol Clin 1990;30:238.

Rothova A et al: Causes and frequency of blindness in patients with intraocular inflammatory disease. Br J Ophthalmol 1996;80:332.

Shields JA: Ocular toxocariasis: A review. Surv Ophthalmol 1984;28:361.

Smith RE, Nozik RA: *Uveitis: A Clinical Approach to Diagnosis and Management,* 2nd ed. Williams & Wilkins, 1989.

Tabbara KF, al Kassimi H: Ocular brucellosis. Br J Ophthalmol 1990;74:249.

Tay-Kearney ML et al: Clinical features and associated systemic diseases of HLA-B27 uveitis. Am J Ophthalmol 1996;121:47.

Yaldo MK, Lieberman MF: The management of secondary glaucoma in the uveitis patient. Ophthalmol Clin North Am 1993;6:147.

TUMORS OF THE UVEAL TRACT

Char DH: *Clinical Ocular Oncology,* 2nd ed. Lippincott-Raven, 1997.

Char DH et al: Helium ion versus iodine 125 brachytherapy in the management of uveal melanoma: A prospective, randomized, dynamically balanced trial. Ophthalmology 1993;100:1547.

Damato BE, Paul J, Foulds WS: Predictive factors of visual outcome after local resection of choroidal melanoma. Br J Ophthalmol 1996;80:102.

Damato BE, Paul J, Foulds WS: Risk factors for metastatic uveal melanoma after trans-scleral local resection. Br J Ophthalmol 1996;80:102.

Naumann GOH, Rummelt V: Block excision of tumours of the anterior uvea: Report on 68 consecutive patients. Ophthalmology 1996;103:2017.

Shields JA et al: Acquired neoplasms of the nonpigmented ciliary epithelium (adenoma and carcinoma). Ophthalmology 1996;103:2007.

Shields JA et al: Congenital neoplasms of the nonpigmented ciliary epithelium (medulloepithelioma). Ophthalmology 1996;103:1998.

Spencer WH (editor): *Ophthalmic Pathology,* 4th ed. 4 vols. Saunders, 1996.

SCLERA

Calthorpe CM, Watson PG, McCartney ACE: Posterior scleritis: A clinical and histopathological survey. Eye 1988;2:267.

Foster SC, Sainz de la Maza M: *The Sclera.* Springer, 1994.

Legmann A, Foster CS. Noninfectious necrotizing scleritis. Int Ophthalmol Clin 1996;36:73.

Sainz de la Maza M, Foster CS, Jabbur NS: Scleritis associated with rheumatoid arthritis and with other systemic immune-mediated diseases. Ophthalmology 1994;101:1281.

Watson P, Ortiz JM. *Scleritis.* Mosby-Wolfe, 1995.

Lens

8

Richard A. Harper, MD, & John P. Shock, MD

The crystalline lens is a remarkable structure that in its normal state, functions to bring images into focus on the retina. It is positioned just posterior to the iris, and is supported by **zonular fibers** arising from the ciliary body. These fibers insert onto the equatorial region of the lens capsule. The lens capsule is a basement membrane that surrounds the lens substance. Epithelial cells at the lens equator continue to be produced throughout life, so that older lens fibers are compressed into a central **nucleus;** younger, less compact fibers around the nucleus make up the **cortex** (see Figures 1–12, 1–14, and 1–15). Because the lens is avascular and has no innervation, it must derive nutrients from the aqueous humor. Lens metabolism is primarily anaerobic owing to the low level of oxygen dissolved in the aqueous.

The eye is able to adjust its focus from distance to near objects because of the ability of the lens to change shape, a phenomenon known as **accommodation.** The inherent elasticity of the lens allows it to become more or less spherical depending on the amount of tension exerted by the zonular fibers on the lens capsule. Zonular tension is controlled by the action of the ciliary muscle, which, when contracted, relaxes zonular tension. The lens then assumes a more spherical shape, resulting in increased dioptric power to bring nearer objects into focus. Ciliary muscle relaxation reverses this sequence of events, allowing the lens to flatten and thus bringing more distant objects into view. As the lens ages, its accommodative power is gradually reduced as lens elasticity decreases.

PHYSIOLOGY OF SYMPTOMS

Symptoms associated with lens disorders are primarily visual. **Presbyopic symptoms** are due to decreased accommodative ability with age and result in diminished ability to perform near tasks. Loss of lens transparency results in blurred vision (without pain) for both near and distance. If the lens is partially dislocated (subluxation), visual blur can be due to a change in refractive error. Complete dislocation of the lens from the visual axis results in an **aphakic refractive state;** severely blurred vision results from loss of over one-third of the eye's refractive power.

The lens is best examined with the pupil dilated. A magnified view of the lens can be obtained with a slit-lamp or by using the direct ophthalmoscope with a high plus (+10) setting.

CATARACT

A cataract is any opacity in the lens. Aging is the most common cause of cataract, but many other factors can be involved, including trauma, toxins, systemic disease, and heredity. Age-related cataract is a common cause of visual impairment. Cross-sectional studies place the prevalence of cataracts at 50% in those age 65–74; the prevalence increases to about 70% for those over 75.

The pathogenesis of cataracts is not completely understood. However, cataractous lenses are characterized by protein aggregates that scatter light rays and reduce transparency. Other protein alterations result in yellow or brown discoloration. Additional findings may include vesicles between lens fibers or migration and aberrant enlargement of epithelial cells. Factors thought to contribute to cataract formation include oxidative damage (from free radical reactions), ultraviolet light damage, and malnutrition. No medical treatment has been found that will retard or reverse the underlying chemical changes that occur in cataract formation. However, some recent evidence suggests a protective effect of estrogen use on the lenses of postmenopausal women.

A **mature cataract** is one in which all of the lens protein is opaque; the **immature cataract** has some transparent protein. If the lens takes up water, it may become **intumescent.** In the **hypermature cataract,** cortical proteins have become liquid. This liquid may escape through the intact capsule, leaving a shrunken lens with a wrinkled capsule. A hypermature cataract in which the lens nucleus floats freely in the capsular bag is called a **morgagnian cataract.**

Most cataracts are not visible to the casual observer until they become dense enough to cause severe vision loss. The ocular fundus becomes increasingly more difficult to visualize as the lens opacity becomes denser, until the fundus reflection is completely absent. At this stage, the cataract is usually mature, and the pupil may be white.

The clinical degree of cataract formation, assuming that no other eye disease is present, is judged primarily by the Snellen visual acuity test. Generally speaking, the decrease in visual acuity is directly proportionate to the density of the cataract. However, some individuals who have clinically significant cataracts when examined with the ophthalmoscope or slitlamp see well enough to carry on with normal activities. Others have a decrease in visual acuity out of proportion to the degree of lens opacification. This is due to distortion of the image by the partially opaque lens. The Cataract Management Guideline Panel recommends reliance on clinical judgment combined with Snellen acuity as the best guide to the appropriateness of surgery but recognizes the need for flexibility, with due regard to a patient's particular functional and visual needs, the environment, and other risks—all of which may vary widely.

AGE-RELATED CATARACT
(FIGURES 8–1 TO 8–3)

The normal condensation process in the lens nucleus results in **nuclear sclerosis** after middle age. The earliest symptom may be improved near vision without glasses ("second sight"). This occurs from an increase in the refractive index of the central lens, creating a myopic shift in refraction. Other symptoms may include poor hue discrimination or monocular diplopia. Most nuclear cataracts are bilateral but may be asymmetric.

Cortical cataracts are opacities in the lens cortex. Changes in the hydration of lens fibers create clefts in a radial pattern around the equatorial region. They also tend to be bilateral, but are often asymmetric. Visual function is variably affected, depending on how near the opacities are to the visual axis.

Posterior subcapsular cataracts are located in the cortex near the central posterior capsule. They tend to cause visual symptoms earlier in their development owing to involvement of the visual axis. Common symptoms include glare and reduced vision under bright lighting conditions. This lens opacity can result also from trauma, corticosteroid use (topical or systemic), inflammation, or exposure to ionizing radiation.

Age-related cataract is usually slowly progressive over years, and death may occur before surgery becomes necessary. If surgery is indicated, lens extraction definitely improves visual acuity in well over 90% of cases. The remainder of patients either have preexisting retinal damage or develop serious postsurgical complications that prevent significant visual improvement, eg, glaucoma, retinal detachment, vitreous hemorrhage, infection, or epithelial downgrowth

into the anterior chamber. Intraocular lenses have made adjustment following cataract operation much easier than was the rule when only thick cataract glasses were available.

CHILDHOOD CATARACT
(FIGURES 8–4 AND 8–5)

Childhood cataracts are divided into two groups: **congenital (infantile) cataracts,** which are present at birth or appear shortly thereafter; and **acquired cataracts,** which occur later and are usually related to a specific cause. Either type may be unilateral or bilateral.

About one-third of cataracts are hereditary, while another third are secondary to metabolic or infectious diseases or associated with a variety of syndromes. The final one-third result from undetermined causes. Acquired cataracts arise most commonly from trauma, either blunt or penetrating. Other causes include uveitis, acquired ocular infections, diabetes, and drugs.

Clinical Findings
A. Congenital Cataract: Congenital lens opacities are common and often visually insignificant. A partial opacification or one out of the visual axis—or not dense enough to interfere significantly with light transmission—requires no treatment other than observation for progression. Dense central congenital cataracts require surgery.

Congenital cataracts that cause significant visual loss must be detected early—preferably in the newborn nursery by the pediatrician or family physician. Large, dense white cataracts may present as leukocoria (white pupil), noticeable by the parents, but many dense cataracts cannot be seen by the parents. Unilateral infantile cataracts that are dense, central, and larger than 2 mm in diameter will cause permanent deprivation amblyopia if not treated within the first 2 months of life and thus require surgical management on an urgent basis. Even then there must be careful attention to avoidance of amblyopia related to postoperative anisometropia. Symmetric (equally dense) bilateral cataracts may require less urgent management, though bilateral deprivation can result from unwarranted delay. When surgery is undertaken, there must be as short an interval as is reasonably possible between the surgery on the two eyes.

B. Acquired Cataract: Acquired cataracts do not require the same urgent care (aimed at preventing amblyopia) as infantile cataracts, because the children are older and the visual system more mature. Surgical assessment is based on the location, size, and density of the cataract, but a period of observation along with subjective visual acuity testing can be part of the decision making process. Because unilateral cataracts in children will not produce any symptoms or signs parents would routinely notice, screening programs are important for case finding.

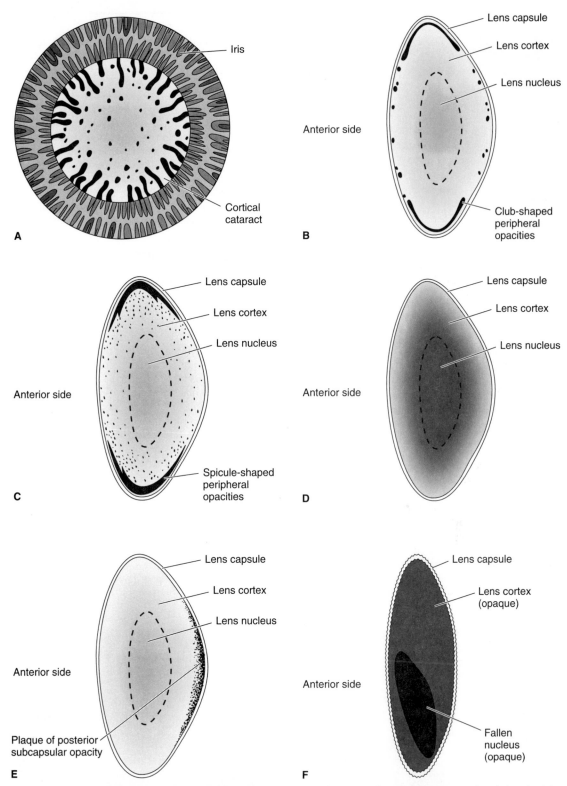

Figure 8–1. Age-related cataract. **A** *and* **B:** "Coronary" type cortical cataract (frontal and cross-sectional views): club-shaped peripheral opacities with clear central lens; slowly progressive. **C:** "Cuneiform" type cortical cataract: peripheral spicules and central clear lens; slowly progressive. **D:** Nuclear sclerotic cataract: diffuse opacity principally affecting nucleus; slowly progressive. **E:** Posterior subcapsular cataract: plaque of granular opacity on posterior capsule; may be rapidly progressive. **F:** "Morgagnian" type (hypermature lens): the entire lens is opaque, and the lens nucleus has fallen inferiorly.

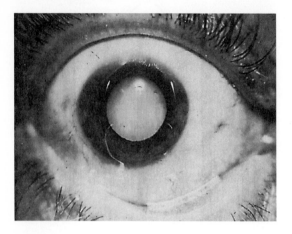

Figure 8–2. Mature age-related cataract viewed through a dilated pupil. (Courtesy of A Rosenberg.)

Treatment

Surgical treatment of infantile and early childhood cataracts involves lens extraction through a 3 mm limbal incision utilizing a mechanical irrigation-aspiration handpiece. Phacoemulsification is rarely required. In contrast to the procedure used for adult lens extraction, the posterior capsule and anterior vitreous are removed by many surgeons using a mechanical vitreous suction-cutting instrument. This prevents formation of secondary capsular opacification, or after-cataract (see below). Primary removal of the posterior capsule thus avoids the necessity for secondary surgery and enhances early optical correction.

Using today's sophisticated surgical techniques, operative and postoperative complications are similar to those reported with adult cataract procedures. Optical correction can consist of spectacles in older bilaterally aphakic children, but most childhood cataract operations should be followed by contact lens correction. The use of intraocular lenses in early childhood is under active investigation and, if successful, may reduce the difficulty in optical rehabilitation associated with contact lenses in children.

Prognosis

The visual prognosis for childhood cataract patients requiring surgery is not as good as that for patients with age-related cataract. The associated amblyopia and occasional anomalies of the optic nerve or retina limit the degree of useful vision that can be achieved in this group of patients. The prognosis for improvement of visual acuity is worst following surgery for unilateral congenital cataracts and best for incomplete bilateral congenital cataracts that are slowly progressive.

TRAUMATIC CATARACT

Traumatic cataract (Figures 8–6 to 8–8) is most commonly due to a foreign body injury to the lens or blunt trauma to the eyeball. Air rifle pellets are a frequent cause; less frequent causes include arrows, rocks, contusions, overexposure to heat ("glassblower's cataract"), and ionizing radiation. Most traumatic cataracts are preventable. In industry, the best safety measure is a good pair of safety goggles.

The lens becomes white soon after the entry of a foreign body, since interruption of the lens capsule allows aqueous and sometimes vitreous to penetrate into the lens structure. The patient is often an industrial worker who gives a history of striking steel upon steel. A minute fragment of a steel hammer, for example, may pass through the cornea and lens at a tremendous rate of speed and lodge in the vitreous or retina.

CATARACT SECONDARY TO INTRAOCULAR DISEASE ("COMPLICATED CATARACT")

Cataract may develop as a direct effect of intraocular disease upon the physiology of the lens (eg, severe

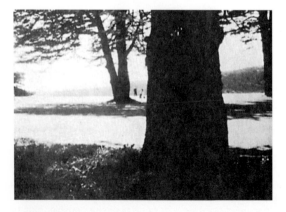
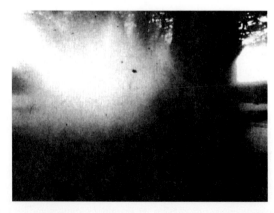

Figure 8–3. Age-related cataract. In the photo at right the scene shown at left is reproduced as if seen by a person with a moderately advanced senile cataract (opacity denser centrally). (Courtesy of E Goodner.)

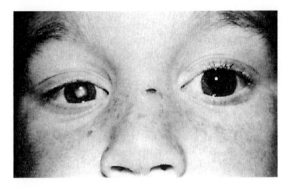

Figure 8–4. Congenital cataract.

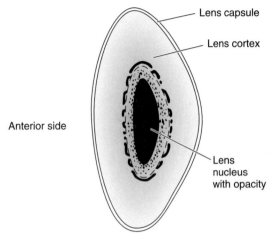

Figure 8–5. Congenital cataract, zonular type. One zone of lens involved. The cortex is relatively clear.

recurrent uveitis). The cataract usually begins in the posterior subcapsular area and eventually involves the entire lens structure. Intraocular diseases commonly associated with the development of cataracts are chronic or recurrent uveitis, glaucoma, retinitis pigmentosa, and retinal detachment. These cataracts are usually unilateral. The visual prognosis is not as good as in ordinary age-related cataract.

CATARACT ASSOCIATED WITH SYSTEMIC DISEASE

Bilateral cataracts may occur in association with the following systemic disorders: diabetes mellitus (Figure 8–9), hypoparathyroidism, myotonic dystrophy, atopic dermatitis, galactosemia, and Lowe's, Werner's, and Down's syndromes. (These entities are discussed in Chapters 15 and 18.)

DRUG-INDUCED CATARACT

Corticosteroids administered over a long period of time, either systemically or in drop form, can cause lens opacities. Other drugs associated with cataract include phenothiazines, amiodarone, and strong miotic drops such as phospholine iodide, used in the treatment of glaucoma.

AFTER-CATARACT (SECONDARY MEMBRANE)

After-cataract (Figure 8–10) denotes opacification of the posterior capsule due to partially absorbed traumatic cataract or following extracapsular cataract extraction. Persistent subcapsular lens epithelium may favor regeneration of lens fibers, giving the posterior capsule a "fish egg" appearance (Elschnig's pearls). The proliferating epithelium may produce multiple layers, leading to frank opacification. These cells may also undergo myofibroblastic differentiation. Their contraction produces numerous tiny wrinkles in the posterior capsule, resulting in visual distortion. All of

these factors may lead to reduced visual acuity following extracapsular cataract extraction.

After-cataract is a significant problem in almost all pediatric patients unless the posterior capsule and anterior vitreous are removed at the time of surgery. Up to one-half of all adult patients develop an opaque secondary membrane after extracapsular cataract extraction. Before the neodymium:YAG laser came into use, this condition was treated by performing a small capsulotomy with a knife or barbed 27-gauge needle, either at the time of the original operation or as a secondary procedure.

The neodymium:YAG laser provides a noninvasive method for discission of the posterior capsule (see Chapter 24). Pulses of laser energy cause small "ex-

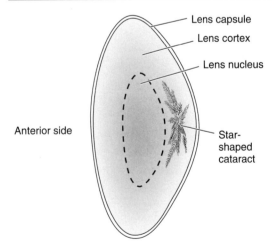

Figure 8–6. Traumatic "star-shaped" cataract in the posterior lens. This is usually due to ocular contusion and is only detectable through a well-dilated pupil.

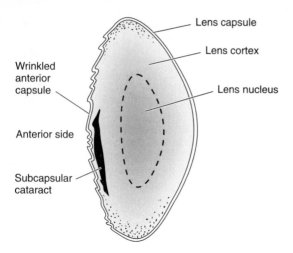

Figure 8–7. Traumatic cataract with wrinkled anterior capsule.

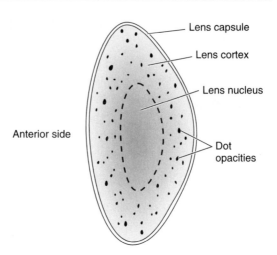

Figure 8–9. Punctate dot cataract. This type of cataract is sometimes seen as an ocular complication of diabetes mellitus. It may also be congenital.

plosions" in target tissue, creating a small hole in the posterior capsule in the pupillary axis. Complications of this technique include a transient rise in intraocular pressure, damage to the intraocular lens, and rupture of the anterior hyaloid face with forward displacement of vitreous into the anterior chamber. The rise in intraocular pressure is usually detectable within 3 hours post treatment and resolves within a few days with treatment. Rarely, the pressure does not return to normal for several weeks. Small pits or cracks may occur on the intraocular lens but usually have no effect on visual acuity. In the aphakic eye, rupture of the vitreous face with anterior displacement of vitreous may predispose to development of rhegmatogenous retinal detachment or cystoid macular edema. No sig-

nificant damage seems to be done to corneal endothelium with the neodymium:YAG laser.

CATARACT SURGERY

Cataract surgery has undergone dramatic change during the past 30 years with the introduction of the operating microscope and microsurgical instruments, improvements in suture materials, the development of intraocular lenses, and alterations in techniques for local anesthesia. Further refinements continue to occur,

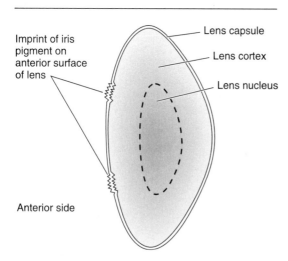

Figure 8–8. Imprint of iris pigment on anterior surface of lens.

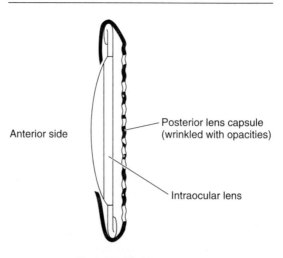

Figure 8–10. After-cataract.

with automated instrumentation and modifications of intraocular lenses allowing surgery through small incisions.

The generally preferred method of cataract surgery in adults and older children preserves the posterior portion of the lens capsule and thus is known as **extracapsular cataract extraction.** Intraocular lens implantation is part of this procedure. An incision is made at the limbus or in the peripheral cornea, usually superiorly but sometimes temporally. An opening is formed in the anterior capsule, and the nucleus and cortex of the lens are removed. The intraocular lens is then placed in the empty "capsular bag," supported by the intact posterior capsule. In the standard form of extracapsular cataract extraction, the nucleus is removed intact, but this requires a relatively large incision. The cortex is removed by manual or automated aspiration. The technique of **phacoemulsification** utilizes a handheld ultrasonic vibrator to disintegrate the hard nucleus such that the nuclear material and cortex can be aspirated through an incision of approximately 3 mm. This same incision size is then adequate for insertion of the recently developed folding lenses. If a rigid intraocular lens is used, the wound needs to be extended to approximately 5 mm. The advantages of small-incision surgery are more controlled operating conditions, avoidance of suturing, rapid wound healing with lesser degrees of corneal distortion, and reduced postoperative intraocular inflammation—all contributing to more rapid visual rehabilitation. The phacoemulsification technique does, however, run the risk of posterior displacement of nuclear material through a posterior capsular tear, which generally necessitates complex vitreoretinal surgery. After all forms of extracapsular cataract surgery there may be secondary opacification of the posterior capsule that requires discission using the neodymium:YAG laser (see After-Cataract, above). Lens extraction through the pars plana during posterior vitrectomy is called **phacofragmentation.** This type of cataract removal is only performed in conjunction with the removal of an opaque or scarred vitreous.

Intracapsular cataract extraction, consisting of removal of the entire lens together with its capsule, is less frequently performed today. The incidence of postoperative retinal detachment and cystoid macular edema is significantly higher than after extracapsular surgery, but intracapsular surgery is still a useful procedure, particularly when facilities for extracapsular surgery are not available.

Intraocular Lens

There are many styles of intraocular lenses, but most prostheses consist of a central biconvex optic and two legs or haptics to maintain the optic in position. The optimal intraocular lens position is within the capsular bag following an extracapsular procedure. This is associated with the lowest incidence of postoperative complications, such as pseudophakic

bullous keratopathy, glaucoma, iris damage, hyphema, and lens decentration. The newest posterior chamber lenses are made of flexible materials such as silicone and acrylic polymers. This flexibility allows the lens implant to be folded, thus decreasing the required incision size. Lens designs that incorporate **multifocal optics** have also been produced. The goal of this design is to provide the patient with good vision for both near and distance without glasses, which current monofocal designs are unable to do.

After intracapsular surgery—or if there is inadvertent damage to the posterior capsule during extracapsular surgery—intraocular lenses can be placed in the anterior chamber or sometimes fixated in the ciliary sulcus.

Methods of calculating the correct dioptric power of an intraocular lens are discussed in Chapter 20. If an intraocular lens cannot be safely placed or is contraindicated, postoperative refractive correction generally requires a contact lens or aphakic spectacles.

Postoperative Care

If a small-incision technique is used, the postoperative recovery period is usually shortened. The patient may be ambulatory on the day of surgery but is advised to move cautiously and avoid straining or heavy lifting for about a month. The eye can be bandaged for a few days, but if the eye is comfortable, the bandage can be removed on the first postoperative day and the eye protected by spectacles or by a shield during the day. Protection at night by a metal shield is required for several weeks. Temporary glasses can be used a few days after surgery, but in most cases the patient sees well enough through the intraocular lens to wait for permanent glasses (usually provided 6–8 weeks after surgery).

DISLOCATED LENS (ECTOPIA LENTIS)

Partial or complete lens dislocation (Figure 8–11) may be hereditary or may result from trauma.

Hereditary Lens Dislocation

Hereditary lens dislocation is usually bilateral and is commonly associated with homocystinuria and Marfan's syndrome (Chapter 15). The vision is blurred, particularly if the lens is dislocated out of the line of vision. If dislocation is partial, the edge of the lens and the zonular fibers holding it in place can be seen in the pupil. If the lens is completely dislocated into the vitreous, it can be seen with the ophthalmoscope.

A partially dislocated lens is often complicated by

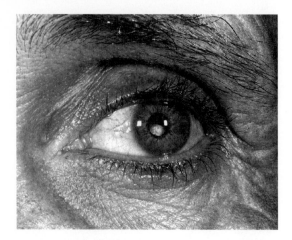

Figure 8–11. Dislocated lens.

cataract formation. If that is the case, the cataract may have to be removed, but this procedure should be delayed as long as possible because vitreous loss, predisposing to subsequent retinal detachment, is likely during surgery. If the lens is free in the vitreous, it may lead in later life to the development of glaucoma of a type that responds poorly to treatment. If dislocation is partial and the lens is clear, the visual prognosis is good.

Traumatic Lens Dislocation

Partial or complete traumatic lens dislocation may occur following a contusion injury such as a blow to the eye with a fist. If the dislocation is partial, there may be no symptoms; but if the lens is floating in the vitreous, the patient has blurred vision and usually a red eye. **Iridodonesis,** a quivering of the iris when the patient moves the eye, is a common sign of lens dislocation and is due to the lack of lens support. This is present both in partially and in completely dislocated lenses but is more marked in the latter.

Uveitis and glaucoma are common complications of dislocated lens, particularly if dislocation is complete. If there are no complications, dislocated lenses are best left untreated. If uveitis or uncontrollable glaucoma occurs, lens extraction must be done despite the poor results possible from this operation. The technique of choice is limbal or pars plana lensectomy using a motor-driven lens and vitreous cutter.

REFERENCES

Al-Ghoul KJ et al: Distribution and type of morphologic damage in human nuclear age-related cataracts. Exp Eye Res 1996;62:237.

Andley U: Photooxidative stress. In: *Principles and Practice of Ophthalmology: Clinical Practice.* Vol 1. Albert DM, Jakobiec FA (editors). Saunders, 1994.

Apple DJ et al: Posterior capsule opacification. Surv Ophthalmol 1992;37:73.

Apple DJ, Sims J: Harold Ridley and the invention of the intraocular lens. Surv Ophthalmol 1996;40:279.

Benitez del Castillo JM et al: Effects of estrogen use on lens transmittance in postmenopausal women. Ophthalmology 1997;104:970.

Birch EE, Stager DR: The critical period for surgical treatment of dense congenital unilateral cataract. Invest Ophthalmol Vis Sci 1996;37:1532.

Bourne WM, Nelson LR, Hodge DO: Continued endothelial cell loss ten years after lens implantation. Ophthalmology 1994;101:1014.

Brady KM et al: Cataract surgery and intraocular lens implantation in children. Am J Ophthalmol 1995;120:1.

Cataract Management Guideline Panel: Cataract in Adults: Management of functional impairment. Clinical Practice Guideline, Number 4. Rockville, MD. U.S. Department of Health and Human Services, Public Health Service, Agency for Health Care Policy and Research. AHCPR Pub. No. 93-0542.

Desai P et al: Gains from cataract surgery: Visual function and quality of life. Br J Ophthalmol 1996;80:868.

Graziosi P et al: Location and severity of cortical opacities in different regions of the lens in age-related cataract. Invest Ophthalmol Vis Sci 1996;37:1698

Halpert M, BenEzra D: Surgery of the hereditary subluxated lens in children. Ophthalmology 1996;103:681.

Hiller R et al: Cigarette smoking and the risk of development of lens opacities: The Framingham studies. Arch Ophthalmol 1997;115;1113.

Javitt JC et al: National Outcomes of Cataract Extraction: Retinal detachment and endophthalmitis after outpatient cataract surgery. Ophthalmology 1994;101:100.

Klein BE et al: Incidence of cataract surgery in the Wisconsin Epidemiologic Study of Diabetic Retinopathy. Am J Ophthalmol 1995;119:295.

Klein BE et al: Incident cataract surgery: The Beaver Dam eye study. Ophthalmology 1997;104:573.

Lambert SR, Drack AV: Infantile cataracts. Surv Ophthalmol 1996;40:427.

Mares-Perlman JA et al: Relation between lens opacities and vitamin and mineral supplement use. Ophthalmology 1994;101:315.

Norregaard JC: International variation in ophthalmologic management of patients with cataracts. Results from the International Cataract Surgery Outcomes Study. Arch Ophthalmol 1997;115:399.

Powe NR et al: Synthesis of the literature on visual acuity and complications following cataract extraction with intraocular lens implantation. Arch Ophthalmol 1994;112:239.

Schein OD et al: Variation in cataract surgery practice and clinical outcomes. Ophthalmology 1994;102:1142.

West SK, Valmadrid CT: Epidemiology of risk factors for age-related cataract. Surv Ophthalmol 1995;39:323

Vitreous

9

Conor O'Malley, MD

EXAMINATION OF THE VITREOUS

Slitlamp Examination

Normal vitreous is not visible by either direct or indirect ophthalmoscopy. The numerous ophthalmoscopically visible features are anomalies attributable either to structural changes, such as the floaters of syneresis and the ring-like form associated with posterior vitreous detachment (Figure 9–1), or to invasive elements, such as blood, white blood cell masses, or fibrovascular proliferations from adjacent tissues. Normal vitreous in situ and many important anomalies (eg, the retraction, condensation, and shrinkage of vitreous characteristic of diabetes or injury) can be viewed only with a slitlamp. The slitlamp (biomicroscope) is a microscope with a specialized illuminating system that make transparent and near-transparent ocular fluids and tissues visible. Although slitlamp examination of the vitreous is quite easy to learn and plays an important role in the management of vitreous disease, too few ophthalmologists make optimal use of this instrument.

Contact Lenses as Aid in Vitreous Examination

The anterior central vitreous is the only part of the inner eye (behind the lens) that can be seen with the slitlamp alone. In order to view other areas, special contact lenses must be placed on the patient's eye. A relatively thin contact lens with a flat front surface allows stereoscopic examination of tissues *on and near the visual axis of the eye*—the optic disk, the posterior retina and choroid, and the axial vitreous. Much thicker contact lenses with built-in mirrors and a flat front surface allow examination of the nonaxial retina and vitreous.

These special contact lenses are also used in therapeutic procedures. Fundus contact lenses with built-in mirrors are widely used in laser photocoagulation of the peripheral retina, such as in the management of retinal neovascularization due to diabetic retinopathy, retinal vein occlusion, or (more rarely) sickle cell anemia. The thinner contact lenses are used in ablation of macular lesions associated with diabetic retinopathy, age-related macular degeneration, and histoplasmosis.

Use of special contact lenses, whether for diagnostic or therapeutic procedures, requires maximum dilation of the pupil with a combination of mydriatic and cycloplegic solutions; use of a topical anesthetic to make the patient more comfortable; and use of a clear viscous solution of methylcellulose to prevent air from entering the lens-cornea interface.

B-Scan Ultrasonography

B-scan ultrasonography is an important diagnostic tool used in many posterior segment problems associated with gross vitreous opacification (Figure 9–2). Where light-dependent ophthalmoscopes and slitlamps provide insufficient information, skillful use of B-scan ultrasonography can provide much information about the vitreous and adjacent structures. For example, it is possible to identify and locate vitreous membranes (Figure 9–3), vitreoretinal relationships and retinal detachments greater than 1 mm in depth (Figures 9–3 to 9–5), scleral ruptures, and intraocular foreign bodies (even nonlucent plastic and glass).

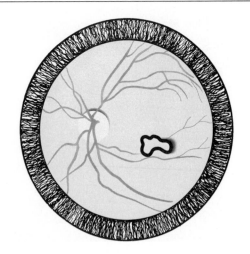

Figure 9–1. Posterior vitreous detachment as seen with the +8 lens of the ophthalmoscope.

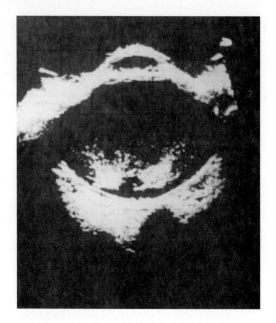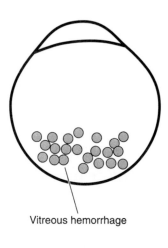

Figure 9–2. Vitreous hemorrhage limited to posterior vitreous region in aphakic eye. (Reproduced, with permission, from Coleman DJ: Ultrasound in vitreous surgery. Trans Am Acad Ophthalmol Otolaryngol 1972;76:469.)

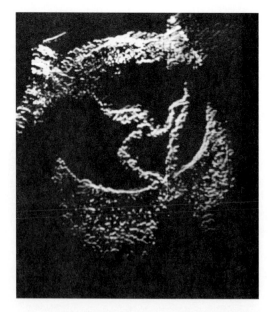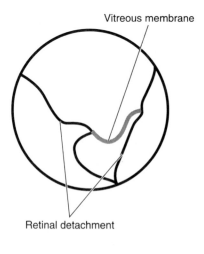

Figure 9–3. Total retinal detachment viewed horizontally below iris plane. A vitreous membrane connecting two leaves of retina is clearly demonstrated. (Reproduced, with permission, from Coleman DJ: Ultrasound in vitreous surgery. Trans Am Acad Ophthalmol Otolaryngol 1972;76:469.)

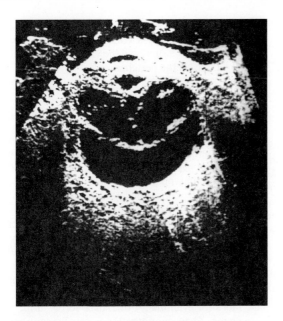 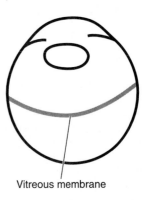

Figure 9–4. Vitreous membrane extending along posterior limiting membrane of vitreous from ora to ora. Retina is in place. (Reproduced, with permission, from Coleman DJ: Ultrasound in vitreous surgery. Trans Am Acad Ophthalmol Otolaryngol 1972;76:469.)

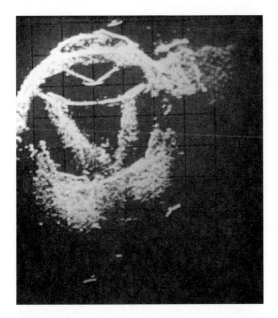 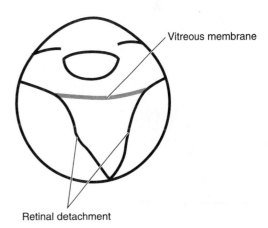

Figure 9–5. Vitreous membrane connecting two leaves of detached retina. Lens is normal. (Reproduced, with permission, from Coleman DJ: Ultrasound in vitreous surgery. Trans Am Acad Ophthalmol Otolaryngol 1972;76:469.)

DISORDERS OF THE VITREOUS

"FLASHING LIGHTS"

"Flashing lights" (**photopsia**) are a common symptom of an abnormal relationship between the retina and the vitreous. The patient is aware of a localized "light," "glow," "streak of light," or "flashing" (as of a neon tube) in the field of vision in the absence of a corresponding light source in the environment. The patient can usually point to the area of the disturbance and often describes an arc-shaped flicker in the periphery of one or two quadrants. The light seldom persists for more than a fraction of a second. It frequently recurs at short intervals for a few minutes and then disappears for hours, days, or even weeks. It is most readily identified on moving the eye and when illumination is dim or absent. Bilateral episodes may occur simultaneously but more commonly are separated by an interval of days to many years.

The light represents a cerebral awareness of the initial physical traction on and excitation of the sensory retina by abnormal vitreous. It is most commonly associated with recent collapse and detachment of the vitreous due to syneresis with focal vitreous traction on vitreoretinal lesions such as lattice degeneration, meridional folds, congenital rosettes, and other vitreoretinal adhesions. A careful history will readily distinguish the light from the scintillating scotoma of migraine, which is characterized by a symmetric quivering scotoma usually in both eyes, of predictable configuration and progression, accompanied by variable nausea or headache.

The vitreoretinal traction may require no treatment.

However, as it can induce retinal tears, retinal detachment (Figure 9–6), or vitreous hemorrhage, every new case requires a survey of the vitreoretinal relationship, especially in the periphery.

VITREOUS FLOATERS

Vitreous floaters are by far the most common symptom of abnormal vitreous. A given floater represents the patient's awareness of the shadow of a mobile vitreous opacity cast upon the retina. The mind projects the corresponding dark form onto the appropriate area of the visual field.

The term "vitreous floaters" denotes a common, potentially serious symptom that was formerly called *muscae volitantes*—Latin for flies that flit, flutter, or fly to and fro.

The onset may be either insidious or acute and unilateral or bilateral. The patient is aware of one or more (or even many) fine, dark forms in the field of vision. Their configuration is usually so pronounced that the patient spontaneously classifies them as "spots," "soot," "particles," "spiders," "cobwebs," "threads," "worms," "dark streaks," "a ring," etc. Combinations are often reported. The objects continue to migrate after the eye comes to rest—hence the name "floaters."

Central, relatively immobile floaters are visually annoying and may even be disabling. Peripheral ones are readily overlooked, as they are intermittent and require large eye motion or special positions merely to be seen. Unlike "flashing lights," they are most readily seen against bright lights or a uniform light background. They are extremely common in myopes and people with syneresis.

Floaters may be caused by small hemorrhages into the vitreous resulting from retinal tears or hemorrhagic diseases such as diabetic retinopathy, hypertension, leukemia, old retinal branch vein occlusions, Eales' disease, Coats' disease, and subacute infective endocarditis. Individual red cells are seen as small round black spots. Recent hemorrhages are often seen as black streaks or cobwebs that later break up into small round spots.

White cell invasion of the vitreous gel associated with pars planitis may also cause "spots before the eyes." Vitreous floaters due to pigment are usually a consequence of long-standing tear-induced detachment of the retina that has not yet reached the macula.

Vitreous floaters should never be dismissed as harmless or imaginary. A careful survey of the vitreous and retina is always indicated in order to identify the nature and origin of floaters and to decide on management. Failure to make such an examination not infrequently leads to missed diagnosis. In the absence of a serious causative pathologic process, the patient may be reassured that the condition is harmless.

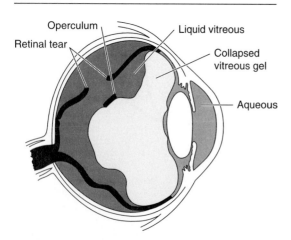

Operculum

Liquid vitreous

Retinal tear

Collapsed vitreous gel

Aqueous

Figure 9–6. Schematic representation of vitreous collapse causing the retina to tear and detach.

ASTEROID HYALOSIS

Asteroid hyalosis is an uncommon condition that occurs in otherwise healthy eyes in elderly people. Unilateral cases are three times as common as bilateral cases. Hundreds of small yellow spheres consisting of calcium soaps are seen in the vitreous. These move when the eyes move but always return to their original positions because they are attached to interlacing fibers. There are no related ocular or systemic diseases. The opacities have little or no effect upon vision but reflect the examiner's light very strongly. If there are enough asteroid bodies, the fundus is not viewable by ophthalmoscopy.

ACUTE VITREOUS COLLAPSE

The vitreous cavity is bounded by the retina, optic disk, pars plana, zonule, and crystalline lens. Normal vitreous fills this cavity and remains firmly attached to the retina and pars plana near the ora serrata.

All types of gels, whether vitreous or gelatin, become increasingly susceptible with the passage of time to a degenerative process known as **syneresis,** involving the drawing together of particles of the dispersed medium, separation of the medium, and shrinkage of the gel. Syneresis affects at least 65% of persons over 60 years of age. Myopes are especially susceptible, even in childhood.

With age, the center of the vitreous may undergo syneresis and become filled with liquid breakdown products of the degenerated gel (Figure 9–7). The liquid contents of the cavity can migrate into the preretinal space. The more solid, heavier vitreous gel collapses downward and forward to create a posterior vitreous detachment (Figure 9–8). The dynamic forces that accompany this collapse can rupture the last vestiges of the adhesions that once connected the vitreous to the disk, blood vessels, and sensory retina in childhood.

The patient and examiner can often see portions of the adhesions that remain attached to the collapsed vitreous as opacities. If they arise from the disk mar-

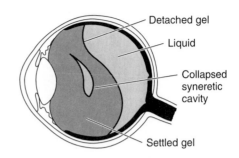

Figure 9–8. Posterior vitreous detachment.

gin, the patient and examiner may note a ring-shaped opacity on the back of the vitreous.

Since the front of the vitreous is attached to the globe and the back of the vitreous is collapsed in on itself, abrupt motions of the eye transmit a whip-like force to the back of the vitreous. The vitreous tends to fill out toward its normal configuration; liquid vitreous is drawn into the syneretic cavity, and the posterior separation tends to disappear (Figure 9–9).

The whip-like motions of the vitreous can give rise to photopsia by causing stimulation of the vitreoretinal juncture and may cause a characteristic floating motion of posterior vitreous opacities, or floaters. The floaters move with the eye and float to a resting position after the eye comes to rest.

Since acute vitreous collapse can also cause asymptomatic retinal tears or detachment, *it should be assumed that patients with new floaters or photopsia have retinal tears or detachment until proved otherwise by thorough examination of the peripheral retina with an indirect ophthalmoscope.*

RETINAL TEARS
(See also Chapter 10.)

While retinal tears can be caused by trauma, vitreous shrinkage, or proliferative vitreoretinopathy, most are caused by acute vitreous collapse. Tears following acute vitreous collapse are the result of a dynamic interaction between a focal vitreoretinal adhesion, collapsed mobile vitreous, and normal eye movement (Figure 9–10).

Since the gel and liquid components of the collapsed vitreous are structurally relatively independent of the retina, they do not move synchronously with the retina. When the eye (and hence the retina) moves, the gel and liquid tend to lag behind the retina, and when the eye stops moving, the gel and liquid tend to continue in motion. The vitreous gel and liquid are said to exhibit inertial lag with respect to the retina. Inertial lag of the gel can cause the vitreous to tear the friable sensory retina at the point where they adhere to

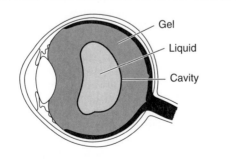

Figure 9–7. Large intravitreal cavity filled with liquid breakdown products of syneresis.

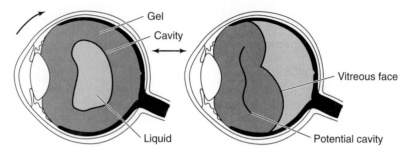

Figure 9–9. Liquid vitreous tends to be drawn into intravitreal cavity on abrupt eye motion **(left)** and expelled at rest **(right)**.

each other (Figure 9–11). The torn retina is seen to be pulled inward as a flap or a detached operculum (Figure 9–12). If retinal vessels are broken, they bleed briefly. A variable amount of blood accumulates in the vitreous cavity.

Some patients are not aware of the onset of retinal tears but often complain of photopsia and floaters. Some present with gross vitreous hemorrhage. Many retinal tears never lead to retinal detachment, but recent symptomatic tears, especially those with symptomatic vitreous hemorrhage, have a strong tendency to cause retinal detachment. Patients with symptoms of acute vitreous collapse or vitreous hemorrhage should therefore undergo careful examination of the retina from the optic disk to the ora serrata to rule out one or more tears. Management of tears by prophylactic laser therapy or cryopexy is relatively simple and very effective compared to the performance of silicone buckling once retinal detachment has occurred.

Retinal tears are usually located anterior to the equator and are more often in the upper quadrants (Figure 9–12 left). Retinal detachment secondary to retinal tear formation is characterized as rhegmatogenous (see Chapter 10), particularly to differentiate it from serous retinal detachment such as that due to choroidal tumor, choroidal or scleral inflammation, or choroidal neovascularization, and from tractional retinal detachment such as that due to retinal neovascularization.

VITREOUS HEMORRHAGE

Vitreous hemorrhage can occur whenever the sensory retina is torn. Retinal neovascularization secondary to diabetic retinopathy, branch or central retinal vein occlusion, and hypertension are also frequent causes of vitreous hemorrhage. Acute collapse of the vitreous with posterior vitreous detachment will sometimes cause bleeding without tear formation. The patient often complains of floaters that suggest red blood cells, a sudden shower of small black dots, or even tiny ring-like forms with clear centers. Visual loss ranges from imperceptible to gross.

The appearance of the retina and its visibility vary with the cause and amount of bleeding in the vitreous cavity (see Chapter 10). Fresh blood is red and tends to be located behind the vitreous gel or within a syneretic cavity (Figure 9–13). Within weeks to months, the blood tends to break down, becomes a pale color, and migrates into the gel (Figure 9–14).

Vitreous hemorrhage in association with rhegmatogenous retinal detachment necessitates urgent retinal surgery. This often requires vitrectomy to allow adequate visualization of the retina. Vitreous hemorrhage associated with tractional retinal detachment involving the macula generally requires early vitrectomy. Traditionally, vitreous hemorrhage not associated with retinal detachment is treated conservatively for 3–6 months in the hope of spontaneous resolution. Improvements in the outcome of vitreous surgery have led to earlier surgery, particularly in patients with proliferative diabetic retinopathy.

Vitrectomy is not indicated for 3–6 months if treatment of the underlying cause can wait, as the vitreous may clear adequately without surgery.

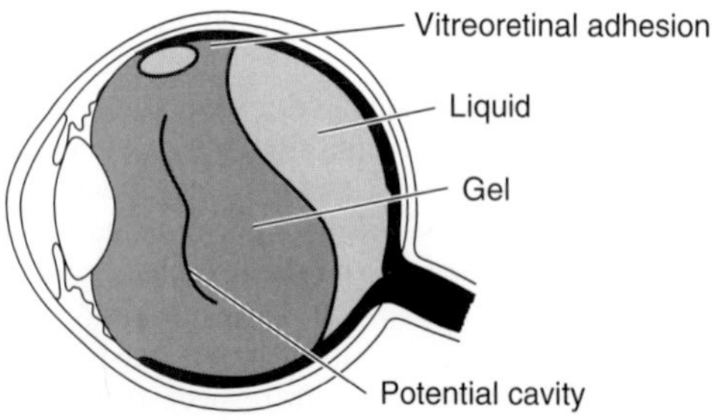

Figure 9–10. Local vitreoretinal adhesion.

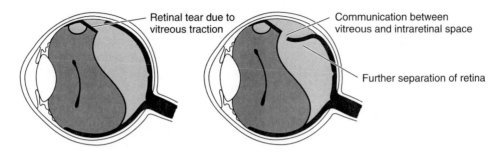

Figure 9–11. *Left:* Retinal tear. *Right:* Retinal detachment.

RHEGMATOGENOUS RETINAL DETACHMENT
(See also Chapter 10.)

In the normal eye, the intact sensory retina is kept opposed to the pigment epithelium by the suction the latter exerts on the watertight space between them. If a retinal tear is present, rapid eye motions and sudden rotation of the globe can readily generate enough inertial force to initiate retinal detachment (Figure 9–15). The space between the two layers of the retina fills with liquid vitreous, and eddy currents develop in this space, further accelerating the detachment process (Figure 9–16). Usually the detachment continues until it is total, particularly if the retinal tear is located superiorly.

Surgery with retinopexy, either by cryotherapy or laser photocoagulation, and usually with silicone buckling, is required (1) to close the hole in the retina, reestablishing a watertight intraretinal space; (2) to restrict the inertial lag of the liquid and gel with respect to the retina; and (3) to approximate and seal together the two layers of the retina around the tear to counter the effects of eddy currents in the vitreous cavity. (See also Chapter 10.)

TRACTION RETINAL DETACHMENT

Traction retinal detachment is detachment of the sensory retina due to vitreoretinal traction, usually secondary to proliferative diabetic retinopathy, proliferative vitreoretinopathy, retinopathy of prematurity, or ocular trauma (Figure 9–17). The detachment typically involves the retina posterior to the equator and has a concave surface. Surgery is indicated if the detachment involves the macula and requires vitrectomy and removal of the tractional elements. Scleral buckling and injection of intraocular gas or silicone oil may also be necessary. In a few cases, tractional retinal detachment is complicated by retinal tear formation, leading to combined rhegmatogenous and tractional detachment. This generally requires early vitreoretinal surgery.

PROLIFERATIVE VITREORETINOPATHY

A number of abnormal conditions of the vitreous and retina are characterized by contractile membranes arising metaplastically from abnormally located retinal pigment epithelial cells and retinal glial cells. The membranes can occur on either the inner or outer surface of the sensory retina or on several vitreous surfaces. The membranes may be weak and subtle or strong, easily seen, and capable of causing great distortion of the host tissues.

The causal retinal pigment epithelial cells and retinal glial cells are pluripotential cells, with great metaplastic potential. They may proliferate at remote sites and take on the characteristics of myofibroblasts. These myofi-

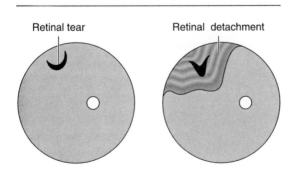

Figure 9–12. *Left:* Ophthalmoscopic view of retinal tear. *Right:* Ophthalmoscopic view of retinal detachment.

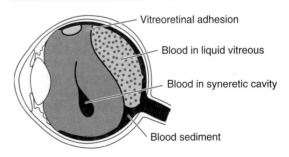

Figure 9–13. Acute vitreous hemorrhage. A retinal vessel ruptures due to vitreous traction.

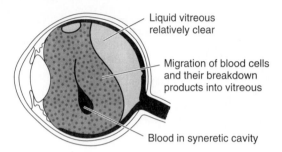

Figure 9–14. Chronic vitreous hemorrhage.

broblast-like cells readily form contractile membranes that may deform the inner and outer surfaces of the retina and the posterior vitreous surfaces (Figure 9–18).

The basic process, or its outcome, is known as massive vitreous retraction, preretinal traction, preretinal vitreous membrane, subretinal fibrosis, macular pucker, or surface wrinkling retinopathy.

Proliferative vitreoretinopathy requires no treatment unless it causes surface wrinkling retinopathy of the macula (also known as macular pucker) or unduly complicates therapy for retinal detachment. While research holds some promise for an antiproliferative pharmaceutical agent, current treatment involves a special surgical procedure that employs dissection, severing, or removal of vitreous tissue (see below).

INJURY TO THE VITREOUS

Contusion

Because the vitreous is inelastic compared with the adjacent tissues, contusions that abruptly though briefly alter the shape of the eye are apt to cause injuries where the vitreous is adherent.

Disinsertion of the vitreous base is not uncommon. It is frequently associated with tearing of the pars plana or retina, vitreous hemorrhage, or detachment of the retina—as long as 20 years later.

Less commonly, photopsia, vitreous floaters, and even vitreous hemorrhage or detachment of the retina may result from stress behind the vitreous base. The affected sites may be previously subclinical anomalous vitreoretinal adhesions (eg, lattice degeneration) or areas of frank vitreoretinal disease such as diabetic retinopathy.

Rupture of the Globe

Rupture of the globe is always a serious injury that may result in early or late blindness or even loss of the eyeball. Prolapse of the vitreous through the wound is a severe complication often associated with acute secondary tearing or detachment of the retina. A seemingly uncomplicated prolapse may be followed by late retinal detachment with or without tears due to fibrous ingrowth from the orbit and subsequent contraction. The latter may be visible as membranes or bands in the vitreous. Various forms of vitreous surgery are used to prevent or treat such complications.

Penetration of the Globe

An almost endless variety of material may accidentally penetrate the globe. Common examples are needles, airgun pellets, and small particles of metal, stone, or plastic that fly into the eye at high velocity.

Prolapse of the vitreous may occur at the site of entry or exit or both. The part traversed by the foreign body is permanently damaged and is often marked by visible condensation, shrinkage, or fibrous elements. Vitreous surgery is increasingly used to prevent or treat complications such as retinal detachment with or without tears.

Vitreous Loss

Vitreous loss is an iatrogenic complication. The vitreous gel prolapses through a surgical wound, usually at (but not limited to) the corneal limbus during the course of operating on the lens, iris, or cornea.

Fibrous tissue invasion and contraction are frequent sequels that are prone to cause traction complications involving the retina. Corneal edema and iris displace-

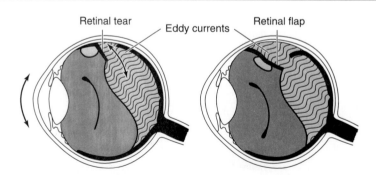

Figure 9–15. Abrupt rotation of globe generates eddy currents in liquid vitreous, a result of inertial lag *(left),* that tends to lift the retinal flap and surrounding sensory retina *(right).*

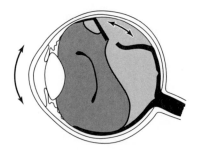

Figure 9–16. Enlargement of retinal detachment due to inertial lag of liquid vitreous within the retina.

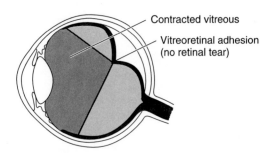

Figure 9–17. Traction detachment of retina.

ment (eg, "updrawn pupil") may also occur. An acute prolapse can be effectively excised. An old prolapse may require surgery for release of vitreous traction.

VITREOUS INFLAMMATION

Vitreous inflammation includes a wide spectrum of disorders ranging from a few scattered white cells to abscess formation. Most commonly, one or more focal inflammatory lesions in the choroid or retina—as in chorioretinitis or retinitis—are responsible for a secondary cellular invasion of the liquid vitreous or relatively resistant gel. There may be a mild localized blurring of the fundus landmarks and lesions that provoke little or no visual complaint except for a possible vitreous floater effect. With greater infiltration, vision is decreased and the fundus is invisible or almost so. The condition may be so marked that the red reflection is lost and the vitreous appears opaque and white. Since these conditions spare the anterior segment, there is no pain and the external eye appears normal. The prognosis and treatment depend upon the underlying condition. The vitreous usually clears when the primary defect is quiescent. Vitreous surgery is used to remove gross residual opacities that show no sign of clearing spontaneously.

Vitreous Abscess (Endophthalmitis)*

Vitreous abscess may occur following penetrating ocular trauma, including ocular surgery or following bloodstream dissemination from elsewhere in the body, such as colonization by *Candida albicans* of an indwelling venous catheter. The vitreous is an excellent culture medium; following bacterial or fungal invasion, it undergoes liquefaction and abscess formation.

The diagnosis of vitreous abscess is confirmed by aspirating 0.5–1 mL of vitreous under local anesthesia through a pars plana sclerotomy using a 20- to 23-gauge needle. The aspirate should be examined microscopically.

Once the organism is identified, immediate medical treatment is indicated (see Table 3–1).

In some cases, vitrectomy is indicated to drain the abscess and allow better visualization of the fundus.

Even with optimal treatment, vitreous abscess carries a grave prognosis.

---

* If all three coats of the eye as well as the vitreous are involved by an inflammatory process, the condition is known as panophthalmitis. The line of demarcation between endophthalmitis and panophthalmitis is usually obscure.

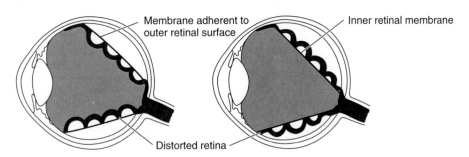

Figure 9–18. Proliferative vitreoretinopathy. *Left:* Contracture of membrane adherent to outer retinal surface. ***Right:*** Contracture of inner retinal membrane.

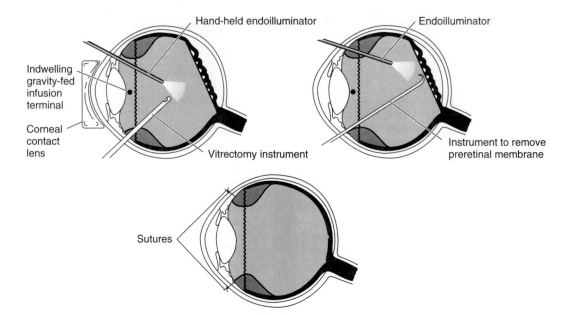

Figure 9–19. Vitreous surgery. ***Top left:*** Position of corneal contact lens and intraocular devices. ***Top right:*** Removal of preretinal membrane. ***Bottom:*** Placement of sutures at completion of procedure.

VITREOUS SURGERY

Vitreous surgery is useful for a broad spectrum of intraocular disorders. Airtight and watertight incisions measuring 1–4 mm are made in the pars plana and sclera (Figure 9–19). One incision is used for an indwelling gravity-fed infusion terminal, which maintains the desired tension and configuration of the globe. Surgical gases and medications are also instilled through this terminal. Another incision is used for a hand-held endoilluminator, which illuminates the contents and all of the walls of the vitreous cavity. The illuminated structures are viewed microscopically through the pupil with the aid of a corneal contact or other lens that neutralizes the light-focusing power of the eye. The remaining incision is used to allow for instrumentation (severing or removal of tissue), diathermy, and laser photocoagulation (Figure 9–19).

Vitreous surgery provides access to virtually all of the intraocular tissues between the endothelium of the cornea and the retinal pigment epithelium. Surgery is most commonly done (1) to remove vitreous opacified by blood (Figure 9–20 top), (2) to remove shrunken vitreous causing traction retinal detachment (Figure 9–20 middle), (3) to treat vitreous contracture complicating retinal detachment (Figure 9–20 bottom) (see preretinal membranes), (4) to remove metaplastic membranes that deform or detach the sensory retina (Figures 9–18 and 9–19), (5) to create an optical opening in recalcitrant pupillary membranes, and (6) to remove infected vitreous in endophthalmitis (so as to dilute the organismal toxins and reduce the population of causal organisms and to instill therapeutic solutions). Vitreous surgery is frequently combined with scleral buckling for retinal detachment.

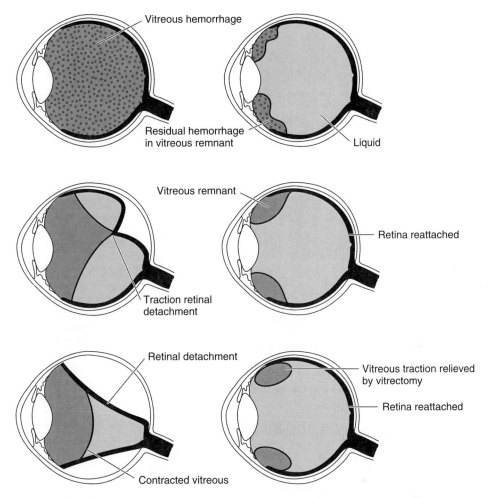

Figure 9–20. Scope of vitreous surgery. ***Top:*** Removal of vitreous hemorrhage. Residual hemorrhage will clear in time from vitreous remnants. ***Middle:*** Reattachment of traction retinal detachment following vitrectomy. ***Bottom:*** Vitreous contracture complicating retinal detachment. Removal of vitreous and repair of retinal detachment.

REFERENCES

Abrams GW et al: Vitrectomy with silicone oil or long-acting gas in eyes with severe proliferative vitreo-retinopathy: Results of additional and long-term follow-up. Silicone Study Report 11. Arch Ophthalmol 1997;115:335.

Bacon AS et al: Infective endophthalmitis following vitreoretinal surgery. Eye 1993;7:529.

Crafoord S et al: Long-term results of macular pucker surgery. Acta Ophthalmol Scand 1997;75:85.

Endophthalmitis Vitrectomy Study Group: Results of the endophthalmitis vitrectomy study. Arch Ophthalmol 1995;113:1479.

Flynn HW Jr et al: Pars plana vitrectomy in the Early Treatment Diabetic Retinopathy Study: ETDRS report number 17. Ophthalmology 1992;99:1351.

Freeman WR et al: Vitrectomy for the treatment of full-thickness stage 3 or 4 macular holes. Results of a multi-centered randomized clinical trial. Arch Ophthalmol 1997;115:11.

Hikichi T, Trempe CL: Ocular conditions associated with posterior vitreous detachment in young patients. Ophthalmic Surg Lasers 1996;27:782.

Lewis H, Ryan SJ (editors): *Medical and Surgical Retina: Advances, Controversies and Management.* Mosby, 1994.

Lindgren G, Sjödell L, Lindblom B: A prospective study of dense spontaneous vitreous hemorrhage. Am J Ophthalmol 1995;119:458.

McCormack P et al: Is surgery for proliferative vitreoretinopathy justifiable? Eye 1994;8:75.

Quinn GE et al: Visual acuity of eyes after vitrectomy for retinopathy of prematurity: Follow-up at five years. Ophthalmology 1996;103:595.

Smiddy WE et al: Vitrectomy for complications of proliferative diabetic retinopathy: Functional outcomes. Ophthalmology 1995;102:1688.

Snead MP et al: Vitreous detachment and the posterior hyaloid membrane: A clinicopathological study. Eye 1994;8:204.

10

Retina

Robert A. Hardy, MD, & J. Brooks Crawford, MD

I. RETINA

Robert A. Hardy, MD

The human retina is a highly organized structure, consisting of alternate layers of cell bodies and synaptic processes. Despite its compact size and apparent simplicity when compared with nervous structures such as the cerebral cortex, the retina has a remarkably sophisticated level of processing power. Visual processing of the retina is elaborated upon by the brain, and the perception of color, contrast, depth, and form occurs in the cortex.

The anatomy of the retina is presented in Chapter 1. Figure 1–17 shows the major cell types and identifies the layers of this tissue. Division of the retina into layers composed of groups of similar cells permits the clinician to localize a function or functional disturbance to a single layer or group of cells. Processing of retinal information proceeds from the photoreceptor layer through the ganglion cell axon to the optic nerve and brain.

PHYSIOLOGY

The retina is the most complex of the ocular tissues. In order to see, the eye must perform as an optical instrument, as a complex receptor, and as an effective transducer. Rod and cone cells in the photoreceptor layer are capable of transforming light stimulus into a nerve impulse that is conducted by the nerve fiber layer of the retina through the optic nerve and ultimately to the occipital visual cortex. The macula is responsible for the best visual acuity and for color vision, and most of its photoreceptor cells are cones. In the central fovea, there is a nearly 1:1 relationship between the cone photoreceptor, its ganglion cell, and the emerging nerve fiber, and this ensures the most acute vision. In the peripheral retina, many photoreceptors are coupled to the same ganglion cell, and a more complex system of relays is necessary. The result of such an arrangement is that the macula is used primarily for central and color vision (photopic vision) while the remaining retina, which is populated mostly by rod photoreceptors, is utilized primarily for peripheral and night (scotopic) vision.

The rod and cone photoreceptors are located in the avascular outermost layer of the sensory retina and are the site of the chemical reaction initiating the visual process. Each rod photoreceptor cell contains rhodopsin, which is a photosensitive visual pigment formed when opsin protein molecules combine with 11-*cis* retinal. As a photon of light is absorbed by rhodopsin, 11-*cis* retinal is immediately isomerized to its all-*trans* form. Rhodopsin is a membrane-bound glycolipid that is partially embedded in the double membrane disks of the photoreceptor outer segment. Peak light absorption by rhodopsin occurs at approximately 500 nm, which is the blue-green region of the light spectrum. Spectral sensitivity studies of cone photopigments have shown peak wavelength absorption at 430, 540, and 575 nm for blue-, green-, and red-sensitive cones, respectively. The cone photopigments are composed of 11-*cis*retinal bound to a variety of opsin proteins.

Scotopic vision is mediated entirely by the rod photoreceptors. With this dark-adapted form of vision, varying shades of gray are seen, but colors cannot be distinguished. As the retina becomes fully light-adapted, the spectral sensitivity of the retina shifts from a rhodopsin-dominated peak of 500 nm to approximately 560 nm, and color sensation becomes evident. An object takes on color when it contains photopigments that absorb specific wavelengths and selectively reflect or transmit certain wavelengths of light within the visible spectrum (400–700 nm). Daylight vision is mediated primarily by cone photoreceptors, twilight by a combination of cones and rods, and night vision by the rod photoreceptors.

EXAMINATION

The examination of the retina is described in Chapter 2 and depicted in Figures 2–12 to 2–18. The retina can be examined with a direct or indirect ophthalmoscope or with a slitlamp (biomicroscope) and contact or handheld biconvex lens. With these instruments, the skilled observer is clinically able to dissect the layers of the retina in order to determine the type, level, and extent of retinal disease. Fundus photography and fluorescein angiography (Figures 2–27 to 2–29) are useful adjuncts to the clinical examination; photography allows pictorial documentation for future comparison, and angiography provides the vascular detail needed for laser treatment of retinal diseases.

The clinical application of visual electrophysiologic and psychophysical tests is described in Chapter 2. Such tests may be helpful in establishing the diagnosis of certain disease entities.

DISEASES OF THE MACULA

AGE-RELATED MACULAR DEGENERATION

Age-related macular degeneration is the leading cause of permanent blindness in the elderly. The exact cause is unknown, but the incidence increases with each decade over age 50. Other associations besides age include race (usually Caucasian), sex (slight female predominance), family history, and a history of cigarette smoking. The disease includes a broad spectrum of clinical and pathologic findings that can be classified into two groups: nonexudative ("dry") and exudative ("wet"). Although both types are progressive and usually bilateral, they differ in their manifestations, prognosis, and management. The more severe exudative form accounts for approximately 90% of all cases of legal blindness due to age-related macular degeneration.

1. NONEXUDATIVE MACULAR DEGENERATION

Nonexudative age-related macular degeneration is characterized by variable degrees of atrophy and degeneration of the outer retina, retinal pigment epithelium, Bruch's membrane and choriocapillaris. Of the ophthalmoscopically visible changes in the retinal pigment epithelium and Bruch's membrane, drusen are the most typical (Figure 10–1). **Drusen** are discrete, round, yellow-white deposits of variable size beneath the pigment epithelium and are scattered throughout the macula and posterior pole. With time, they may enlarge, coalesce, calcify, and increase in number. Histopathologically, most drusen consist of focal collections of eosinophilic material lying between the pigment epithelium and Bruch's membrane; they therefore represent focal detachment of the pigment epithelium. In addition to drusen, clumps of pigment irregularly dispersed within depigmented

areas of atrophy may progressively appear throughout the macula. The level of associated visual impairment is variable and may be minimal. Fluorescein angiography demonstrates irregular patterns of retinal pigment epithelial hyperplasia and atrophy. Electrophysiologic testing in most patients is normal.

There is no generally accepted treatment or means of prevention of this type of macular degeneration. Laser retinal photocoagulation appears to have a beneficial effect on drusen but has not yet been shown to improve visual outcome. Although high plasma levels of antioxidants are associated with a reduced risk of age-related macular degeneration, the use of vitamin supplements does not appear to be preventive. Most patients with macular drusen never experience significant loss of central vision; the atrophic changes may stabilize or progress slowly. However, the exudative stage may develop suddenly at any time, and in addition to regular ophthalmic examinations, patients are given an Amsler grid (Figure 2–22) to help monitor and report any symptomatic changes.

2. EXUDATIVE MACULAR DEGENERATION

Although patients with age-related macular degeneration usually manifest nonexudative changes only, the majority of patients who experience severe vision loss from this disease do so from the development of subretinal neovascularization and related exudative maculopathy. Serous fluid from the underlying choroid can leak through small defects in Bruch's membrane, causing focal detachment of the pigment epithelium. Additional fluid may lead to further separation of the overlying sensory retina, and vision usu-

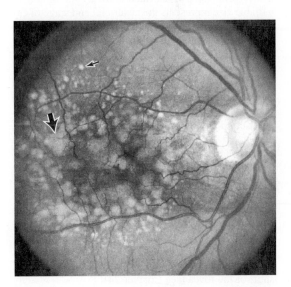

Figure 10–1. Age-related macular degeneration with discrete (small arrow) and large confluent (large arrow) macular drusen.

ally decreases if the fovea is involved. Retinal pigment epithelial detachments may spontaneously flatten, with variable visual results, and leave a geographic area of depigmentation at the involved site.

Ingrowth of new vessels from the choroid into the subretinal space is the most important change that predisposes patients with drusen to macular detachment and irreversible loss of central vision. These new vessels grow in a flat cartwheel or sea-fan configuration away from their site of entry into the subretinal space. The clinical changes of early subretinal neovascularization are subtle and may be easily overlooked; during this occult stage of new vessel formation, the patient is asymptomatic, and the new vessels may not be apparent either ophthalmoscopically or angiographically.

The ophthalmologist must maintain a high index of suspicion that subretinal neovascularization is present whenever a patient with evidence of age-related macular degeneration has sudden or recent central vision loss, including blurred vision, distortion, or a new scotoma. If the fundus examination reveals subretinal blood, exudate, or a grayish-green choroidal lesion in the macula, there is great likelihood that neovascularization is present, and a fluorescein or indocyanine green angiogram should be obtained promptly to determine if a treatable lesion can be identified.

Although some subretinal neovascular membranes may spontaneously regress, the natural course of subretinal neovascularization in age-related macular degeneration is toward irreversible loss of central vision over a variable period of time. The sensory retina may be damaged by long-standing edema, detachment, or underlying hemorrhage. Furthermore, a hemorrhagic detachment of the retina may undergo fibrous metaplasia, resulting in an elevated subretinal mass called a disciform scar. This elevated fibrovascular mound of variable size represents the cicatricial end stage of exudative age-related macular degeneration. It is usually centrally located and results in permanent loss of central vision.

Treatment

In the absence of subretinal neovascularization, no medical or surgical treatment of serous retinal pigment epithelial detachment is of proved benefit. The use of parenteral alpha interferon, for example, has not been effective for this disease. However, if a well-defined extrafoveal (≥ 200 μm from the center of the foveal avascular zone) subretinal neovascular membrane is present, laser photocoagulation is indicated. Angiography defines the precise location and borders of the neovascular membrane, which is then completely ablated by heavy confluent laser burns. Photocoagulation destroys the overlying retina as well but is worthwhile if the subretinal membrane can be halted short of the fovea (see Chapter 24).

Krypton laser photocoagulation of juxtafoveal (<200 μm from the center of the foveal avascular zone) subretinal neovascularization is recommended in nonhypertensive patients. The Macular Photocoagulation Study Group has refined its treatment recommendations for subfoveal disease and shown that selected patients may benefit from laser photocoagulation. The ability to determine the probable rate and direction of growth of a subretinal neovascular membrane would facilitate clinical decisions about if and when to treat a given membrane in cases where treatment indications are unclear. Unfortunately, many patients with exudative macular degeneration present with subretinal neovascularization that is either not sufficiently well defined or is too extensive for laser photocoagulation to be useful.

Following successful photocoagulation of a subretinal neovascular membrane, recurrent neovascularization either contiguous with or remote from the laser scar may occur in one-half of cases by 2 years. Recurrence is often accompanied by severe vision loss, so that careful monitoring with Amsler grids, ophthalmoscopy, and angiography is essential. Low-dose radiotherapy has provided encouraging results in patients with subfoveal neovascularization. Patients with impaired central vision in both eyes may benefit from a variety of low vision aids.

CENTRAL SEROUS CHORIORETINOPATHY

Central serous chorioretinopathy is characterized by serous detachment of the sensory retina as a consequence of focal leakage of fluid from the choriocapillaris through a defect in the retinal pigment epithelium (Figures 10–2 and 10–3). This disease typically affects young to middle-aged men and may be related to life stress events. Most patients present with the sudden

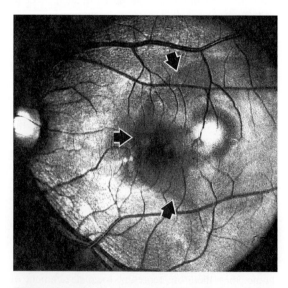

Figure 10–2. Central serous chorioretinopathy with sensory retinal detachment (arrows) extending into the fovea.

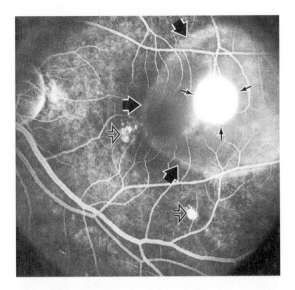

Figure 10–3. Fluorescein angiogram of central serous chorioretinopathy shows active disease with both a retinal pigment epithelial detachment (small arrows) and a sensory retinal detachment (large arrows). Two foci of inactive disease (open arrows) are also present.

onset of blurred vision, micropsia, metamorphopsia, and central scotoma. Visual acuity is often only moderately decreased and may be improved to near-normal with a small hyperopic correction.

The diagnosis is made by slitlamp examination of the fundus; the presence of serous detachment of the sensory retina in the absence of ocular inflammation, subretinal neovascularization, an optic pit, or a choroidal tumor is diagnostic. The retinal pigment epithelial lesion appears as a small, round or oval, yellowish-gray spot that is variable in size and may be difficult to detect without the aid of fluorescein angiography. Fluorescein dye leaking from the choriocapillaris may accumulate below the pigment epithelium or sensory retina, resulting in a variety of patterns including the well-recognized smokestack configuration.

Approximately 80% of eyes with central serous chorioretinopathy undergo spontaneous resorption of subretinal fluid and recovery of normal visual acuity within 6 months after the onset of symptoms. Despite normal acuity, however, many patients have a mild permanent visual defect, such as a decrease in color sensitivity, micropsia, or relative scotoma. Twenty to 30 percent of patients will have one or more recurrences of the disease, and complications—including subretinal neovascularization and chronic cystoid macular edema—have been described in patients with frequent and prolonged serous detachments.

The cause of central serous chorioretinopathy is unknown; there is no convincing evidence that the disease is either infectious or due to retinal pigment epithelial dystrophy. Argon laser photocoagulation

directed to the active leak significantly shortens the duration of the sensory detachment and hastens the recovery of central vision, but there is no evidence that prompt photocoagulation reduces the chance of permanent loss of visual function. Although the complications of retinal laser photocoagulation are few, it is probably not advisable to recommend immediate photocoagulation treatment in all patients with central serous chorioretinopathy. The duration and location of disease, the condition of the fellow eye, and occupational visual requirements are all considerations upon which treatment decisions are based.

MACULAR EDEMA

Retinal edema involving the macula may be associated with a variety of intraocular inflammatory diseases, retinal vascular diseases, intraocular surgery, inherited or acquired retinal degenerations, medications, macular membranes, or unknown causes. Macular edema may be diffuse, with nonlocalized intraretinal fluid causing thickening of the macula. When edema fluid accumulates in honeycomb-like spaces of the outer plexiform and inner nuclear layers, it is called **cystoid macular edema.** On fluorescein angiography, fluorescein dye leaks from the perifoveal retinal capillaries and accumulates in a flower-petal pattern about the fovea (Figure 10–4).

The most widely recognized association with cystoid macular edema is intraocular surgery. Approximately 50% of eyes undergoing uneventful intracapsular cataract extraction and 20% of eyes undergoing extracapsular cataract extraction develop angiographic cystoid macular edema. Clinically significant edema

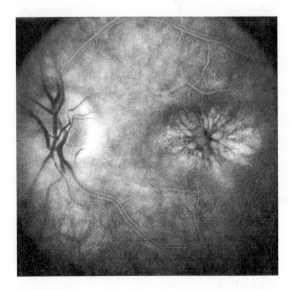

Figure 10–4. Flower-petal pattern of fluorescein dye in a patient with cystoid macular edema after cataract surgery.

usually occurs within 4–12 weeks postoperatively, but in some instances its onset may be delayed for months or years. Many patients with cystoid macular edema of less than 6 months' duration have self-limited leakage that will resolve without treatment. Topical or local (or both) anti-inflammatory therapy may be of value in restoring visual acuity in some patients with chronic postoperative macular edema. YAG laser vitreolysis (see Chapter 24) and surgical vitrectomy may be of benefit when the macular edema is associated with vitreous tissue incarcerated in the cataract wound or adherent to anterior segment structures. When an intraocular lens implant is the cause of postoperative macular edema due to its design, positioning, or inadequate fixation, removal of the lens implant can be considered.

INFLAMMATORY DISORDERS INVOLVING THE MACULA

Presumed Ocular Histoplasmosis Syndrome (Figures 10–5 to 10–7)

In this disease, serous and hemorrhagic detachments of the macula are associated with multiple peripheral atrophic chorioretinal scars and peripapillary chorioretinal scarring (see Chapter 7). The syndrome usually occurs in healthy patients between the third and sixth decades of life, and the scars are probably caused by an antecedent subclinical systemic infection with *Histoplasma capsulatum.* The macular detachments are due to subretinal neovascularization, and the visual prognosis depends on the proximity of the neovascular membrane to the center of the fovea. If the membrane extends inside the foveal avascular zone, only 15% of eyes will retain 20/40 vision. A macular scar may change over time, and 10% of patients with normal maculae will develop new atrophic scars in this region. The relative risk of developing macular subretinal neovascularization in the second eye of an affected patient is significant, and these patients should be instructed in the frequent use of the Amsler grid and the importance of prompt examination when changes are detected.

Argon laser photocoagulation of a subretinal neovascular membrane outside the foveal avascular zone in symptomatic patients is of value in preventing severe vision loss. The surgical removal of submacular membranes may prove useful in preserving vision.

Acute Multifocal Posterior Placoid Pigment Epitheliopathy (AMPPPE)

AMPPPE typically affects healthy young patients who develop rapidly progressive bilateral vision loss in association with ophthalmoscopically visible multifocal flat gray-white subretinal lesions involving the pigment epithelium (Figure 10–8). The cause of this disease, which in many instances is associated with evidence of an influenza-like illness, is unknown; the course and nature of the illness suggests the possibility of viral infection. The characteristic feature of the disease is the rapid resolution of the fundus lesions and a delayed return of visual acuity to near-normal levels. Although the prognosis for visual recovery in this acute self-limited disease is good, many patients will identify small residual paracentral scotomas when carefully tested. Extensive pigmentary changes remaining during the late stages of AMPPPE may mimic widespread retinal degeneration; the clinical history and normal electrophysiologic findings aid in this differential diagnosis.

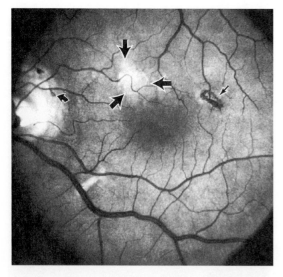

Figure 10–5. Presumed ocular histoplasmosis syndrome with active disease (large arrows) and an inactive pigmented macular scar (small arrow). Peripapillary pigmentation (curved arrow) is also present.

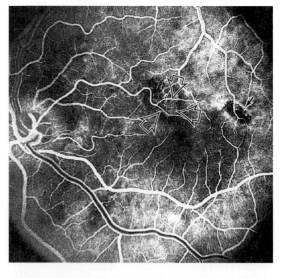

Figure 10–6. The early fluorescein angiogram shows an inactive hypofluorescent scar (small arrow) and the characteristic lacy hyperfluorescence of subretinal neovascularization (open arrows).

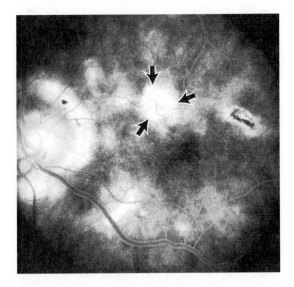

Figure 10–7. Late fluorescein leakage from macular sub-retinal neovascularization in a patient with presumed ocular histoplasmosis syndrome.

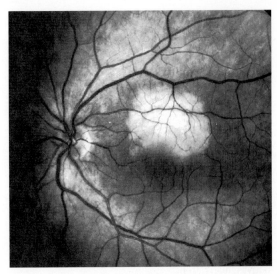

Figure 10–8. Typical macular lesion of acute multifocal posterior placoid pigment epitheliopathy.

Geographic Helicoid Peripapillary Choroidopathy

This is a chronic progressive and recurrent multifocal inflammatory disease of the retinal pigment epithelium, choriocapillaris, and choroid. It characteristically involves the juxtapapillary retina and extends radially to involve the macula and peripheral retina. The active stage manifests itself as sharply demarcated gray-yellow lesions with irregular borders that appear to involve the pigment epithelium and choriocapillaris. Vitritis, anterior uveitis, and subretinal neovascularization have been associated with this disorder. Involvement is usually bilateral, and the cause is unknown. The natural history of this indolent inflammatory disease is variable and may correlate with the presence of disease in the fellow eye. Local or systemic corticosteroid treatment may be of benefit when active inflammation is present; laser photocoagulation is administered as indicated for the complication of subretinal neovascularization.

Vitiliginous Chorioretinitis (Birdshot Retinochoroidopathy)

This is a syndrome characterized by diffuse cream-colored patches at the level of the pigment epithelium and choroid, retinal vasculitis associated with cystoid macular edema, and vitritis. The associations with HLA-A29 and with retinal S-antigen suggest that this disease has a genetic predisposition and that retinal autoimmunity plays a role in its manifestations. In many cases, electroretinography, electro-oculography, and dark adaptation studies are abnormal. The course of the disease is that of exacerbation and remission with variable visual outcomes; visual loss has been at-

tributed to chronic cystoid macular edema, optic atrophy, macular scarring, or subretinal neovascularization. Corticosteroid therapy has not proved effective against this disease.

Acute Macular Neuroretinopathy

Acute macular neuroretinopathy is characterized by the acute onset of paracentral scotomas and mild visual acuity loss accompanied by wedge-shaped parafoveal retinal lesions in the deep sensory retina of one or both eyes. The macular lesions are subtle, reddish-brown, and best seen with a red-free light. The patients are usually young adults with a history of acute viral illness. While the retinal lesions may fade, the scotomas tend to persist and remain symptomatic.

Multiple Evanescent White Dot Syndrome

This is an acute and self-limited unilateral disease that affects mainly young women and is characterized clinically by multiple white dots at the level of the pigment epithelium, vitreal cells, and transient electroretinographic abnormalities. The cause is unknown. There is no evidence of associated systemic disease. The retinal lesions gradually regress in a matter of weeks, leaving only minor retinal pigment epithelial defects.

ANGIOID STREAKS

Angioid streaks appear as irregular, jagged tapering lines that radiate from the peripapillary retina into the macula and peripheral fundus (Figure 10–9). The streaks represent linear crack-like dehiscences in

Bruch's membrane. The lesions are rarely noted in children and probably develop in the second or third decade of life. Early in the disease the streaks are sharply outlined and red-orange or brown. Subsequent fibrovascular tissue growth may partially or totally obscure the streak margins.

Nearly 50% of patients with angioid streaks have an associated systemic disease. Pseudoxanthoma elasticum, Paget's disease of bone, Ehlers-Danlos syndrome, and several hemoglobinopathies and hemolytic disorders have been associated with this retinal disease, but the most common association is with age-related degeneration of Bruch's membrane. Patients with angioid streaks should be warned of the potential risk of choroidal rupture from even relatively mild eye trauma. Older patients with the disease are at risk of developing serous and hemorrhagic detachments of the retina as a consequence of subretinal neovascularization.

Laser treatment may be used to photocoagulate extrafoveal neovascular membranes; however, other neovascular membranes are likely to occur. Prophylactic treatment of angioid streaks before subretinal neovascularization develops is not recommended.

MYOPIC MACULAR DEGENERATION

Pathologic myopia is one of the leading causes of blindness in the United States and is characterized by progressive elongation of the eye with subsequent thinning and atrophy of the choroid and pigment epithelium in the macula. Peripapillary chorioretinal atrophy and linear breaks in Bruch's membrane ("lacquer cracks") are characteristic findings on ophthalmoscopy (Figure 10–10). The degenerative changes of the macular pigment epithelium resemble those found in the older patient with age-related macular degeneration. A characteristic lesion of this disease is a raised, circular, pigmented macular lesion called a Fuchs spot. Most patients are in the fifth decade when the degenerative macular changes cause a slowly progressive loss of vision; rapid loss of visual acuity is usually caused by serous and hemorrhagic macular degeneration overlying a subretinal neovascular membrane.

Fluorescein angiography in patients with pathologic myopia may show delayed filling of choroidal and retinal blood vessels. Angiography is helpful in identifying and locating the site of subretinal neovascularization in patients who develop serous or hemorrhagic detachments of the macula. Because of the frequent close proximity of the subretinal neovascular membrane to the foveola in these patients, laser photocoagulation may not be possible. As subretinal neovascular membranes tend to remain small and because photocoagulation-associated chorioretinal atrophy tends to progress in patients with pathologic myopia, retinal laser treatment is not as beneficial as in other diseases associated with macular subretinal neovascularization.

The chorioretinal changes of pathologic myopia predispose the retina to breaks and thus to retinal detachment. Peripheral retinal findings may include paving stone degeneration, pigmentary degeneration, and lattice degeneration. Retinal breaks usually occur in areas involved with chorioretinal lesions, but they also arise in areas of apparently normal retina. Some of these breaks, particularly those of the "horseshoe" and round retinal tear type, will progress to rhegmatogenous retinal detachment.

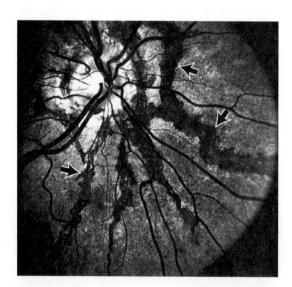

Figure 10–9. Multiple angioid streaks (arrows) extend from the optic nerve. (Courtesy of University of California, San Francisco.)

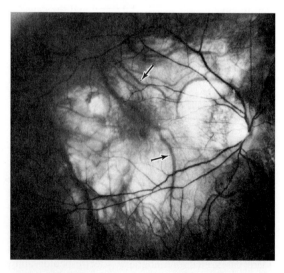

Figure 10–10. Myopic macular degeneration with choroidal vessels (arrows) visible through atrophic retinal pigment epithelium.

MACULAR HOLE

A macular hole is a partial or full-thickness absence of the sensory retina in the macula. This disorder occurs most often in elderly women and is associated with elevated plasma fibrinogen levels. The typical finding on biomicroscopy of the symptomatic eye is a full-thickness, round or oval, sharply defined hole measuring one-third disk diameter in the center of the macula, which may be surrounded by a ring detachment of the sensory retina (Figure 10–11). With a full-thickness macular hole, visual acuity is impaired and metamorphopsia, as well as a central scotoma, are present on the Amsler grid. An operculum of retinal tissue may overlie the macular hole. Tangential traction from epiretinal vitreous cortex plays an important role in the pathogenesis of macular hole. Early stages of macular hole formation, such as a deep foveal yellow spot or ring, may be reversible as the posterior vitreous cortex spontaneously separates from the retina. Therapy for macular hole disease involves reattaching and potentially restoring function to the retina overlying the cuff of subretinal fluid surrounding the hole. While the anatomic results of vitrectomy surgery to close macular holes are encouraging, the clinical benefits are still under study.

EPIRETINAL MACULAR MEMBRANES

Fibrocellular membranes may proliferate on the surface of the retina, either in the macula or peripheral retina. Contraction or shrinkage of these epiretinal membranes may cause varying degrees of visual distortion, intraretinal edema, and degeneration of the underlying retina. Biomicroscopy usually shows retinal wrinkles and vessel tortuosity and may rarely also show retinal hemorrhages, cotton-wool spots, serous retinal detachment, and macular hole; a posterior vitreous detachment is nearly always present (Figure 10–12). Disorders associated with epiretinal membranes include retinal tears with or without rhegmatogenous retinal detachment, vitreous inflammatory diseases, trauma, and a variety of retinal vascular diseases.

Patients with macular distortion and vision loss caused by epiretinal membrane contraction are usually left with stable visual acuity, suggesting that membrane contraction is a short-lived and self-limited process. Surgical peeling of severe epiretinal membranes can be performed successfully, but regrowth of epiretinal tissues occurs in some cases. There is no role for photocoagulation in the treatment of epiretinal macular membrane disease.

TRAUMATIC MACULOPATHY

Blunt trauma to the anterior segment of the eye may cause a contrecoup injury to the retina called **commotio retinae.** The retina develops a gray-white color that affects primarily the outer retina and may be confined to the macular area (Berlin's edema) or may involve extensive areas of the peripheral retina. The retinal whitening in the macular area may clear completely, or impairment of central vision may be permanent and associated with a pigmented retinal scar (Figure 10–13) or a macular hole. Trauma similar to that which causes Berlin's edema may also cause choroidal rupture with subretinal hemorrhage and permanent central vision loss.

In addition to blunt trauma, several other traumatic injuries involving the macula are of importance.

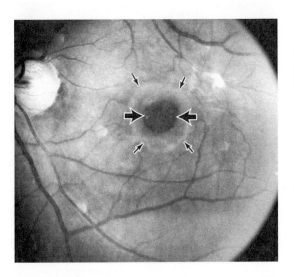

Figure 10–11. Macular hole (large arrows) with surrounding sensory retinal detachment (small arrows).

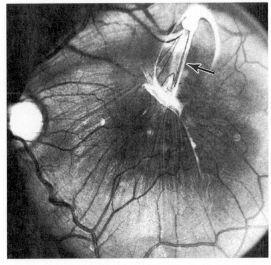

Figure 10–12. Epiretinal macular membrane elevates retinal vessels (arrow) and produces retinal striae.

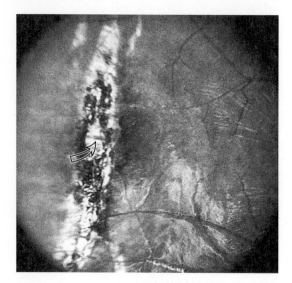

Figure 10–13. Traumatic choroidal rupture resulting in pigmented scar. A choroidal vessel (arrow) is visible through the scar.

Table 10–1. Anatomic classification of macular dystrophies.

Nerve fiber layer
X-linked juvenile retinoschisis
Photoreceptor cells
Cone-rod dystrophy
Retinal pigment epithelium
Fundus albipunctus
Fundus flavimaculatus
Vitelliform dystrophy (Best's disease)

lamp examination, foveal schisis appears as small superficial retinal cysts arranged in a stellate pattern accompanied by radial striae centered in the foveal area (Figure 10–14). Visual acuity is usually between 20/40 and 20/200; peripheral visual field abnormalities are present in the 50% of patients with associated peripheral retinoschisis. The posterior pole appears normal on fluorescein angiography, and this may be helpful in the clinical differentiation from cystoid macular edema. B wave abnormalities on the electroretinogram are consistent with the histopathologic finding of intraretinal splitting in the nerve fiber layer.

Cone-Rod Dystrophies

The cone-rod dystrophies constitute a relatively rare group of disorders that may be regarded as a single entity showing variable expressivity. Most cases are sporadic, but familial cases are usually transmitted by an autosomal dominant inheritance pattern. Cone-rod dystrophy is characterized by predominant involvement of the cone photoreceptors with progressive color vision defects and associated loss of visual acuity. A bilateral and symmetric bulls-eye pattern of depigmentation and a corresponding zone of hyperfluorescence surrounding a central nonfluorescent

Purtscher's retinopathy is characterized by multiple patches of superficial retinal whitening and retinal hemorrhages in each eye of a patient after severe compression injury to the head or trunk. **Terson's syndrome** is seen in approximately 20% of patients after traumatic (or spontaneous) subarachnoid or subdural hemorrhage and is characterized by vitreous and superficial macular hemorrhage. **Solar retinopathy** refers to a specific foveolar lesion that occurs after sun-gazing and is best described as a usually bilateral sharply circumscribed and often irregularly shaped partial-thickness hole or depression in the center of the fovea.

MACULAR DYSTROPHIES

Macular dystrophies differ from degenerations in that the former are inherited, though not necessarily evident at birth, and are not associated with systemic diseases. Most often the disorder is restricted to the macula; it may be symmetric or asymmetric, but eventually both eyes are affected. In the early stages of some of these disorders the visual acuity may be reduced while the macular changes are subtle or absent on ophthalmoscopy, and the patient's complaint may be dismissed as spurious. Conversely, in other macular dystrophies, the ophthalmoscopic changes may be very striking at a time when the patient is free of visual symptoms. One method of classifying the more common macular dystrophies is to consider the presumptive anatomic layer or layers of the retina involved (Table 10–1).

X-Linked Juvenile Retinoschisis

This is a congenital disease of males characterized by a macular lesion called "foveal schisis." On slit-

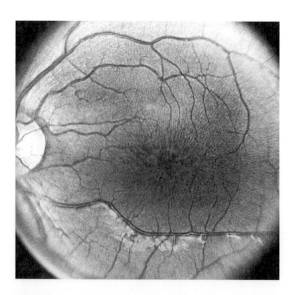

Figure 10–14. X-linked juvenile retinoschisis with typical superficial retinal cysts in the fovea.

spot (similar to that seen in chloroquine retinopathy) are the most commonly described biomicroscopic and angiographic changes in these patients (Figure 10–15). As the disease progresses, the electroretinogram shows marked loss of cone function associated with a slight to moderate loss of rod function. Histopathologic study shows absence of macular and paramacular photoreceptors, and there is associated pigment epithelium degeneration.

Fundus Albipunctatus

Fundus albipunctatus is an autosomal recessive nonprogressive dystrophy characterized by a myriad of discrete small white dots at the level of the pigment epithelium sprinkled about the posterior pole and midperiphery of the retina. Patients are night-blind with normal visual acuity, normal visual fields, and normal color vision. While the electroretinogram and electro-oculogram are usually normal, dark adaptation thresholds are markedly elevated. **Retinitis punctata albescens** is the less common progressive variant of this dystrophy.

Fundus Flavimaculatus (Stargardt's Disease)

This is a bilateral and symmetric autosomal recessive disorder characterized by multiple yellow-white fleck lesions of variable size and shape confined to the retinal pigment epithelium (Figure 10–16). Many patients suffer central visual loss in childhood; however, macular involvement and the ultimate visual outcome are variable. Fluorescein angiography is important in differentiating flecks from drusen; the former are usually hypofluorescent. The electroretinogram and electro-oculogram are usually normal. Histopathologic abnormalities are confined to the pigment epithelium; the yellow flecks seen clinically are dense accumulations of lipofuscin within engorged pigment epithelial cells.

Vitelliform Dystrophy (Best's Disease)

Vitelliform dystrophy is an autosomal dominant disorder with variable penetrance and expressivity with onset usually in childhood. The ophthalmoscopic appearance is variable and ranges from a mild pigmentary disturbance within the fovea to the typical vitelliform or "egg yoke" lesion located within the central macula (Figure 10–17). This characteristic cyst-like lesion is generally quite round and well demarcated and contains homogeneous opaque yellow material lying at the apparent level of the retinal pigment epithelium. The "egg yoke" may degenerate and be associated with subretinal neovascularization, subretinal hemorrhage, and extensive macular scarring. Visual acuity often remains good, and the electroretinogram is normal; the distinctly abnormal electro-oculogram is the hallmark of this disease.

DISEASES OF THE PERIPHERAL RETINA

RETINAL DETACHMENT

The term "retinal detachment" denotes separation of the sensory retina, ie, the photoreceptors and inner tissue layers, from the underlying retinal pigment epithelium. There are three main types: rhegmatogenous

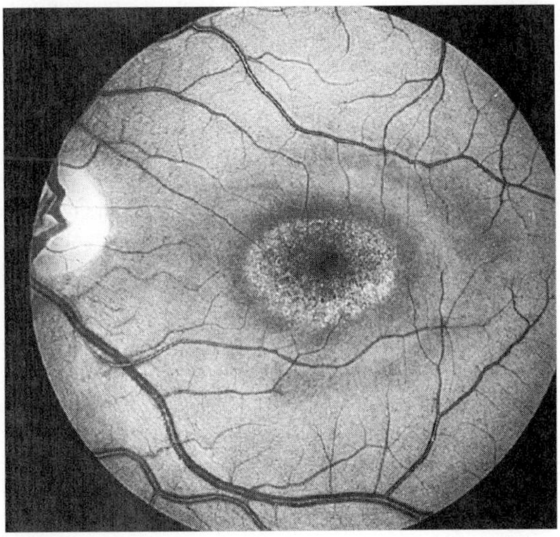

Figure 10–15. Cone dystrophy with depigmentation and a bull's-eye pattern to the macula.

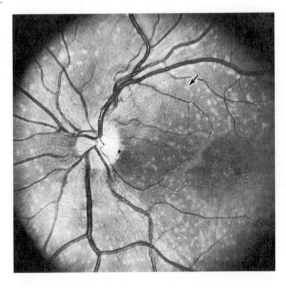

Figure 10–16. Fundus flavimaculatus with multiple irregular fleck lesions (arrow) involving the macula.

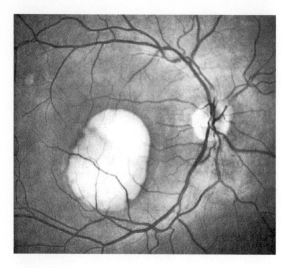

Figure 10–17. Vitelliform dystrophy with a well-demarcated cyst-like macular lesion.

detachment, traction detachment, and serous or hemorrhagic detachment.

1. RHEGMATOGENOUS RETINAL DETACHMENT

The most common of the three major types of retinal detachments is **rhegmatogenous retinal detachment.** The characteristics of a rhegmatogenous detachment are a full-thickness break (a "rhegma") in the sensory retina, variable degrees of vitreous traction, and passage of liquefied vitreous through the sensory retinal defect into the subretinal space. A spontaneous rhegmatogenous retinal detachment is usually preceded or accompanied by a posterior vitreous detachment. Myopia, aphakia, lattice degeneration, and ocular trauma are associated with this type of retinal detachment. Binocular indirect ophthalmoscopy with scleral depression (Figures 2–16 and 2–18) reveals elevation of the translucent detached sensory retina. A careful search usually reveals one or more full-thickness sensory retinal breaks such as a horseshoe tear, round atrophic hole, or anterior circumferential tear (retinal dialysis). The location of retinal breaks varies according to type; horseshoe tears are most common in the superotemporal quadrant, atrophic holes in the temporal quadrants, and retinal dialysis in the inferotemporal quadrant. When multiple retinal breaks are present, the defects are usually within 90 degrees of one another.

Treatment

Scleral buckling or pneumatic retinopexy are the two most popular and effective surgical techniques for the repair of rhegmatogenous retinal detachment. Each procedure requires careful localization of the retinal break and treatment with cryotherapy or laser in order to create an adhesion between the pigment epithelium and the sensory retina. With scleral buckling surgery, the retinal break is mounted on sclera indented by an explant. The scleral indentation can be achieved by a variety of techniques and materials, each of which has inherent advantages and disadvantages. Pneumatic retinopexy involves the intraocular injection of air or an expandable gas in order to tamponade the retinal break while the chorioretinal adhesion forms. An overall reattachment rate of 90% is reported; however, the visual results are dependent on the preoperative status of the macula. If the macula is involved in rhegmatogenous retinal detachment, the likelihood of complete visual recovery is slight.

2. TRACTION RETINAL DETACHMENT

Traction retinal detachment is the second most common type and is most commonly due to proliferative diabetic retinopathy, proliferative vitreoretinopathy, retinopathy of prematurity, or ocular trauma. In contrast to the convex appearance of rhegmatogenous retinal detachment, the typical traction retinal detachment has a more concave surface and is likely to be more localized, usually not extending to the ora serrata. The tractional forces that actively pull the sensory retina away from the underlying pigment epithelium are caused by a clinically apparent vitreal, epiretinal, or subretinal membrane consisting of fibroblasts and of glial and retinal pigment epithelial cells. In diabetic traction retinal detachment, vitreous contraction draws the fibrovascular tissue and underlying retina anteriorly toward the vitreous base. Initially the detachment may be localized along the vascular arcades, but progression may spread to involve the midperipheral retina and the macula. Proliferative vitreoretinopathy is a complication of rhegmatogenous retinal detachment and is the most common cause of failure of surgical repair in these eyes.

The basic pathologic process in eyes with proliferative vitreoretinopathy is growth and contraction of cellular membranes on both sides of the retina and on the posterior vitreous surface. Focal traction from cellular membranes can produce a retinal tear and lead to combined tractional-rhegmatogenous retinal detachment.

Treatment

The primary treatment of traction retinal detachment is vitreoretinal surgery and may involve vitrectomy, membrane removal, scleral buckling, and injection of intraocular gas or silicone oil.

3. SEROUS & HEMORRHAGIC RETINAL DETACHMENT

Serous and hemorrhagic retinal detachment can occur in the absence of either retinal break or vitreoretinal traction. These detachments are the result of a collection of fluid beneath the sensory retina and are caused primarily by diseases of the retinal pigment epithelium and choroid. Degenerative, inflammatory, and infectious diseases limited to the macula, including the multiple causes of subretinal neovascularization, may be associated with this third type of retinal detachment and are described in an earlier section of this chapter. This type of detachment may also be associated with systemic vascular and inflammatory disease as described in Chapters 7 and 15.

RETINOPATHY OF PREMATURITY

Retinopathy of prematurity is a vasoproliferative retinopathy that is the leading cause of childhood blindness in the United States and a major cause of blindness throughout the developed world. An international classification of this disease divides the retina into three zones and characterizes the extent of disease by the number of clock hours involved; the retinal changes are divided into five stages described in Table 10–2.

The demarcation line is a narrow white band that marks the junction of vascular and avascular retina in stage 1; it is the first definite ophthalmoscopic sign of retinopathy of prematurity. As this band increases in height, width, and volume and rises up from the plane of the retina, the ridge of stage 2 is seen. Neovascular proliferation along the posterior aspect of the ridge and extending into the vitreous defines stage 3. Stage 4 is characterized by subtotal retinal detachment, and the clinical sign of stage 5 is a funnel-shaped total retinal detachment.

Treatment

The treatment of retinopathy of prematurity is based on the classification and stage of the disease. It is important to note that a significant number of patients with retinopathy of prematurity undergo spontaneous regression. Peripheral retinal changes of regressed retinopathy of prematurity include avascular retina, peripheral folds, and retinal breaks; associated changes in the posterior pole may include straightening of the temporal vessels, temporal stretching of the macula, and retinal tissue that appears to be dragged over the disk (Figure 10–18). Other ocular findings of regressed retinopathy of prematurity include myopia (which may be asymmetric), strabismus, cataract, and angle-closure glaucoma.

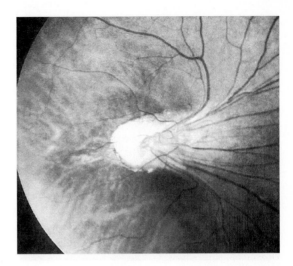

Figure 10–18. Retinopathy of prematurity with stretching of the macula and straightening of retinal vessels.

While stage 1 and stage 2 disease require nothing more than observation, transscleral cryotherapy or laser photocoagulation to the avascular retina should be considered in eyes with stage 3 disease. Vitreoretinal surgery as described above in the section on traction retinal detachment may be appropriate for eyes with stage 4 or stage 5 disease. The etiology and treatment of retinopathy of prematurity as well as the recommended screening protocols are discussed in Chapter 17.

RETINAL DEGENERATIONS

This group of disorders encompasses a number of diseases with various ocular and, in some instances, systemic manifestations. In this section, several specific disorders will be used as prototypes with which to understand the major characteristics of retinal degenerations.

Retinitis Pigmentosa

Retinitis pigmentosa is a group of hereditary retinal degenerations characterized by progressive dysfunction of the photoreceptors and associated with progressive cell loss and eventual atrophy of several retinal layers. The typical form of this disease can be inherited as an autosomal recessive, autosomal dominant, or X-linked recessive trait; one-third of cases will have a negative family history. The hallmark symptoms of retinitis pigmentosa are night blindness (nyctalopia) and gradually progressive peripheral visual field loss. The most characteristic ophthalmoscopic findings are narrowing of the retinal arterioles, mottling of the retinal pigment epithelium, and peripheral retinal pigment clumping, referred to as "bone-spicule formation" (Figure 10–19). While retinitis pigmentosa is a generalized photoreceptor disorder, in most cases

Table 10–2. Stages of retinopathy of prematurity.

Stage	Clinical Findings
1	Demarcation line
2	Intraretinal ridge
3	Ridge with extraretinal fibrovascular proliferation
4	Subtotal retinal detachment
5	Total retinal detachment

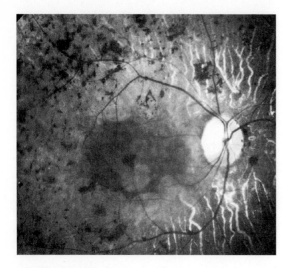

Figure 10–19. Retinitis pigmentosa with arteriolar narrowing and peripheral retinal pigment clumping.

rod function is more severely affected, leading to subjective sensations associated with poor scotopic function. The electroretinogram usually shows either markedly reduced or absent retinal function; the electro-oculogram lacks the usual light rise. The fundus appearance of retinitis pigmentosa may be mimicked by several disorders, including chorioretinitis, trauma, vascular occlusion, and resolved retinal detachment.

The effects of supplemental vitamins on the progression of retinitis pigmentosa require further study before treatment recommendations can be made. Patients with the disease benefit from genetic counseling and appropriate referral to agencies that provide services to the visually impaired.

Leber's Congenital Amaurosis

Leber's congenital amaurosis is a group of disorders characterized by severe visual impairment or blindness from infancy with no discernible cause. The disorders are usually inherited in an autosomal recessive manner and may be associated with mental retardation, seizures, and renal or muscular abnormalities. The ophthalmoscopic findings are variable; most patients show either a normal fundus appearance or only subtle retinal pigment epithelial granularity and mild vessel attenuation. A markedly reduced or absent electroretinogram indicates generalized photoreceptor dysfunction, and in infants this test is the only method by which an absolute diagnosis can be made.

Gyrate Atrophy

Gyrate atrophy is an autosomal recessive disorder caused by reduced activity of ornithine aminotransferase, a mitochondrial matrix enzyme that catalyzes several amino acid pathways. The incidence of this disorder is relatively high in Finland, and the ophthal-

mologic features are the most prominent manifestations of the disease. Patients usually develop nyctalopia within the first decade of life, and progressive peripheral visual field loss follows. Characteristic sharply demarcated circular areas of chorioretinal atrophy develop in the midperiphery of the fundus during the teenage years and become confluent with macular involvement late in the course of the disease. The electroretinogram is decreased or absent, and the electro-oculogram is reduced.

Treatment approaches to this disease have included pyridoxine supplementation, restriction of dietary arginine, and supplemental dietary lysine.

Peripheral Chorioretinal Atrophy

Peripheral chorioretinal atrophy (paving stone degeneration) is a common chorioretinal degeneration found in nearly one-third of adult eyes. Ophthalmoscopically, the lesions appear as isolated or grouped, small, discrete, yellow-white areas with prominent underlying choroidal vessels and pigmented borders. Choroidal vascular insufficiency is thought to be the cause of this benign disorder because the pathologic changes are limited to that portion of the retina supplied by the choriocapillaris. Paving stone degeneration is not of great pathologic significance, though it may be a sign of peripheral vascular disease.

Lattice Degeneration

Lattice degeneration is the most common of the inherited vitreoretinal degenerations, with an estimated incidence of 7% of the general population. Lattice degeneration is more commonly found in myopic eyes and is frequently associated with retinal detachment, occurring in nearly one-third of retinal detachment patients. The ophthalmoscopic appearance may be that of localized round, oval, or linear retinal thinning, with pigmentation, branching white lines, and whitish-yellow flecks; the hallmarks of the disease are the thinned retina punctuated by sharp borders with firm vitreoretinal adhesions at the margins. The mere presence of lattice degeneration is not cause enough for prophylactic therapy. A strong family history of retinal detachments, retinal detachment in the fellow eye, high myopia, and aphakia are risk factors for retinal detachment in eyes with lattice degeneration, and prophylactic treatment with cryosurgery or laser photocoagulation may be warranted.

RETINOSCHISIS

Degenerative retinoschisis, unlike X-linked juvenile retinoschisis described above, is a common acquired peripheral retinal disorder that is believed to develop from preexisting peripheral cystoid degeneration. The cystic changes of peripheral cystoid degeneration are seen to some degree in virtually all adults. This cystoid degeneration is characterized by intraretinal microcysts that often coalesce, giving the appearance of lobulated, irregularly branching, tortuous channels. Peripheral cystoid degeneration may develop into either of two degenerative forms of retinoschisis, each of which is characterized by sharply demarcated and absolute visual field defects.

Typical degenerative retinoschisis occurs in 1% of adults and is a bilateral disease in one-third of affected patients. On clinical examination, the disorder appears as a round or ovoid area of retinal splitting with fusiform elevation of the inner layer and an optically empty schisis cavity. The retinal splitting occurs at the outer plexiform layer. Complications such as hole formation and marked posterior extension are very uncommon and rarely require treatment.

Reticular degenerative retinoschisis is characterized by round or oval areas of retinal splitting in which a bullous elevation of an extremely thin inner layer occurs, most commonly in the lower temporal quadrant. In this form of the disease, the splitting usually occurs in the nerve fiber layer, and typical peripheral cystoid degeneration is usually present anterior to the lesion. When retinal breaks are present in both the inner and the outer layers, progressive rhegmatogenous retinal detachment may develop and threaten the macula, thus requiring treatment.

RETINAL VASCULAR DISEASES

DIABETIC RETINOPATHY

Diabetic retinopathy is one of the leading causes of blindness in the Western world. The view that chronic hyperglycemia of diabetes mellitus is the major determinant of diabetic retinopathy is supported by the observation that retinopathy in young people with type I (insulin-dependent) diabetes does not occur for at least 3–5 years after the onset of this systemic disease. Similar results have been obtained for type II (non-insulin-dependent) diabetes, but in such patients the time of onset and therefore the duration of disease are more difficult to determine precisely. It is recommended that patients with type I diabetes mellitus be referred for ophthalmologic examination within 3 years after diagnosis and reexamined on at least an annual basis. Type II diabetic patients should be referred for ophthalmologic examination at the time of diagnosis and reexamined at least annually. As diabetic retinopathy can become particularly aggressive during pregnancy, any diabetic woman who becomes pregnant should be examined by an ophthalmologist in the first trimester and at least every 3 months thereafter until parturition.

In terms of both prognosis and treatment, it is useful to divide diabetic retinopathy into nonproliferative and proliferative categories. The prevalence of proliferative retinopathy in type I diabetics with 15 years of systemic disease is 50%. While the prevalence of proliferative disease at 15 years is much less in type II diabetics, the prevalence of macular edema as a function of the duration of systemic disease is the same in both groups.

1. NONPROLIFERATIVE DIABETIC RETINOPATHY

Diabetic retinopathy is a progressive microangiopathy characterized by small vessel damage and occlusion. The earliest pathologic changes are thickening of the capillary endothelial basement membrane and reduction of the number of pericytes. **Background diabetic retinopathy** is a clinical reflection of the hyperpermeability and incompetence of involved vessels. The capillaries develop tiny dot-like outpouchings called microaneurysms, while the retinal veins become dilated and tortuous (Figure 10–20).

Multiple hemorrhages may appear throughout different levels of the retina. Flame-shaped hemorrhages are so shaped because of their location within the horizontally oriented nerve fiber layer, while dot and blot hemorrhages are in the deeper retina, where cells and axons are vertically oriented.

Macular edema is the most frequent cause of visual loss among patients with background diabetic retinopathy. The edema is caused primarily by a breakdown of the inner blood-retinal barrier at the level of the retinal capillary endothelium, allowing leakage of fluid and plasma constituents into the surrounding retina. The edema may be focal or diffuse and appears clinically as thickened, cloudy retina with associated microaneurysms and intraretinal exudate. Circinate zones of

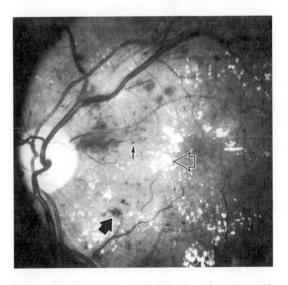

Figure 10–20. Background diabetic retinopathy with abundant macular exudate (open arrow), microaneurysms (small arrow), and intraretinal hemorrhage (large arrow).

yellow, lipid-rich exudate may form around clusters of microaneurysms and are most frequently centered in the temporal portion of the macula. While the prevalence of macular edema is 10% in the diabetic population as a whole, there is a dramatic increase in prevalence in eyes with more severe retinopathy.

With progressive microvascular occlusion, signs of increasing ischemia may be superimposed on the picture of background retinopathy and produce the clinical picture of **preproliferative diabetic retinopathy.** The most typical findings here are multiple cotton-wool spots, beading of the retinal veins, and irregular segmental dilation of the retinal capillary bed (intraretinal microvascular abnormalities). Closure of retinal capillaries surrounding the foveal avascular zone may cause significant ischemia, manifest clinically by the presence of large dark retinal hemorrhages and small thread-like macular arterioles. Eyes with macular edema and significant ischemia have a poorer visual prognosis—with or without laser treatment—than eyes with edema and relatively good perfusion.

The visual and electrophysiologic dysfunctions associated with diabetes probably result from the local vascular abnormalities and the systemic metabolic effects of the disease to which the retina is subjected. A characteristic blue-yellow color vision abnormality develops, and hue discrimination may be impaired. Contrast sensitivity may be reduced in patients, even in the presence of normal visual acuity. Visual field testing may show relative scotomas corresponding to areas of retinal edema and nonperfusion, and abnormalities in dark adaptation have also been described. Electroretinographic abnormalities bear a relationship to the severity of retinopathy and may aid in predicting progression of retinopathy. Fluorescein angiography is invaluable in defining the microvascular abnormalities of diabetic retinopathy (Figures 10–21 and 10–22). Large filling defects of capillary beds—"capillary nonperfusion"—show the extent of retinal ischemia (Figure 10–23) and are usually most prominent in the midperiphery. The fluorescein leakage associated with retinal edema may assume the petaloid configuration of cystoid macular edema or may be diffuse. Other fluorescein abnormalities include vascular loops and intraretinal shunts. The focus of treatment in patients with nonproliferative diabetic retinopathy and no macular edema is treatment of hyperglycemia and intercurrent systemic disease. A controlled clinical trial has shown that aldose reductase inhibitor therapy does not prevent progression of diabetic retinopathy. Focal argon laser treatment of discrete points of retinal leakage in patients with clinically significant macular edema, principally defined as thickening of the retina at or within 500 μm of the center of the macula, reduces the risk of visual loss and increases the likelihood of visual improvement (see Chapter 24). Eyes with diabetic macular edema that is not clinically significant should usually be monitored closely without laser treatment. Since macular edema may be present

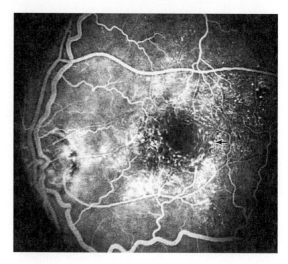

Figure 10–21. Fluorescein angiogram in nonproliferative diabetic retinopathy shows microaneurysms (arrow) and perifoveal retinal vascular changes.

with little or no change in visual acuity and requires slitlamp biomicroscopic retinal examination for full evaluation, primary health care providers should recognize the importance of prompt and early referral of diabetic patients to the ophthalmologist.

2. PROLIFERATIVE DIABETIC RETINOPATHY

The most severe ocular complications of diabetes mellitus are associated with proliferative diabetic retinopathy. Progressive retinal ischemia eventually

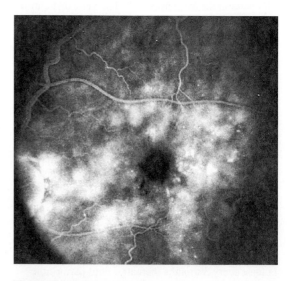

Figure 10–22. Late phase fluorescein angiogram shows hyperfluorescence typical of noncystoid diabetic macular edema.

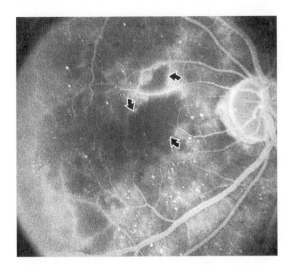

Figure 10–23. Fluorescein angiogram shows hypofluorescence from capillary drop-out (arrows) typical of ischemic diabetic maculopathy.

stimulates the formation of delicate new vessels that leak serum proteins (and fluorescein) profusely. Neovascularization is frequently located on the surface of the disk and at the posterior edge of the peripheral zones of "nonperfusion" (Figures 10–24 and 10–25). Iris neovascularization, or rubeosis iridis, can also result.

The fragile new vessels proliferate onto the posterior face of the vitreous and become elevated once the vitreous starts to contract away from the retina. If the vessels bleed (Figure 10–26), massive vitreous hemorrhage may cause sudden visual loss. Eyes in which

posterior vitreous detachment is complete are at less risk of developing neovascularization and vitreous hemorrhage. In eyes with proliferative diabetic retinopathy and persistent vitreoretinal adhesions, elevated neovascular fronds may undergo fibrous change and form tight fibrovascular bands that tug on the retina and exert continued vitreous contraction. This can cause either a progressive traction retinal detachment or, if a retinal tear is produced, rhegmatogenous retinal detachment. The retinal detachment may be heralded or concealed by vitreous hemorrhage. When vitreous contraction is complete in these eyes, proliferative retinopathy tends to enter the burned-out or "involutional" stage.

Treatment

Argon laser panretinal photocoagulation is usually indicated in proliferative diabetic retinopathy. Patients at greatest risk of significant visual loss are those with preretinal or vitreous hemorrhage or neovascularization of the disk. Panretinal photocoagulation can significantly reduce the chance of massive vitreous hemorrhage and retinal detachment in these patients by causing the regression and, in some cases, the disappearance of new vessels. The technique involves scattering up to several thousand regularly spaced laser burns throughout the retina, sparing the central region bordered by the disk and the major temporal vascular arcades (Chapter 24). Although the mechanism is not precisely understood, panretinal photocoagulation presumably works by reducing the angiogenic stimulus from ischemic retina.

The role of vitreoretinal surgery in proliferative diabetic eye disease continues to evolve. Conservative management of monocular vision impairing diabetic

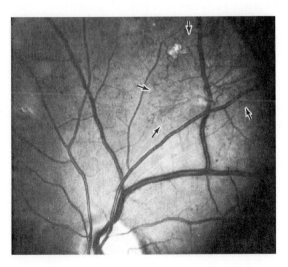

Figure 10–24. A frond of neovascular tissue (arrows) is seen along the superotemporal vascular arcade in this eye with proliferative diabetic retinopathy.

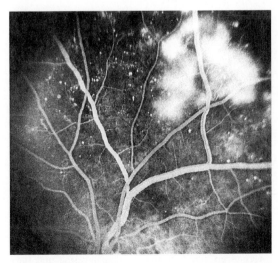

Figure 10–25. Fluorescein angiogram of proliferative diabetic retinopathy shows leakage from the neovascular tissue. The pinpoint areas of hyperfluorescence are microaneurysms.

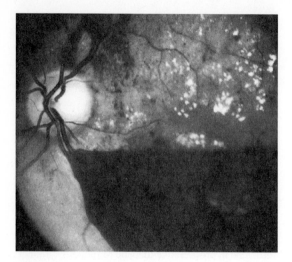

Figure 10–26. Proliferative diabetic retinopathy with pre-retinal hemorrhage obscuring the inferior macula. Macular exudate, microaneurysms, and intraretinal hemorrhages are also present.

vitreous hemorrhage in the binocular patient had been to allow spontaneous resolution over the course of several months. The results of a 4-year study designed to assess the role of early vitrectomy for severe vitreous hemorrhage and proliferative diabetic retinopathy support this surgery as a means by which good vision may be restored or maintained. The role of vitreoretinal surgery in the treatment of diabetic traction retinal detachment is described elsewhere in this chapter.

CENTRAL RETINAL ARTERY OCCLUSION

The patient with central retinal artery occlusion routinely relates a history of painless catastrophic visual loss occurring over a period of seconds; antecedent transient visual loss (amaurosis fugax) may be reported. The visual acuity ranges between counting fingers and light perception in 90% of eyes at the time of initial examination. An afferent pupillary defect can appear within seconds after retinal arterial obstruction, preceding the fundus abnormalities by an hour.

Ophthalmoscopically, the superficial retina becomes opacified except in the foveola, where a cherry-red spot is evident (Figure 10–27). The cherry-red spot is pigment of the choroid and retinal pigment epithelium viewed through the extremely thin overlying foveolar retina and contrasted with the thicker and translucent perifoveolar retina. Twenty-five percent of eyes with central retinal artery occlusion have cilioretinal arteries that spare macular retina and may preserve some central visual acuity. Clinically, the retinal opacification resolves within 4–6 weeks, leaving a pale optic disk as the major ocular finding. In older patients, giant cell arteritis must be excluded

and if necessary treated immediately with high doses of systemic corticosteroids. Other causes of central retinal artery occlusion are arteriosclerosis and emboli from carotid or cardiac sources. These are discussed further in Chapter 15.

Treatment

Because irreversible retinal damage has been shown to occur after 90 minutes of complete central retinal artery occlusion in the subhuman primate model, precious little time is available in which to begin therapy. Anterior chamber paracentesis can be employed in order to decrease intraocular pressure and increase retinal perfusion. This is particularly indicated in embolic central retinal artery occlusion. Intravenous acetazolamide has been used to decrease intraocular pressure, and an inhaled oxygen-carbon dioxide mixture has been employed to induce retinal vasodilation and increase the PO_2 at the retinal surface. Direct infusion of a thrombolytic agent into the ophthalmic artery can result in recovery of vision. It must be performed within 8 hours after onset of the central retinal artery occlusion, requires specific radiologic expertise, and there is a risk of cerebral infarction. Systemic anticoagulants are generally not employed.

BRANCH RETINAL ARTERY OCCLUSION

Branch retinal artery occlusion usually presents with sudden loss of visual field and with reduction in visual acuity if the fovea is involved. Fundus signs of retinal edema with associated cotton-wool spots are limited to the area of retina supplied by the occluded vessel. Embolic causes are proportionately more com-

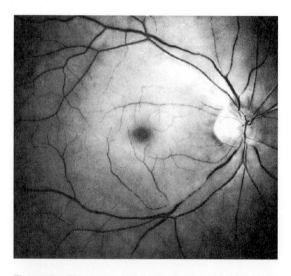

Figure 10–27. Acute central retinal artery occlusion with opaque white retina and attenuated vessels. (Courtesy of University of California, San Francisco.)

mon than in central retinal artery occlusion, and emboli are frequently identified on clinical examination (see Chapter 15). Migraine, oral contraceptive use, and vasculitis must also be considered.

CENTRAL RETINAL VEIN OCCLUSION

Central retinal vein occlusion is a common and easily diagnosed retinal vascular disorder with potentially blinding complications. The patient presents with sudden painless loss of vision. The clinical appearance varies from a few small scattered retinal hemorrhages and cotton-wool spots (Figure 10–28) to a marked hemorrhagic appearance with both deep and superficial retinal hemorrhage, which may rarely break through into the vitreous cavity. Most patients who develop the disease are over 50 years of age, and more than half have associated cardiovascular disease. Predisposing factors and their investigation are discussed in Chapter 15. Chronic open-angle glaucoma should always be excluded (see Chapter 11).

The two major complications associated with central retinal vein occlusion are reduced vision from macular edema and neovascular glaucoma secondary to iris neovascularization. Macular dysfunction occurs in almost all eyes with central vein occlusion. Although some eyes will show spontaneous improvement, most eyes will have persistent decreased central vision as a result of chronic macular edema. Nearly one-third of eyes with central retinal vein occlusion show significant retinal capillary nonperfusion on fluorescein angiography; one-half of these eyes will develop neovascular glaucoma.

Treatment

Careful follow-up evaluation is warranted, and prompt panretinal laser photocoagulation is recommended for eyes that develop anterior segment neovascularization. No treatment for macular edema, including grid pattern photocoagulation, has proved effective to date.

BRANCH RETINAL VEIN OCCLUSION

Branch retinal vein occlusion presents as sudden unilateral vision loss with segmentally distributed intraretinal hemorrhage. The vein occlusion always occurs at the site of an arteriovenous crossing (Figure 10–29), and retinal neovascularization may develop if the occlusion produces an area of retinal capillary nonperfusion that is more than 5 disk diameters in area. Sight-threatening complications of the disease are macular edema, macular ischemia, and vitreous hemorrhage from retinal neovascularization.

Treatment

Once peripheral retinal neovascularization has developed, sectoral laser retinal photocoagulation to the area of ischemic retina reduces the risk of vitreous hemorrhage by one-half. When vision loss due to macular edema persists for several months without spontaneous improvement, grid pattern argon laser macular photocoagulation may be indicated. Anticoagulant therapy has not been shown to be beneficial in either the prevention or the management of branch retinal vein occlusion. Investigation for an underlying systemic cause is discussed in Chapter 15. Important as-

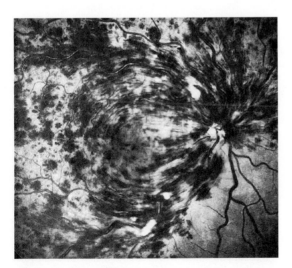

Figure 10–28. Central retinal vein occlusion with extensive superficial retinal hemorrhage obscuring macular and optic nerve detail.

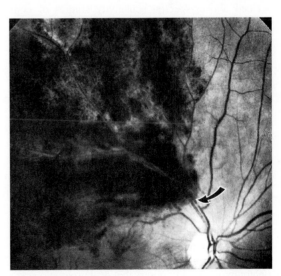

Figure 10–29. Branch retinal vein occlusion involves the superotemporal vein. The point of obstruction (arrow) is at an arteriovenous crossing.

sociated ocular diseases are chronic open-angle glaucoma and uveitis secondary to Behçet's syndrome.

RETINAL ARTERIAL MACROANEURYSM

Retinal macroaneurysms are fusiform or round dilations of the retinal arterioles occurring within the first three orders of arteriolar bifurcation. Most cases are unilateral, and the superotemporal artery is the most commonly involved vessel. Two-thirds of patients have associated systemic arterial hypertension.

The most common clinical symptom is loss of central vision as a result of retinal edema, exudation, or hemorrhage. Macroaneurysms may bleed into the subretinal space, into the retina, beneath the internal limiting membrane, or into the vitreous; the "hourglass" hemorrhage is typical and is due to bleeding beneath and anterior to the retina.

Although no clear indication for treatment with laser photocoagulation has been established, laser treatment of the macroaneurysm should be considered if lipid exudate coming from it threatens the fovea.

COLOR VISION DEFECTS

The perception of color is a cortical response to specific physical stimuli received by the retina. A narrow band of the electromagnetic spectrum, wavelengths between 400 and 700 nm, is capable of being absorbed by visual pigments contained in the outer segments of human cone photoreceptors. As described above, spectral sensitivity studies of cone photopigments have identified blue, green, and red cone photoreceptors. A minimal requirement for color discrimination is the presence of at least two kinds of cone photopigment, and normal color vision requires the presence of all three. Color vision testing is described in Chapter 2. In a broad sense, color vision defects are either congenital or acquired. While hereditary congenital color defects are almost always "red-green," affecting 8% of males and 0.5 % of females, acquired defects are more often of the "blue-yellow"variety and affect males and females equally. Congenital color vision defects affect both eyes equally, while acquired color defects frequently affect one eye more than the other. Most congenital color vision defects are X-linked recessive and are constant in type and severity throughout life. Acquired color vision defects generally vary in type and severity, depending upon the location and source of the usually ophthalmoscopically observable ocular pathology.

Dichromats are individuals whose cone photoreceptors contain only two of the three cone photopigments. Persons with a red-green color deficiency re-

lated to red-sensitive pigment loss were historically described first, and the condition is therefore referred to as **protanopia.** A second type of red-green deficiency involving green-sensitive pigment loss is known as **deuteranopia.** Blue-yellow color blindness is the third form and is referred to as **tritanopia.** While a color vision defect is present, there is no acuity loss in these patients.

Based on a color matching classification, the most common color vision deficit is that of **anomalous trichromats.** These individuals require three primaries for matching an unknown color but—unlike normal **trichromats**—use them in "anomalous" amounts. Each of the anomalous trichromats has a defect analogous to that of the dichromats described above.

There are two forms of monochromatism, and although both leave the affected individual completely without color discrimination, they are two quite separate entities. In **rod monochromatism,** the individual is born without functioning cones in the retina, and such a loss accounts for the associated symptoms of low visual acuity, absent color vision, photophobia, and nystagmus. The generalized loss of cones in this condition is shown unequivocally by the photopic electroretinogram. In **cone monochromatism,** affected individuals with this extremely rare condition have no hue discrimination but do have normal acuity and no photophobia or nystagmus. Cone monochromats do have cone photoreceptors, but all the cones contain the same visual pigment.

II. TUMORS OF THE RETINA

J. Brooks Crawford, MD

PRIMARY BENIGN INTRAOCULAR TUMORS

Retinal Angioma*

Retinal hemangiomas occur as isolated tumors or associated with cerebellar hemangioblastomas, pancreatic cysts and carcinomas, renal cysts and carcinomas, and pheochromocytomas in von Hippel-Lindau syndrome (Figure 10–30). The retinal tumors are pink or red, endophytic, and usually supplied by a large feeder vessel. Juxtapapillary tumors are usually exophytic. Vision is affected by bleeding or exudation from the tumor vessels. Photocoagulation, diathermy, and cryotherapy are used to treat the retinal lesions.

Astrocytic (Glial) Hamartomas

Astrocytic hamartomas are translucent to whitish retinal and optic nerve head tumors most frequently associated with tuberous sclerosis (Bourneville's dis-

---

* See also Retinocerebellar Angiomatosis in Chapter 14.

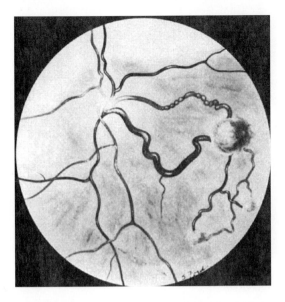

Figure 10–30. Angiomatosis retinae of Von Hippel-Lindau disease (drawing). (Courtesy of F Cordes.)

ease) (Figure 10–31). They may also be associated with neurofibromatosis-1 and -2 or may occur as isolated findings. These tumors are congenital. They may grow slowly and, as they mature, become calcified, acquiring a mulberry configuration.

PRIMARY MALIGNANT TUMORS OF THE RETINA

Retinoblastoma (Figure 10–32)

Retinoblastoma is a rare but life-endangering tumor of childhood. Two-thirds of cases appear before the end of the third year; rare cases have been reported at

almost every age. Bilateral disease occurs in about 30% of cases. This is generally a sign of heritable disease, but up to one-third of heritable cases have purely unilateral disease. An allele within chromosomal band 13q14 controls both the heritable and nonheritable forms of the tumor. The normal retinoblastoma gene, present in every individual, is a suppressor gene or anti-oncogene. Individuals with the heritable form of the disease have one altered allele in every cell of the body; when the other allele in a developing retinal cell is affected by a spontaneous mutation, the tumor develops. In the nonheritable form of the disease, both alleles of the normal retinoblastoma gene in a developing retinal cell are inactivated by spontaneous mutation. Survivors of the heritable form of the disease (those 5% of new cases who had an affected parent or those who have had a germinal mutation) have almost a 50% chance of producing an affected child.

Retinoblastomas may exhibit outward (exophytic) or inward (endophytic) growth—either or both. The latter then extend into the vitreous (Figure 10–33). Both types gradually fill the eye and extend through the optic nerve to the brain and, less commonly, along the emissary vessels and nerves in the sclera to the orbital tissues. Occasionally, they grow diffusely in the retina, discharging malignant cells into the vitreous or anterior chamber, thereby producing a pseudoinflammatory process and mimicking retinitis, vitritis, uveitis, or endophthalmitis. Microscopically, most retinoblastomas are composed of small, closely packed, round or polygonal cells with large, darkly staining nuclei and scanty cytoplasm. They sometimes form characteristic Flexner-Wintersteiner rosettes, which are indicative of photoreceptor differentiation. Degenerative changes are frequent, accompanied by necrosis and calcification. A few will spontaneously resolve.

Retinoblastoma usually remains unnoticed until it has advanced far enough to produce a white pupil (leukocoria), strabismus, or inflammation. All children with strabismus or intraocular inflammation should be evaluated for the presence of retinoblastoma. The tumor is usually seen in the early stages only when sought for, as in children having a heredi-

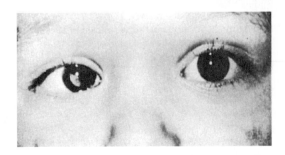

Figure 10–32. Retinoblastoma as viewed through the pupil.

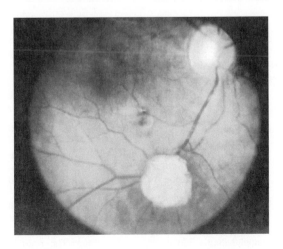

Figure 10–31. Retinal astrocytic hamartoma.

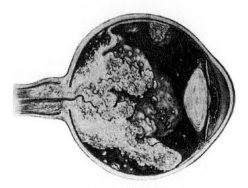

Figure 10–33. Endophytic retinoblastoma.

tary background or in cases where the other eye has been affected.

Retrolental fibroplasia, persistence of the primary vitreous, retinal dysplasia, Coats' disease, and nematode endophthalmitis may simulate retinoblastoma.

In general, the earlier the discovery and treatment of the tumor, the better the chance to prevent spread through the optic nerve and orbital tissues.

Enucleation is the treatment of choice for large retinoblastomas. Eyes with smaller tumors can be effectively treated with plaque or external beam radiotherapy (Figure 10–34), cryotherapy, or photocoagulation. Chemotherapy is being used to reduce the size of large tumors prior to other types of therapy and occasionally as the sole form of therapy. It is also used to treat tumors that have extended into the brain, orbit, or distally and may be used after enucleation in patients at high risk for such widespread disease.

Second primary malignant tumors, especially osteosarcomas, develop in a large number (estimates range from 20% to 90%) of survivors of the heritable form of retinoblastomas after a period of many years.

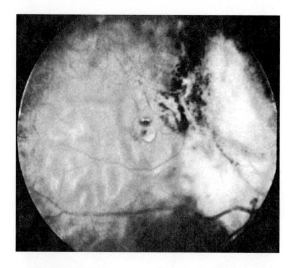

Figure 10–34. Retinoblastoma after radiotherapy.

These patients need to be carefully evaluated for the remainder of their lives.

LYMPHOMA

Intraocular lymphomas rarely occur in association with systemic lymphomas but are not uncommon as primary tumors, most often involving the retina and vitreous. They were formerly called ocular reticulum cell sarcomas but are now considered to be large cell lymphomas. They often mimic retinitis, vitritis, or uveitis; therefore, it is important to consider this tumor in the differential diagnosis of unexplained intraocular inflammation in an older patient.

Central nervous system involvement is the usual cause of death. Radiation plus chemotherapy is the treatment of choice and prolongs survival.

REFERENCES

RETINA & RETINAL DISORDERS

Axer-Siegel R et al: Diabetic retinopathy during pregnancy. Ophthalmology 1996;103:1815.

Bird AC: Retinal photoreceptor dystrophies. Am J Ophthalmol 1995:119:543.

Bird AC et al: An international classification and grading system for age-related maculopathy and age-related macular degeneration. Surv Ophthalmol 1995;39:567.

Bressler NM: Submacular surgery. Arch Ophthalmol 1997;115:1071.

Bressler NM, Bressler SB: Preventative ophthalmology: Age-related macular degeneration. Ophthalmology 1995;102:1206.

Cardillo JA et al: Post-traumatic proliferative vitreoretinopathy. Ophthalmology 1997:104:1166.

Central Vein Occlusion Study Group: Natural history and clinical management of central retinal vein occlusion. Arch Ophthalmol 1997;115:486.

Christensen WG et al: A prospective study of cigarette smoking and risk of age-related macular degeneration in women. JAMA 1996;276:1147.

Cryotherapy for Retinopathy of Prematurity Cooperative Group: Early retinal vessel development and iris vessel dilatation as factors in retinopathy of prematurity. Arch Ophthalmol 1996:114:150.

Cunningham ET et al: Acute multifocal retinitis. Am J Ophthalmol 1997:123:347.

Diabetes Control and Complications Trial: The effect of intensive treatment on long-term complications in insulin-dependent diabetes mellitus. N Engl J Med 1993:329:977.

Early Treatment Diabetic Retinopathy Study Research Group: Focal photocoagulation treatment of diabetic macular edema. Arch Ophthalmol 1995:113:1144.

Endophthalmitis Vitrectomy Study Group: The endophthalmitis vitrectomy study. Ophthalmology 1997:104:261.

EURODIAB IDDM complications Study Group: Retinopathy and vision loss in insulin-dependent diabetes in Europe. Ophthalmology 1997:104:252.

Eye Disease Case-control Study Group: Risk factors for branch retinal vein occlusion. Am J Ophthalmol 1993:116:286.

Freeman WR: Vitrectomy surgery for full-thickness macular holes. Am J Ophthalmol 1993:116:233.

Gass JDM: *Stereoscopic Atlas of Macular Diseases,* 4th ed. 2 vols. Mosby, 1997.

Glacet-Bernard A et al: Prognostic factors for retinal vein occlusion. Ophthalmology 1996;103:551.

Guymer RH et al: Laser treatment in subjects with high-risk clinical features of age-related macular degeneration: Posterior pole appearance and retinal function. Arch Ophthalmol 1997;115:595.

Hart PM et al: Teletherapy for subfoveal choroidal neovascularisation of age-related macular degeneration: Results of follow up in a non-randomised study. Br J Ophthalmol 1996;80:1046.

Hayreh SS et al: Incidence of various types of retinal vein occlusion. Am J Ophthalmol 1994:117:429.

Hilton GF et al: *Retinal Detachment,* 2nd ed. American Academy of Ophthalmology, 1995.

Jampol LM et al: Peripheral proliferative retinopathies. Surv Ophthalmol 1994:38:519.

Klein R et al: Incidence of retinopathy and associated risk factors in insulin-dependent diabetes. Arch Ophthalmol 1997:115:351.

Macular Photocoagulation Study Group: Laser photocoagulation for juxtafoveal choroidal neovascularization. Arch Ophthalmol 1994:112:500.

Martin DF et al: Treatment and pathogenesis of traumatic chorioretinal rupture. Am J Ophthalmol 1994:117:190.

Moss SE et al: Ocular factors in the incidence and progression of diabetic retinopathy. Ophthalmology 1994: 101:77.

Ryan SJ (editor): *Retina,* 2nd ed. 3 vols. Mosby, 1994.

Schaffer DB et al: Prognostic factors in the natural course of retinopathy of prematurity. Ophthalmology 1993;100: 230.

Seddon JM et al: A prospective study of cigarette smoking and age-related macular degeneration in women. JAMA 1996;276:1141.

Silicone Study Group: Vitrectomy with silicone oil for severe proliferative vitreoretinopathy. Arch Ophthalmol 1997:115:335.

Stevens TS et al: Occult choroidal neovascularization in age-related macular degeneration. Arch Ophthalmol 1997:115:345.

Vitrectomy for Treatment of Macular Hole Study Group: Vitrectomy for the treatment of stage 3 or 4 macular holes. Arch Ophthalmol 1997:115:11.

West S et al: Are antioxidants or supplements protective for age-related macular degeneration? Arch Ophthalmol 1994:112:222.

TUMORS OF THE RETINA

Char DH: *Clinical Ocular Oncology,* 2nd ed. Lippincott-Raven, 1997.

Ferris FL, Chew EY: A new era for the treatment of retinoblastoma. Arch Ophthalmol 1996;114:1412.

Gallie BL, Phillips RA: Retinoblastoma: A model of oncogenesis. Ophthalmology 1993;100:666.

Murphree AL et al: Chemotherapy plus local treatment in the management of intraocular retinoblastoma. Arch Ophthalmol 1996;114:1348.

Shields CL et al: Plaque radiotherapy in the management of retinoblastomas: Use as a primary and secondary treatment. Ophthalmology 1993;100:216.

Spencer WH (editor): *Ophthalmic Pathology,* 4th ed. 4 vols. Saunders, 1996.

11

Glaucoma

Daniel Vaughan, MD, & Paul Riordan-Eva, FRCS, FRCOphth

Glaucoma is characterized by elevated intraocular pressure associated with optic disk cupping and visual field loss. In the majority of cases, there is no associated ocular disease (primary glaucoma) (Table 11–1).

Approximately 20,000 Americans are blind from glaucoma, making it the leading cause of preventable blindness in the United States. An estimated 2 million Americans have glaucoma. Primary open-angle glaucoma, the most common form, causes insidious asymptomatic progressive bilateral visual loss that is often not detected until extensive field loss has already occurred. Other forms of glaucoma are responsible for severe visual morbidity in individuals of all ages. Acute (angle-closure) glaucoma comprises 10–15% of cases in Caucasians. This percentage is much higher in Asians, particularly among the Burmese and Vietnamese in Southeast Asia.

The mechanism of raised intraocular pressure in glaucoma is impaired outflow of aqueous resulting from abnormalities within the drainage system of the anterior chamber angle (open-angle glaucoma) or impaired access of aqueous to the drainage system (closed-angle glaucoma) (Table 11–2). Treatment is directed toward reducing the intraocular pressure and, when possible, correcting the underlying cause.

Reducing aqueous production is a method of reducing intraocular pressure used in all forms of glaucoma. Several medications reduce aqueous production. Surgical procedures that reduce aqueous production are available but are generally used only after medical treatment has failed. Facilitating flow of aqueous through the trabecular meshwork is useful in open-angle glaucoma. Improving access of aqueous to the anterior chamber angle in closed-angle glaucoma may be achieved by peripheral laser iridotomy or surgical iridectomy if the cause is pupillary block, miosis if there is angle crowding, or cycloplegia if there is anterior lens displacement. Surgically bypassing the drainage system is useful in open-angle glaucoma and in angle closure that fails to respond to medical treatment. In the secondary glaucomas, consideration must always be given to treating the primary abnormality.

In all patients with glaucoma, the necessity for treatment and its effectiveness are assessed by regular determination of intraocular pressure (tonometry), inspection of optic disks, and measurement of visual fields.

The management of glaucoma is best left to the ophthalmologist, but the magnitude of the problem and the importance of detecting asymptomatic cases call for the cooperation and assistance of all medical personnel. Ophthalmoscopy (noting optic nerve changes) and tonometry should be part of the routine ophthalmologic examination of all patients old enough to cooperate and certainly all patients over 30 years of age. This is especially important in patients with a family history of glaucoma.

PHYSIOLOGY OF AQUEOUS HUMOR

The intraocular pressure is determined by the rate of aqueous production and the resistance to outflow of aqueous from the eye. Some knowledge of the physiology of aqueous humor is necessary for understanding glaucoma.

Composition of Aqueous

The aqueous is a clear liquid that fills the anterior and posterior chambers of the eye. Its volume is about 250 μL, and its rate of production, which is subject to diurnal variation, is about 2.5 μL/min. The osmotic pressure is slightly higher than that of plasma. The composition of aqueous is similar to that of plasma except for much higher concentrations of ascorbate, pyruvate, and lactate and lower concentrations of protein, urea, and glucose.

Formation & Flow of Aqueous

Aqueous is produced by the ciliary body. An ultrafiltrate of plasma produced in the stroma of the ciliary processes is modified by the barrier function and secretory processes of the ciliary epithelium. Entering the posterior chamber, the aqueous passes through the pupil into the anterior chamber (Figure 11–1) and

Table 11–1. Glaucoma classified according to etiology.

A. Primary glaucoma
1. Open-angle glaucoma
   a. Primary open-angle glaucoma (chronic open-angle glaucoma, chronic simple glaucoma)
   b. Normal-pressure glaucoma (low-pressure glaucoma)
2. Angle-closure glaucoma
   a. Acute
   b. Subacute
   c. Chronic
   d. Plateau iris
B. Congenital glaucoma
1. Primary congenital glaucoma
2. Glaucoma associated with other developmental ocular abnormalities
   a. Anterior chamber cleavage syndromes
      Axenfeld's syndrome
      Rieger's syndrome
      Peter's anomaly
   b. Aniridia
3. Glaucoma associated with extraocular developmental abnormalities
   a. Sturge-Weber syndrome
   b. Marfan's syndrome
   c. Neurofibromatosis
   d. Lowe's syndrome
   e. Congenital rubella
C. Secondary glaucoma
1. Pigmentary glaucoma
2. Exfoliation syndrome
3. Due to lens changes (phacogenic)
   a. Dislocation
   b. Intumescence
   c. Phacolytic
4. Due to uveal tract changes
   a. Uveitis
   b. Posterior synechiae (seclusio pupillae)
   c. Tumor
5. Iridocorneoendothelial (ICE) syndrome
6. Trauma
   a. Hyphema
   b. Angle contusion/recession
   c. Peripheral anterior synechiae
7. Postoperative
   a. Ciliary block glaucoma (malignant glaucoma)
   b. Peripheral anterior synechiae
   c. Epithelial downgrowth
   d. Following corneal graft surgery
   e. Following retinal detachment surgery
8. Neovascular glaucoma
   a. Diabetes mellitus
   b. Central retinal vein occlusion
   c. Intraocular tumor
9. Raised episcleral venous pressure
   a. Carotid-cavernous fistula
   b. Sturge-Weber syndrome
10. Steroid-induced
D. Absolute glaucoma: The end result of any uncontrolled glaucoma is a hard, sightless, and often painful eye.

Table 11–2. Glaucoma classified according to mechanism of intraocular pressure rise.

A. Open-angle glaucoma
1. Pretrabecular membranes: All of these may progress to angle-closure glaucoma due to contraction of the pretrabecular membranes.
   a. Neovascular glaucoma
   b. Epithelial downgrowth
   c. ICE syndrome
2. Trabecular abnormalities
   a. Primary open-angle glaucoma
   b. Congenital glaucoma
   c. Pigmentary glaucoma
   d. Exfoliation syndrome
   e. Steroid-induced glaucoma
   f. Hyphema
   g. Angle contusion or recession
   h. Iridocyclitis (uveitis)
   i. Phacolytic glaucoma
3. Posttrabecular abnormalities
   a. Raised episcleral venous pressure
B. Closed-angle glaucoma
1. Pupillary block (iris bombé)
   a. Primary angle-closure glaucoma
   b. Seclusio pupillae (posterior synechiae)
   c. Intumescent lens
   d. Anterior lens dislocation
   e. Hyphema
2. Anterior lens displacement
   a. Ciliary block glaucoma
   b. Central retinal vein occlusion
   c. Posterior scleritis
   d. Following retinal detachment surgery
3. Angle crowding
   a. Plateau iris
   b. Intumescent lens
   c. Mydriasis for fundal examination
4. Peripheral anterior synechiae
   a. Chronic angle closure
   b. Secondary to flat anterior chamber
   c. Secondary to iris bombé
   d. Contraction of pretrabecular membranes

Outflow of Aqueous

The trabecular meshwork is composed of beams of collagen and elastic tissue covered by trabecular cells that form a filter with a decreasing pore size as the canal of Schlemm is approached. Contraction of the ciliary muscle through its insertion into the trabecular meshwork increases pore size in the meshwork and hence the rate of aqueous drainage. Passage of aqueous into Schlemm's canal depends upon cyclic formation of transcellular channels in the endothelial lining. Efferent channels from Schlemm's canal (about 30 collector channels and 12 aqueous veins) conduct the fluid into the venous system. A small amount of aqueous passes between the bundles of the ciliary muscle and through the sclera (uveoscleral flow) (Figure 11–1).

The major resistance to aqueous outflow from the anterior chamber is the endothelial lining of Schlemm's canal and the adjacent portions of the trabecular meshwork—rather than the venous collector system. But the pressure in the episcleral venous network determines the minimum level of intraocular pressure that can be achieved by medical therapy.

then to the trabecular meshwork in the anterior chamber angle. During this period, there is some differential exchange of components with the blood in the iris.

Intraocular inflammation or trauma causes an increase in the protein concentration. This is called plasmoid aqueous and closely resembles blood serum.

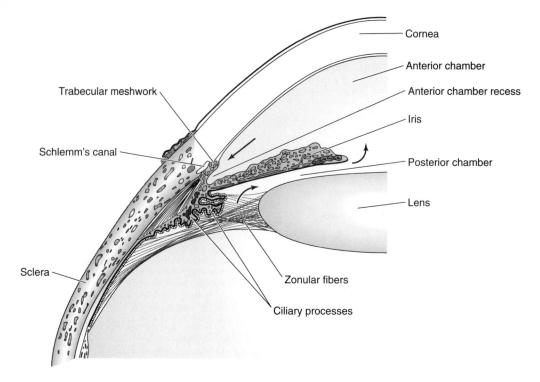

Figure 11–1. Anterior segment structures. Arrows indicate direction of flow of aqueous.

Pressure Dynamics

Intraocular pressure is such an important feature of glaucoma that a review of pressure-tension-strain relationships is desirable for elucidation of the possible mechanisms of neuronal damage.

A. Pressure: Hydrostatic pressure is the force per unit area exerted by a fluid (gas or liquid) within a closed space. With the eye, as with other fluid-filled closed systems, the pressure force is exerted normal to the structural wall (the corneoscleral wall). Average pressure in the eye is about 14 mm Hg. For calculations, centimeters of water is a more convenient unit of pressure than millimeters of mercury. To convert millimeters of mercury to centimeters of water, multiply by 1.36. In more familiar terms, the average eye pressure is about 19 cm (7.5 inches) of water, or 0.25 psi (pounds per square inch). Glaucomatous damage usually begins at roughly double that value, and the eye ruptures at about 240 times average values.

Hydrostatic pressure per se causes no damage to the delicate neurons paralleling the scleral wall. A diver lying on the ocean bottom may be compared to a neuron lying on the uveoscleral bed. The diver will perceive no discomfort at a depth of 43 meters (141 feet) even though the pressure is about 3000 mm Hg, or approximately the pressure within an eye that results in rupture. The diver's body—though subjected to about 10 tons of hydrostatic pressure—will not be pushed against the ocean floor, and a neuron is not pushed against the sclera by hydrostatic pressure.

B. Tension (Tensile Stress): A jack supporting a car is subjected to compressive stress. A towline pulling a car is subjected to tensile stress, or tension. Stresses are assigned a magnitude of force per unit area. Tensile stress, or the tension force vector, acts parallel to the scleral wall (attempting to pull the sclera apart). In the same way, the pressure of the abdomen at right angles to a belt is almost analogous to intraocular pressure, while the tension along the belt acting to pull the belt apart is analogous to scleral tension.

Trampolines and drumheads are examples of pure tension without pressure. The pressure is the same on either side of the tensed membrane. Tension levels in the sclera, cornea, and lamina cribrosa are not equal. The tension equation for thin-walled spheres can be used to obtain a close approximation of tensions in various parts of the corneoscleral wall. Tension in the sclera is directly proportionate to the intraocular pressure multiplied by the radius of curvature of the sclera and inversely proportionate to twice the thickness of the sclera:

$$\text{Tension} = \frac{\text{Pressure} \times \text{Radius}}{2 \times \text{Thickness}}$$

An inflated surgical glove or balloon (Figure 11–2) illustrates this relationship. The palm of the glove has relatively high tension and the thumb relatively low

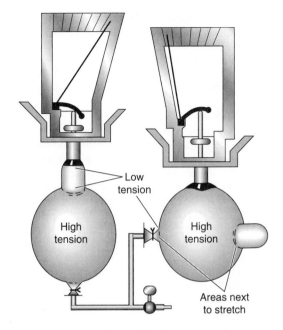

Figure 11–2. Equal-pressure balloons.

tension, though the pressure within the glove is equal at all locations. The thumb has low tension because the radius of curvature is small and the thickness large relative to the same factors at the palm. In the eye, tension is lower in the cornea or optic cup than in the sclera.

An eye under slowly increasing pressure usually ruptures beneath the lateral rectus where the sclera is thinner, as the tension equation would suggest. A precipitous pressure rise due to trauma (eg, a blow from a club) frequently ruptures the eye at the limbus owing to the anvil effect of the more viscous vitreous.

C. Strain: Strain is stretch or displacement per unit length. A strain gauge measures displacement. Strain can result in damage and in the body can cause both pain and damage. Using the belt analogy, strain is the stretch per unit length of the belt resulting from the tension in the belt caused by the pressure of the abdomen.

Young's modulus E is used for determining the elastic properties of structures such as cables, pressure vessels, submarines, biologic cells, unicellular organisms, *and eyes.* E is defined as the tension required to stretch a material of unit cross section to double its original length. This is represented by the following equation:

$$E = \frac{\text{Change in tension of sclera}}{\text{Change in length of sclera per unit length}}$$

Thus, the stretch of the sclera per unit length (strain) is derived by dividing the change in tension of the sclera by Young's modulus of the sclera E.

The belt analogy may now be used to illustrate the way in which neurons are damaged in glaucoma. En-

vision a very obese person wearing a large belt (sclera) with a delicate cloth liner (neurons). After fasting for several days, the obese subject feasts heavily, with the result that there is some ripping of the delicate cloth liner. The progression of the damage process is as follows: (1) The expanding abdomen (intraocular pressure) exerts gentle pressure at right angles to the belt, producing a summation tension parallel to the belt (sclera), tending to pull the belt apart. (2) The tension leads to stretching (strain) of the belt, following the rules of Young's modulus. (3) The stretching (strain) results in damage to the delicate cloth liner (neurons).

PATHOPHYSIOLOGY OF GLAUCOMA

The pathophysiology of intraocular pressure elevation—whether due to open-angle or to angle-closure mechanisms—will be discussed as each disease entity is considered (see below). The effects of raised intraocular pressure within the eye are common to all forms of glaucoma, their manifestations being influenced by the time course and magnitude of the rise in intraocular pressure.

The major mechanism of visual loss in glaucoma is ganglion cell atrophy, leading to thinning of the inner nuclear and nerve fiber layers of the retina and axonal loss in the optic nerve. The optic disk becomes atrophic, with enlargement of the optic cup (see below). The iris and ciliary body also become atrophic, and the ciliary processes show hyaline degeneration.

In acute angle-closure glaucoma, the intraocular pressure reaches 60–80 mm Hg, resulting in ischemic damage to the iris with associated corneal edema and optic nerve damage.

CLINICAL ASSESSMENT IN GLAUCOMA

Tonometry

Tonometry is measurement of intraocular pressure. The most widely used instrument is the Goldmann applanation tonometer, which is attached to the slitlamp and measures the force required to flatten a fixed area of the cornea. Other applanation tonometers are the Perkins tonometer and the Tono-Pen, both of which are portable; and the pneumatotonometer, which is useful when the cornea has an irregular surface and can be used with a soft contact lens in place. The Schiotz tonometer is portable and measures the corneal indentation produced by a known weight. (For further discussion of tonometry, see Chapter 2; for

/ CHAPTER 11

tonometer disinfection techniques, see Chapter 21).

The normal range of intraocular pressure is 10–24 mm Hg. A single normal reading does not rule out glaucoma. In primary open-angle glaucoma, many affected individuals will have a normal intraocular pressure when first measured. Conversely, isolated raised intraocular pressure does not necessarily mean that the patient has primary open-angle glaucoma, since other evidence in the form of a glaucomatous optic disk or visual field changes is necessary for diagnosis. If the intraocular pressure is consistently elevated in the presence of normal optic disks and visual fields (ocular hypertension), the patient may be observed periodically as a glaucoma suspect.

Gonioscopy
(See also Chapter 2)

The anterior chamber angle is formed by the junction of the peripheral cornea and the iris, between which lies the trabecular meshwork (Figure 11–3). The configuration of this angle—ie, whether it is wide (open), narrow, or closed—has an important bearing on the outflow of aqueous. The anterior chamber angle width can be estimated by oblique illumination with a penlight (Figure 11–4) or by slitlamp observation of the depth of the peripheral anterior chamber, but it is best determined by gonioscopy, which allows direct visualization of the angle structures (Figure 11–3). If it is possible to visualize the full extent of the trabecular meshwork, the scleral spur, and the iris processes, the angle is open. Being able to see only Schwalbe's line or a small portion of the trabecular meshwork means that the angle is narrow. Being unable to see Schwalbe's line means that the angle is closed.

Large myopic eyes have wide angles, and small hyperopic eyes have narrow angles. Enlargement of the lens with age narrows the angle and accounts for some cases of angle-closure glaucoma.

Race is also a factor. The angles of Southeast Asians are much narrower than those of Caucasians.

Optic Disk Assessment

The normal optic disk has a central depression—the physiologic cup—whose size depends on the bulk of the fibers that form the optic nerve relative to the size of the scleral opening through which they must pass. In hyperopic eyes, the scleral opening is small, and thus the optic cup is small; the reverse is true in myopic eyes. Glaucomatous optic atrophy produces specific disk changes characterized chiefly by loss of disk substance—detectable as enlargement of the optic disk cup—associated with disk pallor in the area of cupping. Other forms of optic atrophy cause widespread pallor without increased disk cupping.

In glaucoma, there may be concentric enlargement of the optic cup or preferential superior and inferior cupping with focal notching of the rim of the optic disk. The optic cup also increases in depth as the lamina cribrosa is displaced backward. As cupping develops, the retinal vessels on the disk are displaced nasally (Figure 11–5). The end result of glaucomatous cupping is the so-called "bean pot" cup in which no neural rim tissue is apparent (Figures 11–6 and 11–7).

The "cup-disk ratio" is a useful way of recording the size of the optic disk in glaucoma patients. It is the ratio of cup size to disk diameter, eg, a small cup is 0.1 and a large cup 0.9. In the presence of elevated intraocular pressure, a cup-disk ratio greater than 0.5 or significant asymmetry between the two eyes is highly

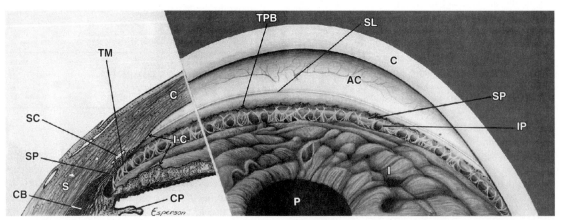

AC = anterior chamber	I = iris	S = sclera	TM = trabecular meshwork
C = cornea	I-C = iris-corneal angle	SC = Schlemm's canal	TPB = trabecular pigment band
CB = ciliary body	IP = iris processes	SL = Schwalbe's line	
CP = ciliary process	P = pupil	SP = scleral spur	

Figure 11–3. Composite illustration showing anatomic *(left)* and gonioscopic *(right)* view of normal anterior chamber angle. (Courtesy of R Shaffer.)

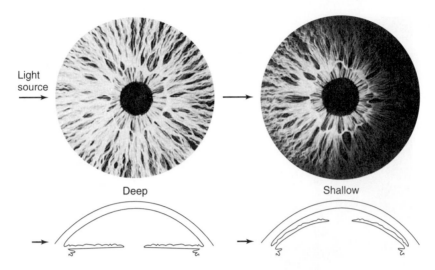

Light
source

Deep

Shallow

Figure 11–4. Estimation of depth of anterior chamber by oblique illumination (diagram). (Courtesy of R Shaffer.)

suggestive of glaucomatous atrophy.

Clinical assessment of the optic disk can be performed by direct ophthalmoscopy or by examination with the 70-diopter lens, the Hruby lens, or special corneal contact lenses that give a three-dimensional view.

Other clinical evidence of neuronal damage in glaucoma is atrophy of the nerve fiber layer. This is detectable (Hoyt's sign) by ophthalmoscopy—particularly when red-free light is used—and precedes the development of optic disk changes.

Visual Field Examination

Regular visual field examination is essential to the diagnosis and follow-up of glaucoma. Glaucomatous field loss is not in itself specific, since it consists of nerve fiber bundle defects that may be seen in other forms of optic nerve disease; but the pattern of field loss, the nature of its progression, and the correlation with changes in the optic disk are characteristic of the disease.

Glaucomatous field loss involves mainly the central 30 degrees of field (Figure 11–8). The earliest change is baring of the blind spot. Contiguous extension into

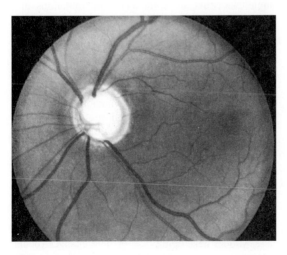

Figure 11–5. Typical glaucomatous cupping. Note the nasal displacement of the vessels and hollowed-out appearance of the optic disk except for a thin border. (Courtesy of S Mettier Jr.)

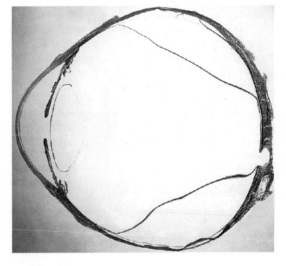

Figure 11–6. Cross-section of an eye with open-angle glaucoma. Note open anterior chamber angle (peripheral iris is not in contact with the posterior corneal surface). Deep glaucomatous cupping ("bean-pot" appearance) shows the process to be well advanced. (Courtesy of R Carriker.)

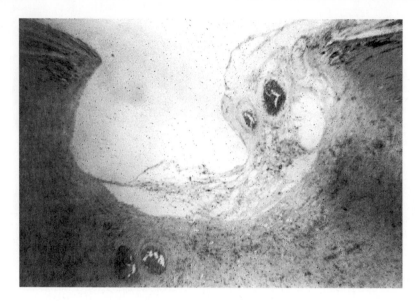

Figure 11–7. Glaucomatous ("bean-pot") cupping of the optic disk.

Bjerrum's area of the visual field—at 15 degrees from fixation—produces a Bjerrum scotoma and then an arcuate scotoma. Focal areas of more pronounced loss within Bjerrum's area are known as Seidel scotomas. Double arcuate scotomas—above and below the horizontal meridian—are often accompanied by a nasal step (of Roenne) because of differences in size of the two arcuate defects. Peripheral field loss tends to start in the nasal periphery as a constriction of the isopters. Subsequently, there may be connection to an arcuate defect, producing peripheral breakthrough. The temporal peripheral field and the central 5–10 degrees are affected late in the disease. Central visual acuity is not a reliable index of progress of the disease. In end-stage disease, there may be normal central acuity but only 5 degrees of visual field in each eye. In advanced glaucoma, the patient may have 20/20 visual acuity and be legally blind.

Various ways of testing the visual fields in glaucoma include the automated perimeter, the Goldmann perimeter, the Friedman field analyzer, and the tangent screen. (For technique and other details, see Chapter 2)

PRIMARY GLAUCOMA

PRIMARY OPEN-ANGLE GLAUCOMA

Primary open-angle glaucoma is the most common form. About 0.4–0.7% of persons over age 40 and 2–3% of persons over age 70 are estimated to have primary open-angle glaucoma. The disease is four times more common and generally more aggressive in blacks. There is a strong familial tendency in pri-

mary open-angle glaucoma, and close relatives of affected individuals should undergo regular screening.

The chief pathologic feature of primary open-angle glaucoma is a degenerative process in the trabecular meshwork, including deposition of extracellular material within the meshwork and beneath the endothelial lining of Schlemm's canal. This differs from the normal aging process. The consequence is a reduction in aqueous drainage leading to a rise in intraocular pressure.

Juvenile-onset open-angle glaucoma (a familial primary open-angle glaucoma with early onset), about 5% of familial cases of primary open-angle glaucoma, and about 3% of nonfamilial cases of primary open-angle glaucoma are associated with mutations in a gene on chromosome 1. This gene causes trabecular meshwork cells to produce an extracellular protein known as TIGR (trabecular meshwork-inducible glucocorticoid response) as a result of its association with glaucoma secondary to steroid therapy. It is suggested that these mutations result in abnormal amounts or types of TIGR. A mutation on chromosome 3 has also been implicated in autosomal dominant adult-onset primary open-angle glaucoma.

Raised intraocular pressure precedes optic disk and visual field changes by months to years. Although there is a clear association between the level of intraocular pressure and the severity and rate of progression of visual loss, there is great variability between individuals in the effect on the optic nerve of a given pressure elevation. Some people tolerate elevated intraocular pressure without developing disk or field changes (ocular hypertension; see below); others develop glaucomatous changes with consistently "normal" intraocular pressure (low-pressure glaucoma; see below).

The mechanism of neuronal damage in primary

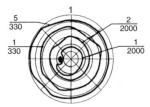

Baring of the blind spot. The earliest nerve fiber bundle defect.

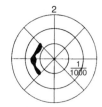

Incipient double nerve fiber bundle defect (Bjerrum scotoma).

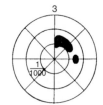

Bjerrum scotoma isolated from blind spot.

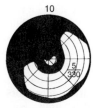

End stages in glaucoma field loss. Remnant of central field still shows nasal step.

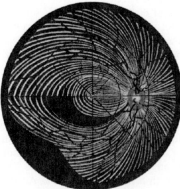

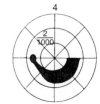

Fully developed nerve fiber bundle defect with nasal step (arcuate scotoma).

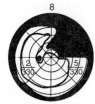

Peripheral depression with double nerve fiber bundle defect. Isolation of central field.

The basic visual field loss in glaucoma is the nerve fiber bundle defect with nasal step and peripheral nasal depression. It is here shown superimposed upon the nerve fiber layer of the retina and the retinal vascular tree. All perimetric changes in glaucoma are variations of these fundamental defects.

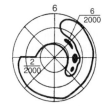

Double arcuate scotoma with peripheral breakthrough and nasal step.

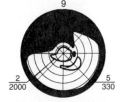

Nasal depression connected with arcuate scotoma. Nasal step of Rönne.

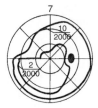

Peripheral breakthrough of large nerve fiber bundle defect with well developed nasal step.

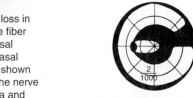

Seidel scotoma. Islands of greater visual loss within a nerve fiber bundle defect.

Figure 11–8. Visual field changes in glaucoma. (Reproduced, with permission, from Harrington DO: *The Visual Fields: A Textbook and Atlas of Clinical Perimetry,* 5th ed. Mosby, 1981.)

open-angle glaucoma and its relationship to the level of intraocular pressure is much debated. The major theories implicate intraocular pressure-dependent changes (as discussed above) or reduction in the vascular supply to the optic nerve head.

Higher levels of intraocular pressure are associated with greater field loss at presentation. When there is glaucomatous field loss on first examination, the risk of further progression is much greater. Since intraocular pressure is the only treatable risk factor, it remains the focus of therapy. There is strong evidence that control of intraocular pressure slows disk damage and field loss.

In the patient with extensive disk changes or field loss, it is advisable to reduce the intraocular pressure as much as possible, whereas a patient with only a suspicion of disk or field changes may need less vigorous treatment. In all cases, the inconveniences and possible complications of treatment must be considered. Many glaucoma patients are old and frail and may not tolerate vigorous treatment. In order to gain a perspective on the need for treatment, an initial period of observation without treatment may be necessary to determine the rate of progression of disk and field changes. There is no justification for subjecting an elderly patient to extremes of treatment when the likelihood of their developing significant visual loss during their lifetime is small.

Diagnosis

The diagnosis of primary open-angle glaucoma is established when glaucomatous optic disk or field changes are associated with elevated intraocular pressures, a normal-appearing open anterior chamber angle, and no other reason for intraocular pressure elevation. Approximately 50% of patients with primary open-angle glaucoma have a normal intraocular pressure when first examined, so repeated tonometry is necessary before the diagnosis can be established.

Screening for Glaucoma

The major problem in detection of primary open-angle glaucoma is the absence of symptoms until relatively late in the disease. When patients first notice field loss, substantial glaucomatous cupping has already occurred. If treatment is to be successful, it must be started early in the disease, and this depends upon an active screening program. Unfortunately, glaucoma screening programs are hampered by the unreliability of a single intraocular pressure measurement in the detection of primary open-angle glaucoma and the complexities of relying on optic disk or visual field changes. At present it is necessary to rely for early diagnosis on regular ophthalmologic assessment of first-degree relatives of affected individuals.

Medical Treatment of Glaucoma

A. Suppression of Aqueous Production: Topical **beta-adrenergic blocking agents** are now the most widely used form of glaucoma therapy. They may be used alone or in combination with other drugs. Timolol maleate 0.25% and 0.5%, betaxolol 0.25% and 0.5%, levobunolol 0.25% and 0.5%, metipranolol 0.3%, and carteolol 1% are the currently available preparations. The major contraindications to their use are chronic obstructive airways disease—particularly asthma—and cardiac conduction defects. Betaxolol, with its relatively greater selectivity for β_1 receptors, less often produces respiratory side effects but is also less effective at reducing intraocular pressure. Depression, confusion, and fatigue may occur with the topical beta-blocking agents.

Apraclonidine is an α_2-adrenergic agonist that decreases aqueous humor formation without effect on outflow. **Epinephrine** and **dipivefrin** have some effect on aqueous production (see below).

Brimonidine 0.2% is a new alpha-adrenergic agonist that primarily inhibits aqueous production and secondarily increases aqueous outflow. It shows promise both as a first-line antiglaucoma drug and as an adjunctive agent.

Dorzolamide hydrochloride 2% is a recently developed topical carbonic anhydrase inhibitor that is especially effective when employed adjunctively, though not as effective as systemic carbonic anhydrase inhibitors. Combining dorzolamide and timolol in the same solution is under investigation.

Systemic **carbonic anhydrase inhibitors**—acetazolamide is the most widely used, but dichlorphenamide and methazolamide are alternatives—are used in chronic glaucoma when topical therapy is insufficient and in acute glaucoma when very high intraocular pressure needs to be controlled quickly. They are capable of suppressing aqueous production by 40–60%. Acetazolamide can be administered orally in a dosage of 125–250 mg up to four times daily or as Diamox Sequels 500 mg once or twice daily, or it can be given intravenously (500 mg). The carbonic anhydrase inhibitors are associated with major systemic side effects that limit their usefulness for long-term therapy.

Hyperosmotic agents influence aqueous production as well as dehydrating the vitreous body (see below).

B. Facilitation of Aqueous Outflow: Parasympathomimetic agents increase aqueous outflow by action on the trabecular meshwork through contraction of the ciliary muscle. **Pilocarpine** is the most commonly used drug in this group. It is given as 0.5–6% solution instilled several times a day or as 4% gel instilled at bedtime. Carbachol 0.75–3% is an alternative cholinergic agent. Irreversible anticholinesterase agents are the longest-acting parasympathomimetics available. These include demecarium bromide, 0.125% and 0.25%, and echothiophate iodide, 0.03–0.25%, which are generally restricted to aphakic or pseudophakic patients because of their cataractogenic potential. *Caution:* The irreversible anticholinesterase agents will potentiate succinylcholine administered during anesthesia, and anesthetists must be appropriately warned prior to surgery.

All parasympathomimetic agents produce miosis with dimness of vision, particularly in patients with cataract, and accommodative spasm that may be disabling to younger patients. Retinal detachment is a serious but rare occurrence.

Latanoprost 0.005%, a prostaglandin $F_{2\alpha}$ analog, acts as an antiglaucoma drug by increasing the uveoscleral outflow of aqueous. It is used once daily in the evening and may work alone or as an adjunct to other antiglaucoma agents. To date there have been no systemic side effects, and once-daily dosing is a distinct advantage. However, it does increase iris pigmentation.

Epinephrine, 0.25–2% instilled once or twice daily, increases aqueous outflow with some decrease in aqueous production. There are a number of external ocular side effects, including reflex conjunctival vasodilation, adrenochrome deposits, follicular conjunctivitis, and allergic reactions. **Dipivefrin** is a prodrug of epinephrine that is metabolized intraocularly to its active state. Neither epinephrine nor dipivefrin should be used in eyes with narrow anterior chamber angles.

C. Reduction of Vitreous Volume: Hyperosmotic agents render the blood hypertonic, thus drawing water out of the vitreous and causing it to shrink. This is in addition to decreasing aqueous production. Reduction in vitreous volume is helpful in the treatment of acute angle-closure glaucoma and in malignant glaucoma when anterior displacement of the crystalline lens (caused by volume changes in the vitreous or choroid) produces angle closure (secondary angle-closure glaucoma).

Oral **glycerin (glycerol),** 1 mL/kg of body weight in a cold 50% solution mixed with lemon juice, is the most commonly used agent, but it should be used with care in diabetics. Alternatives are oral isosorbide and intravenous urea or mannitol (see Chapter 3 for dosages).

D. Miotics, Mydriatics, and Cycloplegics: Constriction of the pupil is fundamental to the management of primary angle-closure glaucoma and the angle crowding of plateau iris. Pupillary dilation is important in the treatment of angle closure secondary to iris bombé due to posterior synechiae.

When angle closure is secondary to anterior lens displacement, cycloplegics (cyclopentolate and atropine) are used to relax the ciliary muscle and thus tighten the zonular apparatus in an attempt to draw the lens backward.

Surgical & Laser Treatment of Glaucoma

A. Peripheral Iridotomy and Iridectomy: Pupillary block in angle-closure glaucoma is most satisfactorily overcome by forming a direct communication between the anterior and posterior chambers that removes the pressure difference between them. This is best done with the neodymium:YAG laser. Surgical peripheral iridectomy is performed if YAG laser iridotomy is ineffective. YAG laser iridotomy is preventive when used in patients with narrow angles before closure attacks occur.

B. Laser Trabeculoplasty: Application of laser (usually argon) burns via a goniolens to the trabecular meshwork facilitates aqueous outflow by virtue of its effects on the trabecular meshwork and Schlemm's canal or cellular events that enhance the function of the meshwork. The technique is applicable to many forms of open-angle glaucoma, and the results are variable depending upon the underlying cause. The pressure reduction usually allows decrease of medical therapy and postponement of glaucoma surgery. Treatments can be repeated (see Chapter 24). Laser trabeculoplasty may be used in the initial treatment of primary open-angle glaucoma. In most cases, the intraocular pressure gradually returns to the pretreatment level 2–5 years later.

C. Glaucoma Drainage Surgery: The increased effectiveness of medical and laser treatment has reduced the need for glaucoma drainage surgery, but surgery is able to produce a more marked reduction in intraocular pressure.

Trabeculectomy is the procedure most commonly used to bypass the normal drainage channels, allowing direct access from the anterior chamber to the subconjunctival and orbital tissues. The major complication is fibrosis in the episcleral tissues, leading to closure of the new drainage pathway. This is most likely to occur in young patients, blacks, in patients with glaucoma secondary to uveitis, and in those who have previously undergone glaucoma drainage surgery or other surgery involving the episcleral tissues. Adjunctive treatment with antimetabolites such as fluorouracil and mitomycin reduces the risk of bleb failure but may lead to other bleb-related complications or maculopathy from persistent ocular hypotony.

Implantation of a silicone tube to form a permanent conduit for aqueous flow out of the eye is an alternative procedure for eyes that are unlikely to respond to trabeculectomy. This includes eyes with secondary glaucoma, particularly neovascular glaucoma, and glaucoma following corneal graft surgery.

Goniotomy is a useful technique in treating primary congenital glaucoma, in which there appears to be an obstruction to aqueous drainage in the internal portion of the trabecular meshwork.

D. Cyclodestructive Procedures: Failure of medical and surgical treatment in advanced glaucoma may lead to consideration of laser or surgical destruction of the ciliary body to control intraocular pressure. Cryotherapy, diathermy, high-frequency ultrasound, and thermal mode neodymium:YAG laser therapy can all be used to cause destruction of the ciliary body.

Course & Prognosis

Without treatment, open-angle glaucoma may be insidiously progressive to complete blindness. If antiglaucoma drops control the intraocular pressure in an eye that has not suffered extensive glaucomatous damage, the prognosis is good (though visual field loss may progress in spite of normalized intraocular pressure). When the process is detected early, most glaucoma patients can be successfully managed medically.

NORMAL-PRESSURE GLAUCOMA
(Low-Pressure Glaucoma)

A minority of patients with glaucomatous optic disk or visual field changes have an intraocular pressure consistently below 25 mm Hg. These patients have normal- or low-pressure glaucoma. The pathogenesis involves an abnormal sensitivity to intraocular pressure because of vascular or mechanical abnormalities at the optic nerve head. Disk hemorrhages are more frequently seen in normal-pressure than in primary open-angle glaucoma and often herald progression of field loss.

Before the diagnosis of low-pressure glaucoma can be established, a number of entities must be excluded:

(1) Prior episode of raised intraocular pressure, such as caused by iridocyclitis, trauma, or topical steroid therapy.

(2) Large diurnal variation in intraocular pressure with significant elevations, usually early in the morning.

(3) Postural changes in intraocular pressure with a marked elevation when lying flat.

(4) Intermittent elevations of intraocular pressure such as in subacute angle closure.

(5) Other causes of optic disk and field changes, including congenital disk abnormalities and acquired optic atrophy due to tumors or vascular disease.

OCULAR HYPERTENSION

Ocular hypertension is elevated intraocular pressure without disk or field abnormalities and is more common than primary open-angle glaucoma. The rate at which such individuals develop glaucoma is approximately 5–10 per 1000 per year. The risk increases with increasing intraocular pressure, increasing age, a positive family history for glaucoma, myopia, diabetes mellitus, and cardiovascular disease. It is also increased in blacks. The development of disk hemorrhages in a patient with ocular hypertension also indicates an increased risk for development of glaucoma.

Patients with ocular hypertension are considered glaucoma suspects and should undergo regular monitoring (one to three times a year) of the optic disk, intraocular pressure, and visual fields.

PRIMARY ACUTE ANGLE-CLOSURE GLAUCOMA

Primary acute angle-closure glaucoma occurs when sufficient iris bombé develops to cause occlusion of the anterior chamber angle by the peripheral iris. This blocks aqueous outflow and the intraocular pressure rises rapidly, causing severe pain, redness, and blurring of vision. Angle-closure glaucoma occurs in eyes with preexisting anatomic narrowing of the anterior chamber angle (found mainly in hyperopes). The acute attack generally occurs in older patients when there has been enlargement of the crystalline lens associated with aging. In angle-closure glaucoma, the pupil is mid-dilated, with associated pupillary block. This usually occurs in the evenings, when the level of illumination is reduced. It may also occur with pupillary dilation for ophthalmoscopy. If pupillary dilation is necessary in a patient with a shallow anterior chamber (easily detected by oblique illumination with a penlight [Figure 11–4] and then confirmed by gonioscopy), it is best to rely on short-acting mydriatics and observe the patient carefully.

Clinical Findings

Acute angle-closure glaucoma is characterized by a sudden onset of severe blurring followed by excruciating pain, halos, and nausea and vomiting. Other findings include markedly increased intraocular pressure, a shallow anterior chamber, a steamy cornea, a fixed, moderately dilated pupil, and ciliary injection. It is important to perform gonioscopy on the fellow eye.

Differential Diagnosis
(See Inside Front Cover)

Acute iritis causes more photophobia than acute glaucoma. Intraocular pressure is usually not elevated; the pupil is constricted; and the cornea is usually not edematous. Marked flare and cells are present in the anterior chamber, and there is deep ciliary injection.

In acute conjunctivitis, there is little or no pain and no visual loss. There is discharge from the eye and an intensely inflamed conjunctiva but no ciliary injection. The pupillary responses and intraocular pressure are normal, and the cornea is clear.

Complications & Sequelae

If treatment is delayed, the peripheral iris may adhere to the trabecular meshwork (anterior synechiae), producing irreversible occlusion of the anterior chamber angle requiring surgery. Optic nerve damage is common.

Treatment

Acute angle-closure glaucoma is an ophthalmic emergency!

Treatment is initially directed at reducing the intraocular pressure. Intravenous and oral acetazolamide—along with hyperosmotic agents and topical beta-blockers—will usually reduce the intraocular pressure. Pilocarpine 4% can then be used intensively, eg, 1 drop every 15 minutes for 1 hour. Epinephrine must not be used because it will accentuate angle closure.

Once the intraocular pressure is under control, peripheral iridectomy should be undertaken to form a permanent connection between the anterior and posterior chambers, thus preventing recurrence of iris bombé. This is most often done with the neodymium:YAG laser. Surgical peripheral iridectomy is indicated if laser treatment is unsuccessful.

In most cases, the fellow eye should undergo prophylactic laser iridotomy.

SUBACUTE ANGLE-CLOSURE GLAUCOMA

The same etiologic factors operate in subacute as in acute angle-closure glaucoma except that episodes of elevated intraocular pressure are of short duration and are recurrent. The episodes of angle closure resolve spontaneously, but there is accumulated damage to the anterior chamber angle, with formation of peripheral anterior synechiae. Subacute angle closure will occasionally progress to acute closure.

There are recurrent short episodes of unilateral pain, redness, and blurring of vision associated with halos around lights. Attacks often occur in the evenings and resolve overnight. Examination between attacks may show only a narrow anterior chamber angle. The diagnosis can be confirmed by gonioscopy.

Treatment is similar to that of primary angle-closure glaucoma.

CHRONIC ANGLE-CLOSURE GLAUCOMA

A small number of patients with the predisposition to a anterior chamber angle closure never develop episodes of acute rise in intraocular pressure but form increasingly extensive peripheral anterior synechiae accompanied by a gradual rise in intraocular pressure. These patients present in the same way as those with primary open-angle glaucoma, often with extensive visual field loss in both eyes. Occasionally, they have attacks of subacute angle closure.

On examination, there is elevated intraocular pressure, narrow anterior chamber angles with variable amounts of peripheral anterior synechiae, and optic disk and visual field changes.

Once again, peripheral iridectomy is an important component of treatment. (Laser iridotomy in these patients is liable to produce a marked rise in intraocular pressure.) Intraocular pressure is then controlled medically if possible, but the extent of peripheral anterior synechia formation and sluggish outflow through the remaining trabecular meshwork make pressure control very difficult, so that drainage surgery is often required. Epinephrine and strong miotics must not be used unless peripheral iridectomy has been performed because they will accentuate angle closure.

PLATEAU IRIS

Plateau iris is an uncommon condition in which the central anterior chamber depth is normal but the anterior chamber angle is very narrow owing to a congenital high insertion of the iris. Such an eye has little pupillary block, but dilation will cause bunching up of the peripheral iris, occluding the angle (angle crowding) even if peripheral iridectomy has been performed. Affected individuals present with acute angle-closure glaucoma at a young age, with recurrences after peripheral iridectomy. Long-term miotic therapy or laser iridoplasty is required.

Pupillary dilation for fundus examination is apt to cause acute angle closure in patients with plateau iris and may precipitate a similar event in other eyes with deep anterior chambers—due to angle crowding rather than the pupillary block mechanism seen in eyes with shallow anterior chambers.

CONGENITAL GLAUCOMA

Congenital glaucoma (rare) can be subdivided into (1) primary congenital glaucoma, in which the developmental abnormalities are restricted to the anterior chamber angle; (2) the anterior segment developmental anomalies—Axenfeld's syndrome, Peter's anomaly, and Rieger's syndrome—in which iris and corneal development are also abnormal; and (3) a variety of other conditions—including aniridia, Sturge-Weber syndrome, neurofibromatosis-1, Lowe's syndrome, and congenital rubella—in which the developmental anomalies of the angle are associated with other ocular or extraocular abnormalities.

Clinical Findings

Congenital glaucoma is manifest at birth in 50%, diagnosed in the first 6 months in 70%, and diagnosed by the end of the first year in 80%. The earliest and most common symptom is epiphora. Photophobia and decreased corneal luster may be present. Increased intraocular pressure is the cardinal sign. Glaucomatous cupping of the optic disk is a relatively early—and the most important—change. Later findings include increased corneal diameter (above 11.5 mm is considered significant), epithelial edema, tears of Descemet's membrane, and increased depth of the anterior chamber (associated with general enlargement of the anterior segment of the eye) as well as edema and opacity of the corneal stroma (Figure 11–9).

Differential Diagnosis

Megalocornea, corneal clouding due to congenital dystrophy or mucopolysaccharidoses, and traumatic

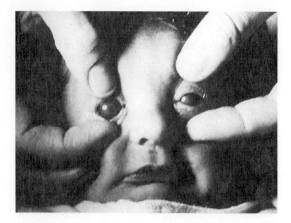

Figure 11–9. Congenital glaucoma (buphthalmos.)

rupture of Descemet's membrane should be ruled out. Measurement of intraocular pressure, gonioscopy, and evaluation of the optic disk are important in making the differential diagnosis. Assessment generally requires examination under general anesthesia.

Course & Prognosis

In untreated cases, blindness occurs early. The eye undergoes marked stretching and may even rupture with minor trauma. Typical glaucomatous cupping occurs relatively soon, emphasizing the need for early treatment.

1. ANTERIOR SEGMENT DEVELOPMENTAL ANOMALIES

These rare diseases constitute a spectrum of maldevelopment of the anterior segment, involving the angle, iris, cornea, and occasionally the lens. Usually there is some hypoplasia of the anterior stroma of the iris, with bridging filaments connecting the iris stroma to the cornea. If these bridging filaments occur peripherally and connect to a prominent, axially displaced Schwalbe's line (posterior embryotoxon), the disease is known as **Axenfeld's syndrome.** This resembles the trabeculodysgenesis of primary congenital glaucoma. If there are broader iridocorneal adhesions associated with the disruption of the iris, with polycoria and, in addition, skeletal and dental anomalies, the disorder is called **Rieger's syndrome** (an example of iridotrabecular dysgenesis). If adhesions are between the central iris and the central posterior surface of the cornea, the disease is known as **Peter's anomaly** (an example of iridocorneal trabeculodysgenesis).

These diseases are usually dominantly inherited, though sporadic cases have been reported. Mutations on chromosomes 4 and 13, probably involving homeobox genes, have been identified in pedigrees with Axenfeld-Rieger syndrome. Glaucoma occurs in ap-

proximately 50% of such eyes and often does not present until late childhood or early adulthood. Goniotomy has a much lower success rate in these cases, and trabeculotomy or trabeculectomy may be recommended. Many such patients require long-term medical glaucoma therapy, and the prognosis is guarded for long-term retention of good visual function.

2. ANIRIDIA

The distinguishing feature of aniridia, as the name implies, is the vestigial iris. In many cases, little more than the root of the iris or a thin iris margin is present. Other deformities of the eye may be present, such as congenital cataracts, corneal dystrophy, and foveal hypoplasia. Vision is usually poor. Glaucoma frequently develops before adolescence and is usually refractory to medical or surgical management.

This rare syndrome is genetically determined. Both autosomal dominant and autosomal recessive inheritance have been reported.

If medical therapy is ineffective, goniotomy or trabeculotomy may occasionally normalize the intraocular pressure. Filtering operations are often necessary, but the long-term visual prognosis is poor.

SECONDARY GLAUCOMA

Increased intraocular pressure occurring as one manifestation of some other eye disease is called secondary glaucoma. These diseases are difficult to classify satisfactorily. Treatment involves controlling intraocular pressure by medical and surgical means but also dealing with the underlying disease if possible.

PIGMENTARY GLAUCOMA

This syndrome seems to be primarily a degeneration of the pigmented epithelium of the iris and ciliary body. The pigment granules flake off from the iris as a result of friction against the underlying packets of zonular fibers, resulting in iris transillumination. The pigment is deposited on the posterior corneal surface (Krukenberg's spindle) and becomes lodged in the trabecular meshwork, impeding the normal outflow of aqueous. The syndrome occurs most often in myopic males between the ages of 25 and 40 who have a deep anterior chamber with a wide anterior chamber angle.

The pigmentary changes may be present without glaucoma (**pigment dispersion syndrome**), but such persons must be considered "glaucoma suspects." A number of pedigrees of autosomal dominant inheritance of pigmentary glaucoma have been reported, and a gene for pigment dispersion syndrome has been mapped to chromosome 7.

The logical treatment in this condition is miotic therapy because it overcomes movement of the iris across the zonules. However, because the patients are usually young myopes, such therapy is poorly tolerated unless administered as pilocarpine once daily, preferably at bedtime. Beta-blockers and epinephrine are also effective.

The major problem, however, is the young age at which the disease develops, which increases the chance that drainage surgery will be necessary and enhances the advisability of combining such surgery with antimetabolite therapy. Laser trabeculoplasty is frequently used in this condition but is unlikely to obviate the need for drainage surgery.

EXFOLIATION SYNDROME
(Pseudo-Exfoliation Syndrome)

In exfoliation syndrome, flake-like deposits of a fibrillary material are seen on the anterior lens surface (in contrast to the true exfoliation of the lens capsule caused by exposure to infrared radiation, ie, "glassblower's cataract"), ciliary processes, zonule, posterior iris surface, loose in the anterior chamber, and in the trabecular meshwork (along with increased pigmentation). These deposits can also be detected histologically in the conjunctiva, suggesting a more widespread abnormality. The disease usually occurs in patients over age 65. Treatment is as for primary open-angle glaucoma.

GLAUCOMA SECONDARY
TO CHANGES IN THE LENS

Lens Dislocation

The crystalline lens may be dislocated as a result of trauma or spontaneously, as in Marfan's syndrome. Anterior dislocation may cause obstruction of the pupillary aperture, leading to iris bombé and angle closure. Posterior dislocation into the vitreous is also associated with glaucoma, though the mechanism is obscure. It may be due to angle damage at the time of traumatic dislocation.

In anterior dislocation, the definitive treatment is lens extraction once the intraocular pressure has been controlled medically. In posterior dislocation, the lens is usually left alone and the glaucoma treated as primary open-angle glaucoma.

Intumescence of the Lens

The lens may take up considerable fluid during cataractous change, increasing markedly in size. It may then encroach upon the anterior chamber, producing both pupillary block and angle crowding and resulting in angle-closure glaucoma. Treatment consists of lens extraction once the intraocular pressure has been controlled medically.

Phacolytic Glaucoma

Some advanced cataracts may develop leakiness of the anterior lens capsule, which allows passage of liquefied lens proteins into the anterior chamber. There is an inflammatory reaction in the anterior chamber, and the trabecular meshwork becomes edematous and obstructed with lens proteins, leading to an acute rise in intraocular pressure. Lens extraction is the definitive treatment once the intraocular pressure has been controlled medically and intensive topical steroid therapy has reduced the intraocular inflammation.

GLAUCOMA SECONDARY
TO CHANGES IN THE UVEAL TRACT

Uveitis

The intraocular pressure is usually below normal in uveitis because the inflamed ciliary body is functioning poorly. However, elevation of intraocular pressure may also occur through a number of different mechanisms. The trabecular meshwork may become blocked by inflammatory cells from the anterior chamber, with secondary edema, or may occasionally be involved in an inflammatory process specifically directed at the trabecular cells (trabeculitis). Chronic or recurrent uveitis produces permanent impairment of trabecular function, peripheral anterior synechiae, and occasionally angle neovascularization, all of which increase the chance of secondary glaucoma. Seclusio pupillae due to 360-degree posterior synechiae produces iris bombé and acute angle-closure glaucoma. The uveitis syndromes that tend to be associated with secondary glaucoma are Fuchs's heterochromic cyclitis, HLA-B27-associated acute anterior uveitis, and uveitis due to herpes zoster and herpes simplex.

Treatment is directed chiefly at controlling the uveitis with concomitant medical glaucoma therapy as necessary, avoiding miotics because of the increased chance of posterior synechia formation. Long-term therapy, including surgery, is often required because of irreversible damage to the trabecular meshwork.

Acute angle closure due to seclusion of the pupil may be reversed by intensive mydriasis but often requires laser peripheral iridotomy or surgical iridectomy. Any uveitis with a tendency to posterior synechia formation must be treated with mydriatics whenever the uveitis is active to reduce the risk of pupillary seclusion.

Tumor

Uveal tract melanomas may cause glaucoma by anterior displacement of the ciliary body, causing secondary angle closure, direct involvement of the anterior chamber angle, blockage of the filtration angle by pigment dispersion, and angle neovascularization. Enucleation is usually necessary.

IRIDOCORNEOENDOTHELIAL (ICE) SYNDROME
(Essential Iris Atrophy, Chandler's Syndrome, Iris Nevus Syndrome)

This rare idiopathic condition of young adults is usually unilateral and manifested by corneal decompensation, glaucoma, and iris abnormalities.

GLAUCOMA SECONDARY TO TRAUMA

Contusion injuries of the globe may be associated with an early rise in intraocular pressure due to bleeding into the anterior chamber (hyphema). Free blood blocks the trabecular meshwork, which is also rendered edematous by the injury. Treatment is initially medical, but surgery may be required if the pressure remains elevated.

Late effects of contusion injuries on intraocular pressure are due to direct angle damage. The interval between the injury and the development of glaucoma may obscure the association. Clinically, the anterior chamber is seen to be deeper than in the fellow eye, and gonioscopy shows recession of the angle. Medical therapy is usually effective, but drainage surgery may be required.

Laceration or contusional rupture of the anterior segment is associated with loss of the anterior chamber. If the chamber is not reformed soon after the injury—either spontaneously, by iris incarceration into the wound, or surgically—peripheral anterior synechiae will form and result in irreversible angle closure.

GLAUCOMA FOLLOWING OCULAR SURGERY

Ciliary Block Glaucoma (Malignant Glaucoma)

Surgery upon an eye with markedly increased intraocular pressure and a closed angle can lead to ciliary block glaucoma. Immediately after surgery, the intraocular pressure increases markedly, and the lens is pushed forward as a result of the collection of aqueous in and behind the vitreous body.

Treatment consists of cycloplegics, mydriatics, aqueous suppressants, and hyperosmotic agents. Hyperosmotic agents are used to shrink the vitreous body and let the lens fall more posteriorly.

Posterior sclerotomy, vitrectomy, and even lens extraction may be needed.

Peripheral Anterior Synechiae

Just as with trauma to the anterior segment (see above), surgery that results in a flat anterior chamber will lead to formation of peripheral anterior synechiae. Early surgical re-formation of the chamber is required if it does not occur spontaneously.

NEOVASCULAR GLAUCOMA

Neovascularization of the iris (rubeosis iridis) and anterior chamber angle is most often secondary to widespread retinal ischemia such as occurs in advanced diabetic retinopathy and ischemic central retinal vein occlusion. Glaucoma results initially from obstruction of the angle by the fibrovascular membrane, but subsequent contraction of the membrane leads to angle closure.

Treatment of established neovascular glaucoma is difficult and often unsatisfactory.

GLAUCOMA SECONDARY TO RAISED EPISCLERAL VENOUS PRESSURE

Raised episcleral venous pressure may contribute to glaucoma in Sturge-Weber syndrome, in which a developmental anomaly of the angle is also often present, and carotid-cavernous fistula, which may also cause angle neovascularization due to widespread ocular ischemia. Medical treatment cannot reduce the intraocular pressure below the level of the abnormally elevated episcleral venous pressure, and surgery is associated with a high risk of complications.

STEROID-INDUCED GLAUCOMA

Topical and periocular corticosteroids may produce a type of glaucoma that simulates primary open-angle glaucoma, particularly in individuals with a family history of the disease, and will exaggerate the intraocular pressure elevation in those with established primary open-angle glaucoma. Withdrawal of the medication usually eliminates these effects, but permanent damage can occur if the situation goes unrecognized too long. If topical steroid therapy is absolutely necessary, medical glaucoma therapy will usually control the intraocular pressure. Systemic steroid therapy is less likely to cause a rise in intraocular pressure.

It is imperative that patients receiving topical or systemic steroid therapy undergo periodic tonometry and ophthalmoscopy, particularly if there is a family history of glaucoma.

Brubaker RF: Delayed functional loss in glaucoma. LII Edward Jackson Memorial Lecture. Am J Ophthalmol 1996;121:473.

REFERENCES

Burke JA et al: New approaches in glaucoma management: A clinical profile of brimonidine. Surv Ophthalmol 1996;41:S3.

Camras CB: Comparison of latanoprost and timolol in patients with ocular hypertension and glaucoma. Ophthalmology 1996;103:138.

Caprioli J: Recognizing structural damage to the optic nerve head and nerve fiber layer in glaucoma. Am J Ophthalmol 1997;124:516.

Coleman AL et al: Interobserver and intraobserver variability in the detection of glaucomatous progression of the optic disc. J Glaucoma 1996;5:384.

Donohue EK, Wilensky JT: Trusopt, a topical carbonic anhydrase inhibitor. J Glaucoma 1996;5:68.

Drance SM: Glaucoma: A look beyond intraocular pressure. Am J Ophthalmol 1997;123:817.

Erie JC, Hodge DO, Gray DT: The incidence of primary angle-closure glaucoma in Olmsted County, Minnesota. Arch Ophthalmol 1997;115:177.

Foster PJ et al: Glaucoma in Mongolia. Arch Ophthalmol 1996;114:1235.

Fraser S, Wormald R, Hitchings R: Blood pressure and glaucoma. Br J Ophthalmol 1996;80:858.

Gordon J, Piltz-Seymour JR: The significance of optic disc hemorrhages in glaucoma. J Glaucoma 1997;6:62.

Graham SL et al: Ambulatory blood pressure monitoring in glaucoma. Ophthalmol 1995;102:61.

Greenfield DS, Liebmann JM, Ritch R: Brimonidine: A new alpha$_2$-adrenoreceptor agonist for glaucoma treatment. J Glaucoma 1997;6:250.

Heijl A et al: A comparison of dorzolamide and timolol in patients with pseudoexfoliation and glaucoma or ocular hypertension. Ophthalmol 1997;104:137.

Higginbotham EJ: Topical β-adrenergic antagonists and quinidine. Arch Ophthalmol 1996;114:745.

Higginbotham EJ: Will latanoprost be the "wonder" drug of the '90's for the treatment of glaucoma? Arch Ophthalmol 1996;114:998.

Hitchings R: Shared care for glaucoma. Br J Ophthalmol 1995;79:626.

Jacobi PC, Dietlein TS, Krieglstein GK: Technique of goniocurettage: A potential treatment for advanced chronic open angle glaucoma. Br J Ophthalmol 1997;81:302.

Jampel HD: Target pressure in glaucoma therapy. J Glaucoma 1997;6:133.

Kanellopoulos AJ, Erickson KA, Netland PA: Systemic calcium channel blockers and glaucoma. J Glaucoma 1996;5:357.

Kaufman PL: Glaucoma Research Foundation meeting summary. J Glaucoma 1997;6:65.

Konstas AGP et al: Effect of timolol on the diurnal intraocular pressure in exfoliation and primary open-angle glaucoma. Arch Ophthalmol 1997;115:975.

Laibovitz R et al: Comparison of quality of life and patient preference of dorzolamide and pilocarpine as adjunctive therapy to timolol in the treatment of glaucoma. J Glaucoma 1995;4:306.

Leske MC: Open-angle glaucoma and blood groups. Arch Ophthalmol 1996;114:205.

Lowe RF: A history of primary angle closure glaucoma. Surv Ophthalmol 1995;40:163.

Mastrobattista JM, Luntz M: Ciliary body ablation: Where are we and how did we get there? 1996;43:193.

Maus TL et al: Comparison of dorzolamide and acetazolamide as suppressors of aqueous humor flow in humans. Arch Ophthalmol 1997;115:45.

Mishima HK: A comparison of latanoprost and timolol in primary open-angle glaucoma and ocular hypertension. Arch Ophthalmol 1996;114:929.

Mitchell P et al: Prevalence of open-angel glaucoma in Australia. Ophthalmol 1996;103:1661.

Moorthy RS et al: Glaucoma associated with uveitis. Surv Ophthalmol 1997;41:361.

Nicolela MT, Drance SM: Various glaucomatous optic nerve appearances. Ophthalmol 1996;103:640.

O'Donoghue E: Beta-blockers and the elderly with glaucoma: Are we adding insult to injury? Br J Ophthalmol 1995;79:794.

Ong K et al: Comparative study of brain magnetic resonance imaging findings in patients with low-tension glaucoma and control subjects. Ophthalmology 1995;102:1632.

Patelska B et al: Latanoprost for uncontrolled glaucoma in a compassionate case protocol. Am J Ophthalmol 1997;124:279.

Quigley HA: Number of people with glaucoma worldwide. Br J Ophthalmol 1996;80:389.

Spaeth GL: Patient self-management skills influence the course of glaucoma. Ophthalmology 1997;104:1065.

Stewart WC, Sine CS, LoPresto C: Surgical vs medical management of chronic open-angle glaucoma. Am J Ophthalmol 1996;122:767.

Stewart WC et al: A 90-day study of the efficacy and side effects of 0.25% and 0.5% apraclonidine vs. 0.5% timolol. Arch Ophthalmol 1996;114:938.

Stone EM et al: Identification of a gene that causes primary open angle glaucoma. Science 1997;275:668.

Strahlman ER et al: The use of dorzolamide and pilocarpine as adjunctive therapy to timolol in patients with elevated intraocular pressure. Ophthalmol 1996;103:1283.

Strahlman ER, Tipping R, Vogel R: A double-masked, randomized 1-year study comparing dorzolamide (Trusopt), timolol, and betaxolol. Arch Ophthalmol 1995;113:1009.

Strohmaier I, Snyder E, Adamsons I: Long-term safety and efficacy of COSOPT, a fixed combination of dorzolamide and timolol. Invest Ophthalmol Vis Sci 1996;37 (3):S1102.

Tezel G et al: Comparative optic disc analysis in normal pressure glaucoma, primary open-angle glaucoma, and ocular hypertension. Ophthalmology 1996;103:2105.

Van Buskirk EM: Glaucomatous optic neuropathy. J Glaucoma 1994;3:S2.

Wyse TB et al: Topical prostaglandins for glaucoma therapy. J Glaucoma 1997;6:180.

12

Strabismus

Taylor Asbury, MD, & Douglas R. Fredrick, MD

Under normal binocular viewing conditions, the image of the object of regard falls simultaneously on the fovea of each eye (bifoveal fixation) and the vertical retinal meridians are both upright. Either eye can be misaligned, so that only one eye at a time views the object of regard. Any deviation from perfect ocular alignment is called "strabismus." Misalignment may be in any direction—inward, outward, up, or down. The amount of deviation is the angle by which the deviating eye is misaligned. Strabismus present under binocular viewing conditions is **manifest strabismus, heterotropia,** or **tropia.** A deviation present only after binocular vision has been interrupted (ie, by occlusion of one eye) is called **latent strabismus, heterophoria,** or **phoria.**

Strabismus is present in about 4% of children. Treatment should be started as soon as a diagnosis is made in order to ensure the best possible visual acuity and binocular visual function. There is no such thing as "outgrowing" strabismus.

DEFINITIONS

Angle kappa: The angle between the visual axis and the central pupillary line. When the eye is fixing a light, if the corneal reflection is centered on the pupil, the visual axis and the central pupillary line coincide and the angle kappa is zero. Ordinarily, the light reflex is 2–4 degrees nasal to the pupillary center, giving the appearance of slight exotropia (positive angle kappa). A negative angle kappa gives the false impression of esotropia.

Conjugate movement: Movement of the eyes in the same direction at the same time.

Ductions: (Figure 12–1.) Monocular rotations with no consideration of the position of the other eye.
Adduction: Inward rotation.
Abduction: Outward rotation.
Supraduction (elevation): Upward rotation.
Infraduction (depression): Downward rotation.

Fusion: Formation of one image from the two images seen simultaneously by the two eyes. Fusion has two aspects:
Motor fusion: Adjustments made by the brain in innervation of extraocular muscles in order to bring both eyes into bifoveal and torsional alignment.
Sensory fusion: Integration in the visual sensory areas of the brain of images seen with the two eyes into one picture.

Heterophoria (phoria): Latent deviation of the eyes held straight by binocular fusion.
Esophoria: Tendency for one eye to turn inward.
Exophoria: Tendency for one eye to turn outward.
Hyperphoria: Tendency for one eye to deviate upward.
Hypophoria: Tendency for one eye to deviate downward. (See Hypotropia.)

Heterotropia (tropia):
Strabismus: Manifest deviation of the eyes that cannot be controlled by binocular fusion.
Esotropia: Convergent manifest deviation ("crossed eyes").
Exotropia: Divergent manifest deviation ("wall-eyes").
Hypertropia: Manifest deviation of one eye upward.
Hypotropia: Manifest deviation of one eye downward. By convention, in the absence of specific causation to account for the lower position of one eye, vertical deviations are designated by the higher eye (eg, right hypertropia, not left hypotropia, when the right eye is higher).
Incyclotropia: Inward rotation of one eye about its anteroposterior axis (ie, clockwise right eye, counterclockwise left eye).
Excyclotropia: Outward rotation of one eye about its anteroposterior axis (ie, counterclockwise right eye, clockwise left eye).

Orthophoria: The absence of any tendency of either eye to deviate when fusion is suspended. This state is rarely seen clinically. A small phoria is normal.

Primary deviation: The deviation measured with the normal eye fixing and the eye with the paretic muscle deviating (Figure 12–2).

Prism diopter (Δ): A unit of angular measurement used to characterize ocular deviations. A 1-diopter prism deflects a ray of light toward the base of the prism by 1 centimeter at 1 meter. One degree of arc equals approximately 1.7^Δ.

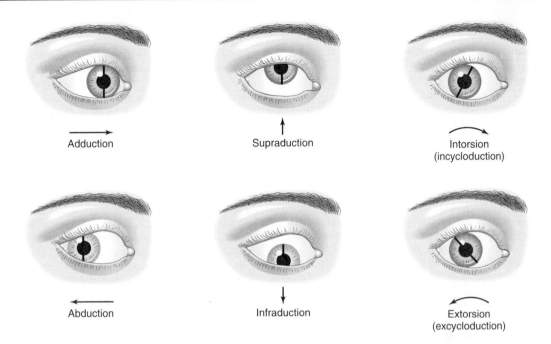

Adduction

Supraduction

Intorsion
(incycloduction)

Abduction

Infraduction

Extorsion
(excycloduction)

Figure 12–1. Ductions (monocular rotations), right eye. Arrows indicate direction of eye movement from primary position.

Secondary deviation: (Figure 12–2.) The deviation measured with the paretic eye fixing and the normal eye deviating.

Torsion: Rotation of the eye about its anteroposterior axis (Figure 12–1).

Intorsion (incycloduction): Rotation of the 12 o'clock meridian of the eye toward the midline of the head.

Extorsion (excycloduction): Rotation of the 12 o'clock meridian of the eye away from the midline of the head.

Vergences (disjunctive movements): Movement of the two eyes in opposite directions.

Convergence: The eyes turn inward.
Divergence: The eyes turn outward.
Versions: Binocular rotations of the eyes in qualitatively the same direction.

PHYSIOLOGY

1. MOTOR ASPECTS

Individual Muscle Functions (Table 12–1)

Each of the six extraocular muscles plays a role in positioning the eye about three axes of rotation. The

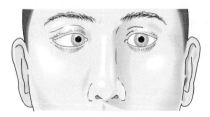

Primary deviation
(left eye fixing)

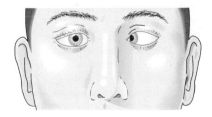

Secondary deviation (right eye fixing;
"overshoot" of sound left eye)

Figure 12–2. Paresis of horizontal muscle (right lateral rectus). Secondary deviation is greater than primary deviation because of Hering's law. With the left eye fixing, the right eye is deviated inward because of the paretic right lateral rectus. For the right eye to fix, the paretic right lateral rectus muscle must receive excessive stimulation. The yoke muscle, the left medial rectus, also receives the same excessive stimulation (Hering's law), which causes "overshoot," shown above.

Table 12–1. Functions of the ocular muscles.

Muscle	Primary Action	Secondary Actions
Lateral rectus	Abduction	None
Medial rectus	Adduction	None
Superior rectus	Elevation	Adduction, intorsion
Inferior rectus	Depression	Adduction, extorsion
Superior oblique	Intorsion	Depression, abduction
Inferior oblique	Extorsion	Elevation, abduction

primary action of a muscle is the principal effect it has on eye rotation. Lesser effects are called secondary or tertiary actions. The exact action of any muscle depends on the direction of the eye in space.

The medial and lateral rectus muscles adduct and abduct the eye, respectively, with little effect on elevation or torsion. The vertical rectus and oblique muscles have vertical rotation and torsional functions. In general terms, the vertical rectus muscles are the main elevators and depressors of the eye, and the obliques are mostly involved with torsional positioning. The vertical effect of the superior and inferior rectus muscles is greater when the eye is abducted. The vertical effect of the obliques is greater when the eye is adducted.

Field of Action

The position of the eye is determined by the equilibrium achieved by the pull of all six extraocular muscles. The eyes are in the **primary position of gaze** when they are looking straight ahead with the head and body erect. To move the eye into another direction of gaze, the agonist muscle contracts to pull the eye in that direction and the antagonist muscle relaxes. The field of action of a muscle is the direction of gaze in which that muscle exerts its greatest contraction force as an agonist, eg, the lateral rectus muscle undergoes the greatest contraction in abducting the eye (Table 12–1).

Synergistic & Antagonistic Muscles (Sherrington's Law)

Synergistic muscles are those that have the same field of action. Thus, for vertical gaze, the superior rectus and inferior oblique muscles are synergists in moving the eye upward. Muscles synergistic for one function may be antagonistic for another. For example, the superior rectus and inferior oblique muscles are antagonists for torsion, the superior rectus causing intorsion and the inferior oblique extorsion. The extraocular muscles, like skeletal muscles, show reciprocal innervation of antagonistic muscles (Sherrington's law). Thus, in dextroversion (right gaze), the right medial and left lateral rectus muscles are inhibited while the right lateral and left medial rectus muscles are stimulated.

Yoke Muscles (Hering's Law)

For movements of both eyes in the same direction, the corresponding agonist muscles receive equal innervation (Hering's law). The pair of agonist muscles with the same primary action is called a yoke pair. The right lateral rectus and the left medial rectus muscles are a yoke pair for right gaze. The right inferior rectus and the left superior oblique muscles are a yoke pair for gaze downward and to the right. Table 12–2 lists the yoke muscle combinations.

Development of Binocular Movement

The neuromuscular system of an infant is immature, so that it is not uncommon in the first few months of life for ocular alignment to be unstable. Transient esodeviations are most common and may be associated with immaturity of the accommodation-convergence system. Gradually improving visual acuity together with maturation of the oculomotor system allows a more stable ocular alignment by age 2 months. Any ocular misalignment after this age should be investigated by an ophthalmologist.

2. SENSORY ASPECTS

Binocular Vision

In each eye, whatever is imaged on the fovea is seen subjectively as being straight ahead. Thus, if two dissimilar objects were imaged on the two foveas, the two objects would be seen superimposed, but the dissimilarities would prevent fusion into a single impression. Because of the different vantage point in space of each eye, the image in each eye is actually slightly different from that in the other. Sensory fusion and stereopsis are the two different physiologic processes that are responsible for binocular vision.

Table 12–2. Yoke muscles in cardinal positions of gaze.

Eyes up and right	RSR and LIO
Eyes up and left	LSR and RIO
Eyes right	RLR and LMR
Eyes left	LLR and RMR
Eyes down and right	RIR and LSO
Eyes down and left	LIR and RSO

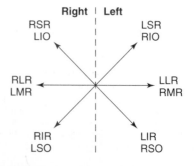

Sensory Fusion & Stereopsis

Sensory fusion is the process whereby dissimilarities between the two images are not appreciated. On the peripheral retina of each eye, there are **corresponding points** that in the absence of fusion localize stimuli in the same direction in space. In the process of fusion, the direction values of these points can be modified. Thus, each point of the retina in each eye is capable of fusing stimuli that strike sufficiently close to the corresponding point in the other eye. This region of fusible points is called **Panum's area.**

Fusion is possible because subtle differences between the two images are ignored, and stereopsis, or binocular depth perception, occurs because of the cerebral integration of these two slightly dissimilar images.

Sensory Changes in Strabismus

Up to age 7 or 8, the brain usually develops responses to abnormal binocular vision that may not occur if the onset of strabismus is later. These changes include diplopia, suppression, anomalous retinal correspondence, and eccentric fixation.

A. Diplopia: If strabismus is present, each fovea receives a different image. The objects imaged on the two foveas are seen in the same direction in space. This process of localization of spatially separate objects to the same location is called **visual confusion.** The object viewed by one of the foveas is imaged on a peripheral retinal area in the other eye. The foveal image is localized straight ahead, while the peripheral image of the same object in the other eye is localized in some other direction. Thus, the same object is seen in two places (diplopia).

B. Suppression: Under binocular viewing conditions, the images seen by one eye become predominant and those seen by the other eye are not perceived (suppression). Suppression takes the form of a **scotoma** in the deviating eye only under binocular viewing conditions. (A scotoma is an area of reduced vision within the visual field, surrounded by an area of less depressed or normal vision.) Suppression scotomas in esotropia are usually approximately elliptical in shape, extending on the retina from just temporal to the fovea to the point in the peripheral retina where the object of regard for the other eye is imaged. In exotropia, the suppression area tends to be larger and extends from the fovea to usually the entire temporal half of the retina. When fixation shifts to the other eye, the suppression scotoma also switches to the newly deviating eye. In the absence of strabismus, a blurred image in one eye may also lead to suppression. The lack of simultaneous perception in the central retina prevents fine stereopsis, though crude stereopsis from the peripheral retina may still be present.

C. Amblyopia: Prolonged abnormal visual experience in a child under the age of 7 years may lead to amblyopia (reduced visual acuity in the absence of detectable organic disease in one eye). The two clinical contexts in which amblyopia occurs are strabismus and any disorder that causes a blurred retinal image in one or both eyes, eg, a significant refractive difference between the eyes (**anisometropia**) or visual deprivation such as that due to congenital cataract.

In strabismus, the eye used habitually for fixation retains normal acuity and the nonpreferred eye often develops decreased vision (amblyopia). If spontaneous alternation of fixation is present, amblyopia does not develop. Suppression and amblyopia are different processes. Amblyopia is present when the affected eye is tested alone. Suppression occurs under binocular conditions and is a process in which the brain "ignores" a portion of the image received from the deviating eye so that the patient avoids diplopia. This visual field defect is termed a facultative scotoma, since no visual deficit can be demonstrated when the suppressing eye is tested alone.

D. Anomalous Retinal Correspondence: Anomalous retinal correspondence is a sensory adaptation that occurs in strabismus under binocular viewing conditions. Heterotropia leads to suppression in the nonfixating eye and a shift in the visual direction of the deviated eye. This shift in visual direction offsets the amount of motor deviation and prevents the perception of diplopia. This binocular phenomenon allows some form of binocular cooperation to occur in patients with strabismus, but stereopsis will remain abnormal.

E. Eccentric Fixation: In eyes with sufficiently severe amblyopia, an extrafoveal retinal area may be used for fixation under monocular viewing conditions. It is always associated with severe amblyopia and unstable fixation. The eccentric fixation point is often not displaced in a direction appropriate to the direction of strabismus (eg, the nasal retina in esotropia). Gross eccentric fixation can be readily identified clinically by occluding the dominant eye and directing the patient's attention to a light source held directly in front. An eye with gross eccentric fixation will not point toward the light source but will appear to be looking in some other direction. More subtle degrees of eccentric fixation can be detected by an ophthalmoscope that projects a small fixation target onto the retina. If any area other than the macula is selected for fixation by the patient, the presence of eccentric fixation has been established.

EXAMINATION

History

A careful history is important in the diagnosis of strabismus.

A. Family History: Strabismus and amblyopia are frequently found to occur in families.

B. Age at Onset: This is an important factor in long-term prognosis. The earlier the onset of strabismus, the worse the prognosis for good binocular function.

C. Type of Onset: The onset may be gradual, sudden, or intermittent.

D. Type of Deviation: The misalignment may be in any direction. It may be greater in certain positions of gaze, including the primary position for distance or near.

E. Fixation: One eye may constantly deviate, or alternating fixation may be observed.

Visual Acuity

Visual acuity should be evaluated even if only a rough approximation or comparison of the two eyes is possible. Each eye is evaluated by itself, since binocular testing will not reveal poor vision in one eye. For the very young child, it may only be possible to establish that an eye is able to follow a moving target. The target should be as small as the child's age, interest, and level of alertness allow. Fixation is described as being normal if it is centrally (foveally) fixated and maintained while the eye follows a moving object. One technique for quantitatively measuring visual acuity in younger children is forced-choice preferential looking.

By the age of $2^1/_2$–3 years, it is possible to perform recognition visual acuity testing using the Allen pictures. By age 4 years, many children will understand the Snellen tumbling "E" game and the HOTV recognition test. By age 5 or 6 years, most children can respond to Snellen alphabet visual acuity testing. At this age, single optotype Snellen acuity has normally developed fully, but Snellen acuity to a line of multiple optotypes (linear acuity) may not develop fully for another 2 years.

Determination of Refractive Error

It is important to determine the cycloplegic refractive error by retinoscopy (see Chapter 20). The standard drug for producing complete cycloplegia in children under age 2 years is atropine, which may be given as 0.5% or 1% eye drops or ointment instilled twice a day for 3 days. Atropine should not be used in older children, since prolonged cycloplegia lasting up to 2 weeks will interfere with near vision. After age 2, cyclopentolate 1% or 2% is the preferred cycloplegic.

Inspection

Inspection alone may show whether the strabismus is constant or intermittent, alternating or nonalternating, and variable or constant. Associated ptosis and abnormal position of the head may also be noted. The quality of fixation of each eye separately and of both eyes together should be noted. Nystagmoid movements indicate unstable fixation and often reduced visual acuity.

Prominent epicanthal folds that obscure all or part of the nasal sclera may give an appearance of esotropia (pseudoesotropia). Although this entity is confusing to lay persons as well as some physicians, these children have a normal corneal light reflection test. Prominent epicanthal folds gradually disappear by 4 or 5 years of age.

Determination of Angle of Strabismus (Angle of Deviation)

A. Prism and Cover Tests: (Figure 12–3.) Cover tests consist of four parts: (1) the cover test, (2) the uncover test, (3) the alternate cover test, and (4) the prism cover test. In all four tests, the patient looks intently at a target, which may be in any direction of gaze at distance or near.

1. Cover test–As the examiner observes one eye, a cover is placed in front of the other eye to block its view of the target. If the observed eye moves to take up fixation, it was not previously fixating the target, and a manifest deviation (strabismus) is present. The direction of movement reveals the direction of deviation (eg, the eye moves outwardly if there is esotropia).

2. Uncover test–As the cover is removed from the eye following the cover test, the eye emerging from under cover is observed. If the position of the eye changes, interruption of binocular vision has allowed it to deviate, and heterophoria is present. The direction of corrective movement shows the type of heterophoria.

3. Alternate cover test–The cover is placed alternately in front of first one eye and then the other. This test reveals the total deviation (heterotropia plus heterophoria if also present).

4. Prism plus cover testing–To quantitatively measure the deviation, an increasing strength of prism is placed in front of one or both eyes until there is neutralization of eye movement on alternate cover testing. For example, to measure full esodeviation, the cover is alternated while prisms of increasing base-out strength are placed in front of one or both eyes until the horizontal refixation movement of the deviated eye is neutralized.

B. Objective Tests: Prism and cover measurements are objective in the sense that no report of sensory observations is required from the patient. However, cooperation and some degree of vision are required. Clinical determinations of eye position that require no sensory observation by the patient (objective tests) are considerably less accurate, although still useful at times. Two methods commonly used depend on observing the position of the corneal reflection of a light. Results by both methods must be modified by allowing for the angle kappa.

1. Hirschberg method–The patient fixates a light at a distance of about 33 cm (13 inches). Decentering of the light reflection is noted in the deviating eye. By allowing 18^Δ for each millimeter of decentration, an estimate of the angle of deviation can be made.

2. Prism reflex method (Krimsky test)–The patient fixates a light. A prism is placed before the deviating eye, and the strength of the prism required to center the corneal reflection measures the angle of deviation.

Ductions (Monocular Rotations)

With one eye covered, the other eye follows a moving target in all directions of gaze. Any decrease of rotation indicates weakness in the field of action of that muscle.

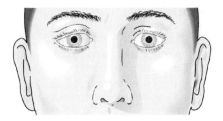

Eyes straight (maintained in position by fusion).

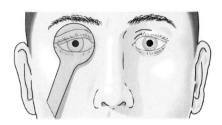

Position of eye under cover in orthophoria (fusion-free position). The right eye under cover has not moved.

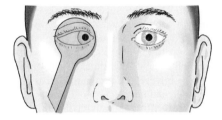

Position of eye under cover in esophoria (fusion-free position). Under cover, the right eye has deviated inward. Upon removal of cover, the right eye will immediately resume its straight-ahead position.

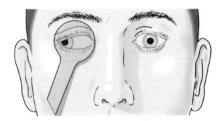

Position of eye under cover in exophoria (fusion-free position). Under cover, the right eye has deviated outward. Upon removal of the cover, the right eye will immediately resume its straight-ahead position.

Figure 12–3. Cover testing. The patient is directed to look at a target at eye level 6 m (20 feet) away. ***Note:*** In the presence of strabismus, the deviation will remain when the cover is removed.

Versions (Conjugate Ocular Movements)

Hering's law states that yoke muscles receive equal stimulation during any conjugate ocular movement. Versions are tested by having the eyes follow a light in the nine diagnostic positions: primary—straight ahead; secondary—right, left, up, and down; and tertiary—up and right, down and right, up and left, and down and left (Table 12–2). Apparent rotation of one eye relative to the other is noted as overaction or underaction. By convention, in the tertiary positions, the oblique muscles are said to be overacting or underacting with respect to the yoke rectus muscle. Fixation in the field of action of a paretic muscle results in overaction of the yoke muscle, since greater innervation is required for contraction of the underacting muscles (Figure 12–4). Conversely, fixation by the normal eye will lead to underaction of the paretic muscle.

Disjunctive Movements

A. Convergence: (Figure 12–5.) As the eyes follow an approaching object, they must turn inward in order to maintain alignment of the visual axes with the object of regard. The medial rectus muscles are contracting and the lateral rectus muscles are relaxing under the influence of neural stimulation and inhibi-

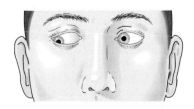

Fixing with normal right eye

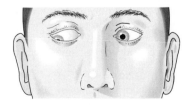

Fixing with paretic left eye

Figure 12–4. Testing versions. Example of paretic left superior oblique.

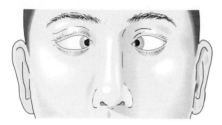

Figure 12–5. Convergence. The position of the eyes at the normal near point of convergence (NPC) is shown above. The break point is within 5 cm of the bridge of the nose.

tion. (Neural pathways of supranuclear control are discussed in Chapter 14.)

Convergence is an active process with a strong voluntary as well as involuntary component. An important consideration in evaluating the extraocular muscles in strabismus is convergence.

To test convergence, a small object is slowly brought toward the bridge of the nose. The patient's attention is directed to the object by saying, "Keep the image from going double as long as possible." Convergence can normally be maintained until the object is nearly to the bridge of the nose. An actual numerical value is placed on convergence by measuring the distance from the bridge of the nose (in centimeters) at which the eyes "break" (ie, when the nondominant eye swings laterally so that convergence is no longer maintained). This point is termed the **near point of convergence,** and a value of up to 5 cm (2 inches) is considered within normal limits.

The ratio of accommodative convergence to accommodation (AC/A ratio) is a way of quantitating the relationship of convergence to accommodation. Accommodative convergence is elicited by viewing an accommodative target, ie, one that has resolvable contours or letters that stimulate accommodation. The result is commonly expressed as prism diopters of convergence per diopter of accommodation. The AC/A ratio is useful as a research tool to further investigate and clarify this relationship and has contributed significantly to our understanding and therefore to the treatment of accommodative esotropia—particularly in using bifocals and miotics, as described later in this chapter.

B. Divergence: Electromyography has established that divergence is an active process, not merely a relaxation of convergence. Clinically, this function is seldom tested except in considering the amplitudes of fusion.

Sensory Examination

While many tests of the status of binocular vision have been devised, only a few need be mentioned here. The tests are for stereopsis, suppression, and fusion potential. All require the simultaneous presentation of two targets separately, one to each eye.

A. Stereopsis Testing: Many stereopsis tests are done with targets and Polaroid glasses to separate the stimuli. The monocularly observed targets have nearly imperceptible clues of depth. **Random dot stereograms** have no monocular depth clues. A field of random dots is seen by each eye, but the dot-to-corresponding-dot correlation between the two targets is such that if stereopsis is present, a form is seen in three dimensions.

B. Suppression Testing: The presence of suppression is readily demonstrated with the **Worth four-dot test.** Glasses containing a red lens over one eye and a green lens over the other are placed on the patient. A flashlight containing red, green, and white spots is viewed. The color spots are markers for perception through each eye, and the white dot, potentially visible to each eye, can indicate the presence of diplopia. The separation of the spots and the distance at which the light is held determine the size of the retinal area tested. Foveal and peripheral areas may be tested at distance and near.

C. Fusion Potential: In individuals with a manifest deviation, the status of binocular fusion potential can be determined by the red filter test. A red filter is placed over one eye. The patient is directed to look at a distance or near fixation light target. A red light and a white light are seen. Prisms are placed over one or both eyes in an attempt to bring the two images together. If fusion potential exists, the two images come together and are seen as a single pink light. If no fusion potential exists, the patient will continue to see one red and one white light.

OBJECTIVES & PRINCIPLES OF THERAPY OF STRABISMUS

The main objectives of strabismus treatment in children are (1) reversal of the deleterious sensory effects of strabismus (amblyopia, suppression, and loss of stereopsis) and (2) best possible alignment of the eyes by medical or surgical treatment. In all cases, the psychologic benefit of cosmetically straight eyes cannot be overestimated.

Timing of Treatment in Children

A child can be examined at any age, and treatment for amblyopia or strabismus should be instituted as soon as the diagnosis is made. Neurophysiologic studies in animals have shown that the infant brain is quite responsive to sensory experience, and the quality of function possible later in life is greatly influenced by early life experiences. It has been shown that overall results are favorably influenced by early alignment of the eyes, preferably by age 2. Good eye alignment can be achieved later, but normal sensory adaptation becomes more difficult as the child grows older. By age 8, the sensory status is generally so fixed that deficient stereopsis and amblyopia cannot be effectively treated.

Medical Treatment

Nonsurgical treatment of strabismus includes treatment of amblyopia, the use of optical devices (prisms and glasses), pharmacologic agents, and orthoptics.

A. Treatment of Amblyopia: The elimination of amblyopia is crucial in the treatment of strabismus and is always one of the first goals. The strabismic deviation may lessen—rarely enlarge—following the treatment of amblyopia. Surgical results are more predictable and stable if there is good visual acuity in each eye preoperatively.

1. Occlusion therapy–The mainstay of amblyopia treatment is occlusion. The sound eye is covered with a patch to stimulate the amblyopic eye. Glasses are also used if there is a significant refractive error.

Two stages of successful amblyopia treatment are identified: initial improvement and maintenance of the improved visual acuity.

a. Initial stage–Full-time occlusion is the standard initial treatment. In some cases only part-time occlusion is used if the amblyopia is not too severe or the child is very young. As a guideline, full-time occlusion may be done for as many weeks as the child's age in years without risk of reduced vision in the sound eye. Occlusion treatment is continued in some form as long as visual acuity improves (occasionally up to a year). It is not worthwhile continuing to patch for more than 4 months if there is no improvement.

Amblyopia is functional (ie, there is no identifiable organic lesion, although the adaptation must be cerebral). In most cases, if treatment is started soon enough, substantial improvement or complete normalization of visual acuity can be achieved. Occasionally, there is no improvement even under ideal conditions. Poor compliance with treatment (peeking around a patch or inadequate enforcement of patching by the parents) can always be a factor.

b. Maintenance stage–Maintenance treatment consists of part-time patching continued after the improvement phase to maintain the best possible vision beyond an age when amblyopia is likely to recur (about age 8).

2. Atropine therapy–A few children are intolerant to occlusion therapy. In such cases that have moderate or high hyperopia, atropine therapy may be effective. Atropine causes cycloplegia and therefore decreased accommodative ability. The sound eye is atropinized, and glasses are used to focus that eye for distance or near fixation only. This forces use of the amblyopic eye at all other times. Atropine 1%, 1 drop every few days, is usually sufficient for sustained cycloplegia.

B. Optical Devices:

1. Spectacles–The most important optical device in the treatment of strabismus is accurately prescribed spectacles. The clarification of the retinal image produced by glasses allows the natural fusion mechanisms to operate to the fullest extent. Small refractive errors need not be corrected. If there is significant hyperopia and esotropia, the esotropia probably is at least partially due to the hyperopia (accommodative esotropia). The prescription compensates for the full cycloplegic findings. If bifocals permit sufficient relaxation of accommodation to allow for near fusion, they should be used.

2. Prisms–Prisms produce optical redirection of the line of sight. Corresponding retinal elements are brought into line to eliminate diplopia. Correct sensory alignment of the eyes is also a form of antisuppression treatment. Used preoperatively, prisms can simulate the sensory effect that will follow successful surgery. In patients with horizontal deviation, prisms will show the patient's ability to fuse a simultaneous small vertical deviation, thus indicating whether surgery also needs to be done for the vertical component. In children with esotropia, prisms can be used preoperatively to predict a postoperative shift in position that might nullify the surgical result, and the planned surgery can be modified accordingly (prism adaptation test).

Prisms can be implemented in several ways. A particularly convenient form is the plastic Fresnel press-on prism. These plastic membranes can be placed on the glasses without the need for an optician and are very useful for diagnostic and temporary therapeutic purposes. For permanent wear, prisms are best ground into the spectacle prescription, but the amount is limited to about 5^Δ per lens since prismatic distortion becomes prominent at higher strengths.

C. Pharmacologic Agents:

1. Miotics–Echothiophate iodide and isoflurophate inactivate acetylcholinesterase at the neuromuscular junction and thus potentiate the effect of every nerve impulse. Accommodation becomes more effective relative to convergence than before treatment. Since accommodation controls the near reflex (the triad of accommodation, convergence, and miosis), less convergence will occur with reduced accommodation and the angle of deviation will be significantly reduced, often to zero.

Miotics have been used extensively for diagnosis and treatment of accommodative esotropia with or without an accompanying high accommodative convergence-to-accommodation (AC/A) ratio. In children who present with acquired esotropia and who have less than +3.00 spherical hyperopia, miotics can be used diagnostically. If after 4–6 weeks the esodeviation is eliminated, the diagnosis of accommodative esotropia is established. Miotic treatment can be continued, or fully corrected hyperopic glasses can be prescribed. Miotics may also be used in association with single vision glasses to avoid bifocals in many patients with a high AC/A ratio. Long-term use of miotics in children can be associated with development of iris cysts; this can be prevented by coadministration with phenylephrine solution.

2. Botulinum toxin–The injection of botulinum toxin type A (Botox) into an extraocular muscle produces a dose-dependent duration of paralysis of that muscle. The injection is given under electromyographic positional control using a bipolar electrode needle. The toxin is tightly bound to the muscle tissue. The doses used are so small that systemic toxicity does not occur. The desired length of paralysis is dependent upon the angle of deviation. The larger the angle of deviation, the longer the duration of paralysis required. Paralysis of the muscle shifts the eye into the field of action of the antagonist muscle. During the time the eye is deviated, the paralyzed muscle is stretched, whereas the antagonist muscle is contracted. As the paralysis resolves, the eye will gradually return toward its original position but with a new balance of forces that permanently reduces or eliminates the deviation. Two or more injections are often necessary to obtain a lasting effect.

D. Orthoptics: An orthoptist is trained in methods of testing and treating patients with strabismus. Orthoptists offer significant help to the ophthalmologist, particularly in diagnosis and to a lesser extent in treatment. Evaluation of the sensory status may be very helpful in determining the fusion potential. An orthoptist may be able to aid in preoperative treatment,

especially with patients who have amblyopia. At times, orthoptic training and instructions for "exercises" to be used at home can supplement and solidify surgical treatment.

Surgical Treatment
(Figure 12–6)

A. Surgical Procedures: A variety of changes in the rotational effect of an extraocular muscle can be achieved with surgery.

1. Resection and recession–Conceptually, the simplest procedures are strengthening and weakening. A muscle is strengthened by a procedure called **resection.** The muscle is detached from the eye, stretched out longer by a measured amount, and then resewn to the eye, usually at the original insertion site. The small amount of extra length is trimmed off. **Recession** is the standard weakening procedure. The muscle is detached from the eye, freed from fascial attachments, and allowed to retract. It is resewn to the eye a measured distance behind its original insertion.

The superior oblique is strengthened by tucking or advancing its tendon. This can be done by a graded

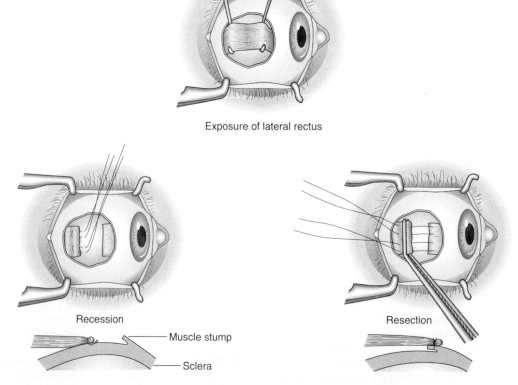

Exposure of lateral rectus

Recession

Resection

— Muscle stump

— Sclera

Figure 12–6. Surgical correction of strabismus (right eye).

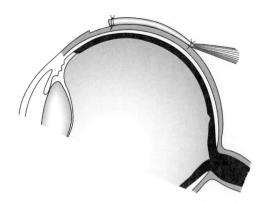

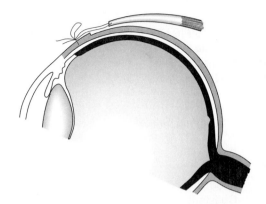

Figure 12–7. Posterior fixation (Faden) procedure. The rectus muscle is tacked to the sclera far posterior to its insertion. This prevents unwrapping of the muscle as the eye turns into the muscle's field of action. The muscle is progressively weakened in its field of action. If this procedure is combined with recession, the alignment in primary position is also affected.

Figure 12–8. Adjustable suture. The suture is placed on the sclera at any point that will be accessible to the surgeon. The bow is untied and the position of the muscle changed as desired.

amount. Superior oblique weakening is accomplished by a tenectomy (complete or partial division of the tendon) or one of several lengthening procedures. There is no effective strengthening procedure on the inferior oblique. The inferior oblique can be weakened by disinsertion, myectomy, or recession, with generally equivalent results.

2. Shifting of point of muscle attachment–In addition to simple strengthening or weakening, the point of attachment of the muscle can be shifted; this may give the muscle a rotational action it did not previously have. For example, a vertical shift of both horizontal rectus muscles on the same eye affects the vertical position of the eye. Vertical shifts of the horizontal rectus muscles in opposite directions affect the horizontal eye position in upgaze and downgaze. This is done for **A** or **V** patterns, in which the horizontal deviation is more of an esodeviation in upgaze or downgaze, respectively.

The torsional effect of a muscle can also be changed. Tightening of the anterior fibers of the superior oblique tendon, known as the Harada-Ito procedure, gives that muscle enhanced torsional action.

3. Faden procedure–A special operation for muscle weakening is called the posterior fixation (Faden) procedure (Figure 12–7). In this operation, a new insertion of the muscle is created well behind the original insertion. This causes mechanical weakening of the muscle as the eye rotates into its field of action. When combined with recession of the same muscle, the Faden operation has a profound weakening effect on the muscle without significant alteration of the primary position of the eye. The procedure can be effective on vertical rectus muscles (dissociated vertical deviation) or horizontal muscles (high AC/A ratio, nystagmus, and other rare incomitant muscle imbalances).

B. Choice of Muscles for Surgery: The decision concerning which muscles to operate on is based on several factors. The first is the amount of misalignment measured in the primary position. Modifications are made for significant differences in distance and near measurements. The medial rectus muscles have more effect on the angle of deviation for near and the lateral rectus muscles more effect for distance. For esotropia greater at near, both medial rectus muscles should be weakened. For exotropia greater at distance, both lateral rectus muscles should be weakened. For deviations approximately the same at distance and near, bilateral weakening procedures or unilateral recession/resection procedures are equally effective.

Surgical realignment affects only the muscular or mechanical part of a neuromuscular imbalance. Although most individuals respond in a predictable manner, variable responses may be due to differing mechanical properties of the muscles and surrounding tissues as well as variable innervational input. For these reasons, more than one operation may be required to obtain a satisfactory result.

C. Adjustable Sutures: (Figure 12–8.) The development of adjustable sutures offers a great advantage in muscle surgery, particularly for reoperations and incomitant deviations. During the operation, the muscle is reattached to the sclera with a slip knot placed so that it is accessible to the surgeon. After the patient has recovered sufficiently from the anesthesia to cooperate in the adjustment process, a topical anesthetic drop is placed in the eye and the suture can be tightened or loosened to change the eye position as indicated by cover testing. Adjustable sutures can be used on any rectus muscle for either recession or resection and on the superior oblique muscle for correction of torsion. Although any patient willing to cooperate is suitable, the method is usually not applicable for children under age 12.

CLASSIFICATION OF STRABISMUS
Esotropia
    Nonparetic
        Nonaccommodative
            Infantile
            Acquired
        Accommodative
        Partially accommodative
    Paretic
Exotropia
    Intermittent
    Constant
"A" and "V" patterns
Hypertropia
    Nonparetic
    Paretic

ESOTROPIA
(Convergent Strabismus, "Crossed Eyes")

Esotropia is by far the most common type of strabismus. It is divided into two types: **paretic** (due to paresis or paralysis of one or both lateral rectus muscles) and **nonparetic** (comitant). Nonparetic esotropia is the most common type in infants and children; it may be accommodative, nonaccommodative, or partially accommodative. Paretic strabismus is uncommon in childhood but accounts for most new cases of strabismus in adults. Most cases of childhood nonaccommodative esotropia are classified as **infantile esotropia,** with onset by age 6 months. The remainder occur after age 6 months and are classified as **acquired nonaccommodative esotropia.**

NONPARETIC ESOTROPIA

Nonaccommodative Esotropia
A. Infantile Esotropia: Nearly half of all cases of esotropia fall into this group. In most cases, the cause is obscure. The convergent deviation is manifest by age 6 months. The deviation is comitant, ie, the angle of deviation is approximately the same in all directions of gaze and is usually not affected by accommodation. The cause, therefore, is not related to the refractive error or dependent upon a paretic extraocular muscle. It is likely that the majority of cases are due to faulty innervational control, involving the supranuclear pathways for convergence and divergence and their neural connections to the me-

dial longitudinal fasciculus. A smaller number of cases are due to anatomic variations such as anomalous insertions of horizontally acting muscles, abnormal check ligaments, or various other fascial abnormalities.

There is also good evidence that strabismus does occur on a genetically determined basis. Esophoria and esotropia are frequently passed on as an autosomal dominant trait. Siblings may have similar ocular deviations. An accommodative element is often superimposed upon comitant esotropia, ie, correction of the hyperopic refractive error reduces but does not eliminate all of the deviation.

The deviation is often large ($\geq 40^\Delta$). Abduction may be limited but can be demonstrated. Vertical deviations may be observed after 18 months of age as a result of overaction of the oblique muscles or dissociated vertical deviation. Nystagmus, manifest or latent, may be present. The most common refractive error is low to moderate hyperopia.

The eye that appears to be straight is the eye used for fixation. Almost without exception, it is the eye with better vision or lower refractive error (or both). If there is anisometropia, there will probably be some amblyopia as well. If at various times either eye is used for fixation, the patient is said to show spontaneous alternation of fixation; in this case, vision will be equal or nearly equal in both eyes. In some cases, the eye preference is determined by the direction of gaze. For example, with large-angle esotropia, there is a tendency for the right eye to be used in left gaze and the left eye in right gaze (cross fixation).

Infantile esotropia is treated surgically. Preliminary nonsurgical treatment may be indicated to ensure the best possible result. It is essential that amblyopia be fully treated prior to surgery. Glasses should be tried in hyperopic refractive errors of 3 D or more to determine if reducing accommodation has a favorable effect on the deviation. A myotic may be used successfully as an alternative to glasses if the refractive error is not above approximately 4 D.

Surgery is usually indicated after medical therapy and treatment of amblyopia have been completed. Once reproducible measurements are obtained, surgery should be performed since there is ample evidence that sensory results are better the sooner the eyes are aligned. Many procedures have been recommended, but the two most popular are (1) weakening of both medial rectus muscles, and (2) recession of the medial rectus and resection of the lateral rectus on the same eye.

B. Acquired Nonaccommodative Esotropia: This type of esotropia develops in childhood, usually after the age of 2 years. There is little or no accommodative factor. The angle of strabismus is often smaller than in infantile esotropia but may increase with time. Otherwise, clinical findings are the same as for congenital esotropia. Treatment is surgical and follows the same guidelines as for congenital esotropia.

Accommodative Esotropia

Accommodative esotropia occurs when there is a normal physiologic mechanism of accommodation with an associated overactive convergence response but insufficient relative fusional divergence to hold the eyes straight. There are two pathophysiologic mechanisms at work, singly or together: (1) sufficiently high hyperopia, requiring so much accommodation (and therefore convergence) to clarify the image that esotropia results; and (2) a high AC/A ratio, which is accompanied by mild to moderate hyperopia (1.5 D or more).

A. Accommodative Esotropia Due to Hyperopia: Accommodative esotropia due to hyperopia typically begins at age 2–3 but may occur earlier or later. Deviation is variable prior to treatment. Glasses with full cycloplegic refraction allow the eyes to become aligned.

B. Accommodative Esotropia Due to High AC/A Ratio: In accommodative esotropia due to a high ratio of accommodative convergence to accommodation (AC/A ratio), a deviation is greater at near than at distance. The refractive error is hyperopic. Treatment is with glasses with full cycloplegic refraction plus bifocals or miotics to relieve excess deviation at near.

Partially Accommodative Esotropia

A mixed mechanism—part muscular imbalance and part accommodative/convergence imbalance—may exist. Although antiaccommodative therapy decreases the angle of deviation, the esotropia is not eliminated. Surgery is performed for the nonaccommodative component of the deviation with the choice of surgical procedure as described for infantile esotropia.

PARETIC (INCOMITANT) ESOTROPIA (Abducens Palsy) (Figures 12–2 and 12–9)

Incomitant strabismus results from paresis or restriction of action of one or more extraocular muscles. Incomitant esotropia is usually due to paresis of one or both lateral rectus muscles as a result of unilateral or bilateral abducens nerve palsy (see Chapter 14). Other causes are fracture of the medial orbital wall with entrapment of the medial rectus muscle, dysthyroid eye disease with contracture of the medial rectus muscles, and Duane's retraction syndrome (see below). Abducens nerve palsy is most frequently seen in adults with systemic hypertension or diabetes, in which case spontaneous resolution usually begins within 3 months. Abducens palsy may also be the first sign of intracranial tumor or inflammatory disease. Associated neurologic signs are then important clues. Head trauma is another frequent cause of abducens palsy.

Incomitant esotropia is also seen in infants and children, but much less commonly than comitant esotropia. These cases result from birth injuries affecting the lateral rectus muscle directly, from injury to the nerve, or, less commonly, from a congenital anomaly of the muscle or its fascial attachments.

Esotropia is characteristically greater at distance than at near and greater to the affected side. Paresis of the right lateral rectus causes esotropia that becomes

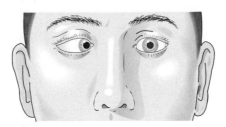

Primary position: right esotropia

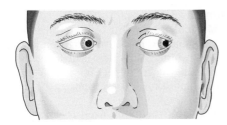

Left gaze: no deviation

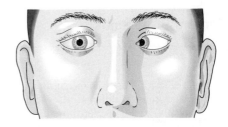

Right gaze: left esotropia

Figure 12–9. Incomitant strabismus (paralytic). Paralysis of right lateral rectus muscle, with left eye fixing.

greater on right gaze and, if paresis is mild, little or no deviation on left gaze. If the lateral rectus muscle is totally paralyzed, the eye will not abduct past the midline.

Acquired abducens palsy is initially managed by occlusion of the paretic eye or with prisms. Botulinum toxin type A injections into the antagonist medial rectus muscle may provide symptomatic relief but do not appear to influence the final outcome. If lateral rectus function in incomplete palsies has not recovered after 6 months, medial rectus botulinum toxin type A injections may be used on a long-term basis to allow fusion—and hence abolition of diplopia—in straight-ahead gaze or to facilitate prism therapy. Horizontal rectus muscle surgery, involving resection of one or both lateral recti and recessions of the medial recti, may also be valuable. Adjustable sutures are useful in achieving the largest possible area of binocular single vision. In complete palsies that have failed to improve after 6 months, surgical transposition of the insertions of the superior and inferior rectus muscles to the insertion of the lateral rectus muscle, combined with temporary paralysis of the medial rectus muscle by botulinum toxin type A, produces the best results. Abduction cannot be restored, but fusion in primary position, with or without the aid of prisms, and a reasonable field of binocular single vision can usually be achieved.

Pseudoesotropia

Pseudoesotropia is the illusion of crossed eyes in an infant or toddler when no strabismus is present. This appearance is usually caused by a flat, broad nasal bridge and prominent epicanthal folds that cover a portion of the nasal sclera, giving the impression that the eyes are crossed. This very common condition may be differentiated from true misalignment by the corneal light reflection appearing in the center of the pupil of each eye when the child fixates a light. With normal facial growth and increasing prominence of the nasal bridge, this pseudoestropic appearance gradually disappears. Of course, true esotropia may be present in association with this common infantile facial configuration.

EXOTROPIA
(Divergent Strabismus)

Exotropia is less common than esotropia, particularly in infancy and childhood. Its incidence increases gradually with age. Not infrequently, a tendency to divergent strabismus beginning as exophoria progresses to intermittent exotropia and finally to constant exotropia if no treatment is given. Other cases begin as constant or intermittent ex-

otropia and remain stationary. As in esotropia, there may be a hereditary element in some cases. Exophoria and exotropia (considered as a single entity of divergent deviation) are frequently passed on as autosomal dominant traits, so that one or both parents of an exotropic child may demonstrate exotropia or a high degree of exophoria.

Alternative Classification of Exotropia

Constant or intermittent exotropia can also be classified on a descriptive basis as being an excess of divergence or an insufficiency of convergence. These descriptive terms do not imply that the cause of the deviation is understood.

A. Basic Exotropia: Distance and near deviations are approximately equal.

B. Divergence Excess: Distance deviation is significantly larger than near deviation.

C. Convergence Insufficiency: Near deviation is significantly larger than distance deviation.

D. Pseudodivergence Excess: Distance deviation is significantly larger than near deviation: however, use of a +3 diopter lens for near measurement will cause the near deviation to become approximately equal to the distance deviation.

INTERMITTENT EXOTROPIA

Clinical Findings

Intermittent exotropia accounts for well over half of all cases of exotropia. The onset of the deviation may be in the first year, and practically all have presented by age 5. The history often reveals that the condition has become progressively worse. A characteristic sign is closing one eye in bright light (Figure 12–10). The manifest exotropia first becomes noticeable with distance fixation. The patient usually fuses at near, overcoming moderate to large angle exophoria. Convergence is frequently excellent. There is no correlation with a specific refractive error.

Since a child fuses at least part of the time, there is usually no gross sensory abnormality. For distance, with one eye deviated, there is suppression of that eye and normal retinal correspondence with little or no amblyopia.

Treatment

A. Medical Treatment: Nonsurgical treatment is largely confined to refractive correction and amblyopia therapy. If the AC/A ratio is high, the use of minus lenses may delay surgery for a while. Occasionally, antisuppression or convergence exercises may be of temporary benefit.

B. Surgical Treatment: Most patients with intermittent exotropia require surgery when their fusional control deteriorates. Deterioration of control is documented over time by an increasing percentage of time the manifest exotropia is observed, an enlarging angle

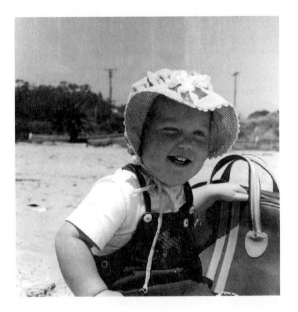

Figure 12–10. Child with intermittent exotropia squinting in sunlight.

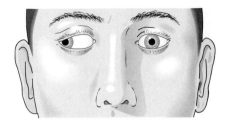

Figure 12–11. Right exotropia.

of deviation, decreasing control for near fixation, and worsening in the patient's measured distance and near stereoscopic abilities. Surgery may also alleviate diplopia or other asthenopic symptoms.

The choice of procedure depends on the measurements of the deviation. Bilateral lateral rectus muscle recession is preferred when the deviation is greater at distance. If there is more deviation at near, it is best to undertake resection of a medial rectus muscle and recession of the ipsilateral lateral rectus muscle. Surgery on one or even two additional horizontal muscles may be necessary for very large deviations ($> 50^\Delta$). It is desirable to obtain slight overcorrection in the immediate postoperative period for best long-term results.

CONSTANT EXOTROPIA
(Figure 12–11)

Constant exotropia is less common than intermittent exotropia. It may be present at birth or may occur when intermittent exotropia progresses to constant exotropia. Because infantile exotropia is commonly seen in children with underlying neurologic impairment, pediatric neurologic consultation is indicated in all such cases. Some cases have their onset later in life, particularly following loss of vision in one eye. Except for cases due to loss of vision, the underlying cause is usually not known.

Clinical Findings

Constant exotropia may be of any degree. With chronicity or poor vision in one eye, the deviation can become quite large. Adduction may be limited, and hypertropia also may be present. There is suppression if the deviation was acquired by age 6–8; otherwise, diplopia may be present. If exotropia is due to very poor vision in one eye, there may be no diplopia. Amblyopia is uncommon in the absence of anisometropia, and spontaneous alternation of the fixating eye is frequently observed.

Treatment

Surgery is nearly always indicated. The choice and amount are as described for intermittent exotropia. Slight overcorrection in an adult may result in diplopia. Most patients adjust to this, especially if they have been forewarned of the possibility. If one eye has reduced vision, the prognosis for maintenance of a stable position is less favorable, with the strong possibility that the deviating eye will gradually become more exotropic. Botulinum toxin type A injections can be useful as primary treatment in small deviations or as supplementary treatment in significant surgical overcorrections or undercorrections.

A & V PATTERNS

A horizontal deviation may be vertically incomitant, ie, the deviation is different in upgaze versus downgaze (A or V pattern). An A pattern shows more esodeviation or less exodeviation in upgaze compared to downgaze. A V pattern shows less esodeviation or more exodeviation in upgaze compared to downgaze. An A pattern is diagnostically significant when greater than 10^Δ and a V pattern when greater than 15^Δ. These patterns are frequently associated with overaction of the oblique muscles, inferior obliques for V patterns and superior obliques for A patterns.

When surgically treating an A or V pattern, oblique muscle overaction must be treated if present. If little or no oblique overaction exists, vertical offsets of one tendon width of the horizontal muscles are utilized to collapse the pattern. The insertions of the medial rectus muscles are displaced toward the narrow end of the pattern (in V esotropia, recessed medial rectus muscles are moved down), and lateral rectus muscles are displaced toward the open end (in V exotropia, the insertions of the recessed lateral rectus muscles are moved up).

HYPERTROPIA
(Figure 12–12)

Vertical deviations are customarily named according to the high eye, regardless of which eye has the better vision and is used for fixation. Hypertropias are less common than horizontal deviations and are usually acquired after childhood.

There are many causes of hypertropia. Congenital anatomic anomalies may result in muscle attachments in abnormal locations. Occasionally, there are anomalous fibrous bands that attach to the eye. Closed head trauma may produce paresis of the superior oblique muscle. Orbital trauma or tumors, brain stem lesions, and systemic diseases such as myasthenia gravis, multiple sclerosis, and Graves' disease can all produce hypertropias. Many of these specific entities are discussed in Chapter 14.

Clinical Findings

The clinical findings may vary, depending on the cause. The history is particularly important in diagnosis of hypertropias. Prism and cover measurements in primary and cardinal positions and head tilts are the mainstay of the clinical evaluation and may often be diagnostic. Observation of ocular rotations for limitations can also be of great value.

Diplopia is almost invariably present if strabismus develops past age 6–8. As in other forms of strabismus, sensory adaptation occurs if the onset is before this age range. Suppression and anomalous retinal correspondence may be present in gaze directions where there is strabismus. In gaze directions without strabismus, there may be no suppression and normal stereopsis.

There may be head tilt, turn, or abnormal posture of the head. The deviation may be of any magnitude and usually changes with the direction of gaze. Most hypertropias are incomitant. The deviation tends to be greatest in the field of action of one of the four vertically acting muscles. There may be an associated **cyclotropia,** especially with superior oblique dysfunction. To measure a cyclotropia, the **double Maddox rod test** is used. In a trial frame, a red and white Maddox rod are aligned vertically, one over each eye. With the patient's head held straight and fixing a light, one rod is gradually turned until the observed lines are parallel to each other and to normal horizontal orientation. The angle of tilt is then read from the angular scale on the trial frame.

The superior oblique is the most commonly paretic vertical muscle. The vertical rectus muscles are commonly involved in trauma, as with entrapment of the inferior rectus in an orbital floor fracture, and in thyroid eye disease, in which the inferior rectus becomes hypertrophied, inelastic, and fibrotic, which pulls the eye downward.

Paresis of the superior oblique is usually present with hypertropia on the involved side with a head tilt to the opposite side. Other motility patterns can be seen when the deviation is of long standing, with contractures of other vertically acting muscles.

The Bielschowsky head tilt test (Figure 12–13) is useful to confirm the diagnosis of superior oblique paresis. The test exploits the differing effects of each vertical muscle on torsion and elevation. Thus, with a paretic right superior oblique when the head is tilted to the right, the superior rectus and superior oblique contract to intort the eye and maintain the position of the retinal vertical meridian as much as possible. The superior rectus elevates the eye, and the superior oblique depresses the eye. Because of weakness of the superior oblique muscle, the vertical forces do not cancel out as they normally would, and right hypertropia increases. In head tilt to the left, the intorting muscles for the right eye relax and the inferior oblique and inferior rectus both contract to extort the eye. Both the paretic superior oblique and the superior rectus relax, and hypertropia is minimized. Hypertropia should be measured by prism plus cover with the head tilted to either side.

Treatment

A. Medical Treatment: For smaller and more comitant deviations, a prism may be all that is required. For constant diplopia, one eye may need to be occluded. Systemic disease must be treated if suspected to be the underlying cause.

B. Surgical Treatment: Surgery is often indicated if the deviation and diplopia persist. The choice of procedure depends on quantitative measurements. The use of adjustable sutures (Figure 12–8) is frequently a great help in fine-tuning the effect of vertical muscle surgery.

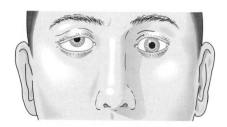

Figure 12–12. Right hypertropia.

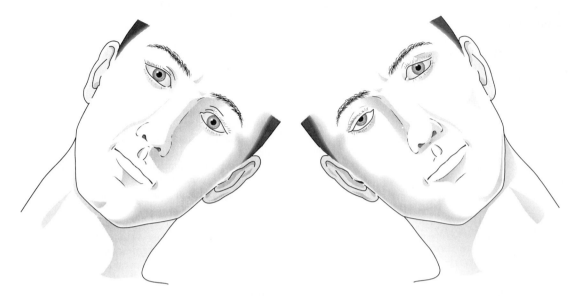

Figure 12–13. Head tilt test (Bielschowsky test). Paresis of right superior oblique. ***Left:*** Hypertropia is minimized on tilting the head to the sound side. The right eye may then extort and the intorting superior oblique and superior rectus relax. ***Right:*** When the head is tilted to the paretic side, the intorting muscles contract together, but their vertical actions do not cancel out as usual, because of superior oblique paresis. Hypertropia is worse with head tilt to the paretic side.

SPECIAL FORMS

DUANE'S RETRACTION SYNDROME

Duane's retraction syndrome is typically characterized by marked limitation of abduction, mild limitation of adduction, retraction of the globe and narrowing of the palpebral fissure on attempted adduction, and, frequently, upshoot or downshoot of the eye in adduction. Usually it is monocular, with the left eye more often affected. Most cases are sporadic, although some families with dominant inheritance have been described. A variety of other anomalies may be associated, such as dysplasia of the iris stroma, heterochromia, cataract, choroidal coloboma, microphthalmos, Goldenhar's syndrome, Klippel-Feil syndrome, cleft palate, and anomalies of the face, ear, or extremities. The causes of the motility defects are varied, and some anomalies of muscle structure have been found. Most cases can be explained by inappropriate innervation to the lateral rectus and sometimes to other muscles as well. Sherrington's law of reciprocal innervation is not obeyed, because nerve fibers to the medial rectus may also go to the lateral rectus. This accounts for simultaneous contraction of the medial and lateral rectus muscles (co-contraction), causing retraction of the globe. Cases with proved absence of the abducens nucleus and nerve have been documented.

Treatment

Only when a primary position misalignment or a significant compensatory head turn exists is surgical treatment indicated. The goal is to obtain straight eyes in the primary position and to horizontally expand the field of single vision. Recession of the medial rectus on the affected side is performed if any esotropia is present in the primary position. For more severe cases, temporal transposition of the vertical rectus muscles accompanied by weakening of the medial rectus muscle, either by adjustable recession or botulinum toxin A, is often indicated.

DISSOCIATED VERTICAL DEVIATION

Dissociated vertical deviation is frequently associated with congenital esotropia and rarely with an otherwise normal muscle balance. The exact cause is not known, though it is logical to assume it is from faulty supranuclear innervation of extraocular muscles.

Clinical Findings

Each eye drifts upward under cover, frequently with extorsion and a small exotropic shift, and then returns to its resting binocular position when the cover is removed. Occasionally, the upward drifting will occur spontaneously, causing a noticeable vertical misalignment. Most cases are bilateral, though asymmetry of involvement is common. There are usually no symptoms.

Treatment

Treatment is indicated if the frequency of the intermittent manifest vertical deviation is unacceptable. Nonsurgical treatment is limited to refractive correction to maximize the potential of motor fusion and therapy for amblyopia. Surgical results have been variable and can be disappointing. Currently, the most popular and successful procedures are very large recession of the superior rectus or recession of the superior rectus combined with the Faden procedure. A new procedure that involves transposing anteriorly the insertion of the inferior oblique muscle has also been effective.

BROWN'S SYNDROME (Superior Oblique Tendon Sheath Syndrome)

Brown's syndrome is due to fibrous adhesions in the superior nasal quadrant involving the superior oblique tendon and trochlea, which mechanically limit elevation of the eye. Limitation of elevation is most marked in the adducted position, and improvement in elevation occurs gradually as the eye is abducted. Differential diagnosis is concerned mainly with paresis of the inferior oblique muscle. Forced duction testing is diagnostic, since there is an upward restriction to elevation in adduction when Brown's syndrome is present. The condition is usually unilateral and idiopathic, though rarely it may be due to trauma or inflammation.

Surgical treatment is limited to those cases where there is an abnormal head position to compensate for hypotropia or cyclotropia of the involved eye. The objective is to free the mechanical adhesions and weaken the superior oblique muscle. Although controversial as to its timing, weakening of the ipsilateral inferior oblique may compensate for the induced fourth nerve palsy. Normalization of the head position may occur, but restoration of full motility is seldom achieved.

HETEROPHORIA

Heterophoria is deviation of the eyes that is held in check by binocular vision. Almost all individuals have some degree of heterophoria, and small amounts are considered normal. Larger amounts may cause symptoms depending on the level of effort required by the individual to control latent muscle imbalance.

Clinical Findings

The symptoms of heterophoria may be clear-cut (intermittent diplopia) or vague ("eyestrain" or as-thenopia). Diplopia may come on only with fatigue or with poor lighting conditions, as in night driving. Usage requirements for the eyes and personality type are additional factors. Thus, there is no degree of heterophoria that is clearly abnormal, though larger amounts are more likely to be symptomatic. Except for hyperopia, high AC/A ratios, and mild cases of muscle paresis not resulting in frank heterotropia, the fundamental causes of heterophorias are unknown.

Asthenopia is sometimes caused by uncorrected refractive errors as well as by muscle imbalance. One possible mechanism is **aniseikonia,** in which an image seen by one eye is a different size and shape from that seen by the other eye. Spectacles with unequal lens powers in the two eyes can cause asthenopia by creating prismatic displacement of the image in one eye for gaze away from the optic axis that is too large to control (induced prism). Another mechanism that may produce symptoms is a change in spatial perception due to the curvature of the lenses or astigmatic corrections. (See Chapter 20.)

The symptoms encountered in asthenopia take a wide variety of forms. There may be a feeling of heaviness, tiredness, or discomfort of the eyes, varying from a dull ache to deep pain located in or behind the eyes. Headaches of all types occur. Easy fatigability, blurring of vision, and diplopia, especially after prolonged use of the eyes, also occur. Symptoms are more common for near visual work than for distance. Frequently, an aversion to reading develops. Symptoms can be brought on by fatigue or illness or following the ingestion of medications or alcohol.

Diagnosis

The diagnosis of heterophoria is based on prism and cover measurements. Relative fusional vergence amplitudes are measured. While the patient views an accommodative target at distance or near, prisms of increasing strength are placed in front of one eye. The fusional vergence amplitude is the amount of prism the patient is able to overcome and still maintain single vision. Measurements are done with base-out, base-in, base-up, and base-down prisms. The important feature is the size of the amplitudes in comparison to the angle of heterophoria. While one cannot give exact norms for normal relative fusion vergence, guidelines for typical normal findings are as follows: at distance, convergence is 14^Δ, divergence is 6^Δ, and vertical is 2.5^Δ; at near, convergence is 35^Δ, divergence is 15^Δ, and vertical is 2.5^Δ.

Treatment

Heterophoria requires treatment only if symptomatic. Untreated heterophoria or asthenopia does not cause any permanent damage to the eyes. Treatment methods are all aimed at reducing the effort required to achieve fusion or at changing muscle mechanics so that the muscle imbalance itself is reduced.

A. Medical Treatment:

1. Accurate refractive correction–Occasionally, poor visual acuity is found in the presence of symptomatic heterophoria. Spectacles providing clear vision are sometimes all that is needed to alleviate symptoms. The clearer image allows the patient's fusional capacity to function to its fullest.

2. Manipulation of accommodation–In general, esophorias are treated with antiaccommodative therapy and exophorias by stimulating accommodation. Plus lenses often work well for esophoria, especially if hyperopia is present, by reducing accommodative convergence. A high AC/A ratio may be effectively treated with plus lenses, sometimes combined with bifocals or miotics.

3. Prisms–The use of prisms requires the wearing of glasses; for some patients, this is unacceptable. A trial of plastic Fresnel press-on prisms should be made before ground-in prisms are ordered. For optical reasons, larger amounts of prismatic correction produce visual distortions limiting the use of prisms in higher strengths. Furthermore, very thick lenses can result. The usual practice is to prescribe about one-third to one-half of the measured deviation, which often allows fusion to occur. Prisms can be useful for esophoria, exophoria, and vertical phorias as well.

4. Botulinum toxin type A (Botox) injection–This treatment is well suited to producing small to moderate shifts in ocular alignment and has been used as a substitute for surgical weakening of one muscle. The main disadvantage is that the resulting effect may be variable or wear off completely months later.

B. Surgical Treatment: Surgery should be done only after medical methods have failed. Muscles are chosen for correction according to the measured deviation at distance and near in various directions of gaze. Sometimes only one muscle needs adjustment. Adjustable sutures can be very helpful (Figure 12–8).

REFERENCES

Atkinson J et al: Two infant vision screening programmes: Prediction and prevention of strabismus and amblyopia from photo- and videorefractive screening. Eye 1996;10:189.

Biglan AW et al: Infantile exotropia. J Pediatr Ophthalmol Strabismus 1996;33:79.

Burke JP, Leach CM, Davis H: Psychosocial implications of strabismus surgery in adults. J Pediatr Ophthalmol Strabismus 1997;34:159.

Eggers HM: Functional anatomy of the extraocular muscles. In: *Biomedical Foundations of Ophthalmology.* Tasman W (editor). Lippincott, 1993.

Epelbaum M et al: The sensitive period for strabismic amblyopia in humans. Ophthalmology 1993;100:323.

Helveston EM: *Surgical Management of Strabismus: An Atlas of Strabismus Surgery,* 4th ed. Mosby, 1993.

Helveston EM: 19th Annual Frank Costenbader Lecture: The origins of congenital esotropia. J Pediatr Ophthalmol Strabismus 1993;30:215.

Ing MR: Outcome study of surgical alignment before six months of age for congenital esotropia. Ophthalmology 1995;102:2041.

Kaban TJ et al: Natural history of presumed congenital Brown syndrome. Arch Ophthalmol 1993;111:943.

Keenan JM, Willshaw HE: The outcome of strabismus surgery in childhood esotropia. Eye 993;7:341.

Kratz RE et al: Anterior tendon displacement of the inferior oblique for DVD. J Pediatr Ophthalmol Strabismus 1989;26:212.

Kushner J: Binocular field expansion in adults after surgery for esotropia. Arch Ophthalmol 1994;112:636.

Lee J et al: Results of a prospective randomized trial of botulinum toxin therapy in acute unilateral sixth nerve palsy. J Pediatr Ophthalmol Strabismus 1994;31:283.

Lipton JR, Willshaw HE: Prospective multicentre study of the accuracy of surgery for horizontal strabismus. Br J Ophthalmol 1995;79:10.

Mruthyunjaya P et al: Subjective and objective outcomes of strabismus surgery in children. J Pediatr Ophthalmol Strabismus 1996;33:167.

Prism Adaptation Study Research Group: Efficacy of prism adaptation in the surgical management of acquired esotropia. Arch Ophthalmol 1990;108:1248.

Rosenbaum AL, Kushner BJ, Kirschen D: Vertical rectus muscle transposition and botulism toxin (Oculinum) to medial rectus for abducens palsy. Arch Ophthalmol 1989;107:820.

Scott AB: *Botulism Toxin: Treatment of Strabismus.* Vol 7, Module 12, in: *Focal Points: Clinical Modules for Ophthalmologists.* American Academy of Ophthalmology, 1989.

Scott MH et al: Prevalence of primary monofixation syndrome in parents of children with congenital esotropia. J Pediatr Ophthalmol Strabismus 1994;31:298.

Shauly Y, Prager TC, Mazow ML: Clinical characteristics and long-term postoperative results of infantile esotropia. Am J Ophthalmol 1994;117:183.

Stoller SH, Simon JW, Lininger LL: Bilateral lateral rectus recession for exotropia: A survival analysis. J Pediatr Ophthalmol Strabismus 1994;31:89.

Tasman W, Jaeger EA (editors): *Duane's Clinical Ophthalmology,* rev ed, vol 1. Lippincott, 1993.

von Noorden GK: *Burian-von Noorden's Binocular Vision and Ocular Motility,* 4th ed. Mosby, 1990.

Wright KW: *Color Atlas of Ophthalmic Surgery: Strabismus.* Lippincott, 1991.

Wright KW et al: High-grade stereo acuity after early surgery for congenital esotropia. Arch Ophthalmol 1994;112:913.

13

Orbit

John H. Sullivan, MD

PHYSIOLOGY OF SYMPTOMS

Owing to the rigid bony structure of the orbit, with only an anterior opening for expansion (Chapter 1), any increase in the orbital contents taking place to the side of or behind the eyeball will displace that organ forward **(proptosis).** Protrusion of the eyeball is the hallmark of orbital disease. Expansive lesions may be benign or malignant and may arise from bone, muscle, nerve, blood vessels, or connective tissue. A mass may be inflammatory, neoplastic, cystic, or vascular. Protrusion is not in itself injurious unless the lids are unable to cover the cornea. The underlying cause, however, is usually serious and sometimes life-threatening. **Pseudoproptosis** is apparent prop-tosis in the absence of orbital disease. Such confusion may arise with high myopia, buphthalmos, and lid retraction.

History and examination provide many clues to the cause of proptosis. The position of the eye is determined by the location of the mass. Expansion within the muscle cone displaces the eye straight ahead **(axial proptosis),** whereas a mass arising outside the muscle cone will also cause sideways or vertical displacement of the globe directly away from the mass **(nonaxial proptosis).** Bilateral involvement generally indicates systemic disease, such as Graves' disease. The term "exophthalmos" is often used when describing proptosis associated with Graves' disease. **Pulsating proptosis** reflects the pulse of an orbital vascular malformation or transmission of cerebral pulsations in the absence of the superior orbital roof, as in neurofibromatosis-1. **Positional proptosis**— which changes with Valsalva's maneuver—is a sign of orbital varices or meningocele. **Intermittent proptosis** may be the result of a sinus mucocele. The Hertel exophthalmometer (see Chapter 2) is the standard method of quantifying the magnitude of proptosis. Serial measurements are most accurate if performed by the same individual with the same instrument.

With the change in position of the eyeball, especially if it takes place rapidly, there may be enough mechanical interference with the movement of the eye to cause dissociation of ocular movements and diplopia (double vision). Pain may occur as a result of rapid expansion, inflammation, or infiltration of sensory nerves. Vision is not usually affected early unless the lesion arises from the optic nerve. Pupillary signs and color vision testing may identify subtle optic nerve compression or involvement before acuity is reduced significantly. Involvement of the superior orbital fissure by trauma or tumor produces a characteristic combination of diplopia resulting from disturbance of function of the oculomotor, trochlear, and abducens nerves and corneal and facial anesthesia (ophthalmic division of trigeminal nerve), known as the **orbital fissure syndrome.** Expanding lesions at the orbital apex result in the **orbital apex syndrome,** characterized by proptosis and optic nerve compression, variably accompanied by the diplopia and corneal and facial anesthesia seen in the orbital fissure syndrome.

DIAGNOSTIC STUDIES

1. IMAGING

CT & MRI

Imaging by **computed tomography (CT scan)** (Figures 13–1 and 13–2) was a major advance in orbital diagnosis. Continued improvement in resolution quality—as well as three-dimensional reconstructions—have made CT the single most important diagnostic study in the investigation of orbital disease. Contrast enhancement with CT during study of vascular lesions sometimes provides additional information. **Magnetic resonance imaging (MRI)** is capable of displaying subtle changes within soft tissue that cannot be imaged with CT, but it is less useful for bony changes. A surface coil applied directly to the orbit enhances image resolution. MRI is contraindicated in the presence of a ferrous intraorbital or intracranial foreign body.

Ultrasonography

The use of ultrasonography in the diagnosis of orbital disease has largely been supplanted by CT and MRI. Although it is a noninvasive and inexpensive form of imaging, its usefulness in both A and B mode is limited to the anterior portion of the orbit. It is of greatest value in the hands of the clinician-

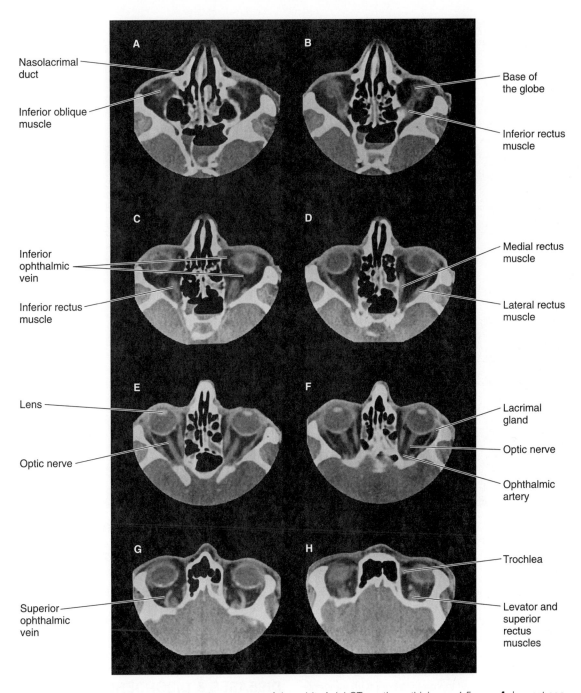

Figure 13–1. Normal CT scan showing the anatomy of the orbit. Axial CT sections, thickness 1.5 mm. **A:** Lowest section. **H:** Highest section. Note clear delineation of individual muscles, optic nerve, and major veins within the orbital fat.

ultrasonographer capable of interpreting "real time" images.

Venography

Venography is occasionally useful in defining the extent of orbital venous disease. Although the diagnosis can be made by MRI, contrast injection into the or-

bital veins via a scalp vein can sometimes reveal the presence of varices that have escaped detection by CT.

Angiography

Selective carotid angiography with bone subtraction is sometimes necessary to make the diagnosis of certain orbital vascular disorders. In spontaneous,

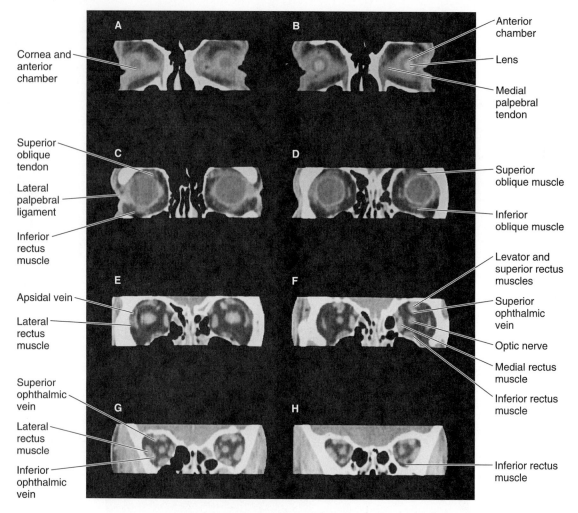

Figure 13–2. Coronal computer reconstructions from axial CT sections. **A:** Most anterior section. **H:** Most posterior section. Note detailed demonstration of ocular and orbital structures.

low-flow dural carotid artery-cavernous sinus fistula, angiography is required for delineation of the extent of involvement and for treatment by embolization.

Radiography

Plain x-rays are sufficient for diagnosis of many orbital disorders such as fractures. However, the thin walls of the orbit are difficult to visualize even with tomography, and CT or MRI imaging is used to determine the extent of injury. Dacryocystography and radionuclide scanning can sometimes be helpful in localizing the site of lacrimal obstructions, but these procedures are seldom used. The results are difficult to interpret, and treatment is seldom altered by the findings. Positive contrast radiography and pneumo-orbitography are no longer used. Orbital thermography is a research procedure.

Fine-Needle Aspiration

Fine-needle aspiration is an invasive procedure that has proved very useful in orbital diagnosis. Cytology

specimens can be aspirated from a lesion the exact location of which is determined by CT imaging. Cytopathology can be inconclusive but is often invaluable.

DISEASES & DISORDERS OF THE ORBIT

INFLAMMATORY DISORDERS

1. GRAVES' OPHTHALMOPATHY

The most common cause of unilateral or bilateral proptosis in adults or children is Graves' disease.

The terminology used to describe ocular involvement in thyroid disease is often confusing. Graves' ophthalmopathy, dysthyroid ophthalmopathy, and dysthyroid eye disease are interchangeable terms. Some degree of ophthalmopathy—usually mild—occurs in a high percentage of hyperthyroid patients. Severe infiltrative orbital myopathy with significant proptosis and restricted motility occurs in about 5% of cases of Graves' disease (Figure 13–3). This severe form, however, can also occur with hypothyroidism or with no detectable thyroid abnormality, in which case the term ophthalmic Graves' disease may be used.

Thyroid ophthalmopathy is thought to be an autoimmune disease. It is often seen in autoimmune (Hashimoto's) thyroiditis. Antithyroglobulin, antimicrosomal, and other antibodies can usually be demonstrated, but their role in pathogenesis is in question.

Clinical Findings

Proptosis associated with thyroid disease is characterized by lid retraction, which serves to distinguish it from other causes of proptosis. Lagophthalmos results from proptosis and lid retraction, and corneal exposure is a factor even in mild cases. Ocular myopathy usually begins with lymphocytic infiltration and edema of the rectus muscles. In time, the inflamed muscles may become fibrotic and permanently restricted. The eye may be tethered so as to raise the intraocular pressure when it is measured in upgaze.

Diplopia usually begins in the upper field of gaze because of infiltrative myopathy involving the inferior rectus muscle. All extraocular muscles may eventually be involved, and there may be no position of gaze free of diplopia. The extraocular muscles may become massively enlarged and—in addition to restricting eye movement—may compress the optic nerve. Compressive optic neuropathy is most common with enlargement of the posterior aspect of the muscles that occurs

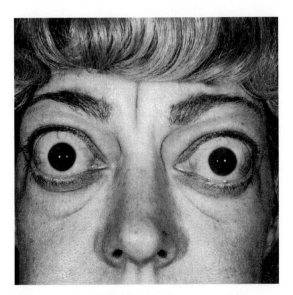

Figure 13–3. Graves' ophthalmopathy.

without severe proptosis. Early signs include an afferent pupillary defect, impairment of color vision, and slight loss of visual acuity. Blindness is liable to occur if compression is unrelieved.

Treatment

The goal of treatment of Graves' ophthalmopathy is initially to maintain corneal protection. As the disease progresses it becomes necessary to address the problems of diplopia, proptosis, and compressive optic neuropathy. Management of severe cases is difficult and multidisciplinary. An endocrinologist should manage the thyroid status, optimal control being crucial to ameliorating the orbital disease. Oral corticosteroids (prednisone, 60–100 mg/d) may be helpful in controlling the acute phase of infiltrative myopathy. Complications and side effects limit the use of corticosteroids in long-term maintenance. Orbital radiation is effective during the active phase of the disease. Soft tissue signs of swelling and chemosis are usually relieved. Diplopia and proptosis may be improved.

Early compression neuropathy may also be relieved by radiation therapy, but neuropathy unresponsive to medical management is an indication for surgical decompression of the orbit. Several approaches have been devised to expand the orbital volume by fracture of the bony walls, usually the orbital floor into the maxillary sinus and the medial wall into the ethmoid sinus, along with removal of the lateral orbital wall in some cases. Proptosis can be reduced by surgery, but there is a risk of intractable diplopia and a lesser risk of orbital infection. For these reasons, decompression for cosmetic reasons is not routinely performed.

Eyelid retraction is often more disturbing than proptosis—both functionally, because of exposure keratitis, and cosmetically. Decompression may relieve lid retraction, but correction of the retraction camouflages proptosis to some extent. Lid retraction is corrected by surgery. The upper and lower lid retractors (aponeurosis and sympathetic muscles) can be lengthened by inserting a spacer such as eye bank sclera. Small amounts (2 mm) of lid retraction can be corrected by simply disinserting the retractors from the upper tarsal border.

Strabismus surgery should not be undertaken until the myopathy has stabilized. The adjustable suture technique is useful. Most patients can achieve at least a small area of binocular single vision in a useful position of gaze. Torsional diplopia, the result of oblique muscle involvement, complicates management.

Some patients have intractable diplopia despite all attempts at correction.

2. PSEUDOTUMOR

A frequent cause of proptosis in adults and children is inflammatory pseudotumor. The term "pseudotumor" was coined to indicate a nonneoplastic process that produces the sentinel sign of an orbital neoplasm, ie, proptosis. In some cases there is an associated systemic vasculitis, such as Wegener's granulomatosis. The site of inflammation is usually diffuse and not amenable to excision. The process can involve any orbital structure (eg, myositis, dacryoadenitis, lymphogranuloma) or cell type (eg, lymphocytes, fibroblasts, histiocytes, plasma cells). Onset is usually rapid, and pain is often present.

Pseudotumor is usually unilateral; when both orbits are involved, it is more often a manifestation of vasculitis. The differential diagnosis includes Graves' ophthalmopathy and orbital lymphoma.

Treatment with systemic NSAIDs, systemic corticosteroids, or radiation is usually effective. Surgery often exacerbates the inflammatory reaction.

ORBITAL INFECTIONS

1. ORBITAL CELLULITIS
(Figure 13–4)

Orbital cellulitis is the most common cause of proptosis in children. Immediate treatment is essential. Fortunately, the diagnosis usually is not difficult, because the clinical findings are characteristic. Although most cases occur in children, aged and immunocompromised individuals may also be affected.

Trauma may be responsible for introduction of contaminated material into the orbit through the skin or paranasal sinuses. In the preantibiotic era, orbital cellulitis frequently led to blindness or death resulting from septic cavernous sinus thrombosis.

The orbit is surrounded by the paranasal sinuses, and part of their venous drainage is through the orbit. Most cases of orbital cellulitis arise from extension of sinusitis through the thin ethmoid bones. The organisms usually responsible are those most frequently found in sinuses: *Haemophilus influenzae, Streptococcus pneumoniae,* other streptococci, and staphylococci.

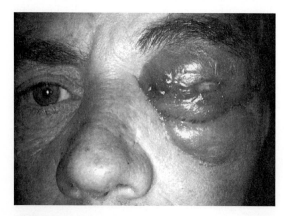

Figure 13–4. Orbital cellulitis. Abscess draining through upper eyelid.

Clinical Findings

Preseptal cellulitis is the most common presentation. CT scan or MRI is helpful in distinguishing between pre- and postseptal involvement as well as identifying and localizing an orbital abscess or foreign body. Plain x-rays alone can only identify the presence of sinusitis.

It is important to distinguish between preseptal and orbital infections. Both present with edema, erythema, hyperemia, pain, and leukocytosis. Chemosis, proptosis, limitation of eye movement, and reduction of vision indicate deep orbital involvement. Extension to the cavernous sinus may cause bilateral involvement of cranial nerves II–VI, with severe edema and septic fever. Erosion of the orbital bones may cause brain abscess and meningitis.

In children, few orbital diseases develop as rapidly as cellulitis. Confusion may exist with rhabdomyosarcoma, pseudotumor, and Graves' ophthalmopathy.

Treatment

Treatment should be initiated before the causative organism is identified. As soon as nasal, conjunctival, and blood cultures are obtained, intravenous antibiotics should be administered. Initial antibiotic therapy should cover staphylococci, *H influenzae,* and anaerobes. Posttraumatic cellulitis—especially following animal bites—must be covered for gram-negative and gram-positive bacilli. Hot compresses help localize the inflammatory reaction. Nasal decongestants and vasoconstrictors help drain the paranasal sinuses. Early surgical drainage is indicated in suppurative preseptal cellulitis. MRI is useful in deciding when and where to drain an orbital abscess. Most cases respond promptly to antibiotics. Those that do not may require drainage of the paranasal sinuses. Early consultation with an otolaryngologist may be helpful.

2. MUCORMYCOSIS

Diabetics and immunocompromised patients have a propensity to develop severe and often fatal fungal infections of the orbit. The organisms are of the Zygomycetes group, which have a tendency to invade vessels and create ischemic necrosis. Infection usually begins in the sinuses and erodes into the orbital cavity. A necrotizing reaction destroys muscle, bone, and soft tissue, frequently without causing signs of orbital cellulitis.

The patient is usually quite ill and presents with pain and proptosis. Examination of the nose and palate often reveals a necrotic area of mucosa, a smear of which shows broad branching hyphae.

Without treatment, the infection gradually erodes into the cranial cavity, resulting in meningitis, brain abscess, and death usually within days to weeks. Treatment is difficult and often inadequate. It consists of correction of the underlying disease combined with surgical debridement and administration of amphotericin B intravenously. Recurrences are common.

CYSTIC LESIONS INVOLVING THE ORBIT

1. DERMOID

Dermoids are not true neoplasms but benign choristomas arising from embryonic tissue not usually found in the orbit. Orbital dermoids arise from surface ectoderm and often contain epithelial structures such as keratin, hair, and even teeth. Most are cystic and filled with an oily fluid that can incite a severe inflammatory reaction if liberated into the orbit. Most dermoids occur in the superior temporal quadrant of the orbit, but they can occur at any bony suture line.

X-rays show a sharp, round bony defect from the pressure of a slowly growing mass affixed to the periosteum.

Epidermoid cyst is a superficial keratin-filled mass, usually near the superior orbital rim. It may be congenital or posttraumatic. Excision is usually not difficult.

A **dermolipoma** is a solid mass of fatty material that occurs below the conjunctival surface. Hair growth on the overlying conjunctiva is not uncommon. Dermolipomas are often much larger than they appear to be, and excision may cause considerable damage to vital structures. If treatment is necessary, limited excision is usually advised.

2. SINUS MUCOCELE

The proximity of the orbit to the paranasal sinuses may lead to invasion of the bony walls and extension of an obstructed sinus into the orbit. Plain x-ray will usually make the diagnosis, but CT or MRI may be required to differentiate sinus mucocele from dermoid cyst and to define the extent of the lesion (Figure 13–5). Otolaryngologic and neurosurgical assistance may be necessary for surgical removal.

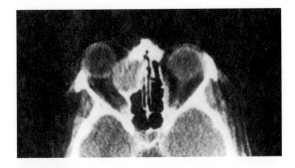

Figure 13–5. CT scan of ethmoid sinus mucocele.

3. MENINGOCELE

Erosion of the meninges into the orbital cavity through a congenital dehiscence in the bony sutures creates a cystic mass filled with cerebrospinal fluid known as a **meningocele.** Both brain and meninges are frequently included in a **meningoencephalocele.** The resultant fluctuant mass in the superior medial orbit typically enlarges with Valsalva's maneuver. Most cases are present at birth, but those arising from the sphenoid bone may not become apparent until adolescence.

VASCULAR ABNORMALITIES INVOLVING THE ORBIT

1. ARTERIOVENOUS MALFORMATION

Arteriovenous malformations are an uncommon cause of proptosis. Varices produce intermittent proptosis, sometimes associated with pain and transient reduction of vision. Some degree of proptosis can be induced with Valsalva's maneuver or by placing the head in a dependent position. MRI scan is usually diagnostic, and venography is seldom indicated.

Surgery is the only method of treatment available and is fraught with hazard. Morbidity following eradication of the varix may jeopardize visual function. Most varices are best left untreated unless vision is at risk.

2. CAROTID ARTERY–CAVERNOUS SINUS FISTULA

Carotid artery-cavernous sinus fistulas with high-flow shunts are easily diagnosed. Although sometimes occurring spontaneously, they usually follow trauma. Physical signs include severe congestion and chemosis, with pulsating proptosis and a loud bruit.

Low-flow shunts (dural carotid cavernous sinus fistula) are usually spontaneous and often misdiagnosed. Mild congestion, venous engorgement and arterialization, elevated intraocular pressure, mild proptosis, and a faint bruit are the usual features. Diagnosis is by contrast MRI or subtraction angiography, and treatment is by selective intra-arterial or transvenous embolization.

PRIMARY ORBITAL TUMORS

CAPILLARY HEMANGIOMA

Capillary hemangiomas are common benign tumors that sometimes involve the eyelids and orbit (Figure 13–6). Superficial lesions are reddish (strawberry nevus), and deeper lesions are more bluish. Over 90% become apparent before the age of 6 months. They tend to enlarge rapidly in the first year of life and regress slowly over 6–7 years. Lesions within the orbit may cause strabismus or proptosis. Involvement of the eyelids may induce astigmatism or occlude vision, resulting in amblyopia.

Small superficial lesions require no treatment and are best allowed to spontaneously regress. Deep orbital lesions are often associated with significant morbidity with or without treatment. The most common dilemma, however, is the rapidly growing lid lesion in a preverbal infant. Parents are often unwilling to wait for spontaneous regression and plead for treatment even if amblyopia is not a threat. The use of intralesional sustained-release corticosteroids has been found to be effective in many instances and has evolved as the preferred method of treatment in most cases. Corticosteroids are thought to have an antiangiogenic effect that inhibits capillary proliferation and induces vascular constriction.

Other forms of treatment are less effective but sometimes necessary. These include prolonged compression, systemic corticosteroids, sclerosing agents, cryotherapy, laser surgery, radiation, and surgical resection.

CAVERNOUS HEMANGIOMA (Figure 13–7)

Cavernous hemangiomas are benign, grow slowly, and usually become symptomatic in middle life. Most occur in women. They most often lie within the muscle cone, producing axial proptosis, hyperopia, and, in many cases, choroidal folds. Unlike capillary hemangiomas, they do not tend to regress spontaneously. Surgical excision is usually successful and is indicated if the patient is symptomatic.

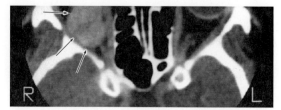

A

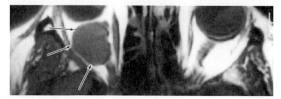

B

Figure 13–7. Cavernous hemangioma (arrows) of the right orbit as demonstrated by both CT scan **(A)** and MRI **(B)**. The left side demonstrates the appearance of a normal orbit and globe. (Courtesy of D Char.)

LYMPHANGIOMA

In its early stages, lymphangioma may be very similar to hemangioma—even histologically such that some authors have suggested a primarily venous origin. Both usually begin in infancy, though lymphangioma may present later in life. Lymphangioma does not regress and is characterized by intermittent hemorrhage and gradual worsening. Large blood cysts may cause proptosis and diplopia and require evacuation.

The tumor is often multifocal and frequently occurs in the soft palate and other areas of the face as well as the orbit. On histologic examination, it consists of large serum-filled channels and lymphoid follicles. Treatment can be for the purpose of either acute decompression of a hemorrhagic blood cyst or eradication of the tumor. Needle aspiration of blood or extirpation of a specific cyst may be temporarily effective. Excision of tumor by any method is seldom satisfactory. The risk of amblyopia is similar to that associated with capillary hemangioma.

RHABDOMYOSARCOMA (Figure 13–8)

Rhabdomyosarcoma is the most common primary malignant tumor of the orbit in childhood. Presentation is before age 10, and rapid growth is characteristic. The tumor may destroy adjacent orbital bone and spread into the brain. The combination of external megavoltage radiation and chemotherapy has improved the survival rate of these patients from less than 50%, when orbital exenteration was used, to over 90% today.

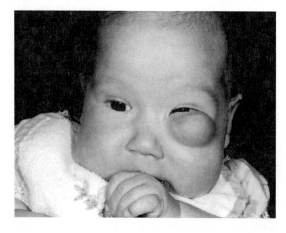

Figure 13–6. Capillary hemangioma.

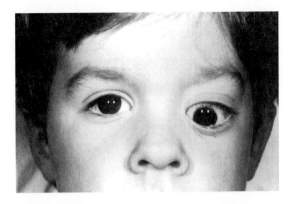

Figure 13–8. Rhabdomyosarcoma.

NEUROFIBROMA

Neurofibromatosis 1 (Recklinghausen's disease) is inherited as an autosomal dominant trait. The responsible gene is on chromosome 17. Plexiform neurofibromas are characteristic and can distort the eyelids (Figure 13–9) and orbit. The presence of café au lait spots helps confirm the diagnosis. The sphenoid bone is often defective; the associated orbital defect may lead to pulsating exophthalmos or enophthalmos. Optic nerve gliomas produce signs (proptosis) and symptoms (visual loss) in 5% of affected individuals; imaging has shown that many more patients harbor asymptomatic optic nerve gliomas. Some of these patients also develop meningiomas and, rarely, malignant peripheral nerve sheath tumors.

OPTIC NERVE GLIOMA

Approximately 75% of symptomatic optic nerve gliomas become apparent before age 10. Twenty-five to 50 percent are associated with neurofibromatosis 1. They are low-grade astrocytomas. Those anterior to the chiasm behave in a benign fashion; those in and posterior to the chiasm may be more aggressive. Visual loss and optic atrophy are the most common signs. Proptosis occurs if the tumor is in the orbit.

Treatment is controversial. There are no compelling statistics to indicate that any form of treatment is applicable to all cases. Some believe that these tumors do not require treatment, others that they require surgical excision, radiotherapy, or chemotherapy. If progressive tumor growth and visual loss can be clearly documented, radiotherapy is often effective in stabilizing or even improving vision. There is a risk of secondary damage to the central nervous system such that chemotherapy is advocated as a better option, but there is little long-term follow-up data. In blind eyes with marked proptosis, the patient's cosmetic appearance can often be improved by excising the tumor through a lateral orbitotomy.

LACRIMAL GLAND TUMORS

Fifty percent of masses presenting in the lacrimal gland are epithelial tumors; one-half of these are malignant. Inflammatory masses and lymphoproliferative tumors comprise the other 50%. The most common epithelial tumor is the pleomorphic adenoma (benign mixed tumor). These tumors should be excised—not biopsied—because of their propensity for recurrence and malignant transformation.

A malignant tumor of the lacrimal gland is suspected when the patient presents with pain and destructive bony changes are evident on x-ray. Biopsy should be performed through the eyelid to avoid tumor seeding in the orbit. Orbital exenteration with ostectomy is required if there is to be any chance of survival. Even with radical treatment, the prognosis is poor.

LYMPHOMA

Lymphomatous tumors of the orbit are divided into malignant lymphomas and reactive lymphoid hyperplasia, or pseudolymphoma. Immunologic and DNA hybridization techniques can help the pathologist determine whether a given lesion is a monoclonal proliferation (and presumably malignant) or a benign polyclonal proliferation. However, malignant lymphomas can have associated benign reactive lesions; benign polyclonal lesions can have small clones of B lymphocytes; and monoclonal tumors often remain localized and behave in a benign fashion.

The differential diagnosis includes orbital infection and pseudotumor, with or without systemic vasculitis. Pain is more common with benign inflammatory processes than with malignant lymphomas.

The prognosis for both polyclonal lymphoid proliferations and well-differentiated B cell monoclonal lesions is excellent. If disease is confined to the orbit, treatment for both monoclonal and polyclonal lesions

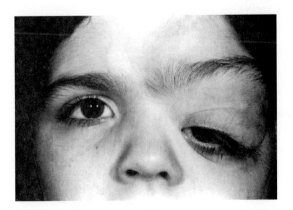

Figure 13–9. Plexiform neurofibroma of upper eyelid in neurofibromatosis 1.

is with radiation. In one study, only 13% of these patients who were free of systemic disease after 6 months developed nonocular lymphomatous lesions.

HISTIOCYTOSIS

Proliferation of Langerhans cells with characteristic cytoplasmic granules comprises a spectrum of disease that includes what were formerly classified as unifocal and multifocal eosinophilic granuloma, Hand-Schüller-Christian disease (multifocal lytic skull lesion, proptosis, and diabetes insipidus), and Letterer-Siwe disease (cutaneous, visceral, and lymph node involvement). The younger the child at the time of diagnosis, the greater the chance of multifocal disease.

The orbital lesions can be treated with surgical curettement, corticosteroid injections, or low-dose radiation.

METASTATIC TUMORS

Metastatic tumors reach the orbit by hematogenous spread, since the orbit is devoid of lymphatics. Metastasis is usually from the breast in women and from the lung in men. In children, the most common metastatic tumor is neuroblastoma, which is often associated with spontaneous periocular hemorrhage as the rapidly growing tumor becomes necrotic. Metastatic tumors are much more common in the choroid than in the orbit, probably because of the nature of the blood supply.

Many metastatic orbital tumors respond to radiation, some to chemotherapy. Small localized tumors that are symptomatic can sometimes be completely or partially excised. Neuroblastomas in children under 11 months have a relatively good prognosis. Adults with metastatic tumors in the orbit have a very limited life expectancy.

SECONDARY TUMORS

Basal cell, squamous cell, and sebaceous gland carcinomas may spread locally into the anterior orbit. Nasopharyngeal carcinomas—most commonly from the maxillary sinus—and meningiomas invade the posterior orbit.

REFERENCES

Bartley GB et al: Long-term follow-up of Graves ophthalmopathy in an incidence cohort. Ophthalmology 1996;103:958.

Bartley GB, Gorman CA: Diagnostic criteria for Graves' ophthalmopathy. Am J Ophthalmol 1995;119:792.

Bonavolonta G et al: Dermoid cysts: 16-year survey. Ophthalmic Plast Reconstr Surg 1995;11:187.

Bron AJ et al (editors): Wolff's Anatomy of the Eye and Orbit, 8th ed. Chapman & Hall, 1997.

Char DH: Clinical Ocular Oncology, 2nd ed. Lippincott-Raven, 1997.

Char DH: Thyroid Eye Disease, 3rd ed. Butterworth-Heinemann, 1997.

De La Paz MA, Boniuk M: Fundus manifestations of orbital disease and treatment of orbital disease. Surv Ophthalmol 1995;40:3.

Dutton J, Slamovits T (editors): Viewpoints: Management of blowout fractures of the orbital floor. Surv Ophthalmol 1991;35:1.

Dutton JJ: Gliomas of the anterior visual pathway. Surv Ophthalmol 1994;38:427.

Farris SR, Grove AS: Orbital and eyelid manifestations of neurofibromatosis: A clinical study and literature review. Ophthalmic Plast Reconstr Surg 1996;12:245.

Fells P et al: Extraocular muscle problems in thyroid eye disease. Eye 1994;8:497.

Goldberg RA et al: Management of cavernous sinus-dural fistulas. Indications and techniques for primary embolization via the superior ophthalmic vein. Arch Ophthalmol 1996;114:707.

Henderson JW et al: Orbital Tumors, 3rd ed. Raven, 1994.

Hutchinson BM, Kyle PM: Long-term visual outcome following orbital decompression for dysthyroid eye disease. Eye 1995;9:578.

Jackson IT, Carreno R et al: Hemangiomas, vascular malformations, and lymphovenous malformations: Classification and methods of treatment. Plast Reconstr Surg 1993;91:1216.

Kronish JW et al: Orbital infections in patients with human immunodeficiency virus infection. Ophthalmology 1996;103:1483.

Lawson CT et al: Definition of the blepharophimosis ptosis epicanthus inversus syndrome critical region at chromosome 3q23 based on the analysis of chromosomal anomalies. Hum Mol Genet 1995;4:963.

Mannor GE et al: Multidisciplinary management of refractory orbital rhabdomyosarcoma. Ophthalmology 1997;104:1198.

Mannor GE et al: Outcome of orbital myositis: Clinical features associated with recurrence. Ophthalmology 1997;104:409.

Mombaerts I et al: Are systemic corticosteroids useful in the management of orbital pseudotumors? Ophthalmology 1996;103:521.

Mombaerts I et al: What is orbital pseudotumor? Surv Ophthalmol 1996;41:66.

Mombaerts I, Koornneef L: Current status in the treatment of orbital myositis. Ophthalmology 1997;104:402.

Perry SR, Rootman J, White VA: The clinical and pathologic constellation of Wegener granulomatosis of the orbit. Ophthalmology 1997;104:683.

Reifler DM et al: Orbital lymphoma associated with acquired immune deficiency syndrome (AIDS). Surv Ophthalmol 1994;38:371.

Rousseau P: Primary chemotherapy in rhabdomyosarcomas and other malignant mesenchymal tumors of the orbit: Results of the International Society of Pediatric Oncology MMT 84 Study. J Clin Oncol 1994;12:516.

Shuper A et al: Visual pathway glioma: An erratic tumor with therapeutic dilemmas. Arch Dis Child 1997;76:259.

Spencer WH (editor): *Ophthalmic Pathology,* 4th ed. 4 vols. Saunders, 1996.

Trobe JD, Gebarski SS: Looking behind the eyes: The proper use of modern imaging. Arch Ophthalmol 1993;111:1185.

Walker RS, Custer PL, Nerad JA: Surgical excision of periorbital capillary hemangiomas. Ophthalmology 1994; 101:1333.

Weber AL, Dallow RL, Sabates NR: Graves' disease of the orbit. Neuroimaging Clin North Am 1996;6:61.

White WL, Ferry JA: Ocular adnexal lymphoma: A clinicopathologic study with identification of lymphomas of mucosa-associated lymphoid tissue type. Ophthalmology 1995;102:1994.

Wilson WB, Prochoda M: Radiotherapy for thyroid orbitopathy. Arch Ophthalmol 1995;113:1420.

Yohai RA et al: Survival factors in rhino-orbital-cerebral mucormycosis. Surv Ophthalmol 1994;39:3.

Paul Riordan-Eva, FRCS, FRCOphth, & William F. Hoyt, MD

The eyes are intimately related to the brain and frequently give important diagnostic clues to central nervous system disorders. Indeed, the optic nerve is a part of the central nervous system. Intracranial disease frequently causes visual disturbances because of destruction of or pressure upon some portion of the optic pathways. Cranial nerves III, IV, and VI, which control ocular movements, may be involved, and nerves V and VII are also intimately associated with ocular function.

THE SENSORY VISUAL PATHWAY

Topographic Overview
(Figures 14–1 and 14–2)

Cranial nerve II subserves the special sense of vision. Light is detected by the rods and cones of the retina, which may be considered the special sensory end organ for vision. The cell bodies of these receptors extend processes that synapse with the bipolar cell, the second neuron in the visual pathway. The bipolar cells synapse, in turn, with the retinal ganglion cells. Ganglion cell axons comprise the nerve fiber layer of the retina and converge to form the optic nerve. The nerve emerges from the back of the globe and travels posteriorly within the muscle cone to enter the cranial cavity via the optic canal.

Intracranially, the two optic nerves join to form the optic chiasm (Figure 14–1). At the chiasm, more than half of the fibers (those from the nasal half of the retina) decussate and join the uncrossed temporal fibers of the opposite nerve to form the optic tracts. Each optic tract sweeps around the cerebral peduncle toward the lateral geniculate nucleus, where it will synapse. All of the fibers receiving impulses from the right hemifields of each eye thus make up the left optic tract and project to the left cerebral hemisphere. Similarly, the left hemifields project to the right cerebral hemisphere. Twenty percent of the fibers in the tract subserve pupillary function. These fibers leave the tract just anterior to the nucleus and pass via the brachium of the superior colliculus to the midbrain pretectal nucleus. The remaining fibers synapse in the lateral geniculate nucleus. The cell bodies of this structure give rise to the geniculocalcarine tract. This tract passes through the posterior limb of the internal capsule and then fans into the optic radiations that traverse parts of the temporal and parietal lobes en route to the occipital cortex (calcarine, striate, or primary visual cortex).

Analysis of Visual Fields in Localizing Lesions in the Visual Pathways

In clinical practice, lesions in the visual pathways are localized by means of central and peripheral visual field examination. The technique (perimetry) is discussed in Chapter 2.

Figure 14–3 shows the types of field defects caused by lesions in various locations of the pathway. Lesions anterior to the chiasm (of the retina or optic nerve) cause unilateral field defects; lesions anywhere in the visual pathway posterior to the chiasm cause contralateral homonymous defects. Chiasmal lesions usually cause bitemporal defects.

Multiple isopters (test objects of different sizes) should be used in order to evaluate the defects thoroughly. A field defect shows evidence of edema or compression when there are areas of "relative scotoma" (ie, a larger field defect for a smaller test object). Such visual field defects are said to be "sloping." This is in contrast to ischemic or vascular lesions with steep borders (ie, the defect is the same size no matter what size test object is used). Such visual field defects are said to be "absolute."

Another important generalization is that the more congruous the homonymous field defects (ie, the more similar the two hemifields in size, shape, and location), the farther posterior the lesion is in the visual pathway. A lesion in the occipital region causes identical defects in each field, whereas optic tract lesions cause incongruous (dissimilar) homonymous field defects. A complete homonymous hemianopia should still have intact visual acuity in the spared visual field since macular function is also spared in the retained visual field. In lesions of the occipital cortex there is a close correlation between the visual field defect and the location of the cortical lesion, the central field being represented posteriorly and the upper field inferiorly (Figure 14–4). Owing to the dual vascular supply to the occipital lobe—from the middle and posterior cerebral circulation—occipital infarcts may spare or

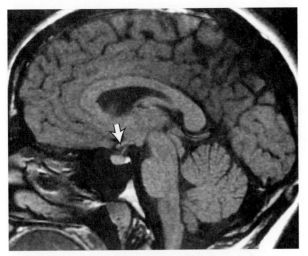
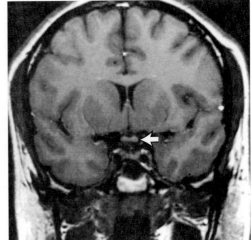
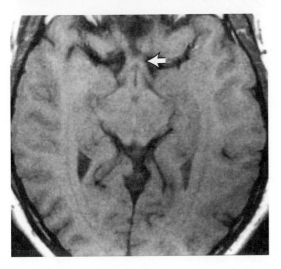

Figure 14–1. Magnetic resonance imaging (MRI) of normal brain in sagittal section *(upper left),* coronal section *(upper right),* and axial section *(lower left).* The white arrows indicate the chiasm.

damage the occipital pole. This leads to sparing or loss of the central field on the side of the hemianopia, the former being referred to as macular sparing (Figure 14–5). Occipital lesions may also produce the phenomenon of residual sight, in which responses to movement, for example, may be demonstrable in the hemianopic field in the absence of form vision.

THE OPTIC NERVE

A wide variety of diseases affect the optic nerve (Table 14–1). Clinical features particularly suggestive of optic nerve disease are an afferent pupillary defect, poor color vision, and optic disk changes. It is important to remember that the optic nerve may be normal in the early stages of disease affecting the retrobulbar optic nerve, particularly compression by an intracranial lesion, even when there has been severe loss of visual acuity and field. Axons can be dysfunctional long before they become atrophic.

Optic disk swelling occurs predominantly in diseases directly affecting the anterior portion of the optic nerve but also occurs with raised intracranial pressure and compression of the intraorbital optic nerve. Optic disk swelling can be a crucial clinical sign, such as in the diagnosis of anterior ischemic optic neuropathy in which optic disk swelling must be present in the acute stage for the diagnosis to be made on clinical grounds. Central retinal vein occlusion, ocular hypotony and intraocular inflammation can produce optic disk swelling and hence the misleading impression of optic nerve disease.

Optic atrophy (Figure 14–6) is a nonspecific response to optic nerve damage from any cause. Since

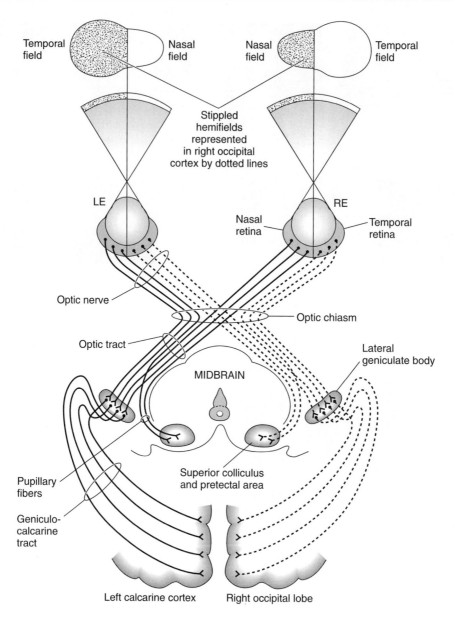

Figure 14–2. The optic pathway. The dotted lines represent nerve fibers that carry visual and pupillary afferent impulses from the left half of the visual field.

the optic nerve consists of retinal ganglion cell axons, optic atrophy may be the consequence of primary retinal disease, such as retinitis pigmentosa or central retinal artery occlusion. Excavation of the optic nerve head (optic disk cupping) is generally a sign of glaucomatous optic neuropathy, but may occur with any cause of optic atrophy. Segmental pallor and attenuated retinal blood vessels are often the consequence of anterior ischemic optic neuropathy. Hereditary optic neuropathies usually produce bilateral temporal segmental disk pallor with preferential loss of papillomacular axons. Peripapillary exudates occur with op-

tic disk swelling, due to papillitis, ischemic optic neuropathy, or papilledema, and may take longer to resolve. (The term "neuroretinitis" for the combination of optic disk swelling and retinal exudates, including a macular star, is a misnomer in that there is no inflammation of the retina, the exudates being a response to the anterior optic nerve disease. This may occur in demyelinative and other types of optic neuritis, anterior ischemic optic neuropathy, and papilledema. The term "neuroretinitis" is more reasonably applied if there is true inflammation of the retina and optic nerve [Figure 14–7].) Other helpful signs of prior disk edema are

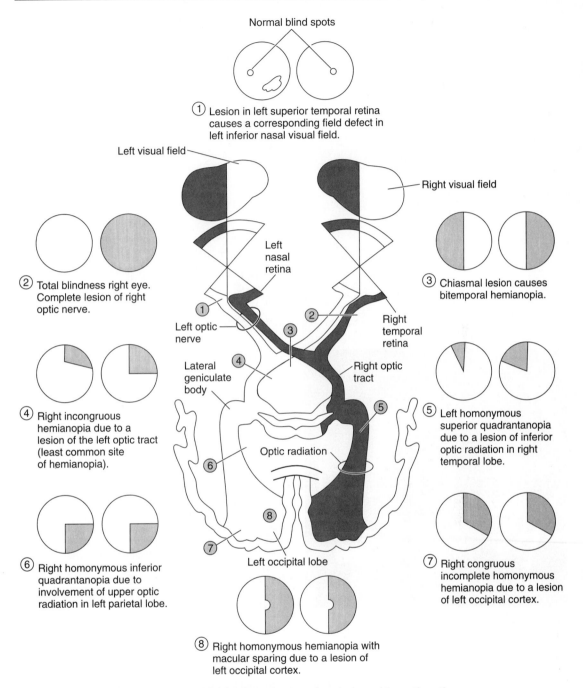

Figure 14–3. Visual field defects due to various lesions of the optic pathways.

peripapillary gliosis and atrophy, chorioretinal folds, and internal limiting membrane wrinkling.

In general there is a correlation between degree of optic disk pallor, and loss of acuity, visual field, color vision and pupillary reactions, but the relationship varies according to the underlying etiology. The major exception to this rule is compressive optic neuropathy in which optic disk pallor is generally a late manifestation.

OPTIC NEURITIS

Optic neuritis may be due to a variety of causes (Table 14–1) but the most common is demyelination. Retrobulbar neuritis is an optic neuritis that occurs far enough behind the optic disk that the disk remains normal during the acute episode. Papillitis is disk swelling caused by inflammation at the nerve head

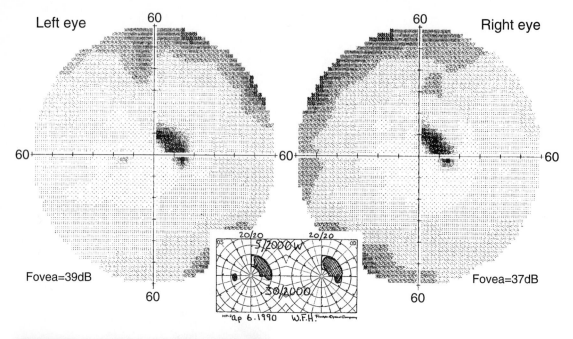

Left eye   60   60   Right eye

Fovea=39dB   Fovea=37dB

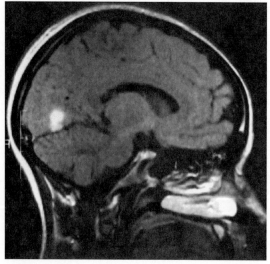

Figure 14–4. Occipital lobe abscess. **Top:** Automated perimetry and tangent screen examination showing homonymous, congruous, paracentral scotoma in right upper visual fields. **Bottom:** Parasagittal MRI showing lesion involving left inferior calcarine cortex. (Reproduced, with permission, from Horton JC, Hoyt WF: The representation of the visual field in human striate cortex. A revision of the classic Holmes map. Arch Ophthalmol 1991;109:816.)

(intraocular optic nerve) (Figure 14–8). Loss of vision is the cardinal symptom of optic neuritis and is particularly useful in differentiating papillitis from papilledema, which it may resemble on ophthalmoscopic examination.

1. DEMYELINATIVE OPTIC NEURITIS

In adults, demyelinative optic neuritis occurs chiefly in women (about 3:1) and in whites. Onset is usually in the third or fourth decade of life. The disorder is associated with multiple sclerosis in 13–85% of patients in different population groups in the world.

The percentage of progression to multiple sclerosis after an episode of optic neuritis tends to be higher with increased length of patient follow-up.

Clinical Features

Visual loss is generally subacute, developing over 2–7 days. Approximately one-third of patients have vision better than 20/40 during their first attack, and slightly more than one-third have vision worse than 20/200. Color vision and contrast sensitivity are correspondingly impaired. In over 90% of cases there is pain in the region of the eye, and about 50% of patients report that the pain is exacerbated by eye movement.

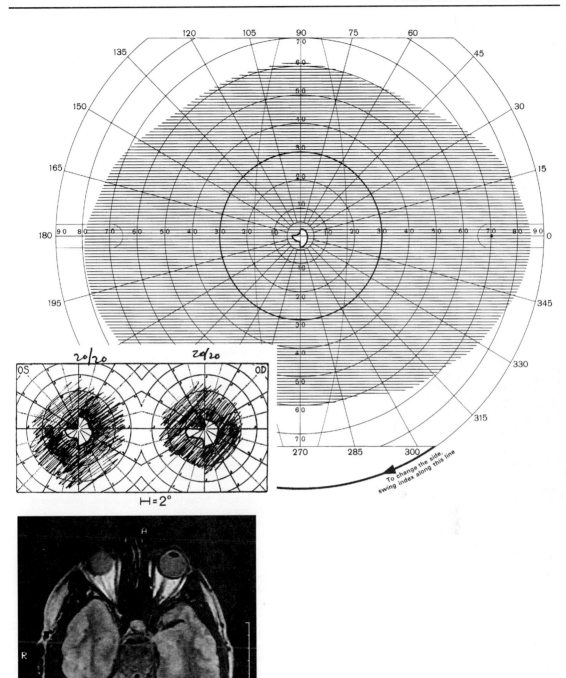

Figure 14–5. Bilateral occipital infarcts with bilateral macular sparing. **Top:** Tangent screen and superimposed Goldmann visual fields of both eyes showing bilateral homonymous hemianopia with macular sparing, greater in the right hemifield. **Bottom:** Axial MRI showing sparing of occipital poles. (Reproduced, with permission, from Horton JC, Hoyt WF: The representation of the visual field in human striate cortex. A revision of the classic Holmes map. Arch Ophthalmol 1991;109:816.)

Table 14–1. Etiologic classification of diseases of the optic nerve.

Inflammatory (optic neuritis)
Demyelinative
  Idiopathic
  Multiple sclerosis
  Neuromyelitis optica (Devic's disease)
Immune-mediated
  Postviral optic neuritis (measles, mumps, chickenpox,
    influenza, infectious mononucleosis)
  Postimmunization optic neuritis
  Acute disseminated encephalomyelitis
  Acute idiopathic polyneuropathy (Guillain-Barré
    syndrome)
  Systemic lupus erythematosus
Direct infections
  Herpes zoster, syphilis, tuberculosis, cryptococcosis,
    cytomegalovirus
Granulomatous optic neuropathy
  Sarcoidosis
  Idiopathic
Contiguous inflammatory disease
  Intraocular inflammation
  Orbital disease
  Sinus disease, including mucormycosis
  Intracranial disease: meningitis, encephalitis
Vascular (ischemic optic neuropathy)
Nonarteritic anterior ischemic optic neuropathy
Giant cell arteritis (arteritic anterior ischemic optic
  neuropathy)
Systemic vasculitis: systemic lupus erythematosus, anti-
  phospholipid antibody syndrome, polyarteritis nodosa,
  Churg-Strauss vasculitis, Sjögren's syndrome,
  Takayasu's disease
Migraine
Inherited coagulation defects: protein C deficiency, protein
  S deficiency, antithrombin III deficiency, activated
  protein C resistance (factor V Leiden mutation)
Diabetic papillopathy
Radiation optic neuropathy
Sudden massive blood loss (eg, bleeding peptic ulcer)
Raised intracranial pressure (papilledema)
Intracranial mass: cerebral tumor, abscess, subdural hem-
  atoma
Arteriovenous malformation
Subarachnoid hemorrhage
Meningitis or encephalitis
Acquired hydrocephalus
Pseudotumor cerebri
  Cerebral venous sinus occlusion
  Secondary pseudotumor cerebri: oral contraceptives,
    tetracyclines, steroid therapy, steroid withdrawal,
    hypervitaminosis A, uremia, hypoparathyroidism,
    respiratory failure
  Idiopathic intracranial hypertension
Spinal tumor
Acute idiopathic polyneuropathy (Guillain-Barré syndrome)
	Mucopolysaccharidosis
	Craniosynostosis
	Optic nerve compression
	Intracranial disease: meningioma, pituitary adenoma,
	  craniopharyngioma, supraclinoid internal carotid
	  aneurysm, meningeal carcinomatosis, basal meningitis
	Orbital disease: dysthyroid eye disease, idiopathic orbital
	  inflammatory disease, orbital neoplasm, orbital abscess
	Optic nerve sheath meningioma
	Nutritional and toxic
	Vitamin deficiencies: vitamin B_{12} deficiency, vitamin B_1
	  (thiamin) deficiency, folate deficiency
	Tobacco-alcohol amblyopia
	Heavy metals: lead, thallium, arsenic
	Drugs: ethambutol, isoniazid, rifampin, disulfiram, quinine,
	  chloramphenicol, amiodarone, digitalis, carmustine,
	  fluorouracil, vincristine, halogenated hydroxyquinolines
	  (eg, iodochlorhydroxyquin, diiodohydroxyquin),
	  hexachlorophene, penicillamine, barbiturates
	Chemicals: methanol, ethylene glycol
	Trauma
	Direct optic nerve injury
	Indirect optic nerve injury
	Optic nerve avulsion
	Hereditary optic atrophy
	Leber's hereditary optic neuropathy (mitochondrial
	  inheritance)
	Autosomal hereditary optic atrophy
	  Autosomal dominant (juvenile) optic atrophy
	  Autosomal recessive (infantile) optic atrophy
	  Wolfram's syndrome (DIDMOAD: diabetes insipidus,
	    diabetes mellitus, optic atrophy, deafness)
	Inherited neurodegenerative diseases
	  Hereditary spinocerebellar ataxia (Friedreich's ataxia)
	  Hereditary motor and sensory neuropathy (Charcot-
	    Marie-Tooth disease)
	  Lysosomal storage disorders
	Neoplastic infiltration
	Glioma, leukaemia, lymphoma, meningeal carcinomatosis,
	  astrocytic hamartoma, melanocytoma, hemangioma
	Optic nerve anomalies
	Hypoplasia
	Dysplasia, including "morning glory syndrome,"
	  coloboma, and optic nerve pit
	Tilted disks, including situs inversus, and scleral
	  crescents
	Megalopapilla
	Myelinated nerve fibers
	Persistent hyaloid system
	Prepapillary vascular loops
	Optic nerve head drusen
	Hyperopic pseudopapilledema
	Glaucomatous optic neuropathy (see Chapter 11)
	Optic atrophy secondary to retinal disease

Almost any field defect is possible, but with manual perimetry a central scotoma is most commonly found. It is usually circular, varying widely in size and density, and may break out to an altitudinal defect. A central scotoma that has broken out to the periphery, however, should make the clinician suspect a compressive lesion. Central visual field testing by automated perimetry most commonly shows diffuse loss. The pupillary light reflex is sluggish, and if the optic nerves are asymmetrically involved a relative afferent pupillary defect will be present.

Papillitis occurs in 35% of cases, with hyperemia of the optic disk and distention of large veins being early signs on ophthalmoscopic examination. Blurring of the disk margins and filling of the physiologic cup are common, and there may be marked edema of the nerve head, but elevations of more than 3 D (1 mm) are unusual. Retinal exudates and edema in the papillomacular bundle may rarely occur and are associated with a lower rate of progression to multiple sclerosis. Flame-shaped hemorrhages in the nerve fiber layer near the optic disk occur in less than 10%

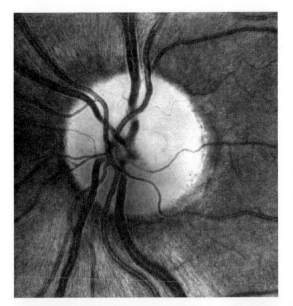
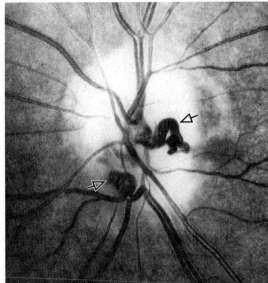
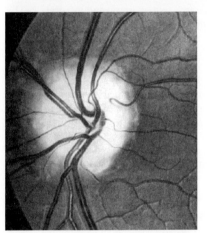
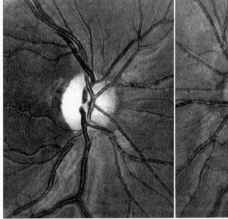
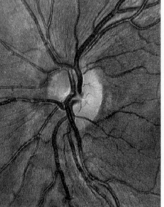

Figure 14–6. Examples of optic atrophy. ***Upper left:*** Primary optic atrophy due to nutritional amblyopia. ***Upper right:*** Secondary optic atrophy with retinochoroidal collaterals (arrows) due to optic nerve sheath meningioma. ***Lower left:*** Optic atrophy with optic disk drusen. ***Lower right:*** Pallor (atrophy) of right optic disk due to nerve compression by sphenoid meningioma. The left disk is normal.

of cases. Vitreous cells can be identified in the prepapillary area in less than 5% of cases.

Investigation & Differential Diagnosis

In typical cases, clinical diagnosis is adequate and no other investigation is required. If there are atypical features—particularly failure of vision to begin to recover by 6 weeks after onset—other diagnoses must be considered especially compressive optic neuropathy, for which MRI or CT scanning should be performed. Other entities to be considered are anterior ischemic optic neuropathy, autoimmune optic neuropathy such as that due to systemic lupus erythematosus, toxic amblyopia, Leber's hereditary optic neuropathy, and vitamin B_{12} deficiency.

Papillitis needs to be differentiated from papilledema (Figure 14–9). In papilledema there is often greater elevation of the optic nerve head, nearly normal visual acuity, normal pupillary response to light, associated intracranial pressure, and an intact visual field except for an enlarged blind spot. If there has been acute papilledema with vascular decompensation (ie, hemorrhages and cotton-wool spots) or chronic papilledema with secondary ischemia of the optic nerve, visual field defects can include nasal nerve fiber bundle defects and nasal quadrantanopias.

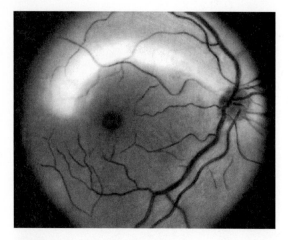

Figure 14–7. Arcuate neuroretinitis due to acute retinal necrosis syndrome. (Reproduced, with permission, from Margolis T et al: Acute retinal necrosis syndrome presenting with papillitis and arcuate neuroretinitis. Ophthalmology 1988;95:937.)

Papilledema is usually bilateral, whereas papillitis is usually unilateral. Despite these obvious differences, differential diagnosis can be difficult because of the similarity of the ophthalmoscopic findings and because papilledema can be quite asymmetric and papillitis bilateral in some postviral events (eg, Devic's disease, or neuromyelitis optica; see below).

During an acute episode of optic neuritis, MRI shows gadolinium enhancement, increased signal on STIR (short tau inversion recovery) sequences, and sometimes swelling of the affected nerve. Brain MRI will show lesions consistent with demyelination in as many as 25% of patients with isolated optic neuritis (Figure 14–10). This does not establish a diagnosis of multiple sclerosis, though it does indicate a significantly increased risk of subsequent development of clinically definite multiple sclerosis. The value of steroid treatment in delaying the development of multiple sclerosis is greater in patients with abnormal brain MRI at presentation. Thus, brain MRI may be indicated in isolated optic neuritis if more precise information is wanted about the risk of multiple sclerosis and the value of systemic steroid treatment.

The visual evoked response from the affected eye may show reduced amplitude or increased latency during the acute episode of optic neuritis. This in itself is not particularly helpful in diagnosis except in distinguishing retrobulbar optic neuritis from subclinical maculopathy, in which the visual evoked response will be relatively preserved in comparison with the pattern and cone-derived ERG. Following recovery of vision after an episode of optic neuritis, the visual evoked response will continue to show an increased latency in about one-third of cases, and this finding can be useful in the identification of past episodes of

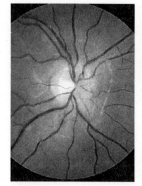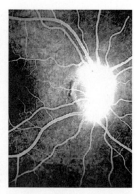

Figure 14–8. Mild disk swelling in demyelinative papillitis, with disk leakage on fluorescein angiography.

demyelinative optic neuritis in patients undergoing investigation for possible multiple sclerosis.

Treatment

Steroid therapy, either intravenous, oral, or by retrobulbar injection, accelerates recovery of vision but does not influence the ultimate visual outcome. Oral steroids may increase the risk of recurrent optic neuritis. Intravenous methylprednisolone (1 g/d for 3 days) followed by oral prednisolone (1 mg/kg/d for 11 days) has been shown to produce a greater than 50% reduction (compared with placebo treatment) in the development of clinically definite multiple sclerosis, but only for a period of 2 years. This effect was most apparent in patients with multiple brain lesions on MRI at presentation.

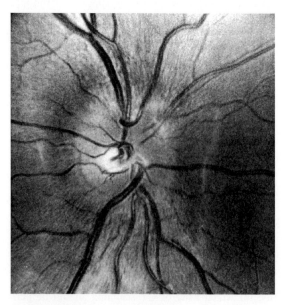

Figure 14–9. Mild papilledema. The disk margins are blurred superiorly and inferiorly by the thickened layer of nerve fibers entering the disk.

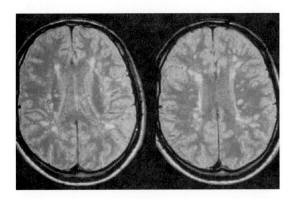

Figure 14–10. Cerebral hemisphere white matter lesions on MRI associated with acute demyelinative optic neuritis.

Prognosis

Without treatment, vision characteristically begins to improve 2–3 weeks after onset and sometimes returns to normal within a few days. Improvement may continue slowly over many months, with recovery to 20/40 or better occurring in over 90% of cases at 1 year from onset. Poorer vision during the acute episode is correlated with poorer visual outcome, but even loss of all perception of light can be followed by complete return of vision. A poor visual outcome is also associated with longer lesions in the optic nerve, especially if there is involvement of the nerve within the optic canal. In gen-

eral there is close correlation between recovery of visual acuity, contrast sensitivity, and color vision. If the disease process is sufficiently destructive, retrograde optic atrophy results, nerve fiber bundle defects appear in the retinal nerve fiber layer (Figure 14–11), and the disk loses its normal pink color and becomes pale. In very severe or recurrent cases, a chalky white disk with sharp outlines results, though disk pallor does not necessarily correlate with poor visual acuity.

Factors that correlate with subsequent development of multiple sclerosis include female sex, HLA-DR2 and -DR3, associated retinal perivenous sheathing, brain MRI abnormalities, and cerebrospinal fluid oligoclonal bands. Optic neuritis in children more commonly affects both eyes simultaneously and produces papillitis than in adults, but the risk of progression to multiple sclerosis is lower.

2. MULTIPLE SCLEROSIS

Multiple sclerosis is typically a chronic relapsing and remitting demyelinating disorder of the central nervous system. The cause is unknown. Some patients develop a chronically progressive form of the disease, either following a period of relapses and remissions or, less commonly, from the outset. Characteristically, the lesions occur at different times and in noncontiguous locations in the nervous system—ie, "lesions are disseminated in time and space." Onset is usually in

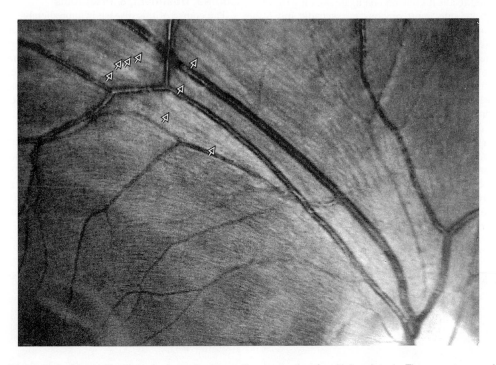

Figure 14–11. Retinal nerve fiber layer in demyelinating optic neuropathy of multiple sclerosis. The upper temporal nerve fiber bundles show multiple slit-like areas of thinning (arrows) representing retrograde axonal atrophy from subclinical disease in the optic nerve. Vision in the eye was 20/20.

young adult life; this disease rarely begins before 15 years or after 55 years of age. There is a tendency to involve the optic nerves and chiasm, brainstem, cerebellar peduncles, and spinal cord, though no part of the central nervous system is protected. The peripheral nervous system is seldom involved.

Clinical Findings

A. Symptoms and Signs: Clinically, there are a variety of symptoms and signs that may vary in number and character from time to time. In addition to ocular disturbances, there may be motor weakness with pyramidal signs, ataxia, urinary disturbances, paresthesias, dysarthria, and intention tremors. Sensory hyperesthesias and urinary incontinence are common early signs. Other problems can evolve over months to years.

Optic neuritis may be the first manifestation. Because of the transient nature of the visual defect and the relative absence of physical findings, the complaint is sometimes diagnosed as hysteria. There may be recurrent episodes, and the other eye usually becomes involved. The overall incidence of optic neuritis in multiple sclerosis is 90%, and the identification of symptomatic or subclinical optic nerve involvement is an important diagnostic clue.

Diplopia is a common early symptom, due most frequently to internuclear ophthalmoplegia. This condition, caused by a lesion of the medial longitudinal fasciculus, is characterized by paresis of the ipsilateral medial rectus muscle on conjugate lateral gaze to the opposite side, most obvious on saccadic movements, and nystagmus in the opposite (abducting) eye; thus, diplopia can occur on lateral gaze. In multiple sclerosis, the medial longitudinal fasciculus lesions are commonly bilateral (Figure 14–12). Medial rectus function can be normal for convergence if its nucleus is not involved by the demyelinating lesion. Less common causes of diplopia are lesions of the sixth or third cranial nerve within the brainstem.

Nystagmus is a common early sign, and—unlike most manifestations of the disease (which tend toward remission)—it is often permanent (70%).

Intraocular inflammation is associated with multiple sclerosis, particularly subclinical peripheral retinal venous sheathing, which can be highlighted by fluorescein angiography.

B. Laboratory Findings: The cerebrospinal fluid gamma globulin concentration is frequently high, and oligoclonal bands can be elevated, representing local production of immunoglobulins. CD8 levels in the cerebrospinal fluid may also be abnormal. Some patients with multiple sclerosis have no spinal fluid abnormalities, especially if their disease process is in a less acute or milder phase.

Pathologically, multiple areas of demyelination are present in the white matter. Early, there is degeneration of myelin sheaths and relative sparing of the axons. Glial tissue overgrowth and complete nerve fiber destruction with some round cell infiltration are seen later.

C. Special Examinations: Retinal nerve fiber layer defects consistent with a subclinical optic neuritis can be detected in 68% of multiple sclerosis patients. The visual evoked response (VER) may help confirm involvement of the visual pathway. The VER has been reported to be abnormal in 80% of definite, 43% of probable, and 22% of suspected cases of multiple sclerosis. A normal VER in cases with suspected multiple sclerosis makes the diagnosis questionable, but with positive oligoclonal bands or abnormal contrast sensitivity the diagnosis can be made with more certainty. CT scan and especially MRI can detect subclinical white matter demyelinating lesions even in the optic nerve and can confirm that there are disseminated lesions compatible with the diagnosis of multiple sclerosis.

Course, Treatment, & Prognosis

The course of this disease is unpredictable. Remissions and relapses are characteristic. Elevation of body temperature may cause temporary exacerbations (Uhthoff's phenomenon). Pregnancy or the number of pregnancies has no effect on disability, but there is an increased risk of relapse just after delivery. Onset during pregnancy has a more favorable outcome than onset unrelated to pregnancy.

Steroid treatment, particularly intravenous methylprednisolone, is useful in hastening recovery from acute relapses in multiple sclerosis but does not influence the final disability or the rate of further relapses. Systemic interferon beta reduces the rate of relapses by one-third but has no effect on long-term disability. There is no treatment that definitely influences the course of chronic progressive disease.

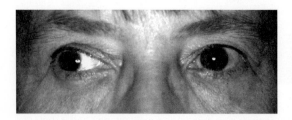 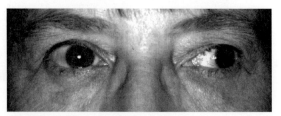

Figure 14–12. Bilateral internuclear ophthalmoplegia due to multiple sclerosis.

3. NEUROMYELITIS OPTICA
(Devic's Disease)

This rare demyelinating disease of the central nervous system—considered by many to be a severe and acute form of multiple sclerosis—is characterized by bilateral optic neuritis and transverse myelitis. It presents with a subacute onset of loss of vision in one eye, followed soon by involvement of the other eye and paraplegia. Approximately 50% of patients progress to death within the first decade due to the paraplegia, but the remainder may have a prolonged remission and, ultimately, a better prognosis than patients with chronic demyelinating disease or multiple sclerosis.

Treatment may begin with a loading dose of intravenous methylprednisolone followed by a 2-month tapering course of oral steroids. With early institution of this treatment, visual recovery can be excellent. Systemic vasculitis and sarcoidosis should always be excluded.

4. OTHER TYPES OF OPTIC NEURITIS

Particularly in children, 1–2 weeks following a viral infection or immunization there may be an episode of optic neuritis, often with simultaneous bilateral involvement. The clinical course mirrors that of idiopathic demyelinative optic neuritis, suggesting a similar pathogenesis, but there is no association with subsequent development of multiple sclerosis. In some cases the acute disease causes more extensive neurologic involvement manifesting as an encephalomyelitis, which overlaps with acute disseminated encephalomyelitis. Optic nerve involvement may also occur in acute idiopathic polyneuropathy (Guillain-Barré syndrome). In systemic lupus erythematosus the optic nerve involvement may be immune-mediated or due to small blood vessel occlusion.

Herpes zoster—particularly herpes zoster oph- thalmicus—may be complicated by optic neuropathy. This is probably due to vasculitis as well as direct neural invasion, and the prognosis is poor even with antiviral and steroid therapy. Other types of primary infection of the optic nerve, such as by syphilis, tuberculosis, cryptococcosis, and cytomegalovirus, are becoming more common with the increasing numbers of severely immunocompromised individuals such as those with AIDS. Lyme disease and cat-scratch disease are important causes of optic neuritis associated with macular star formation. Optic nerve involvement, often requiring long-term steroid therapy, is a recognized manifestation of sarcoidosis. A similar entity, idiopathic granulomatous optic neuropathy, also appears to occur in individuals in whom no evidence of sarcoidosis or other systemic disease can be identified.

Intraocular inflammation may lead to direct invasion of the anterior optic nerve with visual loss or to optic disk swelling without apparent reduction in optic nerve function. Optic nerve involvement is an important cause of permanent visual loss in cellulitis or vasculitis of the orbit. The association between sinusitis and optic neuritis is less strong than once thought, but the occurrence of visual loss in the presence of sphenoid or posterior ethmoid sinus disease may indicate a causal relationship, particularly if there is a sinus mucocele. In diabetic or immunocompromised patients, mucormycosis is an important cause of rapidly progressive sinus disease with optic and other cranial nerve involvement.

ANTERIOR ISCHEMIC OPTIC NEUROPATHY

Anterior ischemic optic neuropathy is characterized by pallid disk swelling associated with acute loss of vision: often there are one or two peripapillary splinter hemorrhages (Figure 14–13). The disorder is

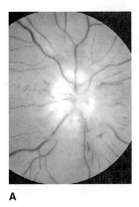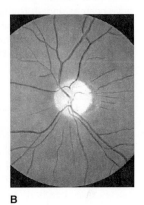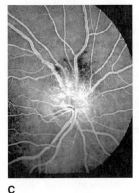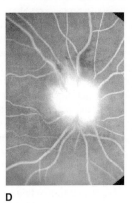

A   B   C   D

Figure 14–13. Pseudo-Foster Kennedy syndrome due to sequential anterior ischemic optic neuropathy. *A:* Swollen right optic disk with hemorrhages due to current ischemic episode. *B:* Atrophy of left optic disk due to previous ischemia. *C:* Early phase of fluorescein angiogram of right eye showing poor perfusion of optic disk and dilated superficial disk capillaries. *D:* Late phase of fluorescein angiogram showing disk leakage.

due to infarction of the retrolaminar optic nerve (the region just posterior to the lamina cribrosa) from occlusion or decreased perfusion of the short posterior ciliary arteries. Fluorescein angiography in the acute stage shows decreased perfusion of the optic disk, often segmental in the nonarteritic form but usually diffuse in the arteritic form, and disk leakage in the late phase. There may be associated perfusion defects in the peripapillary choroid.

Nonarteritic ischemic optic neuropathy occurs generally in the sixth or seventh decade and is associated with arteriosclerosis, diabetes, hypertension, and hyperlipidemia, but any thrombotic condition capable of producing intracranial stroke can affect the posterior ciliary arteries as well. Systemic hypotension during the early morning may be an important etiologic factor. In younger patients, vasculitis (eg, systemic lupus erythematosus, antiphospholipid antibody syndrome, and polyarteritis nodosa), migraine, and inherited prothrombotic states (deficiencies of protein C, protein S, or antithrombin III and activated protein C resistance) should be explored and appropriately treated. A significantly reduced cup:disk ratio with crowding of axons in a relatively small scleral canal, optic nerve head drusen, and increased intraocular pressure may be predisposing factors. The visual loss in nonarteritic anterior ischemic optic neuropathy is generally abrupt, but it may be progressive over 1–2 weeks. Impairment of visual acuity varies from slight to no light perception; visual field defects are commonly altitudinal (inferior defects more common than superior ones). In over 40% of cases, there is spontaneous improvement in visual acuity. No treatment has been shown to provide long-term benefit. The previously advocated optic nerve sheath fenestration procedure has been shown to be potentially harmful. Low-dose aspirin therapy may reduce the risk of involvement of the fellow eye, which occurs in up to 40% of individuals. Recurrences in the same eye are rare, presumably related to decompression of the scleral canal due to infarction of axons. As the acute process resolves, a pale disk with or without "glaucomatous" cupping results.

It is particularly important to identify the **arteritic anterior ischemic optic neuropathy,** due to giant cell arteritis. This causes severe visual loss with the risk of complete blindness if treatment is delayed. It occurs in elderly people and is associated with a high sedimentation rate, painful and tender temporal arteries, pain on mastication, general malaise, and muscular aches and pains (polymyalgia rheumatica). It may represent an autoimmune response to internal elastic lamina that is bared to the systemic circulation by ulcerated arteriosclerotic plaques. The diagnosis is usually based upon an anterior ischemic optic neuropathy and a high ESR in an elderly patient, with or without associated systemic features. Other ocular manifestations of giant cell arteritis are central retinal artery occlusion, cilioretinal artery occlusion, retinal cotton-wool spots, ophthalmic artery occlusion, and diffuse ocular ische-

emia. Diagnosis is established by temporal artery biopsy, looking particularly for inflammatory cell infiltration, often but not always including giant cells, and prominent disruption of the internal elastic lamina.

Treatment with high-dose systemic steroids should be started as soon as a clinical diagnosis of arteritic anterior ischemic optic neuropathy has been made without waiting for the result of temporal artery biopsy, which should be performed within 1 week after starting treatment. Oral prednisolone, 80–100 mg/d, is usually adequate as a starting dose, but intravenous methylprednisolone should be considered in patients with bilateral disease—including those with transient episodes of visual loss in the second eye—and in patients whose visual loss progresses or whose systemic manifestations and high ESR do not respond despite oral therapy. Steroid dosage can usually be reduced to about 40 mg prednisolone per day over two weeks but then should be more gradually tapered and discontinued after about 6 months overall as long as there has been no recurrence of disease activity. Thirty percent of patients require long-term steroid therapy.

Diabetics occasionally develop mild, chronic, usually bilateral disk swelling with little change in visual function, so-called **diabetic papillopathy.** This is thought to represent microvascular disease affecting the optic disk circulation. It is sometimes confused with optic disk neovascularization because of the leakage of dye from the disk on fluorescein angiography. Radiation damage, usually from radiotherapy treatment for skull base or sinus tumors 12–18 months previously, and massive blood loss, such as from a bleeding peptic ulcer, are two causes of ischemic optic neuropathy in which there may be no optic disk swelling during the acute stage of the disease. This is sometimes referred to as posterior ischemic optic neuropathy. Other causes are giant cell arteritis and mucormycosis. In general the diagnosis of posterior ischemic optic neuropathy should not be considered until other causes, particularly a compressive lesion, have been excluded. Radiation optic neuropathy produces characteristic changes of tissue swelling and focal gadolinium enhancement on MRI and may be helped by hyperbaric oxygen therapy.

PAPILLEDEMA
(Figures 14–9 and 14–14
to 14–16)

Papilledema (choked disk) is by definition a noninflammatory congestion of the optic disk due to raised intracranial pressure, of which the most common causes are cerebral tumors, abscesses, subdural hematoma, arteriovenous malformations, subarachnoid hemorrhage, acquired hydrocephalus, meningitis, and encephalitis.

In an ophthalmology practice where patients come in and are usually healthy except for visual complaints, papilledema is often due to idiopathic intracranial hypertension. This is characterized by papilledema, no neurologic abnormality except for perhaps sixth or more rarely seventh cranial nerve palsy, normal neuroimaging studies, including brain MRI, and normal cerebrospinal fluid studies apart from increased intracranial pressure. It is, however, a diagnosis of exclusion, and a number of other causes of this syndrome of pseudotumor cerebri must be excluded, such as cerebral venous sinus occlusion, oral contraceptive use, steroid or tetracycline therapy, uremia, and respiratory failure.

Less common causes of papilledema are spinal tumors, acute idiopathic polyneuropathy (Guillain-Barré syndrome), mucopolysaccharidoses, and craniosynostoses, in which various factors, including decreased cerebrospinal fluid absorption, abnormalities of spinal fluid flow, and reduced cranial volume, contribute to the raised intracranial pressure.

For papilledema to occur, the subarachnoid spaces around the optic nerve must be patent and connect the retrolaminar optic nerve through the bony optic canal to the intracranial subarachnoid space, thus allowing increased intracranial pressure to be transmitted to the retrolaminar optic nerve. There slow and fast axonal transport is blocked, and axonal distention, particularly noticeable at the superior and inferior poles of the optic disk, occurs as the first sign of papilledema. Hyperemia of the disk, dilated surface capillary telangiectases, blurring of the peripapillary disk margin, and loss of spontaneous venous pulsations are the signs of mild papilledema. Edema around the disk can cause a decreased sensitivity to small isopters on visual field testing, but circumferential retinal folds with changes in the internal limiting membrane reflexes (Paton's lines) will eventually become evident as the retina is pushed away from the choked disk; when the retina is pushed away, the blind spot will be enlarged to large isopters on visual field testing as well. In acute papilledema, probably as a consequence either of markedly elevated or rapidly increasing intracranial pressure, there are hemorrhages and cotton-wool spots, indicating vascular and axonal decompensation with the attendant risk of acute optic nerve damage and visual field defects (Figure 14–14). There may also be peripapillary edema (which can extend to the macula) and choroidal folds. In chronic papilledema (Figure 14–15), which is likely to be the consequence of prolonged moderately raised intracranial pressure, a process of compensation appears to limit the optic disk changes such that there are few if any hemorrhages or cotton-wool spots. With persistent raised intracranial pressure, the hyperemic elevated disk gradually becomes gray-white as a result of astrocytic gliosis and neural atrophy with secondary constriction of retinal blood vessels, thus leading to the stage of atrophic papilledema (Figure 14–16). There may also be retinochoroidal collaterals (previously known as opticociliary shunts) linking the central retinal vein and

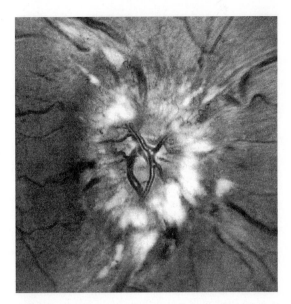

Figure 14–14. Acute papilledema with cotton-wool spots and hemorrhages.

the peripapillary choroidal veins, which develop when the retinal venous circulation is obstructed in the prelaminar region of the optic nerve. (Other causes of retinochoroidal collaterals are central retinal vein occlusion, optic nerve sheath meningioma, optic nerve glioma, and optic nerve head drusen.) Vintage papilledema is characterized by the presence of drusen-like deposits within the swollen optic nerve head.

It takes 24–48 hours for early papilledema to occur and 1 week to develop fully. It takes 6–8 weeks for fully developed papilledema to resolve during adequate treatment. Acute papilledema may reduce visual acuity by causing hyperopia and occasionally is associated with optic nerve infarction, but in most cases vision is normal apart from blind spot enlargement. Chronic atrophic and vintage papilledema are associated with gradual constriction of the peripheral visual field, particularly inferonasal loss, and transient visual obscurations. Sudden reduction of intracranial pressure or systolic perfusion pressure may precipitate severe visual loss in any stage of papilledema.

Papilledema is often asymmetric. It may even appear to be unilateral, though fluorescein angiography in such cases usually shows leakage from both disks. Papilledema occurs late in glaucoma, but it will not occur at all if there is optic atrophy or if the optic nerve sheath on that side is not patent. Foster Kennedy's syndrome is papilledema on one side with optic atrophy on the other (optic nerve and sheath compressed by neoplasm). This is commonly due to meningiomas of the sphenoid wing and classically to meningiomas of the olfactory groove. However, this clinical presentation can be mimicked (pseudo-Foster Kennedy syndrome) by ischemic optic neuropathy

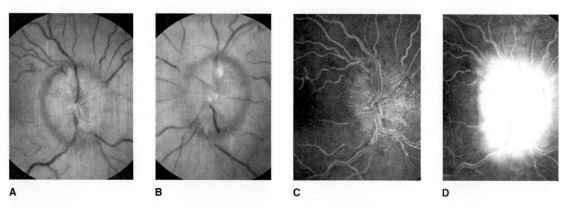

A   B   C   D

Figure 14–15. Chronic papilledema with prominent disk swelling, capillary dilation, and retinal folds but few hemorrhages or cotton-wool spots **(A)** and **(B)**. Fluorescein angiography demonstrates the capillary dilation in its early phase **(C)** and marked disk leakage in its late phase **(D)**.

when an old ischemic optic neuropathy with atrophy is associated with a new hyperemic ischemic optic neuropathy (Figure 14–13).

Papilledema can be mimicked by buried drusen of the optic nerve, small hyperopic disks, and myelinated nerve fibers (Figure 14–17). The treatment of papilledema must be directed to the underlying cause. In idiopathic intracranial hypertension, weight loss and oral acetazolamide (250 mg one to four times daily) are usually effective, but lumboperitoneal shunting or optic nerve sheath fenestration may become necessary if there is severe or progressive visual loss.

OPTIC NERVE COMPRESSION

Optic nerve compression is often amenable to treatment, and early recognition is vital to optimal outcome. The possibility of optic nerve compression should be considered in any patient with signs of optic neuropathy or visual loss not explained by an intraocular lesion. Optic disk swelling may occur with intraorbital optic nerve compression but in many cases, particularly when the optic nerve compression is intracranial, the optic disk shows no abnormality until optic atrophy develops or there is papilledema from associated raised intracranial pressure. (Examination for signs of optic nerve disease, particularly a relative afferent pupillary defect, is thus crucial in assessment of the patient with unexplained visual loss.) Investigation of possible optic nerve compression requires early imaging by MRI or CT. If no structural lesion is identified and meningeal disease is suspected, it may be necessary to proceed to cerebrospinal fluid examination.

Intracranial meningiomas that may compress the optic nerve include those arising from the sphenoid wing, the tuberculum sellae (suprasellar meningioma), and the olfactory groove. Sphenoid wing meningiomas also produce proptosis, ocular motility disturbance,

and trigeminal sensory loss (Figure 14–18). Surgical excision is generally effective in debulking intracranial meningiomas, but complete excision is often very difficult to achieve and recurrence rates are relatively high. Radiotherapy may be indicated as adjuvant or primary treatment. Pituitary adenoma and craniopharyngioma are discussed in the section on chiasmal disease (see below). The management of orbital causes of optic nerve compression is discussed in Chapter 13.

Primary optic nerve sheath meningioma is a rare tumor most commonly presenting, like other types of

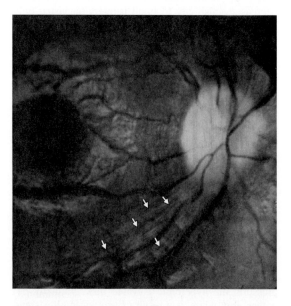

Figure 14–16. Atrophic papilledema in a child with a cerebellar medulloblastoma. The disk is pale and slightly elevated and has blurred margins. The white areas surrounding the macula are reflected light from the vitreoretinal interface. The inferior temporal nerve fiber bundles are partially atrophic (arrows).

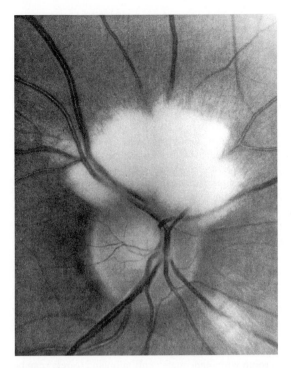

Figure 14–17. Large patch of myelinated nerve fibers originating from superior edge of disk. Another smaller patch is present near the inferior nasal border of the disk. (Right eye.)

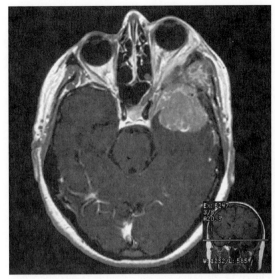

Figure 14–18. Axial MRI of sphenoid wing meningioma causing proptosis.

meningioma, in middle-aged women (Figure 14–19). Five percent of cases are bilateral. Visual loss is slowly progressive. The classic clinical features are a pale, slightly swollen optic disk with retinochoroidal collaterals, but in most cases the collateral vessels are not present (Figure 14–6). Surgical excision invariably leads to complete loss of vision and is generally reserved for blind eyes to prevent intracranial spread of tumor. Focal radiotherapy is becoming more popular.

NUTRITIONAL & TOXIC OPTIC NEUROPATHIES

The usual clinical features of nutritional or toxic optic neuropathy are subacute, progressive, symmetrical visual loss, with central field defects (Figure 14–20), poor color vision, and the development of temporal disk pallor (Figure 14–6).

1. VITAMIN DEFICIENCY

Optic nerve involvement is relatively uncommon in vitamin B_{12} deficiency, but it may be the first manifestation of pernicious anemia. Thiamin (vitamin B_1) deficiency is generally a feature of severe malnutrition, and, as discussed below, there is an overlap with tobacco-alcohol amblyopia. Whether folate deficiency alone can produce an optic neuropathy is not entirely clear.

2. TOBACCO-ALCOHOL AMBLYOPIA

Nutritional amblyopia is another term for this entity. It occurs more commonly in males with poor dietary habits, particularly if the diet is deficient in thiamine.

Heavy drinking with or without heavy smoking is most often associated with a poor nutritional state. Bilateral loss of central vision is present in over 50% of patients, reducing visual acuity to less than 20/200, but can be asymmetric. Central visual fields reveal scotomas that nearly always include both fixation and the blind spot (centrocecal scotoma) (Figure 14–20).

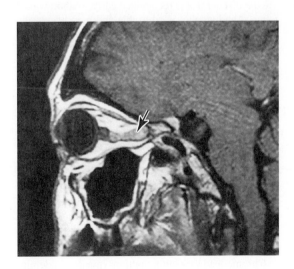

Figure 14–19. MRI of tubular optic nerve sheath meningioma.

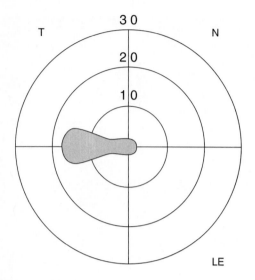

Figure 14–20. Nutritional amblyopia showing centrocecal scotoma. VA = 20/200.

Centrocecal scotomas are usually of constant density, but when density of the scotoma varies, the most dense portion usually lies between fixation and the blind spot in the papillomacular bundle.

Much consideration has been given in the literature to other toxic causes such as cyanide from tobacco, producing low vitamin stores and low levels of sulfur-containing amino acids, but experimental studies with cyanide in primates have not confirmed this theory. Leber's hereditary optic neuropathy, pernicious anemia, methanol poisoning, retrobulbar neuritis, or macular degeneration may cause diagnostic confusion.

Adequate diet plus thiamine, folic acid, and vitamin B_{12} is nearly always effective in completely curing the disease if it is recognized early. Withdrawal of tobacco and alcohol is advisable and may hasten the cure, but innumerable cases are known in which adequate nutrition or vitamin B_{12} supplements effected the cure despite continued excessive intake of alcohol or tobacco. Improvement usually begins within 1–2 months, though in occasional cases significant improvement may not occur for a year. Visual function can but may not return to normal; permanent optic atrophy or at least temporal disk pallor can occur depending upon the stage of disease at the time treatment was started (Figure 14–6). Loss of the ganglion cells of the macula and destruction of myelinated fibers of the optic nerve—and sometimes of the chiasm as well—are the main histologic changes.

3. HEAVY METAL POISONING

Chronic lead exposure, thallium (present in depilatory cream), or arsenic poisoning can produce a toxic effect on the optic nerve.

4. DRUG-INDUCED OPTIC NEUROPATHY

Ethambutol, isoniazid (INH), rifampin, and disulfiram can all produce retrobulbar neuritis or papillitis, which will improve with prompt cessation of the drug with or without nutritional supplements. Serial color vision screening is the most sensitive clinical test and must be done prophylactically.

Quinine is toxic to ganglion cells and will cause optic neuropathy with severely narrowed retinal arteries. Chloramphenicol in high doses causes optic neuropathy. Amiodarone toxicity can produce bilateral disk edema, but it characteristically also induces a verticillate keratopathy as well as other central nervous system signs.

5. CHEMICAL-INDUCED OPTIC NEUROPATHY: METHANOL POISONING

Methanol is used widely in the chemical industry as antifreeze, solvent varnish, or paint remover; it is also present in fumes of some industrial solvents such as those used in old photocopier machines. Significant systemic absorption can occur from fumes inhaled in a room with inadequate ventilation and (rarely) can be absorbed through the skin.

Clinical Findings

Visual impairment can be the first sign and begins with mild blurring of vision that progresses to contraction of visual fields and sometimes to complete blindness. The field defects are quite extensive and nearly always include the centrocecal area.

Hyperemia of the disk is the first ophthalmoscopic finding. Within the first 2 days, a whitish, striated edema of the disk margins and nearby retina appears (Figure 14–21). Disk edema can last up to 2 months and is followed by optic atrophy of mild to severe degree.

Decreased pupillary response to light occurs in proportion to the amount of visual loss. In severe cases, the pupils become dilated and fixed. Extraocular muscle palsies and ptosis may also occur.

Treatment

Treatment consists of correction of the acidosis with intravenous sodium bicarbonate and oral or intravenous administration of ethanol to compete with and thus prevent the slower metabolism of methanol into its by-products. Hemodialysis is indicated for blood methanol levels over 50 mg/dL.

OPTIC NERVE TRAUMA

Direct optic nerve injury occurs in penetrating orbital trauma, including local anesthetic injections for ocular surgery, and in fractures involving the optic canal. Visual loss due to indirect optic nerve trauma,

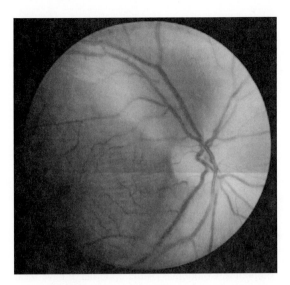

Figure 14–21. Methanol poisoning. Note edema of the retina and optic disk.

which refers to optic nerve damage secondary to distant skull injury, occurs in approximately 1% of all head injuries. The site of injury is usually the forehead, often without skull fracture, and the probable mechanism of optic nerve injury is transmission of shock waves through the orbital walls to the orbital apex. Optic nerve avulsion usually results from an abrupt rotational injury to the globe, such as from being poked in the eye with a finger.

High-dose systemic steroids may be beneficial in both direct and indirect optic nerve injuries. Surgery may be indicated to relieve orbital, subperiosteal, or optic nerve sheath hemorrhage or to treat orbital fractures. Decompression of the bony optic canal has also been advocated for indirect optic nerve trauma but its value is uncertain. There is no effective treatment for optic nerve avulsion.

HEREDITARY OPTIC ATROPHY

1. LEBER'S HEREDITARY OPTIC NEUROPATHY

Leber's hereditary optic neuropathy is a rare disease characterized by sequential subacute optic neuropathy in males aged 11–30 years. The underlying genetic abnormality is a point mutation in mitochondrial DNA (mtDNA), over 90% of affected families harboring a mutation at position 11778, 14484, or 3460. mtDNA is exclusively derived from the mother and thus, in accordance with the general pattern of mitochondrial (maternal) inheritance (see Chapter 18), the mutation is transmitted through the female line—but for unexplained reasons the disease rarely manifests in carrier females. Once an individual is known to have the dis-

order, it is possible without further genetic testing to predict which other family members are at risk, matrilineal nephews, ie, sons of the affected individual's sisters, being particularly at risk.

Blurred vision and a central scotoma appear first in one eye and later—within days, weeks, or months—in the other eye. During the acute episode, there may be swelling of the optic disk and peripapillary retina with dilated telangiectatic small blood vessels on their surface, but characteristically there is no leak from the optic disk during fluorescein angiography. Both optic nerves eventually become atrophic, and vision is usually between 20/200 and counting fingers. The 14484 mutation is associated with recovery of vision but not until many months after the initial onset of visual loss. Total loss of vision or recurrences of visual loss usually do not occur. Leber's neuropathy may be associated with a multiple sclerosis-like illness (particularly in affected females), cardiac conduction defects, and dystonia.

Diagnosis is by identification of one of the three mtDNA point mutations. There is no known treatment. Because high tobacco and alcohol consumption may precipitate visual loss in susceptible individuals, carriers of a pathogenic point mutation, particularly males, should be advised not to smoke and to avoid high alcohol consumption.

Optic atrophy also occurs in other mitochondrial disorders, either as a manifestation of primary optic neuropathy—eg, MERRF (myoclonic epilepsy and ragged red fibers) and MELAS (mitochondrial myopathy, lactic acidosis and stroke-like episodes)—or secondary to retinal degeneration, eg, Kearns-Sayre syndrome. Wolfram's syndrome (see below) is also probably the result of a mitochondrial disorder.

2. AUTOSOMAL HEREDITARY OPTIC ATROPHY

Autosomal dominant (juvenile) optic atrophy generally has an insidious onset in childhood, with slow progression of visual loss throughout life. It is often detected as mild reduction in visual acuity by childhood vision screening programs. There is characteristically a centrocecal scotoma with impaired color vision. Temporal optic disk pallor is usually present, though often mild, and mild disk cupping is occasionally seen. Diagnosis is by identification of other affected family members. The genetic defect has been mapped to the long arm of chromosome 3, and for that reason there may soon be a specific genetic test. Rarely, the disease is associated with congenital or progressive deafness or ataxia.

Autosomal recessive (infantile) optic atrophy manifests as severe visual loss, present at birth or within 2 years and accompanied by nystagmus. It can be associated with progressive hearing loss, spastic quadriplegia, and dementia, though an inborn error of metabolism must first be considered. Wolfram's syndrome consists of juvenile diabetes insipidus, diabetes mellitus, optic atrophy, and deafness (DID-MOAD). Although there is a recessive pattern of inheritance, with the gene defect localized to chromosome 4, the underlying metabolic abnormality is probably a defect in cellular energy production, as in the mitochondrial diseases.

3. OPTIC ATROPHY WITH INHERITED NEURODEGENERATIVE DISEASES

Various neurodegenerative diseases with onset in the years from childhood to early adult life are manifested by steadily progressive neurologic and visual signs. Examples are hereditary spinocerebellar ataxias (Friedreich's ataxia), hereditary motor and sensory neuropathy (Charcot-Marie-Tooth disease), and the lysosomal storage disorders. Most of the sphingolipidoses late in their course are associated with optic atrophy. The leukodystrophies (Krabbe's, metachromatic leukodystrophy, adrenoleukodystrophy, globoid dystrophy, Pelizaeus-Merzbacher disease, Schilder's disease) are associated with optic atrophy earlier. Canavan's spongy degeneration and glioneuronal dystrophy (Alper's disease) are associated with optic atrophy as well. Peroxisome disorders (Zellweger's disease, Refsum's disease, etc) can have optic atrophy with cataract, glaucoma, and a pigmentary retinopathy. Optic atrophy can occur in the mucopolysaccharidoses due to hydrocephalus from mucopolysaccharides in the meninges or due to mucopolysaccharides in glial cells of the optic nerve.

Optic atrophy secondary to retinal ganglion cell atrophy can also occur in Alzheimer's disease. Large retinal ganglion cells project to the superior colliculus, and eye movement abnormalities occur as well.

NEOPLASTIC OPTIC NERVE INFILTRATION

Optic nerve glioma is discussed below, together with chiasmal glioma. In leukemia (usually acute leukemia), non-Hodgkin's lymphoma, and disseminated carcinoma, optic nerve infiltration with marked visual loss and optic disk swelling may develop. Primary neoplasms of the optic nerve include the astrocytic hamartoma of tuberous sclerosis, melanocytoma, and hemangioma, all rarely causing any visual disturbance.

OPTIC NERVE ANOMALIES

There are a large number of congenital optic nerve anomalies. They may be associated with other anomalies of the head since closure of the fetal fissure, ocular melanogenesis, and disk development occur at the same time as development of the skull and face.

Optic nerve hypoplasia, dysplasia, and coloboma have all been associated with basal encephaloceles as well and with varying intracranial anomalies, from Duane's retraction syndrome to agenesis of the corpus callosum (de Morsier's syndrome) and pituitary-hypothalamic dysfunction (especially growth hormone deficiency). Hypoplastic optic nerves are small, with normal-sized retinal blood vessels (Figure 14–22). They are associated with a wide range of visual acuities, astigmatism, a peripapillary halo that may have a pigmented rim also (double-ring sign), and various visual field defects. Dysplastic optic disks usually are associated with poor vision and show abnormal vasculature, retinal pigment epithelium, and glial tissue. They are often surrounded by a chorioretinal pigmentary disturbance. Dysplastic disks have been reported with trisomy 4q. The papillorenal syndrome has been reported with dysplastic disks and colobomas. Colobomas of the optic nerve have been called "pseudoglaucoma" because of their resemblance to glaucomatous cupping (Figure 14–23). Disk colobomas or hypoplasia when associated with chorioretinal lacunae, absence of the corpus callosum, and focal seizures constitute Aicardi's syndrome. This can also include retrobulbar cysts. Optic disk pits are usually not associated with any visual symptoms but they can be mistaken for glaucomatous cupping, particularly if there is an associated field defect. Occasionally, optic disk pits present later in life as a consequence of serous detachment of the macula.

Tilted disks, which occur in 3% of normals, may also be seen with hypertelorism or the craniofacial dysostoses (Crouzon's disease, Apert's disease). They are oval disks with usually an inferior scleral crescent and an associated area of fundus hypopigmentation (Figure 14–24). They may be mistaken for papilledema. They may also produce predominantly upper temporal field defects, which may be mistaken for bitemporal loss due to chiasmal dysfunction. Scleral crescents are particularly common in myopic eyes.

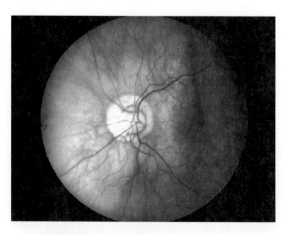

Figure 14–22. Optic nerve hypoplasia.

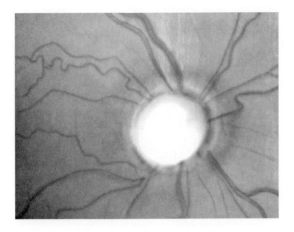

Figure 14–23. Optic disk coloboma.

Megalopapilla may be mistaken for optic atrophy due to the prominence of the lamina cribrosa. Myelinated nerve fibers usually extend into the retina from the disk, but occasionally are just seen in the retinal periphery (Figure 14–17). They always follow the course of the retinal nerve fiber layer. Remnants of the embryonic hyaloid system range from tissue fragments on the optic disk (Bergmeister's papilla) to strands extending to the posterior lens capsule. Prepapillary vascular loops are distinct from the hyaloid system and occasionally become obstructed, leading to branch retinal artery occlusion.

Optic nerve head drusen are clinically apparent in about 0.3% of the population but are found on ultrasound or histopathologic studies in 1% or more. In children, they are usually buried within the disk substance and thus are not visible on clinical examination but cause elevation of the disk surface and mimic papilledema. The optic disk is characteristically small, with no physiologic cup and an anomalous pattern of exit of the retinal vessels. With increasing age and loss of overlying axons, optic nerve head drusen

become exposed, being apparent as "lumpy-bumpy" yellow crystalline excrescences, highlighted by retroillumination of the disk substance (Figure 14–6). On fluorescein angiography, exposed drusen are autofluorescent and result in accumulation of dye within the disk substance (Figure 14–25). Buried drusen are best diagnosed by orbital ultrasound or thin slice CT scanning, which detect their associated calcification. Optic nerve head drusen are usually bilateral. They can rarely cause visual loss, either by optic neuropathy, choroidal neovascularization, or vitreous hemorrhage. Hyperopic eyes may also have small elevated disks, resembling buried optic nerve head drusen and similarly mimicking papilledema.

THE OPTIC CHIASM

In general, lesions of the chiasm cause bitemporal hemianopic defects. Early, these defects are typically incomplete and are often asymmetric. However, as compression progresses, the temporal hemianopia becomes complete, the inferior and superior nasal fields will then be involved, and central visual acuity will decrease. Most diseases that affect the chiasm are neoplastic, with vascular or inflammatory processes only occasionally producing chiasmatic visual field loss.

PITUITARY TUMORS

The anterior lobe of the pituitary gland is the site of origin of pituitary tumors (Figure 14–26). Symptoms and signs include loss of vision, field changes, pituitary dysfunction, extraocular nerve palsies, and evidence on CT scan or MRI of sellar and suprasellar tumor.

Combination therapy with radiation and surgery has been challenged by medical treatment with bromocriptine, which has been effective not only in tumors associated with galactorrhea but also in some null cell (or endocrinologically inactive) tumors. Visual loss or endocrine dysfunction is an indication for treatment. Visual acuity and visual fields may improve dramatically after pressure has been removed from the chiasm. The initial appearance of the optic nerve head does not predict the ultimate visual outcome.

CRANIOPHARYNGIOMA

Craniopharyngiomas are an uncommon group of tumors arising from epithelial remnants of Rathke's pouch (80% of the population normally have such

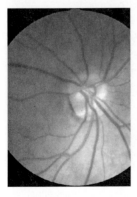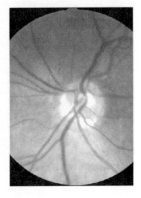

Figure 14–24. Bilateral tilted optic disks.

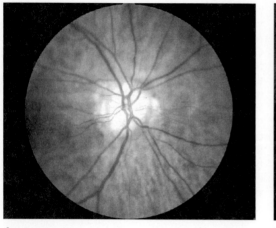

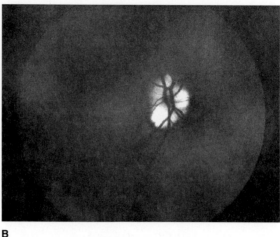

A   B

Figure 14–25. Optic nerve head drusen **(A)** exhibiting autofluorescence **(B).**

remnants) and characteristically become symptomatic between the ages of 10 and 25 years but occasionally not until the 60s and 70s. They are usually suprasellar (Figure 14–27), occasionally intrasellar. The signs and symptoms vary tremendously with the age of the patient and the exact location of the tumor as well as its rate of growth. When a suprasellar tumor occurs, asymmetric chiasmatic or tract field defects are prominent. Papilledema is more common than in pituitary tumors. Optic nerve hypoplasia can be seen in those tumors presenting in infancy. Pituitary deficiency may result, and involvement of the hypothalamus may cause stunted growth. Calcification of parts of the tumor contributes to a characteristic radiologic appearance, especially in children.

Treatment consists of surgical removal—as complete as possible at the first procedure, since reopera-tion tends to involve the hypothalamus, and patients then do poorly. Adjunctive radiotherapy is often used, particularly if there has been incomplete surgical removal.

SUPRASELLAR MENINGIOMAS

Suprasellar meningiomas arise from the meninges covering the tuberculum sellae and the planum sphenoidale, with a high proportion of patients being female. The tumor is usually anterior and superior to the chiasm. Visual field changes due to involvement of the optic nerves and chiasm often occur early (but asymmetrically) followed by slowly progressive damage to the visual pathway. CT scans with contrast enhancement easily demonstrate these tumors. Hyperos-

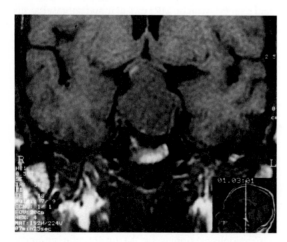

Figure 14–26. Coronal MRI showing large pituitary adenoma elevating and distorting the optic chiasm.

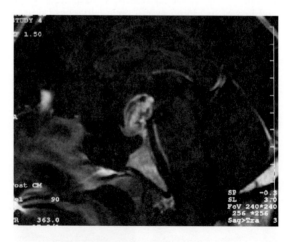

Figure 14–27. Sagittal MRI showing contrast enhanced suprasellar craniopharyngioma.

toses associated with bony erosion and a dense calcified tumor are the radiologic hallmarks of meningioma. Treatment consists of surgical removal, often combined with adjuvant radiotherapy if there has been incomplete excision.

CHIASMATIC & OPTIC NERVE GLIOMAS

Optic nerve and chiasm gliomas are rare, usually indolent disorders of children that sometimes occur as part of the clinical picture of neurofibromatosis 1. Onset may be sudden, with rapid loss of vision. Optic atrophy occurs, and visual field defects reveal an optic nerve or chiasmatic syndrome. Neuroimaging may reveal enlarged optic nerves and a mass in the region of the chiasm and hypothalamus. Treatment depends on the location of the tumor and its clinical course. Irradiation can be given during a tumor growth spurt, and optic nerve resection is sometimes done when an optic nerve tumor aggressively starts to extend intracranially toward the chiasm.

Malignant glioma of the anterior visual pathways is a rare disease of elderly men. There is a rapid clinical course to bilateral blindness and death due to invasion of the base of the brain. There is no effective treatment.

THE RETROCHIASMATIC VISUAL PATHWAYS

Cerebrovascular disease and tumors are responsible for most lesions of the retrochiasmatic visual pathways, though almost any intracranial disease process can involve these structures. Retrochiasmatic visual field defects are homonymous. Partial lesions in the optic tract and lateral geniculate nucleus produce incongruous (or dissimilar) visual field defects due to a 90-degree medial rotation of axons in each tract and the decussation of half of the axons through the chiasm. Thus, there may be more involvement of a nasal hemifield than of its corresponding temporal hemifield. Once the lesion becomes complete, however, incongruity cannot be assessed, and this sign loses its localizing ability. Retrochiasmatic visual field defects should spare visual acuity since the visual pathway from the other hemibrain is intact. The optic tracts and lateral geniculate nucleus are infrequently affected. After several weeks to months, the disks may appear pale, and the retinal nerve fiber layer is deficient. The optic tract and lateral geniculate nucleus have at least a dual blood supply, so that primary vascular lesions are uncommon. Most cases are due to trauma, tumors, arteriovenous malformations, abscesses, and demyelinating diseases.

Lesions involving the geniculocalcarine pathway to the occipital cortex produce homonymous field defects but do not result in optic atrophy (due to the synapse at the geniculate nucleus). Generally, the more posterior a lesion is located, the more congruous the homonymous visual field defect. The inferior geniculocalcarine pathway passes through the temporal lobe and the superior pathway through the parietal lobe, with macular function between them. Lesions of the inferior pathway result in superior visual field defects. Processes affecting the anterior and midtemporal lobes are commonly neoplastic; posterior temporal lobe and parietal processes can be either vascular or neoplastic. An insidious onset with mild and multiple neurologic deficits would be more typically neoplastic, whereas an acute cataclysmic neurologic event would be more typically vascular. Vascular lesions of the occipital lobe, on the other hand, are common and account for over 80% of cases of isolated homonymous visual field loss in patients over age 50 years. The most posterior tip of each occipital lobe projects to homonymous macular fields. Anterior to the macular representation lies the peripheral field; thus, vascular occlusions can selectively involve the posterior occipital cortex and produce homonymous defects with congruous macular scotomas or spare the posterior cortex, and homonymous defects with macular sparing will result. The cortical centers involved in the generation of optokinetic nystagmus lie in the area between the occipital and temporal lobes and in the posterior parietal area, which are within the vascular territory of the middle cerebral artery. Optokinetic nystagmus asymmetry characteristically occurs in parietal lesions but not in occipital lesions. An asymmetric optokinetic nystagmus combined with an occipital visual field defect indicates a process not respecting vascular territories and thus suggests a tumor (Cogan's sign). CT scans and MRI demonstrate cerebral lesions with remarkable clarity (Figures 14–4, 14–5, 14–28, and 14–29).

THE PUPIL

The size of the normal pupil varies at different ages, from person to person, and with different emotional states, levels of alertness, degrees of accommodation, and ambient room light. The normal pupillary diameter is about 3–4 mm, smaller in infancy, and tending to be larger in childhood and again progressively smaller with advancing age. Pupillary size relates to varying interactions between the sympathetically innervated iris dilator, with supranuclear control from the frontal (alertness) and occipital lobes (accommodation). The pupil also normally responds to respirations (ie, hippus). Twenty to 40 percent of normal patients have a slight difference in pupil size (physiologic anisocoria),

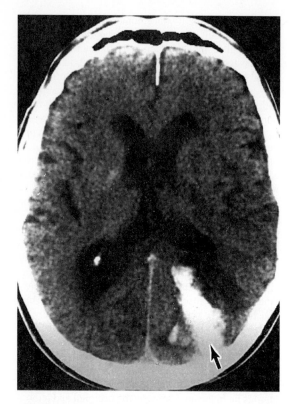

Figure 14–28. Occipital hematoma (arrow) resulting from a bleeding arteriovenous malformation. This lesion produced homonymous hemianopia and headache.

usually of about 0.5 mm. Mydriatic and cycloplegic drugs work more effectively on blue eyes than on brown eyes.

Neuroanatomy of the Pupillary Pathways

Evaluation of the pupillary reactions is important in localizing lesions involving the optic pathways. The examiner should be familiar with the neuroanatomy of

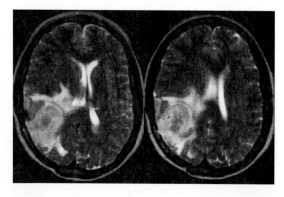

Figure 14–29. Axial MRI showing parietal meningioma with secondary cerebral edema.

the pathway for reaction of the pupil to light and the miosis associated with accommodation (Figure 14–30).

A. Light Reflex: The pathway for the light reflex is entirely subcortical. The afferent pupillary fibers are included within the optic nerve and visual pathways until they exit the optic tract just prior to the lateral geniculate nucleus. They enter the midbrain through the brachium of the superior colliculus and synapse in the pretectal nucleus. Each pretectal nucleus decussates neurons dorsal to the cerebral aqueduct to the ipsilateral and contralateral Edinger-Westphal nucleus via the posterior commissure and the periaqueductal gray matter. A synapse then occurs in the Edinger-Westphal nucleus of the oculomotor nerve. The efferent pathway is via the third nerve to the ciliary ganglion in the lateral orbit. The postganglionic fibers go via the short ciliary nerves to innervate the sphincter muscle of the iris.

B. The Near Reflex: When the eyes look at a near object, three reactions occur—accommodation, convergence, and constriction of the pupil—bringing a sharp image into focus on corresponding retinal points. There is convincing evidence that the final common pathway is mediated through the oculomotor nerve with a synapse in the ciliary ganglion. The afferent pathway enters the midbrain ventral to the Edinger-Westphal nucleus and sends fibers to both sides of the cortex. Although the three components are closely associated, the near reflex cannot be considered a pure reflex, since each component can be neutralized while leaving the other two intact—ie, by prism (neutralizing convergence), by lenses (neutralizing accommodation), and by weak mydriatic drugs (neutralizing miosis). It can occur even in a blind person who is instructed to look at his nose. Bilateral overaction of the near reflex is accommodative spasm. Bilateral accommodative paresis occurs in botulism poisoning and in the Fisher variant of Guillain-Barré syndrome.

ARGYLL ROBERTSON PUPIL

A typical Argyll Robertson pupil is strongly suggestive of central nervous system syphilis associated with tabes dorsalis or general paresis. The pupil is less than 3 mm in diameter (miotic) and does not respond to light stimulation but does accommodate; this finding is nearly always bilateral. The pupils are commonly irregular, eccentric, and dilate poorly with mydriatics as a consequence of concomitant iris atrophy. Less commonly, the sign is incomplete (slow response to light) or unilateral or associated with tonic pupils (mimicking Adie's syndrome). Some degree of Argyll Robertson pupil is present in over 50% of patients with central nervous system syphilis. A wide variety of other central nervous system diseases infrequently cause incomplete Argyll Robertson pupil. These include diabetes, chronic alcoholism, encephalitis, multiple sclerosis, central nervous system degenerative

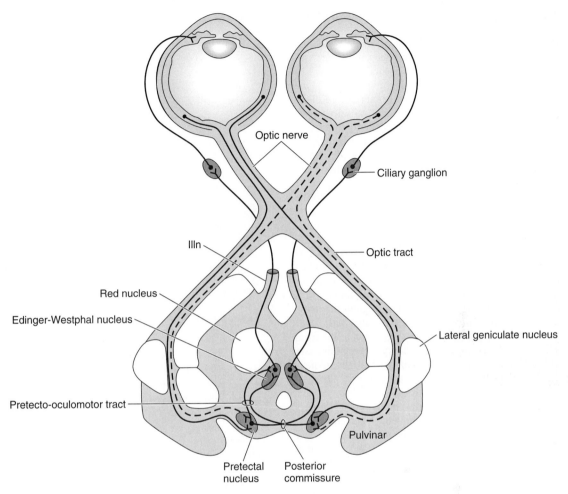

Figure 14–30. Diagram of the path of the pupillary light reflex. (Reproduced, with permission, from Walsh FB, Hoyt WF: *Clinical Neuro-ophthalmology,* 3rd ed. Vol 1. Williams & Wilkins, 1969.)

disease, and tumors of the midbrain. The periaqueductal gray matter of the midbrain is the usual site of the lesion and thus affects the light reflex. The near reflex pathway is more ventral and thus is spared.

TONIC PUPIL

Tonic pupil occurs because of an abnormal pupillary constrictor mechanism in which all or a segment of the sphincter muscle contracts slowly (tonically) to near stimulation and relaxes even more slowly, but either response is better than the light response. It is usually associated with loss of deep tendon reflexes (Adie's syndrome). It results from damage to the ciliary ganglion, which carries 30 nerves destined for the ciliary body to one destined for the iris sphincter. Thus, accommodation is more apt to be preserved by a ciliary body lesion and is also—as a consequence of preferential innervation—more likely to reinnervate

after an injury. This can produce segmental pupillary innervation. A weak (0.1%) solution of pilocarpine instilled into the conjunctival sac causes a tonic pupil to constrict as a result of denervation hypersensitivity; normal pupils are not affected. Some preganglionic oculomotor nerve lesions have, however, been shown to have denervation hypersensitivity probably related to a direct iris pathway that does not synapse at the ciliary ganglion. Bilateral tonic pupils should raise a question of autonomic neuropathy.

HORNER'S SYNDROME

Horner's syndrome is caused by a lesion of the sympathetic pathway, either (1) in its **central portion,** which extends from the posterior hypothalamus through the brainstem to the upper spinal cord (C8–T2); or (2) in its **preganglionic portion,** which exits the spinal cord and synapses in the superior cervical (stellate) ganglion; or (3) in its **postganglionic portion,** from the superior cervical ganglion via the carotid plexus and the ophthalmic division of the trigeminal nerve, by which it enters the orbit. The sympathetic fibers then follow the nasociliary branch of the ophthalmic division of the trigeminal nerve and the long ciliary nerves to the iris and innervate Müller's muscle and the iris dilator. Iris dilator muscle paresis causes miosis, which is more evident in dim light. Melanocyte maturation in the iris of a neonate depends upon sympathetic innervation; thus, less pigmented (bluer) irides occur if a congenital sympathetic lesion is present. Unilateral miosis, ptosis, and absence of sweating on the ipsilateral face and neck make up the complete syndrome. Postganglionic fibers to the face for sweating and vasoconstriction follow the external carotid. Causes of Horner's syndrome include cervical vertebral fractures, tabes dorsalis, syringomyelia, cervical cord tumor, cervical rib, Lyme disease, apical bronchogenic carcinoma, aneurysm of the carotid or subclavian artery, brachial plexus injuries, and injuries to or dissection of the carotid artery high in the neck. Pharmacologic testing with topical cocaine in the conjunctival sac can differentiate Horner's syndrome from physiologic anisocoria, and hydroxyamphetamine can further localize the process to the postganglionic neuron, thus assisting in defining the cause of the syndrome.

Raeder's paratrigeminal syndrome is Horner's syndrome associated with unilateral headache or facial pain in the distribution of the trigeminal nerve. If associated with a sixth, third, fourth, or second cranial nerve palsy, complete neurologic evaluation for basilar skull tumor is required. Without these additional cranial nerves, Raeder's syndrome is a benign condition perhaps related to cluster headache.

AFFERENT PUPILLARY DEFECT

Optic nerve fibers from the right eye decussate at the chiasm to enter the left tract as well as continuing into the right tract, and the same is true on the left side. The pupillary light pathways enter the midbrain through the brachium of the superior colliculus to synapse in the pretectal nucleus; here, they decussate also, as each pretectal nucleus connects to the ipsilateral and contralateral Edinger-Westphal nucleus. For this reason, light shone into the right eye produces an immediate direct response in the right and an immediate indirect consensual response in the left eye (Figure 14–31). The intensity of this response in each eye is proportionate to the light-carrying ability of the directly stimulated optic nerve.

One of the most important assessments to make for the patient complaining of decreased vision is whether it is due to a local ocular problem, eg, cataract, or to a more serious optic nerve problem. Even dense cataracts do not change the light afferent

Light stimulus

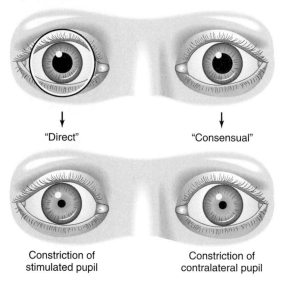

"Direct" "Consensual"

Constriction of stimulated pupil   Constriction of contralateral pupil

Figure 14–31. Normal pupillary light reactions test.

pathways to the brain; hence, a comparison is possible. If an optic nerve lesion is present, the direct light response in the involved eye is less intense than the consensual response (in the involved eye) evoked when the normal eye is stimulated. This phenomenon is called a relative afferent pupillary defect (RAPD) (Figure 14–32). It will be positive also if there is a large retinal lesion. Causes of unilateral decreased vision without an afferent pupillary defect include refractive error, cloudy media (cataract), amblyopia, hysteria or malingering, a macular lesion, and chiasmatic problems. It is anatomically possible for a relative afferent defect with normal visual function to occur if the brachium of the superior colliculus is damaged by a thalamic hemorrhage.

Amaurotic pupillary defect is the term applied to an eye that does not even see light owing to severe unilateral retinal or optic nerve disease. Obviously, a blind eye would not have a direct light response, nor could it induce a consensual response in the normal eye. However, a light shown directly into the normal eye would induce a direct response there and a consensual response in the blind eye (Figure 14–33).

EXTRAOCULAR MOVEMENTS

This section deals with the neural apparatus that controls eye movements and causes them to move simultaneously, up or down and side to side, as well as in convergence or divergence.

Diffuse illumination

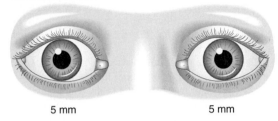

5 mm   5 mm

Light on normal eye

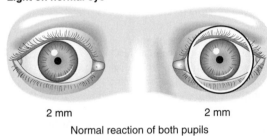

2 mm   2 mm

Normal reaction of both pupils

Light on eye with afferent defect

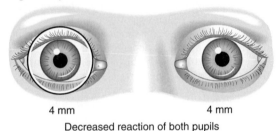

4 mm   4 mm

Decreased reaction of both pupils

Figure 14–32. Afferent pupillary defect (Marcus Gunn pupil).

The neural control of eye movements is ultimately effected by alterations in activity in the nuclei and nerve fibers of the oculomotor, trochlear and abducens nerves. These are referred to as the nuclear and infranuclear pathways. Coordination of eye movements requires connections between these ocular motor nuclei; the internuclear pathways. The supranuclear pathways are responsible for generation of the commands necessary for the execution of the appropriate movement, whether it be voluntary or involuntary.

Classification & Examination of Eye Movements

Eye movements are either fast or slow. Fast eye movements include voluntary or involuntary refixation movements (saccades) and the fast phases of vestibular and optokinetic nystagmus (see below). The fast eye movement system is tested by command refixation movements and by the fast phase of vestibular and optokinetic nystagmus.

Slow eye movements include pursuit movements, which track a slowly moving target once the saccadic system has placed the target on the fovea, and which are tested by asking a patient to follow a slow, smoothly moving target, the slow phase movements generated by vestibular stimuli, the slow phase of optokinetic nystagmus, and vergence movements which—unlike all the other forms of eye movements—involve dysconjugate movements of the two eyes.

Under physiologic conditions, vestibular stimulation occurs from head movements. The resulting slow eye movements, known as the **vestibulo-ocular responses (VOR),** compensate for the head motion such that the position of the eyes in space remains static and steady visual fixation can be maintained. The **doll's head maneuver** is a clinical method of testing the vestibulo-ocular response. The patient is asked to fixate on a target while the examiner moves the head in a horizontal or vertical plane. If the vestibulo-ocular response is deficient, the compensatory eye movements are insufficient and must be supplemented by saccadic movements to maintain fixation. The head motion must be rapid—otherwise, pursuit mechanisms dominate the ocular motor response. In the unconscious patient, the doll's head maneuver is used to assess brainstem function. Since the pursuit and saccadic systems are not operative, the head movements can be slow. Absence of the vestibulo-ocular response leads to failure of the eyes to move within the orbit. Other methods of vestibular stimulation are whole body rotation and caloric testing (see below).

Normal eye

Contralateral pupil constricted

Blind eye

Contralateral pupil not constricted

Figure 14–33. Amaurotic pupillary response.

Generation of Eye Movements

A. Physiology:

1. Fast eye movements–Understanding of the control of eye movements is most complete in the case of saccadic movements. Similar mechanisms are thought to apply to the fast phases of nystagmus. The generation of a saccade involves a **pulse** of increased innervation to move the eye in the required direction and a **step** increase in tonic innervation to maintain the new position in the orbit by counteracting the visco-elastic forces working to return the eye to the primary position. The pulse is produced by the **burst cells of the saccadic generator.** The step change in tonic innervation is produced by the **tonic cells of the neural integrator,** so-called because it effectively integrates the pulse to produce the step. Saccades are ballistic movements—ie, once initiated, their trajectory can not be altered—and there is a close relationship between the amplitude of movement and its peak velocity, larger movements having greater peak velocities. Loss of the saccadic generator function leads to slowing of saccades. Loss of the neural integrator function leads to a failure of maintenance of the desired final position, ie, a failure of gaze holding. Clinically, this usually manifests as a gaze-evoked nystagmus, with a drift of the eyes toward the primary position followed by a corrective saccade back to the desired position of gaze.

2. Slow eye movements–The slow phase movements generated by vestibular stimuli are a direct response to the detection of movement by the semicircular canals. The canals are acceleration detectors, but their output is integrated to produce a velocity signal which is then conveyed to the ocular motor nuclei. The generation of pursuit movements is less well understood. The slow phase of optokinetic nystagmus is in part a pursuit movement, but there is also an additional specific optokinetic movement generated by the perception of movement of the background of the visual scene. This optokinetic movement appears to be generated by the pathways involved in generating slow phase vestibular movements but with an input from the retina, either via cortical centers or directly via a subcortical pathway. Vergence eye movements are generated in response to retinal disparity, ie, stimulation of noncorresponding retinal loci by the object of regard. Electromyography has established divergence as an active process, not a relaxation of convergence.

B. Anatomy:

1. Brainstem centers for fast eye movements–The saccadic generator for horizontal eye movements lies in the paramedian pontine reticular formation. The output from this structure is channeled through the abducens nucleus, which contains both the motor neurons for the abducens nerve and the cell bodies of interneurons which pass via the medial longitudinal fasciculus to innervate the motor neurons in the contralateral medial rectus subnucleus of the oculomotor nerve. The neural integrator for horizontal eye movements appears to be located close to the paramedian pontine reticular formation in the nucleus prepositus hypoglossi.

The saccadic generator for vertical movements is in the rostral interstitial nucleus of the medial longitudinal fasciculus in the rostral midbrain. The pathway to the ocular motor nuclei for upward movements involves the posterior commissure, dorsal to the cerebral aqueduct, and its nucleus. The corresponding pathway for downward eye movements is less well defined. Neural integration for vertical eye movements seems to take place in both the interstitial nucleus of Cajal, close to the rostral interstitial nucleus of the medial longitudinal fasciculus in the midbrain and in the vestibular nuclei in the medulla.

2. Cortical centers for fast eye movements–Voluntary saccades are initiated in the frontal lobe (frontal eye field area 8). The pathway descends through the basal ganglia and the anterior limb of the internal capsule into the brainstem, terminating in the midbrain pretectal area for vertical movements and crossing to the paramedian pontine reticular formation in the opposite side of the pons for horizontal movements. The generation of involuntary (reflexive) saccades, in response to a target appearing in the peripheral field of vision, depends upon activity within the superior colliculus, which receives information from the occipital cortex and also directly from the retina in a purely subcortical pathway.

3. Brainstem centers for slow eye movements–The processing of information from the semicircular canals occurs in the vestibular nuclei, which then connect directly to the ocular motor nuclei. These pathways from the vestibular nuclei in the medulla to the pons and midbrain pass in a number of fiber tracts, including the medial longitudinal fasciculus.

4. Cortical centers for slow eye movements–Pursuit movements originate in the occipital cortex. The pathway descends through the posterior limb of the internal capsule to the midbrain and ipsilateral paramedian pontine reticular formation. The slow phase of optokinetic nystagmus is likely to be generated at least in part in area V5 (or MT) at the junction of the occipital and temporal lobes, which is involved in motion detection. The descending pathway probably accompanies the pathway for pursuit movements. Vergence eye movements are generated in the occipital cortex, and the pathway also probably descends via the posterior limb of the internal capsule, together with the pathway for pursuit movements, to terminate in the rostral midbrain near or in the oculomotor nucleus. Impulses then pass directly to each medial rectus subnucleus and via the medial longitudinal fasciculus to the abducens nuclei. It is not clear whether convergence and divergence are controlled by the same or separate brainstem centers.

ABNORMALITIES
OF EYE MOVEMENTS

Owing to the multiplicity of pathways involved in the supranuclear control of eye movements, with origins in different areas of the brain and an anatomic separation in the brainstem of the horizontal and vertical eye movement systems, disorders of the supranuclear pathways characteristically produce a dissociation of effect upon the various types of eye movements. Thus, the clinical clues to a supranuclear lesion are a differential effect on horizontal and vertical eye movements or upon saccadic, pursuit, and vestibular eye movements. In diffuse brainstem disease, such features may not be apparent, and differentiation from disease at the neuromuscular junction or within the extraocular muscles on clinical grounds can be difficult.

Disease of the internuclear pathways results in a disruption of the conjugacy of eye movements. In infranuclear disease, the pattern of eye movement disturbance usually complies with that expected of a lesion involving one or more cranial nerves or their nuclei.

1. LESIONS
OF THE SUPRANUCLEAR PATHWAYS

Frontal Lobe

A seizure focus in the frontal lobe may cause involuntary turning of the eyes to the opposite side. Destructive lesions cause transient deviation to the same side, and the eyes cannot be turned quickly and voluntarily (saccadic movement) to the opposite side. This is called frontal gaze palsy, and recovery occurs when the opposite frontal eye field substitutes. Ocular pursuit to the opposite side is retained. There is no diplopia. Phenytoin can significantly affect saccades.

Occipital Lobe

Smooth ocular pursuit may be lost with posterior lesions of the hemispheres. The patient is unable to follow a slowly moving object in the direction of the gaze palsy. The command (fast) eye movement is not lost, so pursuit is "saccadic." Sedative agents and carbamazepine can alter smooth pursuit eye movements.

Midbrain

Lesions of the posterior commissure cause impairment of conjugate upgaze. Lesions dorsal and medial to the red nuclei produce a downgaze paresis (trauma, infarcts).

Parinaud's syndrome (pretectal syndrome) is characterized by loss of voluntary upward gaze and convergence-retraction nystagmus and (usually) loss of the pupillary light response with retention of miosis in response to the near reflex. Convergence-retraction movements of the globe on attempted upward gaze is due to simultaneous firing of the rectus muscles due to loss of supranuclear control. There may also be an apparent accommodative spasm, a loss of conjugate voluntary downward gaze associated with loss of convergence and accommodation, ptosis or lid retraction, papilledema, or third nerve palsy. Surrounding structures may also be involved depending on the size and location of the lesion. Conjugate horizontal ocular movements are usually not affected. The syndrome results from tectal or pretectal lesions affecting the periaqueductal area. Pinealomas, infiltrating gliomas, vascular lesions (arteriovenous malformations), demyelinating disease, and trauma may produce this picture.

Pons

Lesions of the paramedian pontine reticular formation produce an ipsilateral horizontal gaze palsy affecting saccadic and pursuit movements. Vestibular slow phase movements are preserved owing to the direct pathway from the vestibular nuclei to the abducens and oculomotor nuclei.

Lesions of the brain stem that cause gaze palsies include vascular accidents, arteriovenous malformations, multiple sclerosis, tumors (pontine gliomas, cerebellopontine angle tumors), and encephalitis.

2. SUPRANUCLEAR SYNDROMES INVOLVING
DISJUNCTIVE OCULAR MOVEMENTS

Spasm of the Near Reflex

The near reflex consists of three components: convergence, accommodation, and constriction of the pupil. Spasm of the near reflex is usually caused by hysteria, though encephalitis, tabes dorsalis, and meningitis may cause spasm by irritation of the supranuclear pathway. It is characterized by convergent strabismus with diplopia, miotic pupils, and spasm of accommodation (induced myopia).

If hysteria is the cause, atropine 1%, 2 drops in each eye twice daily, or minus (concave) lenses may give temporary relief. Psychiatric consultation is indicated for treatment of an underlying mental cause.

Convergence Paralysis

Convergence paralysis is characterized by a sudden onset of diplopia for near vision, with absence of any individual extraocular muscle palsy. It is caused by hysteria or destructive lesions of the supranuclear pathway for convergence. The combination of motor convergence failure and pupillary miosis confirms patient effort and an organic lesion. Multiple sclerosis, myasthenia gravis, head trauma, encephalitis, tabes dorsalis, tumors, aneurysms, minor cerebrovascular accidents, and Parkinson's disease are the most common organic causes.

INTERNUCLEAR OPHTHALMOPLEGIA

The medial longitudinal fasciculus is an important fiber tract extending from the rostral midbrain to the spinal cord. It contains many pathways connecting nuclei within the brainstem, particularly those concerned with extraocular movements. The most common manifestation of damage to the medial longitudinal fasciculus is an internuclear ophthalmoplegia, in which conjugate horizontal eye movements are disrupted owing to failure of coordination between the abducens nerve nucleus in the pons and the oculomotor nerve nucleus in the midbrain. The lesion in the brainstem is ipsilateral to the eye with the adduction failure or opposite to the direction of horizontal gaze that is abnormal. In the mildest form of internuclear ophthalmoplegia, the clinical abnormality is restricted to a slowing of saccades in the adducting eye. In the most severe form, there is a complete loss of adduction on horizontal gaze (Figure 14–12). Convergence is characteristically preserved in internuclear ophthalmoplegia except when the lesion is in the midbrain, when the convergence mechanisms may also be affected. Another feature of internuclear ophthalmoplegia is nystagmus in the abducting eye on attempted horizontal gaze, which is at least in part a result of compensation for the failure of adduction in the other eye. In bilateral internuclear ophthalmoplegia, there may also be an upbeating nystagmus on upgaze due to failure of control of gaze holding in the upward direction, and the eyes may be divergent; this is known as the WEBINO (wall-eyed bilateral internuclear ophthalmoplegia) syndrome.

Internuclear ophthalmoplegia may be due to multiple sclerosis (particularly in young adults), brainstem infarction (particularly in older patients), tumors, arteriovenous malformations, Wernicke's encephalopathy, and encephalitis. Bilateral internuclear ophthalmoplegia is most commonly due to multiple sclerosis.

A horizontal gaze palsy combined with an internuclear ophthalmoplegia, due to a lesion of the abducens nucleus or paramedian pontine reticular formation extending into the ipsilateral medial longitudinal fasciculus, affects all horizontal eye movements in the ipsilateral eye and adduction in the contralateral eye. This is known as a "one-and-a-half syndrome," or paralytic pontine exotropia.

NUCLEAR & INFRANUCLEAR CONNECTIONS

Oculomotor Nerve (III)

The motor fibers arise from a group of nuclei in the central gray matter ventral to the cerebral aqueduct at the level of the superior colliculus. The midline central caudal nucleus innervates both levator palpebrae superioris muscles. The paired superior rectus subnuclei innervate the contralateral superior rectus. The efferent fibers decussate immediately and pass through the opposite superior rectus subnucleus. The subnuclei for the medial rectus, inferior rectus, and inferior oblique muscles are also paired structures but innervate the ipsilateral muscles. The fascicle of the oculomotor nerve courses through the red nucleus and the inner side of the substantia nigra to emerge on the medial side of the cerebral peduncles. The nerve runs alongside the sella turcica, in the outer wall of the cavernous sinus, and through the superior orbital fissure to enter the orbit.

The parasympathetics arise from the Edinger-Westphal nucleus just rostral to the motor nucleus of the third nerve and pass via the inferior division of the third nerve to the ciliary ganglion. From there the short ciliary nerves are distributed to the sphincter muscle of the iris and to the ciliary muscle.

A. Oculomotor Paralysis: Lesions of the third nerve nucleus affect the ipsilateral medial and inferior rectus and inferior oblique muscles, both levator muscles, and both superior rectus muscles. There will be bilateral ptosis and bilateral limitation of elevation as well as limitation of adduction and depression ipsilaterally. From the fascicle of the nerve in the midbrain to its eventual termination in the orbit, all other lesions produce purely ipsilateral results. Just before entering the orbit, the nerve divides into a superior and inferior branch; the former innervates the levator palpebrae and superior rectus muscles and the latter all other muscles and the sphincter.

If the lesion involves the third nerve anywhere from the nucleus (midbrain) to the peripheral branches in the orbit, the eye is turned out by the intact lateral rectus muscle and slightly depressed by the intact superior oblique muscle. (Incyclotorsion from the action of the intact superior oblique muscle can be observed by watching a small blood vessel on the medial conjunctiva as depression of the eye is attempted.) There can be a dilated fixed pupil, absent accommodation, and ptosis of the upper lid, often severe enough to cover the pupil. The eye may only be moved laterally. Trauma, aneurysm, viral infections, and vascular disease are the most common causes. Aneurysm usually arises from the junction of the internal carotid and posterior communicating arteries. Vascular disease includes diabetes mellitus, migraine, hypertension, and the collagenoses. The common location for vascular palsies is in the cavernous sinus region, where the pupillary fibers are peripheral and nourished better by the vasa vasorum. Compressive lesions such as aneurysms involve the external pupillary fibers early and produce pupillary dilation. Thus, aneurysm and vascular disease can be differentiated clinically, since in vascular lesions the pupillary responses are usually spared, whereas aneurysmal compression causes a completely fixed and dilated pupil. Less than 5% of vascular third nerve palsies are associated with complete pupillary palsy, and in only 15% is there partial pupillary palsy.

Some apparently vascular oculomotor palsies with or without pupillary sparing can be seen on MRI to have focal mesencephalic infarcts without the usual rubral tremor or other local signs. In compressive lesions, the pupil may become constricted because of aberrant regeneration (see below), or a concomitant Horner's syndrome (sympathetic paresis) can produce a "frozen" pupil of 3–4 mm.

Bilateral nuclear third nerve palsies can also be associated with sparing of the lids. Bilateral peripheral third nerve palsies can occur secondary to interpeduncular lesions such as basilar artery aneurysm or a herniated hippocampus of the temporal lobe.

Monocular elevator paralysis or inability to elevate in both abduction (superior rectus) and adduction (inferior oblique) can occur as a congenital defect or as a complication of thyroid ophthalmopathy, orbital myositis, orbital floor fracture, myasthenia gravis, paresis of the superior division of the third nerve (tumor, sinusitis, postviral), or midbrain stroke.

Third nerve palsies in children may be congenital or may be due to ophthalmoplegic migraine, meningitis, or postviral.

B. Oculomotor Synkinesis (Aberrant Regeneration of the Third Nerve): This phenomenon is characterized by (1) lid dyskinesias on horizontal gaze (ie, the levator palpebrae superioris fires when the medial rectus fires); (2) adduction on attempted upgaze (ie, the medial rectus fires when the superior rectus fires); (3) retraction on attempted upgaze (ie, co-firing of recti, which are retractors); (4) pseudo-Argyll Robertson pupil (ie, no light response, no near response in the primary position but a "near" response on adduction or adduction-depression—pupillary innervation from medial or inferior rectus); (5) pseudo-Graefe's sign (ie, no lid lag on downgaze but lid retraction due to lid innervation from the inferior rectus); and (6) a monocular vertical optokinetic nystagmus response (due to co-firing muscles fixing the involved eye, allowing only the normal eye to respond to the moving target). This oculomotor synkinesis probably occurs not only as a combination of misdirection of sprouting axons into the wrong sheaths and subsequent muscle co-firing but also as a consequence of ephaptic transmission or cross-talk between axons without covering myelin sheaths.

Oculomotor synkinesis can occur secondary to severe trauma or compression of the third nerve by a posterior communicator artery aneurysm, or primarily due to an internal carotid aneurysm or meningioma in the cavernous sinus. If compression lasts several weeks, strabismus surgery is often required to achieve binocular single vision.

C. Cyclic Oculomotor Palsy: Cyclic oculomotor palsy can complicate a congenital third nerve palsy; it is a rare predominantly unilateral event with a typical third nerve paresis showing cyclic spasms every 10–30 seconds. During these intervals, ptosis improves and accommodation increases. This phenome-

non continues unchanged throughout life but decreases with sleep and increases with greater arousal. It is probably a periodic discharge by damaged neurons of the oculomotor nucleus which summate subthreshold stimuli until a discharge occurs.

D. Marcus Gunn Phenomenon (Jaw-Winking Syndrome): This rare congenital condition consists of elevation of a ptotic eyelid upon movement of the jaw. Acquired cases occur after damage to the oculomotor nerve with subsequent innervation of the lid (levator palpebrae superioris) by a branch of the fifth cranial nerve. Muscular palsies may be present.

Trochlear Nerve (IV)

Motor (entirely crossed) fibers arise from the trochlear nucleus just caudal to the third nerve at the level of the inferior colliculus; they then run posteriorly, decussate in the anterior medullary velum, and wind around the cerebral peduncles. The fourth nerve travels near the third nerve along the wall of the cavernous sinus to the orbit, where it supplies the superior oblique muscle. The fourth nerve is unique among the cranial nerves in arising from the dorsal brainstem.

A. Trochlear Paralysis: Lesions of the fourth nerve are commonly vascular, traumatic, or idiopathic (congenital or developmental with later decompensation). However, cerebellar tumors can also present with a fourth nerve lesion as an early sign. The nerve is vulnerable to injury at the site of exit from the dorsal aspect of the brainstem. Both nerves may be damaged by severe trauma as they decussate in the anterior medullary velum, resulting in bilateral superior oblique palsies.

Superior oblique palsy results in upward deviation (hypertropia) of the eye. The hypertropia increases when the patient looks down and with adduction. In addition, there is excyclotropia; therefore, one of the diplopic images will be tilted with respect to the other. Torsional symptoms suggest an acquired late-onset superior oblique palsy: correspondingly, the lack of torsional symptoms suggest an early onset of the deviation. Tilting the head toward the involved side increases the deviation. Tilting the head away from the side of the involved eye may relieve the diplopia, and patients frequently present with a head tilt. Miscellaneous causes include multiple sclerosis, a brainstem arteriovenous malformation, orbital pseudotumor, and myasthenia gravis. Strabismus surgery is effective in patients who fail to improve with time.

B. Superior Oblique Myokymia: A monocular microtremor of the superior oblique muscle can rarely occur. It is an acquired, haphazard, and episodic overaction of the superior oblique muscle characterized by rapid torsional movements of one eye. Patients notice oscillopsia when this occurs, and the symptoms can be improved by carbamazepine. The cause may be compression of the trochlear nerve by an aberrant artery.

Abducens Nerve (VI)

Motor (entirely uncrossed) fibers arise from the nucleus in the floor of the fourth ventricle in the lower portion of the pons near the internal genu of the facial nerve. Piercing the pons, the fibers emerge anteriorly, the nerve running a long course over the tip of the petrous portion of the temporal bone into the cavernous sinus. It enters the orbit with the third and fourth nerves to supply the lateral rectus muscle.

A. Abducens Nucleus Lesion: The abducens nucleus contains the motor neurons to the ipsilateral lateral rectus and the cell bodies of interneurons innervating the motor neurons to the contralateral medial rectus. It is the final common relay point for all horizontal conjugate eye movements, and a lesion within the nucleus will produce an ipsilateral horizontal gaze palsy affecting all types of eye movement including vestibular movements. This contrasts with a lesion of the paramedian pontine reticular formation, in which vestibular movements are preserved.

B. Abducens Nerve Paralysis: (See also Chapter 12.) This is the most common single muscle palsy. Abduction of the eye is reduced or absent; esotropia is present in the primary position and increases upon gaze to the affected side. Movement of the eye to the opposite side is normal. Möbius' syndrome (congenital facial diplegia) can be associated with a sixth nerve or conjugate gaze palsy. Vascular disorders (arteriosclerosis, diabetes, migraine, and hypertension) are common causes. However, dural arteriovenous fistula, basilar artery disease, increased intracranial pressure, lumbar puncture, tumors at the base of the skull, meningitis, and trauma are other frequent causes. Arnold-Chiari malformation (congenital downward displacement of the cerebellar tonsils) can also produce brainstem traction and sixth nerve palsies. Lyme disease can produce an isolated sixth nerve palsy as well as those that occur secondary to meningeal involvement. A child with a sixth nerve palsy should be evaluated for a brainstem tumor (glioma) or inflammation if trauma was not present or if trauma was minimal. Pseudo-sixth nerve palsies can occur in Duane's retraction syndrome, spasm of the near reflex, thyroid eye disease, myasthenia, dorsal midbrain compression (Parinaud's syndrome), or long-standing strabismus and in medial rectus entrapment by an ethmoid fracture.

C. Duane's Syndrome: Duane's syndrome is uncommon (< 1% of cases of strabismus) and in almost all cases congenital. It is a stationary, nearly always unilateral condition consisting of deficient horizontal ocular motility characterized by complete or partial deficiency of abduction. Evidence based on pathologic studies has determined that Duane's syndrome can be due to congenital absence of the sixth nerve with coinnervation of the lateral rectus by a branch of the third nerve. Therefore, attempted adduction movements result in retraction of the globe and narrowing of the lid fissure. The visual handicap is seldom severe. Visual acuity can be normal, and the eye is oth-

erwise normal. Unless the deviation is very large, strabismus surgery is best avoided.

Cochlear nucleus lesions producing sensorineural hearing loss occur in 6.8% of cases of Duane's syndrome. Congenital malformations may also include the facial and skeletal bones, the ribs, and the external ear. Ocular anomalies can include epibulbar dermoids. Acquired Duane's syndrome is a rare event occurring after a peripheral nerve palsy.

D. Gradenigo's Syndrome: Gradenigo's syndrome is characterized by pain in the face (from irritation of the trigeminal nerve) and abducens palsy. The syndrome is produced by meningeal inflammation at the tip of the petrous bone and most often occurs as a rare complication of otitis media with mastoiditis or petrous bone tumors.

Symptoms and Signs of Extraocular Muscle Palsies

Diplopia occurs when the visual axes are not aligned. This is especially true when the onset of strabismus is after age 6 (suppression and abnormal retinal correspondence do not develop). Dizziness or dysequilibrium may be associated but disappears with monocular patching. Head tilt occurs, especially in paresis of the superior oblique muscle, when the tilt is to the opposite side to avoid diplopia by moving the eye out of the field of action of the paralyzed muscle. Vertical saccadic velocity can differentiate a superior oblique palsy from inferior rectus palsy. Horizontal saccadic velocity can differentiate a restricted globe with pseudo-sixth nerve from sixth nerve paresis. Forced duction tests should also be done, since a paresis could be simulated by a restricted yoke muscle.

Ptosis is caused by weakness or paralysis of the levator muscle. Any extraocular muscle palsy that occurs with minor head trauma (subconcussive injuries) should be investigated for a basal tumor. The minimally positive edrophonium test is unreliable because it can be nonspecific. Fascicular lesions involving the portion of a cranial nerve within the brainstem resemble peripheral nerve lesions but can be differentiated on the basis of other brainstem signs and their subsequent poor recovery. For vascular causes of cranial nerve palsies, recovery by 4 months is the rule. Palsies that persist longer than 6 months—especially those involving the sixth nerve—should be evaluated for an underlying structural compressive lesion (tumor, arteriovenous fistula, aneurysm).

Syndromes Affecting Cranial Nerves III, IV, & VI

A. Superior Orbital Fissure Syndrome: All extraocular peripheral nerves pass through the superior orbital fissure and can be involved by trauma or by tumor encroaching on the fissure.

B. Orbital Apex Syndrome: This syndrome is similar to the superior orbital fissure syndrome with the addition of optic nerve signs and usually greater proptosis and less pain. It is caused by an orbital tumor, inflammation, or trauma that damages the optic and extraocular nerves.

C. Complete Ophthalmoplegia (Sudden): Complete ophthalmoplegia of sudden onset can be due to brainstem vascular disease, Wernicke's encephalopathy, pituitary apoplexy, Fisher's syndrome, myasthenia crisis, bulbar poliomyelitis, diphtheria, botulism, meningitis, and syphilitic or arteriosclerotic basilar aneurysm.

THE CEREBELLUM

The cerebellum has an important modulating influence on the function of the neural integrators. Thus, it is involved in gaze holding and the control of saccades, particularly the relationship between the pulse and the step of saccade generation. Cerebellar dysfunction produces gaze-evoked nystagmus, by its influence on gaze holding, and abnormalities of saccades, including saccadic dysmetria, in which the saccadic amplitude is inaccurate, and postsaccadic drift due to a mismatch between the pulse and step of the saccade.

The cerebellum is also important in the control of pursuit eye movements, and cerebellar dysfunction may thus result in broken (saccadic) pursuit.

MYASTHENIA GRAVIS

Myasthenia gravis is characterized by abnormal fatigability of striated muscles after repetitive contraction which improves after rest and often is first manifested by weakness of the extraocular muscles. Unilateral fatiguing ptosis is a frequent first sign, with subsequent bilateral involvement of extraocular muscles, so that diplopia is often an early symptom. Unusual ocular presentations may simulate gaze palsies, internuclear ophthalmoplegias, vertical nystagmus, and progressive external ophthalmoplegia. Generalized weakness of the arms and legs, difficulty in swallowing, weakness of jaw muscles, and difficulty in breathing may follow rapidly in untreated cases. This weakness shows diurnal variations and often worsens as the day progresses but can be improved by a nap. There are no sensory changes.

The incidence of the disease is in the range of 1:30,000 to 1:20,000. Myasthenia gravis usually affects young adults aged 20–40 (70% are under 40 years of age), though it may occur at any age and is often misdiagnosed as hysteria, especially because the weakness can be greater in exciting or embarrassing situations. Older patients are more commonly male and are more likely to have a thymoma.

The onset may follow an upper respiratory infec-

tion, stress, pregnancy, or any injury, and the disease has been noted as a transitory condition in newborn infants of myasthenic mothers. Myasthenia gravis has been associated with hyperthyroidism (5%), thyroid abnormalities (15%), autoimmune diseases (5%), and diffuse metastatic carcinoma (7%).

In about one-third of cases, the disease is confined to the extraocular muscles at onset. In about two-thirds of these cases, the disease will become generalized with time, usually within the first year.

The differential diagnosis includes progressive external ophthalmoplegia, brainstem lesions, epidemic encephalitis, bulbar and pseudobulbar palsy, postdiphtheritic paralysis, botulism, multiple sclerosis, and toxic reactions to the beta-blockers (eg propranolol) or penicillamine. Many other drugs may unmask or exacerbate myasthenia gravis; they include lithium, aminoglycoside antibiotics, chloroquine, and phenytoin.

The disease has its origin at the neuromuscular junction, especially at the postsynaptic site, probably due to antibodies against it and the presynaptic site. A commercial test of anti-acetylcholine receptor antibodies can diagnose the disease in 80–90% of patients with systemic myasthenia and 40–60% of patients with pure ocular myasthenia; the titers do not correlate with severity of disease, however.

Most patients have merely histologic thymic hyperplasia, often apparent on lateral oblique chest x-rays or CT scans of the mediastinum or noted at surgical removal of the thymus. Thymomas occur in 15% of patients.

Cholinesterase destroys acetylcholine at the myoneural junction, and cholinesterase-inhibiting drugs improve the condition by increasing the amount of acetylcholine available to the damaged postsynaptic site. The edrophonium chloride test is used in addition to the neostigmine diagnostic test. Edrophonium, 2 mg (0.2 mL), is given intravenously over 15 seconds. Relief of ptosis constitutes a positive response and confirms the diagnosis of myasthenia gravis. If no response occurs in 30 seconds, an additional 5–7 mg (0.5–0.7 mL) is given. The test is most helpful when marked ptosis is present, but myasthenia can affect any muscle or combination of muscles, and significant improvement in function is also helpful. Slightly positive edrophonium tests can occur in neurogenic palsies, however, and there may be false-negative results when myasthenia is complicated by muscle wasting.

Repetitive nerve stimulation, especially of the facial or proximal muscles, can also demonstrate abnormal muscle fatigability (a more than 10% decrease in the response is diagnostic of myasthenia). Variation in size and shape of motor unit potentials is noted on needle electromyography of affected muscles, and single-fiber studies show increased variability (jitter) in the temporal pattern of action potentials from muscle fibers of the same motor unit.

Myasthenia can be treated with pyridostigmine, systemic steroids, azathioprine, cyclosporine, immunoglobulins, and plasmapharesis according to the severity of disease. During severe exacerbations, artificial ventilation may be necessary. Thymectomy may be indicated in patients with thymoma (though it may not influence the severity of the myasthenia) and in patients with early-onset generalized disease without evidence of thymoma—in one third of whom it may produce complete remission without the need for immunosuppressants. Ocular myasthenia tends to respond less well to anticholinesterase agents than generalized disease, but the response to systemic steroids is usually good. Extraocular muscle surgery can be undertaken but should be delayed until the ocular motility deficit has been stable for a long time.

Myasthenia is generally a chronic disease with a tendency to pursue a relapsing and remitting course. The prognosis depends upon the extent of the disease, the response to medication and thymectomy, and the careful management of severe exacerbations.

CHRONIC PROGRESSIVE EXTERNAL OPHTHALMOPLEGIA

This rather rare disease is characterized by a slowly progressive inability to move the eyes and severe early ptosis yet normal pupillary reactions and accommodation. It may begin at any age and progresses over a period of 5–15 years to complete external ophthalmoplegia. It is a form of mitochondrial myopathy and may be associated with other manifestations of mitochondrial disease such as pigmentary degeneration of the retina, deafness, cerebellar-vestibular abnormalities, seizures, cardiac conduction defects, and peripheral sensorimotor neuropathy, in which case the term "ophthalmoplegia-plus" may be applied. Onset before 15 years of age of chronic progressive external ophthalmoplegia, heart block, and pigmentary retinopathy constitutes the Kearns-Sayre syndrome. Chronic progressive external ophthalmoplegia is associated with deletions of mitochondrial DNA, which are more frequent and more extensive in the cases with nonocular manifestations.

NYSTAGMUS

Nystagmus is defined as repetitive, rhythmic oscillations of one or both eyes in any or all fields of gaze, initiated by a slow eye movement. The waveform may be pendular, in which the movements in each direction have equal speed, amplitude, and duration; or jerk, in which the slow movement in one direction is followed by a rapid corrective return to the original position (fast component). By convention, the direction of jerk nystagmus is given as the direction of the corrective fast phase and not the direction of the primary slow phase.

Jerk nystagmus is classified as grade I, present only with the eyes directed toward the fast component; grade II, present also with the eyes in primary position; or grade III, present even with the eyes directed toward the slow component. The movements of pendular or jerk nystagmus may be horizontal, vertical, torsional, oblique, circular, or a combination of these. The direction may change depending upon the direction of gaze.

The **amplitude** of nystagmus is the extent of the movement; the **rate** of nystagmus is the frequency of oscillation. Generally speaking, the faster the rate, the smaller the amplitude and vice versa. Nystagmus is usually conjugate but is occasionally dysconjugate, as in physiologic end-gaze nystagmus, convergence-retraction nystagmus, and seesaw nystagmus.

Nystagmus is also occasionally dissociated (more marked in one eye than the other), as in internuclear ophthalmoplegia, spasmus nutans, seesaw nystagmus, monocular visual loss, and acquired pendular nystagmus and with asymmetric muscle weakness in myasthenia gravis.

Physiology of Symptoms

Reduced visual acuity is caused by inability to maintain steady fixation. False projection is evident in vestibular nystagmus, where past-pointing is present. Head tilting is usually involuntary, to decrease the nystagmus. The head is turned toward the fast components in jerk nystagmus or set so that the eyes are in a position that minimizes ocular movement in pendular nystagmus. The patient sometimes complains of illusory movements of objects (oscillopsia). This is more apt to be present in nystagmus due to lesions of lower centers, such as the labyrinth, or associated with the sudden onset of nystagmus in an adult. The apparent movement of the environment occurs during the slow component and causes an extremely distressing vertigo, so that the patient is unable to stand. Head nodding is most apt to accompany congenital nystagmus and spasmus nutans. Nystagmus is noticeable and cosmetically disturbing except when excursions of the eye are very small.

PHYSIOLOGIC NYSTAGMUS

Three types of nystagmus can be elicited in the normal person.

End Point (End-Gaze) Nystagmus

Normal individuals have a wide null or quiet zone but can have horizontal nystagmus on end-horizontal gaze (ie, pupillary light reflex just on both corneas); physiologic end-gaze nystagmus disappears as the

---

CLASSIFICATION OF NYSTAGMUS

Physiologic nystagmus
  End-point nystagmus
  Optokinetic nystagmus
  Stimulation of semicircular canals (physiologic vestibular nystagmus)
    Rotatory
    Caloric
  Voluntary nystagmus

Pathologic nystagmus
  Congenital nystagmus
    With sensory abnormality
    Without sensory abnormality (congenital idiopathic motor nystagmus)
    Latent nystagmus (LN)
    Manifest latent nystagmus (MLN)
  Acquired pendular nystagmus
    Infantile visual deprivation
    Spasmus nutans
    Oculopalatal myoclonus
  Vestibular nystagmus
    Peripheral vestibular nystagmus
    Central vestibular nystagmus
      Downbeat nystagmus
      Upbeat nystagmus
  Gaze-evoked nystagmus
  Gaze-paretic nystagmus
  Convergence-retraction nystagmus
  Seesaw nystagmus
  Periodic alternating nystagmus

Mimics of nystagmus
  Saccadic intrusions
  Spontaneous eye movements in coma

---

eyes move in a few degrees. It is primarily horizontal but may have a slight torsional component and greater amplitude in the abducting eye; it is a normal form of gaze-evoked nystagmus.

Optokinetic Nystagmus

This type of nystagmus may be elicited in all normal individuals, most easily by means of a rotating drum with alternating black and white lines but in fact by any repetitive targets in the visual field such as repetitive telephone poles as seen from a window of a fast-moving vehicle. The slow component follows the object and the fast component moves rapidly in the opposite direction to fixate on each succeeding object. A unilateral or asymmetric horizontal response usually indicates a deep parietal lobe lesion, especially a tumor. It occurs as a result of a deficit in the slow (pursuit) phase. Anterior cerebral (ie, frontal lobe) le-

sions may inhibit this response only temporarily when an acute saccadic gaze palsy is present, which suggests the presence of a compensatory mechanism that is much greater than for lesions situated farther posteriorly. Asymmetry of response in the vertical plane suggests a brainstem lesion. Since it is an involuntary response, this test is especially useful in detecting hysteria or malingering. A large mirror filling the patient's central field at near can be rotated from side to side and will induce an optokinetic nystagmus if vision is present.

Stimulation of Semicircular Canals

The three semicircular canals of each inner ear sense movements of the head in space, being primarily sensitive to acceleration. The neural output of the vestibular system, after processing within the vestibular and related brainstem nuclei, is a velocity signal. This is transmitted, principally via the medial longitudinal fasciculus on each side of the brainstem, to the ocular motor nuclei to produce the necessary compensatory eye movements (vestibulo-ocular responses) for maintaining a stable position of the eyes in space and hence optimal vision. Vestibular signals also pass to the cerebellum and cerebral cortex.

Stimulation of the semicircular canals results in a compensatory eye movement. In the unconscious subject with an intact brainstem, this leads to a tonic deviation of the eyes, whereas in the conscious subject a superimposed corrective fast phase movement, returning the eyes back toward the straight-ahead position, results in a jerk nystagmus. These tests are useful methods of investigating vestibular function in conscious subjects and, in the case of caloric stimulation, brainstem function in comatose patients.

A. Rotatory Physiologic Nystagmus (Bárány Rotating Chair): When the head is tilted 30 degrees forward, the horizontal semicircular canals lie horizontally in space. Rotation, such as in a Bárány, then leads to a horizontal jerk nystagmus with the compensatory slow phase eye movement opposite to the direction of turning and the corrective fast phase in the direction of turning. Owing to impersistence of the vestibular signal during continued rotation, the nystagmus abates. Once the rotation stops, there is a vestibular tone in the opposite direction, which results in a jerk nystagmus with the fast phase away from the original direction of turning (postrotatory nystagmus). Since the subject is stationary, postrotatory nystagmus is often easier to analyze than the nystagmus during rotation.

B. Caloric Stimulation: With the head tilted 60 degrees backward, the horizontal semicircular canals lie vertically in space. Water irrigation of the auditory canal then generates convection currents predominantly within the horizontal rather than the vertical semicircular canals. Cold water irrigation induces a predominantly horizontal jerk nystagmus with a fast phase opposite to the side of irrigation, and warm water irrigation induces a similar jerk nystagmus with a fast phase toward the side of irrigation. (The mnemonic device is "COWS": cold-opposite, warm-same.) Caloric nystagmus is made more obvious by the patient wearing Frenzel's spectacles, which eliminate patient fixation and provide a magnified view for the examiner. It is important to verify that the tympanic membrane is intact before performing irrigation of the external auditory canal.

Voluntary Nystagmus

About 5% of normal individuals can generate short bursts of ocular oscillation that resemble small-amplitude, fast, horizontal pendular nystagmus. Eye movement recordings show the movements to be rapidly alternating saccades. Recognition of the entity is important to avoid unnecessary investigation.

PATHOLOGIC NYSTAGMUS

Congenital Nystagmus

Congenital nystagmus is nystagmus present within 6 months after birth. Ocular instability is usual at birth, due to poor visual fixation, but this abates during the first few weeks of life. The presence of spontaneous nystagmus is always pathologic.

Congenital impairment of vision or visual deprivation due to lesions in any part of the eye or optic nerve can result in nystagmus at birth or soon thereafter. Causes include corneal opacity, cataract, albinism, achromatopsia, bilateral macular disease, aniridia, and optic atrophy. By definition, congenital idiopathic motor nystagmus has no associated underlying sensory abnormality, though visual performance is limited by the ocular instability. Typically it is not present at birth but becomes apparent between 3 and 6 months of age.

At one time it was thought that congenital pendular nystagmus was indicative of an underlying sensory abnormality whereas congenital jerk nystagmus was not. Eye movement recordings have shown this not to be true, both pendular and jerk waveforms being seen whether there is a sensory abnormality or not. Indeed, in many cases a mixed pattern of alternating pendular and jerk waveforms is seen. Congenital nystagmus, particularly the idiopathic motor type with its potential for better visual fixation, generally undergoes a progressive change in its waveform during early childhood. There is development of periods of relative ocular stability, ie, relatively slow eye velocity, known as foveation periods since they are thought to be an adaptive response to maximize the potential for fixation and hence to improve visual acuity. In addition, congenital nystagmus with a jerk nystagmus has a characteristic waveform in which the slow phases have an exponentially increasing velocity. This is known as CN type waveform, and with

very few exceptions its presence signifies that the nystagmus has been present since early childhood. This can be a particularly useful feature in determining that nystagmus noted in adulthood is not of recent onset.

Congenital nystagmus is usually horizontal and conjugate. Vertical and torsional components are only occasionally present. The direction of any jerk component often varies with the direction of gaze, but an important feature in comparison to many forms of acquired nystagmus is that there is no additional vertical component on vertical gaze. In most patients with congenital nystagmus, there is a direction of gaze (null zone) in which the nystagmus is relatively quiet. If this null zone is away from primary position, a head turn may be adopted to place the eccentric position straight ahead. In a few cases, the position of the null zone varies to produce one type of periodic alternating nystagmus. Congenital nystagmus is usually decreased in intensity by convergence, and some patients will adopt an esotropia (nystagmus blockage). Anxiety and increased "effort to see" will often increase the intensity of congenital nystagmus and thus reduce visual acuity.

Once congenital nystagmus has been noted, it is important to identify any underlying sensory abnormality, if only to determine the visual potential. This may require electrodiagnostic studies. Extraocular muscle surgery is predominantly indicated for patients with a marked head turn. Supramaximal recessions of the horizontal rectus muscles reduce the intensity of congenital nystagmus, but the effect may be only temporary.

In general, **latent nystagmus** means nystagmus which increases in intensity when one eye is covered, and this is a characteristic feature of congenital nystagmus. There is also a specific type of latent nystagmus, known as **LN,** which is predominantly seen in infantile esotropia. LN is a horizontal jerk nystagmus with the fast phase toward the side of the fixing eye—with the left eye covered, there is a rightward nystagmus and with the right eye covered a leftward nystagmus. LN also becomes more marked when one eye is covered, only then being apparent on clinical examination, but eye movement recordings show that the nystagmus is always present. **Manifest latent nystagmus (MLN)** is a particular type of LN in which the nystagmus is always apparent on clinical examination. It occurs in patients with LN when binocular function is lost, ie, the equivalent of one eye being covered. This may be because of loss of sight in one eye or even from the development of a divergent squint. If binocular function is restored, MLN will revert to LN.

Acquired Pendular Nystagmus

Any child who develops bilateral visual loss before 6 years of age may also develop a pendular nystagmus, and indeed the acquisition of a pendular nystagmus during infancy necessitates further investigation. A specific syndrome of acquired pendular nystagmus in childhood is **spasmus nutans.** This is a bilateral, generally horizontal (occasionally vertical), fine, dissociated pendular nystagmus, associated with head nodding and an abnormal head posture. There is a benign form, which may be familial, with onset before age 2 and spontaneous improvement during the third or fourth year. Spasmus nutans may also rarely be the first manifestation of an anterior visual pathway glioma.

In adults, acquired pendular nystagmus is a feature of brainstem disease, usually multiple sclerosis or brainstem stroke. There may be horizontal, vertical, or torsional components or even a combination of components to produce oblique or elliptical trajectories. The syndrome of **oculopalatal myoclonus** characteristically develops several months after a brainstem stroke. There is a pendular nystagmus with synchronous movements variably involving the soft palate, larynx, and diaphragm as well as producing head titubation. (The term "myoclonus" is a misnomer since the abnormal movements are a form of tremor.) The associated hypertrophy of the inferior olivary nucleus in the medulla and other evidence suggest a disruption of the dentato-rubro-olivary pathway between the brainstem and the cerebellum as the underlying pathogenesis. Various drug treatments have been tried for adult acquired pendular nystagmus, of which baclofen, clonazepam, isoniazid, and gabapentin have produced the best though still limited results. Baseout prisms may also be tried.

Vestibular Nystagmus

Abnormalities of vestibular tone result in abnormal activation of the vestibulo-ocular pathways and abnormal neural drive to the extraocular muscles. Loss of function in the left horizontal semicircular canal is equivalent to activation of the right horizontal semicircular canal, as would normally be produced by a rightward head turn. The oculomotor response is conjugate leftward slow phase movement of the eyes. The corrective fast phase response is rightward in direction, and a right-beating horizontal nystagmus is thus generated. The pattern of response to dysfunction of one or more semicircular canals can be similarly derived to give the full possible range of **peripheral vestibular nystagmus,** though in clinical practice it is the effect of dysfunction of the horizontal canals that usually predominates. As a general rule, peripheral vestibular lesions are destructive and the fast phase of the resulting nystagmus is away from the side of the lesion. Since the neural signal of the vestibulo-ocular pathways is a velocity signal, the slow phase of peripheral vestibular nystagmus has a constant velocity. This gives rise to the characteristic saw-tooth waveform on eye movement recordings.

Peripheral vestibular nystagmus is not dependent upon visual stimuli and thus is still present in the dark, or with the eyes closed, as well as in blind individuals. It is, however, inhibited by visual fixation or, conversely, accentuated by wearing Frenzel's spectacles, and this is an important factor in the normal dampening over 2–3 weeks of peripheral vestibular nystagmus. Head position does not usually influence peripheral vestibular nystagmus except in benign paroxysmal positional vertigo, in which elicitation of the characteristic pattern of nystagmus with the Hallpike maneuver is a specific diagnostic feature. Other clinical features associated with peripheral vestibular disease are vertigo, tinnitus, and deafness, the latter two reflecting the close association between the vestibular and auditory systems. Causes of peripheral vestibular disease are labyrinthitis, Meniere's disease, trauma (including surgical destruction of one labyrinth), and vascular, inflammatory, or neoplastic lesions of the vestibular nerves.

Central vestibular nystagmus is an acquired jerk nystagmus due to disease in the central vestibular pathways of the brainstem and cerebellum. It has a variety of forms, but characteristic types are a purely torsional or vertical jerk nystagmus and the syndromes of downbeat and upbeat nystagmus, which are probably the result of imbalance in vestibular tone from the vertical semicircular canals. Central vestibular nystagmus is frequently elicited or enhanced by specific head positions, presumably as a result of modulation by input from the peripheral vestibular apparatus. It is not dampened by visual fixation and does not spontaneously abate in intensity with time. Other clinical features reflect the associated brainstem and cerebellar dysfunction and include abnormalities of smooth pursuit eye movements other than those due to the nystagmus itself. Causes of central vestibular nystagmus include lesions of the vestibular nuclei (brainstem demyelination, including multiple sclerosis, inflammation, and stroke, particularly thrombosis of the posteroinferior cerebellar artery leading to lateral medullary infarction—Wallenberg's syndrome).

Downbeat nystagmus is a downward-beating nystagmus, usually present in primary position. It is often most obvious on gaze down and to the side, when the nystagmus becomes oblique, with the horizontal component in the direction of lateral gaze. Downbeat nystagmus is characteristically associated with lesions at the cervicomedullary junction, notably Arnold-Chiari malformation and basilar invagination, and all patients should undergo MRI to exclude such lesions. Other causes are cerebellar degeneration, demyelinating disease, hydrocephalus, anticonvulsants, and lithium.

Upbeat nystagmus is characterized by an upwardbeating nystagmus in primary position which usually increases though it may reduce in intensity on upgaze. It is virtually always the result of brainstem disease but occasionally reflects cerebellar disease. It is seen in brainstem encephalitis, demyelination, and tumors and also as a toxic side effect of barbiturates, alcohol, and anticonvulsants.

Gaze-Evoked & Gaze-Paretic Nystagmus

Maintenance of steady eccentric gaze is dependent upon the neural integrator system, which produces the tonic extraocular muscle activity necessary to overcome the viscous and elastic orbital forces acting to return the globe to primary position. Reduction in activity of the neural integrator results in eccentric gaze being negated by a slow drift of the globe toward primary position. Since the force acting to produce this central drift reduces with decreasing eccentricity, this slow drift has an exponentially decreasing velocity. Additional corrective fast eye movements, returning the eye to the desired eccentric position, result in nystagmus beating in the direction of gaze, whether it be horizontal, vertical, or oblique.

End-point nystagmus (see above) is the physiologic manifestation of the inability of the neural integrator to maintain steady eye position in extreme eccentric gaze. Gaze-evoked nystagmus is the result of pathologic failure of the neural integrator system. In its mildest form it manifests only on moderate horizontal gaze, whereas in its most severe form nystagmus is present with any movement away from primary position. In many cases of gaze-evoked nystagmus, there is also **rebound nystagmus**—following return of the eyes to primary position from a position of eccentric gaze, a jerk nystagmus beating away from the direction of the eccentric gaze develops after a latent period and lasts for a short period.

The neural integrator is situated in the brainstem but is highly dependent upon cerebellar inputs. Thus, gaze-evoked nystagmus may be a manifestation of either brainstem or, especially, cerebellar disease. Often there are other cerebellar eye movement abnormalities such as saccadic dysmetria and disruption of smooth pursuit. The most common causes of gaze-evoked nystagmus are cerebellar diseases, sedatives, and anticonvulsants. Cerebellopontine angle neoplasms, such as vestibular schwannomas (acoustic neuromas), may produce a combination of gaze-evoked nystagmus and a peripheral vestibular nystagmus beating toward the opposite side (Brun's nystagmus).

Reduction in the supranuclear input into the neural integrator or in the ability of the peripheral oculomotor system to facilitate its function will lead to nystagmus with the same basic characteristics as gaze-evoked nystagmus. Thus, conditions ranging from gaze palsy through oculomotor cranial nerve palsies and myasthenia gravis to extraocular muscle disease can manifest with nystagmus on eccentric gaze in the direction of the affected eye movements. This is termed gaze-paretic nystagmus and should be excluded whenever the possibility of a gaze-evoked nystagmus is being considered so as to avoid misdirected investigation.

Convergence-Retraction Nystagmus

Convergence-retraction nystagmus is a feature of the dorsal midbrain (Parinaud's) syndrome either from intrinsic lesions (tumor, hemorrhage, infarction, or inflammation) or extrinsic lesions, particularly pineal tumors and hydrocephalus. On attempted upgaze, which is usually defective, the eyes undergo rapid convergent movements with retraction of the globes. This is best elicited as the patient watches downward-moving stripes on an optokinetic tape or drum. Electromyographic studies have shown cocontraction of extraocular muscles and loss of normal agonist-antagonist reciprocal innervation. Convergence-retraction nystagmus may represent asynchronous, opposed, adducting saccades due to inappropriate activation of the medial rectus muscles.

Seesaw Nystagmus

Seesaw nystagmus is characterized by rising intorsion of one eye and falling extorsion of the other—and then the reverse. It may have a pendular or jerk waveform. Although it is uncommon, it occurs with acquired and congenital chiasmal lesions in association with a bitemporal hemianopia, and midbrain lesions. There does not appear to be a single underlying pathogenesis, but it is likely that dysfunction of the interstitial nucleus of Cajal or the rostral interstitial nucleus of the medial longitudinal fasciculus is important in the cases with midbrain disease.

Periodic Alternating Nystagmus

This is a direction-reversing nystagmus in which each direction can take 1–2 minutes before reversing. The acquired form occurs in pontomedullary junction disease (Arnold-Chiari malformation), multiple sclerosis, and cerebellar degeneration and may respond to baclofen. It may also occur with bilateral blindness and be suppressed if vision is restored. Periodic alternation may also be a feature of congenital nystagmus (see above).

MIMICS OF NYSTAGMUS

Abnormal spontaneous eye movements may be the result of unwanted saccadic eye movements (saccadic intrusions), which include square-wave jerks, macrosaccadic oscillations, ocular flutter, and opsoclonus. These are generally due to cerebellar disease. There is also a variety of abnormal eye movements that occur in coma, including ocular bobbing, ocular dipping, and ping-pong gaze. Superior oblique myokymia is a tremor of the superior oblique muscle leading to episodic monocular vertical oscillopsia.

CEREBROVASCULAR DISORDERS OF OPHTHALMOLOGIC IMPORTANCE

Vascular Insufficiency & Occlusion of the Internal Carotid Artery

Amaurosis fugax is a fleeting or transient loss of vision that is usually associated clinically with carotid occlusive disease, though it can occur with any microembolic or thrombotic disorder, including cardiac valvular disease, cardiac arrhythmia, temporal arteritis, migraine, severe hypotension or shock, papilledema, orbital tumors, and hyperviscosity states. Antiphospholipid antibodies have been associated with transient and permanent cerebral and retinal vascular occlusions in patients younger than the usual stroke population. These antibodies may be the key determinant in patients with existing structural lesions of the carotid artery, mitral valve, etc. In embolization, vision can be suddenly lost or slowly disappear like a curtain rising or falling. In hypotension, the visual field constricts from the periphery to the center.

Perhaps 95% of episodes of amaurosis fugax occur as a result of atherosclerotic lesions of the ipsilateral internal carotid artery. Cerebral and retinal disturbances occur as a result of small emboli breaking loose from the sclerotic plaque and lodging in cerebral or retinal arterioles (occlusion of the central retinal artery or a major branch can occur). Cholesterol emboli (Hollenhorst plaques) may be visible with the ophthalmoscope as small, glistening, yellow-red crystals situated at bifurcations of the retinal arteries. The nonreflective gummy white plugs filling retinal vessels, which characterize platelet-fibrin emboli, are less commonly seen because they quickly disperse and traverse the retinal circulation. In patients with amaurosis fugax, high-grade (70–99%) stenosis of the internal carotid artery, as determined by ultrasound or angiographic studies, is an indication for carotid endarterectomy to reduce the risk of cerebral hemisphere stroke. Low-grade (0–29%) and probably medium-grade (30–69%) stenosis are best treated medically, usually with low-dose (81 mg/d) aspirin. Incidentally noted cholesterol retinal emboli in asymptomatic individuals are associated with a tenfold increased risk of cerebral infarction, but the role of carotid endarterectomy in such individuals is uncertain.

Retinal arterial occlusions occur from calcific or platelet-fibrin emboli. (Cholesterol emboli lodge in retinal vessels but do not usually occlude them.) Calcific emboli, which originate from damaged cardiac valves, have a duller, white-gray appearance compared with cholesterol emboli. In the acute stages of embolic retinal arterial occlusion, treatment with ocular massage, anterior chamber paracentesis, rebreathing into a paper bag to increase inhaled CO_2 level, and intravenous acetazolamide may lead to displacement of the embolus and recovery of vision. After 12 hours, the clinical picture is usually irreversible, though many exceptions to this rule have been reported. Visual acuity better than counting fingers on presentation has a better prognosis with vigorous treatment. Central retinal or branch artery occlusion, especially when due to Hollenhorst plaques, has a poorer 5-year survival rate due to attendant cardiac disease or stroke than does occlusion due to thrombotic disease.

Slow flow (venous stasis) retinopathy is a sign of internal carotid artery occlusion. It is characterized by venous dilation and tortuosity, retinal hemorrhages, macular edema, and eventual neovascular proliferation. It resembles diabetic retinopathy, but the changes occur more in the retinal midperiphery than the posterior pole. In more severe cases, there may be vasodilation of the conjunctiva, iris neovascularization, neovascular glaucoma, and frank anterior segment ischemia with corneal edema, anterior uveitis, and cataract. Diagnosis is most easily confirmed by demonstration of reversal of blood flow in the ipsilateral ophthalmic artery using orbital ultrasound, but further investigation by angiography is usually required to determine the full extent of arterial disease. Carotid endarterectomy may be indicated but carries a risk of precipitating or exacerbating intraocular neovascularization. The role of panretinal laser photocoagulation in treating intraocular neovascularization is uncertain.

Occlusion of the Middle Cerebral Artery

This disorder may produce severe contralateral hemiplegia, hemianesthesia, and homonymous hemianopia. The lower quadrants of the visual fields (upper radiations) are most apt to be involved. Aphasia may be present if the dominant hemisphere is involved.

Vascular Insufficiency of the Vertebrobasilar Arterial System

Brief episodes of transient bilateral blurring of vision commonly precede a basilar artery stroke. An attack seldom leaves any residual visual impairment, and the episode may be so minimal that the patient or doctor does not heed the warning. The blurring is described as a graying of vision just as if the house lights were being dimmed at a theater. Episodes seldom last more than 5 minutes (often only a few seconds) and may be associated with other transient symptoms of vertebrobasilar insufficiency. Antiplatelet drugs can decrease the frequency and severity of vertebrobasilar symptoms.

Occlusion of the Basilar Artery

Complete or extensive thrombosis of the basilar artery nearly always causes death. With partial occlusion or basilar "insufficiency" due to arteriosclerosis, a wide variety of brainstem and cerebellar signs may be present. These include nystagmus, supranuclear oculomotor signs, and involvement of cranial nerves III, IV, VI, and VII.

Prolonged anticoagulant therapy has become the accepted treatment of partial basilar artery thrombotic occlusion.

Occlusion of the Posterior Cerebral Artery

Occlusion of the posterior cerebral artery seldom causes death. Occlusion of the cortical branches (most common) causes homonymous hemianopia, usually superior quadrantic (the artery supplies primarily the inferior visual cortex). Lesions on the left in right-handed persons can cause aphasia, agraphia, and alexia if extensive with parietal and occipital involvement. Involvement of the occipital lobe and splenium of the corpus callosum can cause alexia (inability to read) without agraphia (inability to write); such a patient would not be able to read his or her own writing. Occlusion of the proximal branches may produce the thalamic syndrome (thalamic pain, hemiparesis, hemianesthesia, choreoathetoid movements) and cerebellar ataxia.

Subdural Hemorrhage

Subdural hemorrhage results from tearing or shearing of the veins bridging the subdural space from the pia mater to the dural sinus. It leads to an encapsulated accumulation of blood in the subdural space, usually over one cerebral hemisphere. It is nearly always caused by head trauma. The trauma may be minimal and may precede the onset of neurologic signs by weeks or even months.

In infants, subdural hemorrhage produces progressive enlargement of the head with bulging fontanelles. The diagnosis is established by the finding of bloody spinal fluid on tapping the subdural space and by enlarged head measurements. Ocular signs include strabismus, pupillary changes, papilledema, and retinal hemorrhages.

In adults, the symptoms of chronic subdural hematoma are severe headache, drowsiness, and mental confusion, usually appearing hours to weeks (even months) after trauma. Symptomatology is similar to that of cerebral tumors. Papilledema is present in 30–50% of cases. Retinal hemorrhages occur in association with papilledema. Ipsilateral dilation of the pupil is the most common and most serious pupillary sign and is an urgent indication for immediate surgical evacuation of blood. Unequal, miotic, or mydriatic pupils can occur, or there may be no pupillary signs. Other signs, including vestibular nystagmus and cranial nerve palsies, also occur. Many of these signs result from herniation and compression of the brainstem and therefore often appear late with stupor and coma.

Skull films may show a shift of a calcified pineal gland. CT scan or MRI frequently confirms the diagnosis.

Treatment of acute large subdural hematoma consists of surgical evacuation of the blood; small hematomas may be treated with steroids or simply followed with careful observation. Without treatment, the course of large hematomas is progressively downhill to coma and death. With early and adequate treatment, the prognosis is good.

Subarachnoid Hemorrhage

Subarachnoid hemorrhage most commonly results from ruptured congenital berry aneurysms of the circle of Willis in the subarachnoid space. It may also result from trauma, birth injuries, intracranial hemorrhage, hemorrhage associated with tumors, arteriovenous malformations, or systemic bleeding disorders.

The most prominent symptom of subarachnoid hemorrhage is sudden, severe headache, usually occipital and often associated with signs of meningeal irritation (eg, stiff neck). Drowsiness, loss of consciousness, coma, and death may occur rapidly once an aneurysm ruptures and produces a subarachnoid hemorrhage. Ocular symptoms are not always present. A posterior communicating artery aneurysm may produce a third nerve palsy with pupillary involvement by distention of an aneurysmal sac before the aneurysm ruptures and produces a subarachnoid hemorrhage. Oculomotor palsy with associated numbness and pain in the distribution of the ipsilateral trigeminal nerve is pathognomonic of a supraclinoid, internal carotid, or posterior communicating artery aneurysm. Papilledema usually appears late when it does occur and after there has been a subarachnoid hemorrhage. Various types of intraocular hemorrhage occur infrequently (preretinal hemorrhages are the most common—Terson's syndrome) and carry a poor prognosis for life when they are both early and extensive, since they reflect rapid severe elevation of intracranial pressure.

Exophthalmos may occur as a result of extravasation of blood into orbital tissues. Pressure of an aneurysm on the optic nerve may cause blindness in one eye.

Arteriography following injection of radiopaque substances may help to demonstrate and localize the aneurysms. Blood is present in the cerebrospinal fluid.

Ligation of aneurysmal vessels or of parent arterial trunks may be advisable. Supportive treatment, including control of blood pressure, is all that can be offered during the acute phase of subarachnoid hemorrhage. Thus, it is important to diagnose the posterior communicating artery aneurysm when it first produces a third nerve palsy with pupillary involvement.

Migraine

Migraine is a common episodic illness of unknown cause and varied symptomatology characterized by severe unilateral headache (which alternates sides), visual disturbances, nausea, and vomiting. The neurologic symptoms that usually precede the headache occur in the vasoconstrictive phase; the headache follows in the vasodilative phase. There is usually a family history of a similar disorder. The disease usually becomes manifest between ages 15 and 30 years. It is more common and more severe in women. Many factors, particularly emotional ones, may predispose or contribute to the attacks. Prodromal symptoms are common and include drowsiness, paresthesias, "scintillating" scotomas, blurred vision, and other symptoms. In some patients, homonymous hemianopia can be accurately recorded on the tangent screen during attacks. There are no other objective findings. Visual symptoms usually last only 15–30 minutes. Antiphospholipid antibodies have been associated with migrainous headaches and severe atypical migraine.

Ergotamine tartrate, when given early in an attack, is often effective. Once the attack is well under way, treatment is of little value. Sumatriptan is effective in the acute and well-established migraine attack. The headaches last several hours to several days. Bed rest is often helpful and sometimes essential for relief of discomfort.

PHAKOMATOSES

The phakomatoses (Gr *phakos* "birthmark" + *-oma* "swelling") are a group of diseases characterized by multiple hamartomas occurring in various organ systems and at variable times.

NEUROFIBROMATOSIS

Neurofibromatosis is a generalized hereditary disease characterized by multiple tumors of the skin, central nervous system, peripheral nerves, and nerve sheaths. Other developmental anomalies, particularly of the bones, may be associated. There are two distinct dominant conditions. Neurofibromatosis 1 (peripheral) (Recklinghausen's disease) consists of multiple café au lait spots (99%), peripheral neurofibromas, and Lisch nodules (iris hamartomas) (93%), and its gene lies on the pericentromeric region of chromosome 17. The frequency is 1:3000 live births, with 100% penetrance. In neurofibromatosis 2 (central), there may be few or no café au lait spots or peripheral neurofibromas, but bilateral acoustic neuromas (vestibular schwannomas) are present (Figure 14–34) and its gene lies on chromosome 22. The frequency is 1:35,000. Neurofibromatosis 1 is associated with tumors primarily of astrocytes and neurons, whereas neurofibromatosis 2 is associated with tumors of the meninges and Schwann cells. There is no racial predominance. Signs may be present at birth

but are activated during pregnancy, during puberty, and at menopause.

Clinical Findings

Tumors may occur anywhere in the body, including the eye. Café au lait spots (small pigmented areas of skin) tend to enlarge and darken with age. A few may occur in 5–10% of the normal population, but in neurofibromatosis 1 there are five or six such spots greater than 1.5–2 cm in diameter; axillary freckles are especially significant. Cutaneous neurofibromatosis occurs especially on the trunk and spares the palms and soles. Tumors of the lids can be isolated cutaneous neurofibromas or plexiform (rubbery "bag of worms") neurofibromas. The latter may be associated with glaucoma.

Tumors of the optic nerve, meninges (meningioma), and glial cells (astrocytomas) also occur. Bilaterally thickened optic nerves are pathognomonic of neurofibromatosis 1, and many are asymptomatic (30–80%). A subgroup with nerves having a thickened nerve core and a low-density perineural proliferation are often symptomatic, with proptosis and decreased visual acuity. This latter group may represent a low-grade astrocytoma or optic nerve glioma. About 70% of optic nerve gliomas present before the age of 7 years. MRI shows lengthening and kinking of the optic nerve, and bright spots in brain parenchyma can be seen on T2-weighted images. Optic nerve glioma can cause disk swelling or optic atrophy. There may be Lisch nodules and enlarged corneal nerves. About 75% of patients with neurofibromatosis 2 have early posterior subcapsular lens opacities. Pigment epithelial and retinal hamartomas also occur with increased frequency in neurofibromatosis 2.

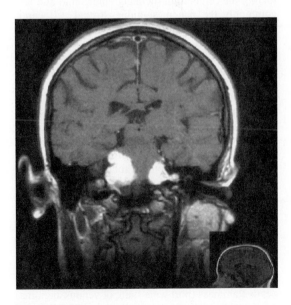

Figure 14–34. Coronal MRI of bilateral acoustic neuromas in neurofibromatosis 2.

Treatment & Prognosis

Visual function in optic nerve gliomas does not change much after diagnosis. Chiasmal gliomas are less aggressive in neurofibromatosis than when they occur in its absence. The risk is greatest during the early follow-up period, and survival relates to the surrounding brain involvement.

When lesions are confined to the skin, the prognosis is good. Intracranial and intraspinal lesions are usually multiple and have a poor prognosis. The disease tends to be fairly stationary, with only slow progression over long periods of time. Neurofibromas of the peripheral nerves occur also and may undergo sarcomatous degeneration (5%).

RETINOCEREBELLAR ANGIOMATOSIS
(Von Hippel–Lindau Disease)

This rare disease occurs most commonly in men in the third decade but can appear at any time up to age 60. Its incidence is 1:10,000, and there is neither gender nor racial predilection. About 25% of patients show autosomal dominant inheritance. The earliest signs are dilation and tortuosity of the retinal vessels, which later develop into an angiomatous formation with hemorrhages and exudates (retinal capillary angioblastomas) (Figure 10–30). A stage of massive exudation, retinal detachment, and secondary glaucoma occurs later and will cause blindness if untreated. The disease is unilateral in 65% of cases. Patients must be followed expectantly with periodic, presymptomatic screening because in up to 25% of cases the retinal angiomatosis is associated with a similar generalized process, most often affecting the cerebellum (hemangioblastoma) and less commonly the pancreas, kidney (renal cell carcinoma), adrenal gland, and other organs. The evidence at present suggests that this is all one genetically determined disease showing autosomal dominant inheritance with variable expression.

Treatment & Prognosis

Early treatment of retinal lesions with photocoagulation, diathermy, or cryotherapy has been effective in some cases. Cerebral and cerebellar tumors have been successfully removed, but recurrences are common. MRI scanning revolutionizes follow-up of these patients, since it can be done without radiation hazard and detects presymptomatic lesions.

STURGE-WEBER SYNDROME

This uncommon nonfamilial disease with unknown inheritance is recognizable at birth by a characteristic nevus flammeus (port wine stain, or venous angioma) on one side of the face following the distribution of one or more branches of the fifth cranial nerve. There

is corresponding angiomatous involvement (leptomeningeal angiodysplasia) of the meninges and brain, which causes jacksonian seizures (85%), mental retardation (60%), and cerebrocortical atrophy. Since these cortical lesions calcify, they can be seen on plain skull x-rays after infancy. Unilateral infantile glaucoma on the affected side frequently develops if there is extensive involvement of the conjunctiva with hemangioma of the episclera and anterior chamber anomalies. Lid or conjunctival involvement nearly always implies ultimate intraocular involvement and glaucoma. Forty percent of patients with a port wine stain on the face develop choroidal hemangioma on the same side. There is at least one cytogenic study reporting trisomy 22.

Treatment & Prognosis

There is no effective treatment for Sturge-Weber syndrome, though the glaucoma can be controlled in rare cases by surgery.

WYBURN-MASON SYNDROME

Wyburn-Mason syndrome is a rare disorder of multiple arteriovenous malformations, variably involving the retina, other portions of the anterior visual pathway, the midbrain, the maxilla, and the mandible, all on the same side of the head.

Headaches and seizures are common central nervous system presenting signs. Large, tortuous, dilated vessels covering extensive areas of the retina are an important diagnostic clue and can cause cystic retinal degeneration with decreased vision. Optic atrophy without retinal lesions can also occur.

ATAXIA-TELANGIECTASIA

Ataxia-telangiectasia is an autosomal recessive disorder characterized by skin and conjunctival telangiectases, cerebellar ataxia, and recurrent sinopulmonary infections. All signs and symptoms are progressive with time, but the ataxia appears first as the child begins to walk, and the telangiectases appear between 4 and 7 years of age. Mental retardation also occurs. The recurrent infections relate to thymic deficiencies and corresponding T cell abnormalities as well as to decreased or absent immunoglobulins. Saccadic and eventual pursuit abnormalities produce a supranuclear ophthalmoplegia.

TUBEROUS SCLEROSIS
(Bourneville's Disease)

Tuberous sclerosis is characterized by the triad of adenoma sebaceum, epilepsy, and mental retardation, though 30–50% of affected individuals have normal intelligence. Adenoma sebaceum (angiofibromas) occur in 90% of patients over the age of 4 years, and the number of lesions increases with puberty. These flesh-colored papules are 1–2 mm in diameter and have a butterfly distribution on the nose and malar area; they can also occur in the subungual and periungual areas. Ashleaf-shaped hypopigmented ovals can be present on the skin even of neonates but are best seen under Wood's (ultraviolet) light.

Retinal hamartomas appear as oval or circular white areas in the peripheral fundus and, like optic nerve hematomas, characteristically have a mulberry-like appearance (Figure 10–31). Renal hamartomas occur in 80% of patients. Subependymal nodules in the periventricular areas of the brain can calcify and appear as candle wax gutterings or drippings on radiologic studies (25–30% of skull x-rays and 90% of CT scans) in patients with clinical tuberous sclerosis. MRI can show actively growing subependymal nodules. These can become astrocytomas. Seizures occur in 90% of patients, usually within the first 3 years of life.

The disease is inherited sporadically (80%) or as an autosomal dominant with low penetrance. The prevalence may be 1:9400 if patients with the incomplete form of the disease are included. Vision is generally normal, and progression of retinal hamartomas is rare. The prognosis for life relates to the degree of central nervous system involvement. In severe cases, death can occur in the second or third decade; if there is minimal central nervous system involvement, life expectancy should be normal.

CEREBROMACULAR DEGENERATION

Genetically determined (autosomal recessive) neuronal lipid storage disease of the brain may affect the neural elements of the retina as well. The clinical forms are classified by the age at onset and the enzyme deficiency. The pathologic changes are present prenatally. Clinical manifestations occur as a critical level of intraneuronal lipidosis is reached, resulting in a progressive disease with dementia, visual disturbances, and neuromotor signs. A definitive diagnosis can be established readily by conjunctival biopsy, rectal biopsy, or appendectomy showing ganglioside accumulation even before clinical signs are present.

The striking ocular finding of a cherry-red spot in the macula is seen in congenital and infantile cases. A halo occurs from loss of transparency of the ganglion cell ring of the macula, which accentuates the central red or the normal choroidal vasculature. A cherry-red spot will occur in central retinal artery occlusion, sphingolipidosis, mucolipidosis, commotio retinae, and methanol toxicity. The sphingolipidoses include Niemann-Pick disease type A and type B, Tay-Sachs disease, Sandhoff's disease, neuronal ceroid lipofuscinosis, and generalized gangliosidosis. Optic atrophy will occur early in Tay-Sachs disease, and the cherry-red spot can be pigmented in dark retinas.

Extraocular muscle involvement can occur in juvenile sphingolipidoses, Refsum's disease, and betalipoproteinemia, the latter two disorders being associated with retinitis pigmentosa.

REFERENCES

Acheson JF, Green WT, Sanders MD: Optic nerve sheath decompression for the treatment of visual failure in chronic raised intracranial pressure. J Neurol Neurosurg Psychiatry 1994;57:1426.

Baker RS, Epstein AD: Ocular motor abnormalities from head trauma. Surv Ophthalmol 1991;35:245.

Barrett TG et al: Optic atrophy in Wolfram (DIDMOAD) syndrome. Eye 1997;11:882.

Basta L, Ormerod LD, Rowsey JJ: Optic disc drusen defined by β-scan ultrasonography. Ann Ophthalmol 1997; 29:181.

Beck RW et al: The course of visual recovery after optic neuritis. Experience of the Optic Neuritis Treatment Trial. Ophthalmology 1994;101:1771.

Beck RW for the Optic Neuritis Study Group: The Optic Neuritis Treatment Trial: Three-year follow-up results. Arch Ophthalmol 1995;113:136.

Beck RW, Trobe JD, for the Optic Neuritis Study Group: What we have learned from the Optic Neuritis Treatment Trial. Ophthalmology 1995;102:1504.

Brey RL et al: Antiphospholipid antibodies and cerebral ischemia in young people. Neurology 1990;40:1190.

Brodsky MV: Congenital optic disk anomalies. Surv Ophthalmol 1994;39:89.

Brown GC, Shields JA: Tumors of the optic nerve head. Surv Ophthalmol 1985;29:239.

Brown J et al: Clinical and genetic analysis of a family affected with dominant optic atrophy *(OPA1).* Arch Ophthalmol 1997;115:95.

Bruno A et al: Vascular outcome in men with asymptomatic retinal cholesterol emboli. Ann Intern Med 1995;122:249.

Burde RM: Optic disk risk factors for nonarteritic anterior ischemic optic neuropathy. Am J Ophthalmol 1993; 116:759.

De Potter P, Zografos L: Survival prognosis of patients with retinal artery occlusion and associated carotid artery disease. Graefes Arch Clin Exp Ophthalmol 1993;231:212.

deGroot J, Chusid JG: *Correlative Neuroanatomy,* 20th ed. Appleton & Lange, 1988.

Dutton JJ: Glioma of the anterior visual pathway. Surv Ophthalmol 1994;38:427.

Eggenberger ER, Miller NR, Vitale S: Lumboperitoneal shunt for the treatment of pseudotumor cerebri. Neurology 1996;46:1524.

Farris BK, Pickard DR: Bilateral postinfectious optic neuritis and intravenous steroid therapy in children. Ophthalmology 1990;97:339.

Frederiksen JL: Bilateral acute optic neuritis—prospective clinical, MRI, CSF, neurophysiological and HLA findings. Neuroophthalmology 1997;17:175.

Gass A et al: High resolution magnetic resonance imaging of the anterior visual pathway in patients with optic neuropathies using fast spin echo and phased array local coils. J Neurol Neurosurg Psychiatry 1995;58:562.

Gradstein L et al: Congenital periodic alternating nystagmus: Diagnosis and management. Ophthalmology 1997;104:918.

Gross-Jendroska M et al: Kearns-Sayre syndrome: A case report and review. Eur J Ophthalmol 1992;2(1):15.

Guy M et al: Gadolinium-DTPA-enhanced magnetic resonance imaging in optic neuropathies. Ophthalmology 1990;97:592.

Halliday AM, McDonald WI: Visual evoked potentials. In *Clinical Neurophysiology*. Stalberg E, Young RR (editors). Butterworths, 1981.

Hardwig P, Robertson DM: Von Hippel-Lindau disease: A familial, often lethal, multisystem phakomatosis. Ophthalmology 1984;91:263.

Harrington DO, Drake MV: *The Visual Fields: Text and Atlas of Clinical Perimetry,* 6th ed. Mosby, 1990.

Hayreh SS et al: Giant cell arteritis: Validity and reliability of various diagnostic criteria. Am J Ophthalmol 1997;123:285.

Hayreh SS et al: Systemic diseases associated with nonarteritic anterior ischemic optic neuropathy. Am J Ophthalmol 1994;118:766.

Hopf HC, Gutmann L: Diabetic 3rd nerve palsy: Evidence for a mesencephalic lesion. Neurology 1990;40:1041.

Horn AKE, Büttner-Enever JA, Büttner U: Saccadic premotor neurones in the brainstem: Functional neuroanatomy and clinical implications. Neuroophthalmology 1996; 10:229.

Hoyt WF: Ophthalmoscopy of the retinal nerve fiber layer in neuro-ophthalmologic diagnosis. Aust NZ J Ophthalmol 1976;4:14.

Huber A: *Eye Signs and Symptoms in Brain Tumors,* 3rd ed. Mosby, 1976.

IFNB Multiple Sclerosis Study Group and The University of British Columbia MS/MRI Analysis Group: Interferon beta-1b in the treatment of multiple sclerosis: Final outcome of the randomized controlled trial. Neurology 1995;45:1277.

Ikeda H, Yoshimoto T: Visual disturbances in patients with pituitary adenoma. Acta Neurol Scand 1995;92:157.

Imes RK, Hoyt WF: Childhood chiasmal gliomas: Update on the fate of patients in the 1969 San Francisco Study. Br J Ophthalmol 1986;70:179.

Ischemic Optic Decompression Trial Research Group: Optic nerve decompression surgery for nonarteritic anterior ischemic optic neuropathy (NAION) is not effective and may be harmful. JAMA 1995;273:625.

Ishibashi Y, Hori Y (editors): Tuberous sclerosis and neurofibromatosis: Epidemiology, pathophysiology, biology and management. Proceedings of the International Symposium on Neurocutaneous Syndrome. Excerpta Medica, 1990.

Jacobs LD et al: Intramuscular interferon beta-1a for disease progression in relapsing multiple sclerosis. Ann Neurol 1996;39:285.

Johnston RL et al: Dominant optic atrophy, Kjer type: Linkage analysis and clinical features in a large British pedigree. Arch Ophthalmol 1997;115;100.

Jonasdottir A et al: Refinement of the dominant optic atrophy locus *(OPA1)* to a 1.4-cM interval on chromosome 3q28-3q29, within a 3-Mb YAC contig. Hum Genet 1997;99:115.

Joseph MP et al: Extracranial optic nerve decompression for traumatic optic neuropathy. Arch Ophthalmol 1990; 108:1091.

Keltner JL et al: Visual field profile of optic neuritis: One-year follow-up in the Optic Neuritis Treatment Trial. Arch Ophthalmol 1994;112:946.

Kheterpal S et al: Imaging of optic disc drusen: A comparative study. Eye 1995;9:67.

King AJ et al: Spontaneous recovery rates for unilateral sixth nerve palsies. Eye 1995;9:476.

Kupersmith MJ et al: Aspirin reduces the incidence of second eye NAION: A retrospective study. J Neuroophthalmol 1997;17:250.

Kupersmith MJ, Rosenberg C, Kleinberg D: Visual loss in pregnant women with pituitary adenomas. Ann Intern Med 1994;121:473.

Lam BL, Weingeist TA: Corticosteroid-responsive traumatic optic neuropathy. Am J Ophthalmol 1990;109:99.

Landau K et al: 24-hour blood pressure monitoring in patients with anterior ischemic optic neuropathy. Arch Ophthalmol 1996;114:570.

Leigh JR, Zee DS: *The Neurology of Eye Movement.* Vol 23 of *Contemporary Neurology Series.* Davis, 1983.

Levine SR et al: Cerebrovascular and neurologic disease associated with antiphospholipid antibodies: 48 cases. Neurology 1990;40:1181.

Lindenberg R, Walsh FB, Sacks JG: *Neuropathology of Vision: An Atlas.* Lea & Febiger, 1973.

Masuyama Y et al: Clinical studies on the occurrence and the pathogenesis of opticociliary veins. J Clin Neuroophthalmol 1990;10:1.

McDonald WI: Optic neuritis and its significance. Clin Exp Neurol 1989;26:1.

McHenry JC, Spoor TC: Spontaneous improvement of progressive anterior ischemic optic neuropathy. Arch Ophthalmol 1993;111:1602.

Mizener JB, Podhajsky P, Hayreh SS: Ocular ischemic syndrome. Ophthalmology 1997;104:859.

Newman NJ: Mitochondrial disease and the eye. Ophthalmol Clin N Am 1992;5(3):405.

Nikoskelainen EK et al: Leber's "plus": Neurological abnormalities in patients with Leber's hereditary optic neuropathy. J Neurol Neurosurg Psychiatry 1995; 59:160.

North American Symptomatic Carotid Endarterectomy Trial Collaborators: Beneficial effect of carotid endarterectomy in symptomatic patients with high-grade carotid stenosis. N Engl J Med 1991;325:445.

Nucci P, Mets MB, Gabianelli EB: Trisomy 4q with morning glory disc anomaly. Ophthalmic Paediatr Genet 1990;2:143.

O'Riordan JI et al: Clinical, CSF, and MRI findings in Devic's neuromyelitis optica. J Neurol Neurosurg Psychiatry 1996;60:382.

Optic Neuritis Study Group: The clinical profile of optic neuritis: Experience of the Optic Neuritis Treatment Trial. Arch Ophthalmol 1991;109:1673.

Patel U, Gupta SC: Wyburn-Mason syndrome: A case report and review of the literature. Neuroradiology 1990; 31:544.

Ragge NK: Clinical and genetic patterns of neurofibromatosis 1 and 2. Br J Ophthalmol 1993;77:662.

Ragge NK et al: Ocular abnormalities in neurofibromatosis 2. Am J Ophthalmol 1995;120:634.

Regillo CD et al: Diabetic papillopathy: Patient characteristics and fundus findings. Arch Ophthalmol 1995; 113:889.

Riordan-Eva P: Optic nerve sheath fenestration. Current Medical Literature (Ophthalmology) 1994;4:67.

Riordan-Eva P et al: The clinical features of Leber's hereditary optic neuropathy defined by the presence of a pathogenic mitochondrial DNA mutation. Brain 1995; 118:319.

Riordan-Eva P, Harding AE: Leber's hereditary optic neuropathy—the clinical relevance of different mitochondrial DNA mutations. J Med Genet 1995;32:81.

Riordan-Eva P, Wood NW: Mitochondrial disorders in neuro-ophthalmology. Curr Opin Neurol 1996;9:1.

Riordan-Eva P et al: Orbital ultrasound in the ocular ischaemic syndrome. Eye 1994;8:93.

Rivero A et al: Single fiber electromyography of extraocular muscles: A sensitive method for the diagnosis of ocular myasthenia gravis. Muscle Nerve 1995;18:943.

Robb R: Idiopathic superior oblique palsies in children. J Pediatr Ophthalmol Strabismus 1990;27:66.

Rodriguez M et al: Optic neuritis: A population-based study in Olmsted County, Minnesota. Neurology 1995;45:224.

Rush JA et al: Optic glioma: Long-term follow-up of 85 histopathologically verified cases. Ophthalmology 1982;89:1213.

Sadun AA: The optic neuropathy of Alzheimer's disease. Metab Pediatr Syst Ophthalmol 1989;12:64.

Sanders MD: Papilloedema: "The pendulum of progress." Eye 1997;11:267.

Spoor TC et al: Treatment of pseudotumor cerebri by primary and secondary optic nerve sheath decompression. Am J Ophthalmol 1991;112:177.

Stahl JS et al: A pilot study of gabapentin for acquired nystagmus. Neuroophthalmology 1996;16:107.

Thompson DS et al: The effects of pregnancy in multiple sclerosis: A retrospective study. Neurology 1986; 36:1097.

Traccis S et al: Successful treatment of acquired pendular elliptical nystagmus in multiple sclerosis with isoniazid and base-out prisms. Neurology 1990;40:492.

Van Dorp DB, Kwee ML: Tuberous sclerosis. Ophthalmic Paediatr Genet 1990;2:95.

Vargas ME et al: Endovascular treatment of giant aneurysms which cause visual loss. Ophthalmology 1994;101:1091.

15

Ocular Disorders Associated With Systemic Diseases

Michael D. Sanders, FRCP, FRCS, FRCOphth, & Elizabeth M. Graham, FRCP, FRCOphth

Examination of the eye provides the ophthalmologist an opportunity to make a unique contribution to the diagnosis of systemic disease. Nowhere else in the body can a microcirculatory system be investigated with such precision, and nowhere else are the results of minute focal lesions so devastating. Many systemic diseases involve the eyes, and therapy demands some knowledge of the vascular, rheologic, and immunologic nature of these diseases.

VASCULAR DISEASE

NORMAL ANATOMY & PHYSIOLOGY

The blood supply to the eye is from the ophthalmic artery, which is the first branch of the internal carotid artery (see Chapter 1). The first branches of the ophthalmic artery are the central retinal artery and the long posterior ciliary arteries. The retina is perfused by retinal and choroidal vessels that provide contrasting anatomic and physiologic circulations. The retinal arteries correspond to arterioles in the systemic circulation. They function as end arteries and feed a capillary bed consisting of small capillaries (7 μm) with tight endothelial junctions. Dependent on this anatomic arrangement is the maintenance of the blood-retina barrier, and this system is autoregulated, since there are no autonomic nerve fibers. Most of the blood within the eye, however, is in the choroidal circulation, which is characterized by a high flow rate, autonomic regulation, and an anatomic arrangement with collateral branching and large capillaries (30 μm), all of which have fenestrations in juxtaposition to Bruch's membrane. Examination of the retinal vessels is facilitated by the use of red-free light and fluorescein angiography, whereas indocyanine green angiography gives further information about the choroidal vessels.

PATHOLOGIC APPEARANCES IN RETINAL VASCULAR DISEASE

Hemorrhages

Retinal hemorrhages result from diapedeses from veins or capillaries, and the morphologic appearances depend upon the size, site, and extent of damage to the vessel (Figure 15–1). Hemorrhages may be caused by any condition that alters the integrity of the endothelial cells. They usually indicate some abnormality of the retinal vascular system, and systemic factors should be considered in relation to (1) vessel wall disease (eg, hypertension, diabetes), (2) blood disorders (eg, leukemia, polycythemia), and (3) reduced perfusion (eg, carotid cavernous fistula, acute blood loss).

A. Preretinal Hemorrhages: These result from

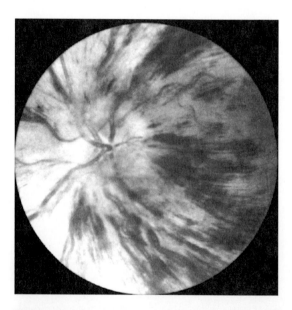

Figure 15–1. Flame-shaped retinal hemorrhages in the nerve fiber layer radiate out from the optic disk. Three days before the photograph was taken, the patient experienced sudden loss of vision, which left him with light perception only.

damage to the superficial disk or retinal vessels and are usually large, producing a gravity-dependent fluid level.

B. Linear Hemorrhages: These usually small hemorrhages lie in the superficial nerve fiber layers and hence have a characteristic linear appearance, conforming to the alignment of nerve fibers in any particular area of the fundus.

C. Punctate Hemorrhages: Hemorrhages situated deeper in the substance of the retina are punctate and derived from capillaries and smaller venules. The circular appearance is related to the anatomic arrangement of structures in the retina.

D. Subretinal Hemorrhages: These hemorrhages are less common because normally there are no blood vessels between the retina and the choroid. Such hemorrhages are large and red, with a well-defined margin and no fluid level. They are seen in relation to the disk and in any condition where abnormal vessels pass from the choroidal circulation into the retina.

E. Hemorrhages Under the Pigment Epithelium: Hemorrhages situated under the pigment epithelium are usually dark and large, so that they must be differentiated from choroidal melanomas and hemangiomas.

F. White Central Hemorrhages (Roth's Spots): Superficial retinal hemorrhages with pale or white centers are not pathognomonic of any disease process but may arise in a variety of circumstances: (1) retinal infarction (cotton-wool spot) with surrounding hemorrhage; (2) retinal hemorrhage in combination with extravasation of white corpuscles (eg, leukemia); and (3) retinal hemorrhage with central resolution.

Acute Ocular Ischemia

A. Optic Disk Infarction (Anterior Ischemic Optic Neuropathy): Impairment of the blood supply to the optic disk produces sudden visual loss, usually with an altitudinal field defect and pallid swelling of the optic disk. The primary abnormality is complete or partial interruption of the choroidal blood supply to the disk, while the retinal capillaries on the surface of the disk appear dilated. Fluorescein angiography confirms the circulatory alterations (Figure 15–2). Pathologic studies show infarction of the retrolaminar region of the optic nerve. The explanation for the vulnerability of the short posterior ciliary vessels supplying this region is unknown. Optic disk infarction is often caused by giant cell arteritis in old age and by hypertension and arteriosclerotic disease in middle age. Small optic disks are particularly prone to infarction.

B. Choroidal Infarction: This is extremely rare, though certain clinical appearances have been attributed to ciliary vessel occlusion. These include small pale areas in the equatorial region that resolve to leave mottled pigmentary areas (Elschnig's spots) due to necrosis of the pigment epithelium. Larger infarcts may occur and may be triangular or linear (Figure 15–3).

C. Retinal Infarction: The funduscopic appearance of arteriolar occlusion depends on the size of the vessel occluded, the duration of occlusion, and the time course. Occlusion of major arterioles produces a total, hemispheric, or segmental pallid swelling of the retina. Occlusion of a precapillary retinal arteriole produces the pathognomonic appearance of a cotton-wool spot (Figure 15–4). This consists of a pale,

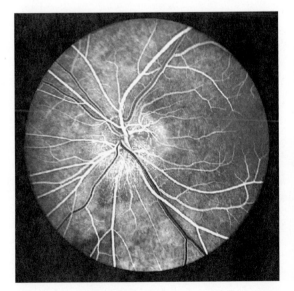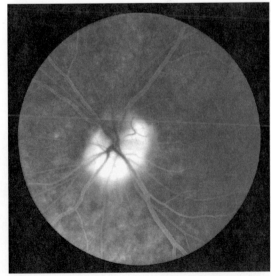

Figure 15–2. Ischemic optic neuropathy. Sudden visual loss in a 48-year-old man produced a complete inferior altitudinal field loss. **Left:** Fluorescein angiogram shows impaired filling of the upper part of the disk with dilation of retinal capillaries at the lower part of the disk. **Right:** Photograph 10 minutes after injection shows leakage of dye mainly at the lower part of the disk.

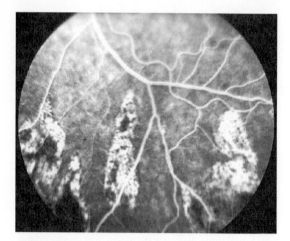

Figure 15–3. Anti-phospholipid antibody syndrome. Fluorescein angiogram demonstrates choroidal infarcts in a patient who presented with multiple strokes.

slightly elevated swelling usually one-fourth to one-half the size of the optic disk. Pathologic examination shows distention of neurons, with cytoid bodies (Figure 15–5); electron microscopy shows the accumulation of axoplasm and organelles. Occlusion of arterioles, whether due to intrinsic vessel wall disease or to intramural factors, may produce these pathognomonic signs.

D. Transient Retinal Ischemia (Amaurosis Fugax): Transient episodes of monocular visual loss lasting 5–10 minutes are characteristic of amaurosis fugax. Patients often describe a curtain coming down from above or across their vision, usually with complete return of vision within seconds or minutes. Paresthesias in the contralateral limbs localize the disorder to the carotid artery and suggest involvement of the ophthalmic artery and middle cerebral artery. It is important for the ophthalmologist to auscultate the carotid for a systolic bruit and to search the fundus for emboli. Amaurosis fugax is most com-

monly due to retinal emboli, of which there are three main types.

1. Cholesterol emboli–These so-called Hollenhorst plaques usually arise from an atheromatous plaque in the carotid artery and consist of cholesterol and fibrin. They lodge at the bifurcation of retinal arterioles, are refractile, and may appear larger than the vessel that contains them (Figure 15–6).

2. Calcific emboli–Originating from damaged cardiac valves, these emboli lodge within the arteriole, producing complete occlusion and infarction of the distal retina. Calcific emboli are solid and calcified and occur in younger patients with a variety of cardiac lesions.

3. Platelet-fibrin emboli–Most cases of amaurosis fugax are probably due to the transit of platelet aggregates through the retinal and choroidal circulations. The emboli are usually broken up as they traverse the retinal circulation and hence are rarely seen, though occasionally they produce retinal infarction. Arising from abnormalities of the heart or great vessels, they may be reduced by drugs that reduce platelet aggregation (eg, aspirin).

Retinal emboli most commonly arise from carotid artery disease (see Chapter 14). A cardiac origin such as atrial fibrillation, mitral valve prolapse, or subacute infective endocarditis needs to be considered, particularly in patients under 40 years of age or those with a history of cardiac disease.

There are several other causes of amaurosis fugax, including factors that induce temporary reduction in ocular perfusion, eg, arterial disease, cardiac disorders, hematologic disorders, retinal or choroidal migraine, and, rarely, elevation of intraocular pressure (Table 15–1).

Central Retinal Vein Occlusion (Figure 15–7)

Central retinal vein occlusion is an important cause of visual morbidity in elderly people, particularly those with hypertension or glaucoma.

Fundus examination shows dilated tortuous veins with retinal and macular edema, hemorrhages all over

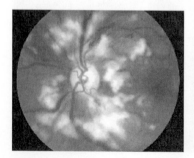
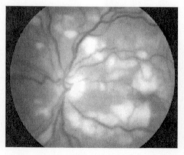
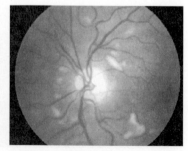

Figure 15–4. Cotton-wool spots. Numerous cotton-wool spots are seen in the posterior poles in three patients. **Left:** A young woman with acute systemic lupus erythematosus and neurologic disease. **Center:** A young man with pancreatitis. **Right:** A patient with AIDS. Cotton-wool spots resolve over 6 weeks regardless of their cause.

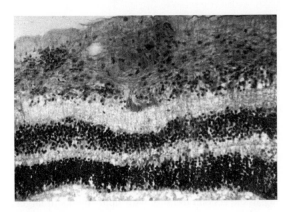

Figure 15–5. Cotton-wool spot. Histologic examination shows cytoid bodies and distended neurons in the superficial retinal layers. Deeper retinal layers are normal. (Courtesy of N Ashton.)

Table 15–1. Causes of amaurosis fugax.

Retinal emboli	Cholesterol emboli Calcific emboli Platelet-fibrin emboli

Arterial disease	Carotid artery stenosis
	Carotid artery ulceration
	  Bifurcation
	  Carotid siphon

Cardiac disease	Dysrhythmias (eg, atrial fibrillation)
	Valvular disease (eg, mitral leaflet
	  prolapse)
	Left ventricular aneurysm or mural
	  thrombus secondary to myocardial
	  infarction

Hematologic disease	Anemia Polycythemia Macroglobulinemia Sickle cell disease

Other	Mechanical compression of vertebral
	  or carotid arteries
	Hypertensive episode
	Hypotensive episode
	  Drugs
	  Spontaneous (eg, diabetes mellitus,
	    Addison's disease)
	Arteritis
	Retinal or choloidal migraine
	Raised intraocular pressure

the posterior pole, and cotton-wool spots. The arterioles are usually attenuated, indicating generalized microvascular disease.

The prognosis for vision is poor. Fluorescein angiography demonstrates two types of response: a nonischemic type, with dilation of retinal vessels and edema; and an ischemic type, with large areas of capillary nonperfusion or evidence of retinal or anterior segment neovascularization. In 93% of ischemic and 50% of nonischemic central retinal vein occlusions, the ultimate visual acuity is less than 20/200.

Central retinal vein occlusion has an increased incidence in certain systemic conditions such as diabetes mellitus, hypertension, collagen vascular diseases, and hyperviscosity syndromes (eg, Waldenström's macroglobulinemia, angioimmunoblastic lymphadenopathy). However, the prevalence of cerebrovascular or cardiovascular disease is not increased compared to the general population. Investigations in-

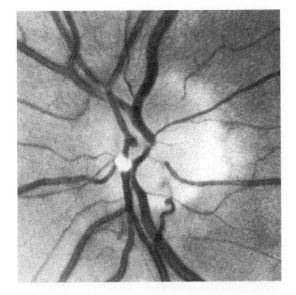

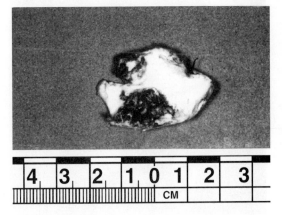

Figure 15–6. Cholesterol embolus (Hollenhorst plaque). ***Left:*** A cholesterol embolus at the optic disk, which is refractile and appears larger than the vessel that contains it. A collateral vessel is seen at the lower border of the disk. ***Right:*** Surgical specimen from a patient with a similar embolus shows an atheromatous ulcer at the bifurcation of the common carotid artery.

clude measurement of serum lipids, plasma proteins, plasma glucose, and assessment of blood viscosity by hemoglobin, hematocrit, and fibrinogen estimations. In young patients, protein C, activated protein C resistance, protein S, and antithrombin III levels should be measured to exclude abnormalities of the thrombolytic system. If hypertension is present, simple renal function tests, including urea and electrolytes, estimation of creatinine clearance, microscopic examination of the urine, and renal ultrasound are indicated.

Treatment of retinal vein occlusion is unsatisfactory. Trials with anticoagulants and fibrinolytic agents have not been successful. In ischemic central retinal vein occlusion, panretinal laser photocoagulation is effective in preventing and treating secondary neovascular glaucoma.

Occasionally, central retinal vein occlusion occurs in young people and may be associated with cells in the vitreous. Rheologic investigations are usually negative, and the prognosis for vision is good.

Retinal Branch Vein Occlusion (Figure 15–8)

Occlusion of a branch vein should be viewed as part of the spectrum of central retinal vein occlusion. Investigations are similar in the two conditions, but arterial disease—particularly hypertension—is common. Branch retinal vein occlusion occurs more frequently in the superotemporal and inferotemporal regions and particularly at sites where arteries cross over veins, and only rarely where veins cross over arteries.

The value of laser treatment in the management of the complications of branch retinal vein occlusion is discussed in Chapters 10 and 24.

ATHEROSCLEROSIS & ARTERIOSCLEROSIS

The process of atherosclerosis occurs in larger arteries and is due to fatty infiltration of a patchy nature occurring in the intima and associated with fibrosis. Involvement of smaller vessels (ie, < 300 μm) by diffuse fibrosis and hyalinization is termed arteriosclerosis. The retinal vessels beyond the disk are less than 300 μm; therefore, involvement of the retinal arterioles should be termed arteriosclerosis, whereas involvement of the central retinal artery is properly termed atherosclerosis.

Atherosclerosis is a progressive change developing in the second decade, with lipid streaks in larger vessels, progressing to a fibrous plaque in the third decade. In the fourth and fifth decades, ulceration, hemorrhages, and thrombosis occur, and the lesion may be calcified. Destruction of the elastic and muscular elements of the media produces ectasia and rupture of the large vessels, though in smaller vessels obstruction is usually seen. The clinical results of atherosclerosis are seen several decades after the onset of the process. Factors contributing to atheroma include hyperlipidemia, hypertension, and obesity.

Arteriosclerosis is characterized by an enhanced light reflection, focal attenuation, and irregularity of caliber. These signs may also be seen in the arterioles of normotensive individuals in middle age. In elderly individuals with arteriosclerosis and associated mild hypertension, it is difficult to differentiate the changes of arteriosclerosis from those due to hypertension.

Appearance of Retinal Vessels

A normal arteriolar wall is transparent, so that what is actually seen is the column of blood within the vessel.

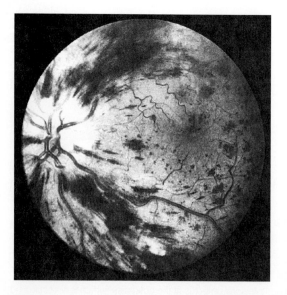 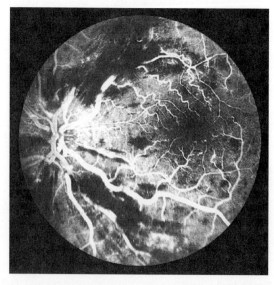

Figure 15–7. Central retinal vein occlusion. **Left:** Photograph shows linear hemorrhages in the nerve fiber layer and punctate hemorrhages in the deeper retinal layers. **Right:** Fluorescein angiogram shows dilation of the veins.

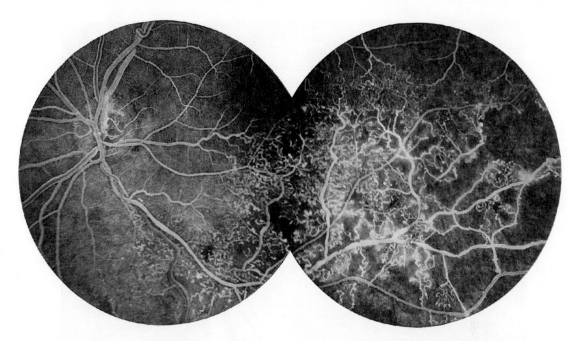

Figure 15–8. Retinal branch vein occlusion. The affected segment of retina shows changes of reduced perfusion. This results in irregularity of the arterioles and veins, areas of capillary closure, and dilated capillaries with microaneurysms.

A thin, central light reflection in the center of the blood column appears as a yellow refractile line about one-fifth the width of the column. As the walls of the arterioles become infiltrated with lipids and cholesterol, the vessels become sclerotic. As this process continues, the vessel wall gradually loses its transparency and becomes visible; the blood column appears wider than normal, and the thin light reflection becomes broader. The grayish yellow fat products in the vessel wall blend with the red of the blood column to produce a typical "copper wire" appearance. This indicates moderate arteriosclerosis. As sclerosis proceeds, the blood column-vessel wall light reflection resembles "silver wire," which indicates severe arteriosclerosis; at times, even occlusion of an arteriolar branch may occur.

Red-free light (a white light with a green filter) allows details of hemorrhages, focal irregularity of blood vessels, and nerve fibers to be seen more clearly (Figure 15–9).

HYPERTENSIVE RETINOPATHY

Wagener and Keith in 1939 classified patients with hypertensive retinopathy into four groups. Stages I and II were restricted to arteriolar changes with attenuation and an increased light reflection ("copper" or "silver" wiring). More emphasis has been placed on stages III and IV, which include cotton-wool spots, hard exudates, hemorrhages, and extensive microvascular changes. Stage IV is differentiated by the additional feature of edema of the optic disk.

The appearance of the fundus in hypertensive retinopathy is determined by the degree of elevation of the blood pressure and the state of the retinal arterioles. Thus, in young patients with accelerated hypertension, an extensive retinopathy is seen, with hemorrhages, retinal infarcts (cotton-wool spots), choroidal infarcts (Elschnig's spots), and occasionally serous detachment of the retina (Figure 15–10). Severe disk edema is a prominent feature. Vision may be impaired but is restored if blood pressure is reduced with caution.

In contrast, elderly patients with arteriosclerotic vessels are unable to respond in this manner, and their vessels are thus protected by the arteriosclerosis. It is for this reason that elderly patients seldom exhibit florid hypertensive retinopathy (Figure 15–11).

Fluorescein angiography has made possible accurate documentation of these microcirculatory changes. In young patients with hypertension, arteriolar attenuation and occlusion are seen, and capillary nonperfusion can be verified in relation to a cotton-wool spot, which is surrounded by abnormal dilated capillaries and microaneurysms with increased permeability on fluorescein angiography.

Resolution of the cotton-wool spots and the arteriolar changes occurs with successful hypotensive therapy. In elderly patients, the underlying arteriosclerotic changes are irreversible.

Other Forms of Hypertensive Retinopathy

A severe retinopathy may be seen in advanced renal disease, in patients with pheochromocytoma, and in preeclampsia-eclampsia. All such patients should

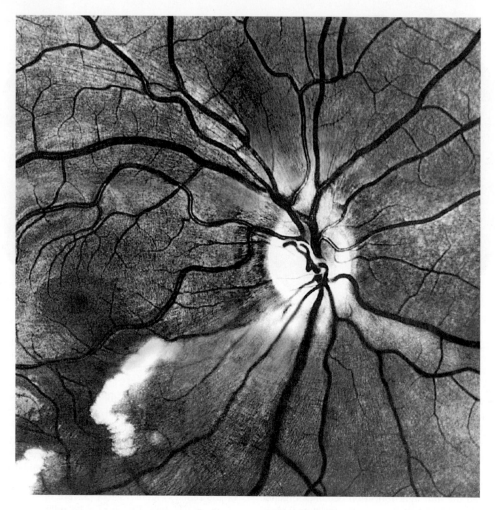

Figure 15–9. Acute retinal infarction. Red-free photograph shows acute arterial occlusion in a congenitally anomalous vessel at the disk. The inferior retina is infarcted, but axoplasm has accumulated beneath the fovea in an irregular pattern owing to preserved neuronal function of the distal ganglion cells.

receive a complete medical workup to establish the nature of the hypertension.

CHRONIC OCULAR ISCHEMIA

Reduction in the retinal arteriovenous pressure gradient may produce acute signs of ocular ischemia (see preceding pages) or the less frequently recognized chronic changes.

Carotid Occlusive Disease

Carotid occlusive disease usually presents in middle-aged and elderly patients and is due to involvement of both the carotid artery and its smaller branches. Contributory factors include hypertension, smoking, and hyperlipidemia.

In anterior segment ischemia, patients develop iritis, intraocular pressure changes, and pupillary abnor-malities. In retinal ischemia (Figure 15–12A), patients show evidence of capillary dilation and hemorrhages, capillary occlusion, new vessels at the optic disk, and cotton-wool spots.

Carotid Cavernous Fistula

Carotid cavernous fistula results from a communication between the carotid artery or its branches and the cavernous sinus, producing characteristic vascular signs. Direct carotid fistulas are usually acute, florid, and posttraumatic, whereas fistulas from dural vessels are usually chronic, mild, and not associated with trauma. Clinical features include elevated intraocular pressure, dilated conjunctival vessels, dilated retinal vessels with hemorrhages and fluorescein leakage (Figure 15–12B), ophthalmoplegia (usually lateral rectus), and bruit. CT and MRI show thickened ocular muscles and a dilated superior ophthalmic vein. The

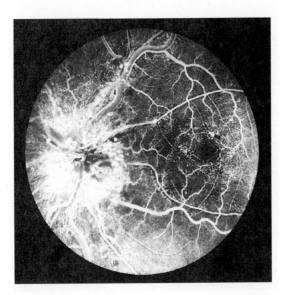

Figure 15–10. Accelerated hypertension. Fluorescein angiogram in a young man showing arteriolar constriction, dilation of capillaries with microaneurysms, and areas of closure. Marked disk edema is present.

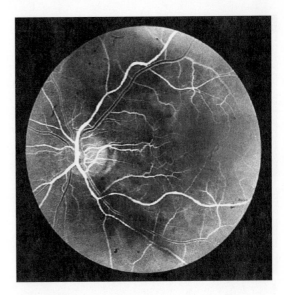

Figure 15–11. Accelerated hypertension. Fluorescein angiogram in an elderly wom.an showing marked arteriolar constriction and irregularity but few signs of florid retinopathy.

condition must be differentiated from thyroid eye disease, and interventional radiology is the ultimate diagnostic and therapeutic resource.

IDIOPATHIC (BENIGN) INTRACRANIAL HYPERTENSION (Pseudotumor Cerebri)

Idiopathic intracranial hypertension is raised intracranial pressure without other cerebrospinal fluid abnormalities and with normal radiologic studies. Patients present with headache, tinnitus, and dizziness; blurred vision, and diplopia are the ophthalmologic features. Etiologic factors include (1) drug therapy, particularly oral contraceptives, nalidixic acid, tetracyclines, sulfonamides, vitamin A, and prolonged steroid therapy or steroid withdrawal in children; (2) endocrine abnormalities; and (3) blood dyscrasias. In many cases there is no obvious cause; in this (idiopathic) group, the patients are usually young overweight women with irregular menstrual cycles. Idiopathic intracranial hypertension is very rare in men.

The cause of the increased intracranial pressure is unknown, though diminished absorption of cerebrospinal fluid due to impaired venous sinus drainage is suspected.

On examination, visual fields are initially normal apart from enlarged blind spots due to papilledema. Generalized field constriction and inferonasal and arcuate defects occur in advanced cases. Cerebrospinal fluid pressure is raised. MRI shows distended nerve sheaths, an empty sella, and absence of a mass lesion. MR angiography complements the examination and detects any venous sinus occlusion. The aims of treatment are to reduce spinal fluid pressure and prevent permanent visual loss associated with optic atrophy, which occurs in up to 50% of patients. Treatment includes strict diet, oral acetazolamide, optic nerve sheath decompression, and lumboperitoneal shunt procedures. Optic nerve sheath decompression functions either as a fistula or by producing subarachnoid fibrous tissue in the nerve sheath and thus protects the disk from the raised sheath pressure. This procedure is relatively free of side effects and complications.

SUBACUTE INFECTIVE ENDOCARDITIS

Inflammatory changes on the cardiac valves may produce multiple embolization with frequent ocular manifestations that range from retinal and choroidal infarction to a mild infective vitritis. The emboli may arise from vegetations on the cardiac valves and may be composed of platelet and fibrinogen aggregates or calcified endocardial vegetations (Figure 15–13).

HEMATOLOGIC & LYMPHATIC DISORDERS

LEUKEMIA

The ocular changes of leukemia occur primarily in those structures with a good blood supply, including the retina, the choroid, and the optic disk (Figure

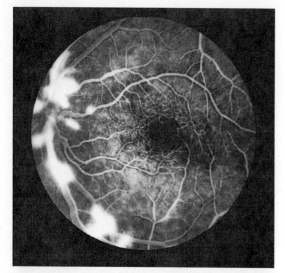

A

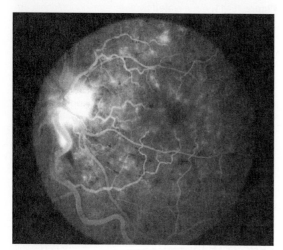

B

Figure 15–12. ***A:*** Fluorescein angiogram of left fundus in a patient with chronic ocular ischemia secondary to Takayasu's disease. Note capillary dilation, leakage of dye, retinal hemorrhages, cotton-wool spots, and neo-vascularization of the optic nerve head. ***B:*** Fluorescein angiogram, showing leakage at optic disk and macula in a patient with chronic ocular ischemia secondary to dural arteriovenous fistula.

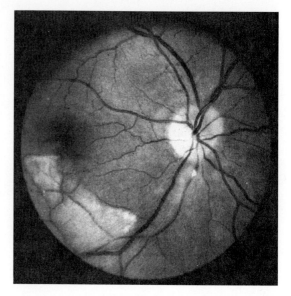

Figure 15–13. Subacute bacterial endocarditis. Calcific embolus impacted in arteriole below the disk, producing a distal area of retinal infarction.

15–14). Changes are most common in the acute leukemias, where hemorrhages are seen in the nerve fiber and preretinal layers.

HYPERVISCOSITY SYNDROMES

Increased viscosity results in a reduced flow of blood through the eye. This produces a characteristic dilation of the retinal arteries and veins, hemorrhages, microaneurysms, and areas of capillary closure (Figure 15–15). Polycythemia, either primary or secondary, may produce a hyperviscosity syndrome; the other main causes are macroglobulinemia and multiple myeloma. Reduction of the abnormalities producing hyperviscosity can reverse the retinal changes.

SICKLE CELL DISEASE

Sickle cell hemoglobinopathies are heritable disorders in which the normal adult hemoglobin is replaced by sickle hemoglobin in the red cell. This causes "sickle-shaped" deformity of the red cell on deoxygenation.

Ocular abnormalities include conjunctival changes, with "comma-shaped capillaries," and retinal changes, including arterial occlusions and peripheral capillary closure which leads to new vessel formation, particularly a sea fan pattern. Retinal detachment may develop. Laser therapy is rarely needed, since the complexes fibrose and reperfusion can occur.

NEOPLASTIC DISEASE
(Figure 15–16)

Neoplastic disease may involve the eye and optic pathways by direct spread, by metastases, or by immunologic mechanisms.

The consequences of metastatic spread depend upon the size and site of the metastatic tumor and the site of the primary lesion. The most frequent primary tumor metastasizing to the eye is carcinoma of the breast in women and bronchial carcinoma in men. Visual loss may occur from nonmetastatic disease with consequent

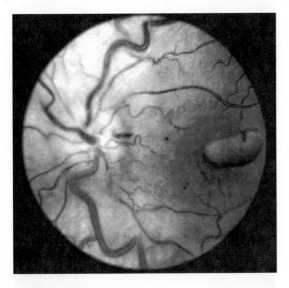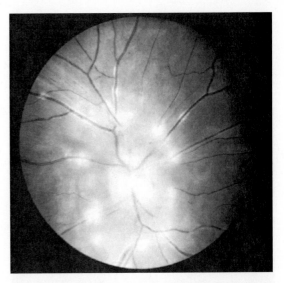

Figure 15–14. *Left:* Retinal changes in chronic myeloid leukemia, where dilated veins and hemorrhages may be seen. *Right:* In acute lymphoblastic leukemia, infiltration of the disk may be seen.

retinal degeneration. The syndromes are called cancer-associated retinopathy, melanoma-associated retinopathy, both associated with specific retinal autoantibody, and diffuse uveal melanocytic proliferation.

METABOLIC DISORDERS

DIABETES MELLITUS

Diabetes mellitus is a complex metabolic disorder that also involves the small blood vessels, often causing widespread damage to tissues, including the eyes.

The ocular complications occur approximately 20 years after onset despite apparently adequate diabetic control. Improved treatment measures (eg, improved insulins, antibiotics) that have lengthened the life span of diabetics have actually resulted in a marked increase in the incidence of retinopathy and other ocular complications. The visual outlook for adult (maturity-onset) diabetics is considerably better than for juvenile diabetics.

The possibility of diabetes should be considered in all patients with unexplained retinopathy, cataract, extraocular muscle palsy, optic neuropathy, or sudden changes in refractive error. Absence of glycosuria or a normal fasting blood glucose level does not exclude a diagnosis of diabetes.

Diabetic Retinopathy
(Figures 15–17 to 15–20)

Diabetic retinopathy is a common cause of blindness and now accounts for almost one-fourth of blind registrations in the western world.

The presence and degree of retinopathy seem to be more closely related to the duration of the disease than to its severity. Good diabetes control retards the development of retinopathy and other diabetic complications.

The juvenile diabetic develops a severe form of retinopathy within 20 years in 60–75% of cases even if under good control. The retinopathy is usually proliferative. In older diabetic patients, retinopathy is more often nonproliferative, with the risk of severe central visual loss from maculopathy.

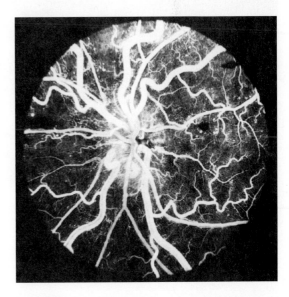

Figure 15–15. Hyperviscosity syndrome. Dilated arteries and veins, with hemorrhages and microaneurysms in a patient with hyperviscosity due to elevated IgM levels.

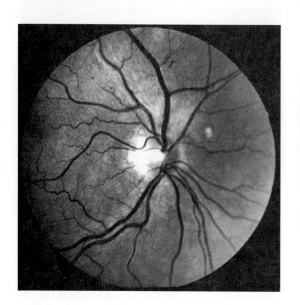

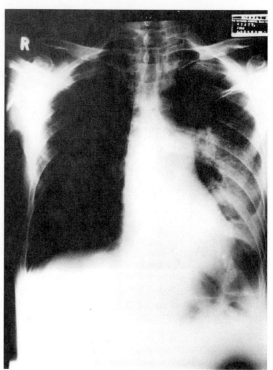

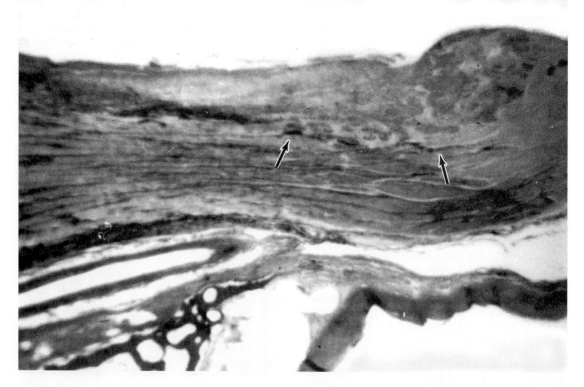

Figure 15–16. Neoplastic disease. ***Top left:*** Normal fundus of a patient with rapid visual loss in his only eye. ***Top right:*** Chest x-ray showed left lower lobe consolidation and a hilar mass. ***Bottom:*** Carcinoma of the bronchus was confirmed at autopsy, and metastasis was found in the optic nerve in the region of the canal (arrows).

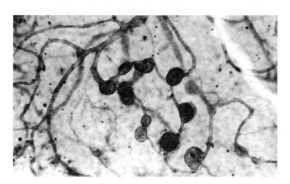

Figure 15–17. Diabetic retinopathy stage I. Trypsin-digested whole mount showing microaneurysms of the retinal capillaries.

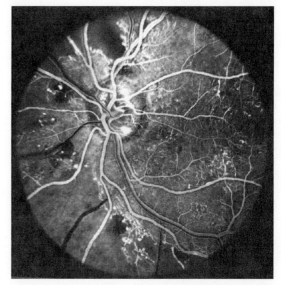

Figure 15–19. Diabetic retinopathy. Fluorescein angiogram shows florid retinopathy of diabetes with extensive areas of capillary closure, dilated capillaries with microaneurysms, and early new vessel formation at the optic disk.

The details of characteristics and treatment of diabetic retinopathy are presented in Chapter 10.

Lens Changes

A. True Diabetic Cataract (Rare): Bilateral cataracts occasionally occur with a rapid onset in severe juvenile diabetes. The lens may become completely opaque in several weeks.

B. Senile Cataract in the Diabetic (Common): Typical senile nuclear sclerosis, posterior subcapsular changes, and cortical opacities occur earlier and more frequently in diabetics.

C. Sudden Changes in the Refraction of the Lens: Especially when diabetes is not well controlled, changes in blood glucose levels cause changes in refrac-

tive power by as much as 3 or 4 diopters of hyperopia or myopia. This results in blurred vision. Such changes do not occur when the disease is well controlled.

Iris Changes

Glycogen infiltration of the pigment epithelium and sphincter and dilator muscles of the iris may cause di-

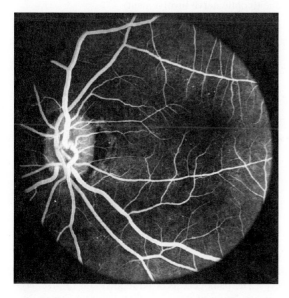

Figure 15–18. Diabetic retinopathy. Fluorescein angiogram shows earliest stage with microaneurysm in the macular region.

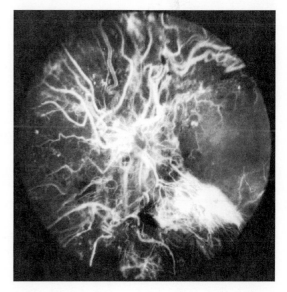

Figure 15–20. Proliferative diabetic retinopathy. Fluorescein angiogram shows extensive growth of vessels into the vitreous with marked fluorescein leakage.

minished pupillary responses. The reflexes may also be altered by the autonomic neuropathy of diabetes.

Rubeosis iridis is a serious complication of the retinal ischemia that is also the stimulus to retinal neovascularization in severe diabetic retinopathy. Numerous small intertwining blood vessels develop on the anterior surface of the iris. Spontaneous hyphema may occur. The formation of peripheral anterior synechiae is aided by the vascularization of anterior chamber structures, eventually blocking aqueous outflow sufficiently to cause secondary glaucoma.

Extraocular Muscle Palsy (Figure 15–21)

This common occurrence in diabetes is manifested by a sudden onset of diplopia caused by paresis of an extraocular muscle. This may be the presenting sign and is due to infarction of the nerve. When the third nerve is involved, pain may be a prominent symptom. Differentiation from a posterior communicating aneurysm is important; in diabetic third nerve palsy, the pupil is usually spared. Recovery of ocular motor function begins within 3 months after onset and usually is complete. The fourth and sixth nerves may be similarly involved.

Optic Neuropathy

Visual loss is usually due to infarction of the optic disk or nerve. A characteristic telangiectatic pattern is visible at the optic disk in some younger diabetics with sudden visual loss.

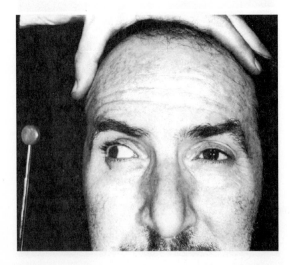

Figure 15–21. Pupil-sparing third nerve palsy in diabetes mellitus. Sudden painful ophthalmoplegia, left ptosis, failure of adduction, and normal pupillary responses.

ENDOCRINE DISEASES

Disturbances of the endocrine glands have a number of important ocular manifestations. By far the most important of these are due to disturbances of the thyroid gland, though parathyroid and pituitary abnormalities also produce significant ocular changes.

THYROID GLAND DISORDERS

1. GRAVES' DISEASE

The general term Graves' disease has been used to denote hyperthyroidism due to an autoimmune process. Patients with the eye signs of Graves' disease but without clinical evidence of hyperthyroidism are referred to as having ophthalmic Graves' disease. Apart from signs of hyperthyroidism, patients may have pretibial myxedema and clubbing of the fingers, and when these signs occur in combination with the ocular signs, the condition is termed thyroid acropachy.

Various laboratory tests are used in the diagnosis of thyroid disease (Table 15–2).

Clinical Findings

Patients may present with nonspecific complaints such as dryness of the eyes, discomfort, or prominence of the eyes. The American Thyroid Association has graded the ocular signs in order of increasing severity from 0 (no signs or symptoms) to 6 (sight loss due to optic nerve involvement).

Class	Signs
0	No signs or symptoms
1	Only signs, which include upper lid retraction, with or without lid lag, or proptosis to 22 mm. No symptoms.
2	Soft tissue involvement
3	Proptosis > 22 mm
4	Extraocular muscle involvement
5	Corneal involvement
6	Sight loss due to optic nerve involvement

Lid retraction is almost pathognomonic of thyroid disease, particularly when associated with exophthalmos. Lid retraction may be unilateral or bilateral and involve the upper and lower lids. It is often accompanied by restrictive myopathy, initially involving the inferior rectus and resulting in impaired elevation of the eyes. The pathogenesis of lid retraction is diverse. Hyperstimulation of the sympathetic nervous system has long been considered a prime element. Direct inflammatory infiltration of the levator muscle is also believed

Table 15–2. Thyroid function tests.

	Hyper-thyroid	Hypo-thyroid	Comments
Plasma T_4	+	–	
T_3 resin uptake	–	+	Thyopac technique. Other tests may vary.
Free thyroxine index	+	–	
Plasma TSH levels	–	+	In pituitary hypothyroidism, TSH is reduced.
Autoanti-bodies	May be present	May be present (Hashimoto's)	

to be a factor. Restrictive myopathy of the inferior rectus muscle can cause lid retraction from the increased stimulation of the levator on attempted upgaze.

A. Exophthalmos: (Figure 15–22.) The degree of exophthalmos may be extremely variable. Measurements using the Hertel or Krahn exophthalmometer range from minimal (20 mm) to excessive (28 mm or more). The condition is usually asymmetric and may be unilateral, and it is important clinically to assess the resistance to manual retropulsion of the globe. The increase in orbital contents that produces the exophthalmos is largely due to an increase in the bulk of the ocular muscles. Visualization of the ocular muscles by CT scan (Figure 15–22) can differentiate exophthalmos from an orbital tumor. In some cases, thickening of the ocular muscles may be restricted to certain muscles only (eg, medial or inferior rectus muscles).

B. Ophthalmoplegia: This is seen more commonly in ophthalmic Graves' disease, which usually affects older people and may be grossly asymmetric. Limitation of elevation is the most frequent finding, and this is mainly due to adhesions between the inferior rectus and inferior oblique muscles. Confirmation may be gained by measuring the intraocular pressure on elevation, when a substantial increase in the intraocular pressure suggests tethering. Often there is mild limitation of ocular movements in all positions of gaze. Patients complain of diplopia, which may be relieved by corticosteroid treatment, may spontaneously return to normal, or, if it remains static for 6–12 months, can frequently be relieved by operation on one or more extraocular muscles.

C. Retinal and Optic Nerve Changes: Compression of the globe by the orbital contents may produce elevation of the intraocular pressure and retinal or choroidal striae. The optic disk may become swollen and progress to visual loss from optic atrophy. Optic neuropathy associated with Graves' disease occasionally occurs as a result of compression and ischemia of the optic nerve as it traverses the tense orbit, particularly at the orbital apex.

D. Corneal Changes: In some patients, a superior limbic keratoconjunctivitis may be seen, though this is not specific for thyroid disease. In severe exophthalmos, corneal exposure and ulceration may occur.

Pathogenesis of the Ocular Signs

The main feature is gross distention of the ocular muscles due to the deposition of mucopolysaccharides. The mucopolysaccharides are strongly hygroscopic, which accounts for the increased water content of the orbits.

The pathogenesis of Graves' disease remains unknown, though an immunologic disorder involving both

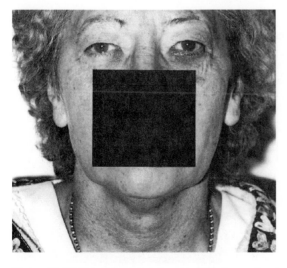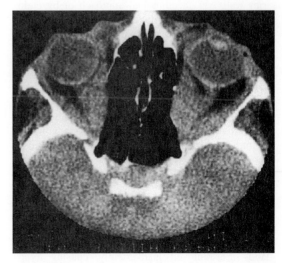

Figure 15–22. Thyroid ophthalmopathy. *Left:* Proptosis, visual loss, and ophthalmoplegia occurred in this elderly woman with a history of thyroid disease. *Right:* CT scans showed gross thickening of the ocular muscles, particularly in relation to the orbital apex. The increased intraorbital pressure is producing convexity of the medial orbital wall.

cellular and humoral elements has been implicated. Long-acting thyroid stimulator (LATS) is unlikely to be of significance in humans, because it is not always found in patients with ocular signs. There has, however, been good correlation between hyperthyroidism and human-specific thyroid stimulator, previously known as LATS protector, although this correlation is not seen in patients with Graves' disease. Thyroid autoantibodies against thyroglobulin and the microsome fraction of thyroid cells are frequently found in Hashimoto's disease and less often in Graves' disease. There are now thought to be two pathogenetic components to Graves' disease: (1) immune complexes of thyroglobulin-antithyroglobulin bind to extraocular muscles and produce a myositis; and (2) exophthalmos-producing substance acts with ophthalmic immunoglobulins to displace thyroid-stimulating hormones from the retro-orbital membranes, which results in the increase of retro-orbital fat.

Treatment

A. Medical Treatment: Medical treatment includes adequate control of the hyperthyroidism as a primary measure. However, thyroid ophthalmopathy may occur in the euthyroid or hypothyroid states. Severe cases with visual loss, disk edema, or corneal ulceration merit urgent medical treatment with corticosteroids in high doses (eg, prednisolone, 100 mg); low doses are ineffective. Plasmapheresis is occasionally used with good results in the treatment of refractory cases, but full immunosuppression must follow plasmapheresis to prevent rebound increase of immunoglobulins and recurrence of disease. Immunosuppressive agents (eg, azathioprine) may play a supportive role and allow a lower maintenance dose of corticosteroids. Orbital radiotherapy may be useful to avoid operation or as a sequel to surgical decompression.

B. Surgical Treatment: Decompression of the orbit may be performed by removing the medial and inferior walls via an ethmoidal approach or by endoscopic techniques. Decompression of the orbital apex is essential for a successful outcome.

2. HYPOTHYROIDISM (Myxedema)

Significant ocular signs are not common in myxedema, though the signs of thyroid ophthalmopathy may be seen. Hyperthyroid patients who subsequently become hypothyroid are at greater risk of ophthalmic involvement.

HYPOPARATHYROIDISM

Occasionally at thyroidectomy, the parathyroid glands are removed inadvertently, causing hypoparathyroidism. Spontaneous cases of hypoparathyroidism, though rare, should be suspected in young patients with cataracts. The blood calcium decreases,

and serum phosphates are increased. Tetany may ensue and can be severe enough to cause generalized convulsions. The ocular manifestations consist of blepharospasm and twitching eyelids. Small, discrete, punctate opacities of the lens cortex develop that may eventually require lens extraction.

Treatment with calcium salts, calciferol, and dihydrotachysterol usually prevents further development of lens opacities, but any that have occurred prior to treatment remain.

VITAMINS & EYE DISEASE

VITAMIN A

Vitamin A is essential for the maintenance of epithelium throughout the body. Ocular changes resulting from vitamin A deficiency (see Figure 15–23) are described in Chapter 6.

VITAMIN B

Vitamin B_1 (thiamin) deficiency produces **beriberi,** and 70% of patients with beriberi have ocular abnormalities. Epithelial changes in the conjunctiva and cornea produce dry eyes. Visual loss may occur as a result of optic atrophy.

Treatment is by correction of dietary deficiency with liver, whole wheat bread, cereals, eggs, and yeast, or with parenteral injection of thiamine.

Nicotinic acid deficiency (pellagra) is quite common in alcoholics and is characterized by dermatitis,

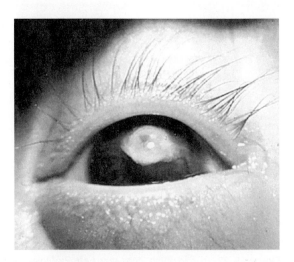

Figure 15–23. Keratomalacia. Case of xerophthalmia in a 5-month-old child.

diarrhea, and dementia. Ocular involvement is rare, but optic neuritis or retinitis may develop.

Riboflavin deficiency has been said to cause a number of ocular changes. Rosacea keratitis, vascularization of the limbal cornea, seborrheic blepharitis, and secondary conjunctivitis have all been attributed to riboflavin deficiency.

VITAMIN C

In vitamin C deficiency (scurvy), hemorrhages may develop in a variety of sites, eg, skin, mucous membranes, body cavities, the orbits, and subperiosteally in the joints. Hemorrhages may also occur into the lids, subconjunctival space, anterior chamber, vitreous cavity, and retina.

Treatment of vitamin C deficiency is with proper diet, particularly adequate amounts of citrus juice.

GRANULOMATOUS DISEASES

Many of the so-called granulomatous infectious diseases, including tuberculosis, brucellosis, leprosy, and toxoplasmosis, undergo a chronic course with frequent exacerbations and remissions. The eye is often involved, particularly by anterior uveitis. The following paragraphs deal with other ocular complications of these systemic diseases.

TUBERCULOSIS

Ocular tuberculosis results from endogenous spread from systemic foci. The incidence of eye involvement is less than 1% in known cases of pulmonary tuberculosis; granulomatous panuveitis and retinal "cold" abscesses may occur (Figure 15–24). There has been a recent increase in the incidence of tuberculosis as a result of the spread of AIDS infection.

Tuberculosis of the Uveal Tract

A. Iritis (Anterior Uveitis): (See Chapter 7.) Local treatment of iritis with mydriatics and corticosteroids is indicated. Systemic tuberculosis therapy is useful in the treatment of established cases of tuberculous uveitis.

B. Miliary Tuberculosis: In this usually fatal form of tuberculosis, many small discrete yellowish nodules are visible ophthalmoscopically in the choroid at the posterior pole of the eye.

SARCOIDOSIS
(Figures 15–25 and 15–26)

Sarcoidosis is a multisystem disease with pulmonary, ocular (uveitis), cutaneous, and reticuloendothelial system manifestations. A granulomatous uveitis may be accompanied by cells in the vitreous periphlebitis, disk swelling, retinal neovascularization, and choroidal disease. New vessels may require photocoagulation. The systemic disease is controlled by the administration of oral corticosteroids and occasionally immunosuppressants. Infiltrative optic neuropathy is a rare cause of progressive severe visual loss.

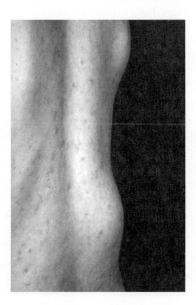
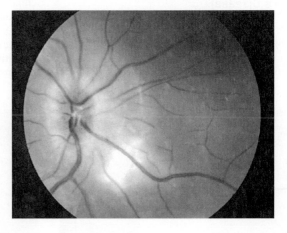

Figure 15–24. Tuberculosis. Cold abscess. A young man presented with a swelling on his back *(left)* and a choroidal lesion *(right).* Aspiration of the abscess revealed *Mycobacterium tuberculosis.*

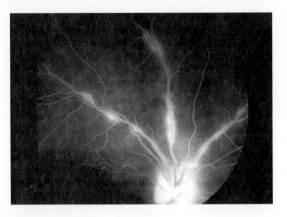 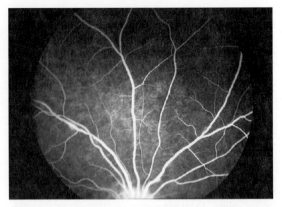

Figure 15–25. Sarcoidosis. Focal periphlebitis and disk leakage may respond dramatically to systemic corticosteroids. *Left:* Before treatment. *Right:* After 6 weeks of treatment with prednisolone, 30 mg daily.

EALES' DISEASE

This disease was originally reported to occur in young men in poor general health who experienced recurrent vitreous hemorrhages from areas of retinal neovascularization. However, such symptoms are also known to occur in tuberculosis, sarcoidosis, systemic lupus erythematosus, sickle cell disease, and diabetes. Extensive investigations are therefore indicated to exclude these conditions in patients with consistent clinical features. If test results are negative, Eales's disease is then appropriate as a diagnosis arrived at by exclusion. Photocoagulation of the new vessels can reduce the chance of further vitreous hemorrhage.

LEPROSY
(Hansen's Disease)

Leprosy is a chronic granulomatous disorder caused by *Mycobacterium leprae,* an acid-fast bacillus. It is estimated that 12–15 million people in the world have leprosy and that of this number, 20–50%

(2.4 million to 6 or 7 million) have ocular involvement. In tropical countries, the infection is endemic.

Three major types of leprosy are recognized: lepromatous, tuberculoid, and dimorphous. The eye may be affected in any type of leprosy, but ocular involvement is more common in the lepromatous type. Ocular lesions are due to direct invasion by *M leprae* of the ocular tissues or of the nerves supplying the eye and adnexa. Since the organism appears to grow better at lower temperatures, infection is more apt to involve the anterior segment of the eye than the posterior segment.

Clinical Findings

The early clinical signs of ocular leprosy are lagophthalmos, loss of the lateral portions of the eyebrows and eyelashes (madarosis), conjunctival hyperemia, and superficial keratitis (Figure 15–27), with interstitial keratitis—beginning typically in the superior temporal quadrant of the cornea—often supervening.

Scarring of the cornea from interstitial or exposure keratitis (or both) causes blurred vision and often blindness. Granulomatous iritis with lepromas (iris

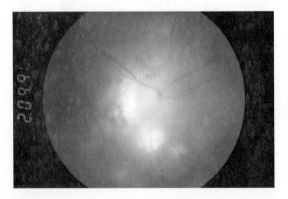 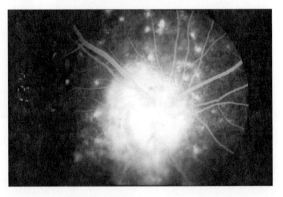

Figure 15–26. Sarcoidosis. Retinal pigment epithelial and choroidal disease may be very distinctive *(left)* and highlighted by fluorescein angiography *(right).*

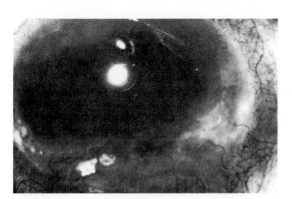

Figure 15–27. Leprosy keratitis, left eye. (Courtesy of W Richards.)

pearls) is common, and a low-grade iritis associated with iris atrophy and a pinpoint pupil may also occur. Hypertrophy of the eyebrows with deformities of the lids and trichiasis late in the course of the disease, and exposure keratitis, typically in the inferior and central cornea, can result from facial motor nerve palsy and absence of corneal sensation.

Ocular leprosy can be diagnosed on the basis of characteristic signs combined with a characteristic skin biopsy.

Treatment

Leprosy is now treated with multidrug therapy, which includes dapsone, rifampin, and clofazimine, and the results in patients with early disease have been encouraging.

SYPHILIS

Congenital Syphilis

The most common eye lesion in congenital syphilis is interstitial keratitis (discussed in Chapter 6). Chorioretinitis unassociated with interstitial keratitis may occur. Congenital syphilis is treated with large doses of penicillin.

Acquired Syphilis

Ocular chancre (primary lesion) occurs rarely on the lid margins and follows the same course as a genital chancre.

Iritis and iridocyclitis occur in the secondary stage of syphilis along with the rash in about 5% of cases. The inflammation may involve the posterior segment, including the pigment epithelium and the retinal capillaries (Figure 15–28).

TOXOPLASMOSIS

This disease is of great ocular importance. The etiologic organism is a protozoal parasite that infects a

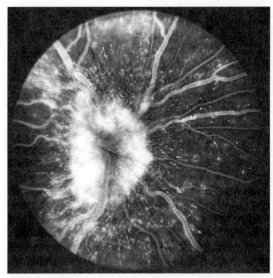

Figure 15–28. Secondary syphilis. Bilateral visual loss occurred in a 24-year-old man. Late fluorescein photographs showed disk leakage with dilation and leakage of peripapillary capillaries.

great number of animals and birds and has worldwide distribution. Felids are the definitive host.

Congenital Toxoplasmosis (Figure 15–29)

Infection occurs in utero, and one-third of infants born to mothers who acquired toxoplasmosis during pregnancy—particularly during the third trimester—will be affected.

A focal choroiditis is seen, usually in the posterior pole, and an active lesion is often related to an old healed lesion. Episodes of posterior uveitis and chori-

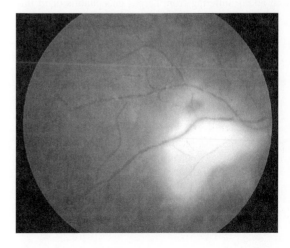

Figure 15–29. Toxoplasmosis. Active area of chorioretinitis adjacent to scar with reaction in adjacent retinal arteriole.

oretinitis usually represent reactivation of a congenital infection. Rarely, panuveitis may occur, or optic neuritis progressing to optic atrophy. Isolated anterior uveitis does not occur. Peripheral vision is usually preserved, but because of macular involvement in at least 50% of cases, central vision is reduced.

Treatment with systemic corticosteroids and antibiotics reduces inflammation but does not prevent scar formation. Subconjunctival or retrobulbar injection of corticosteroids is contraindicated, because it may cause severe exacerbation of disease. Other forms of treatment are discussed in Chapter 7.

Acquired Toxoplasmosis

Acquired toxoplasmosis affects young adults and is characterized by general malaise, lymphadenopathy, sore throat, and hepatosplenomegaly similar to that seen in infectious mononucleosis. It is endemic in South America. Toxoplasmic retinochoroiditis may rarely follow acquired systemic toxoplasmosis. The diagnosis is confirmed by the finding of both IgG and IgM antibodies.

VIRAL DISEASES

HERPES SIMPLEX

The most common manifestation of herpes simplex is fever blisters on the lips. The most common and serious eye lesion is keratitis (see Chapter 6). Vesicular skin lesions can also appear on the skin of the lids and the lid margins. Herpes simplex may cause iridocyclitis and may rarely cause severe encephalitis.

There are two morphologic strains of the virus: type 1 and type 2. Ocular infections are usually produced by type 1, whereas genital infections are caused by type 2. Retinitis due to herpes simplex virus type 1 or 2 occurs in adults suffering from herpes encephalitis or in immunosuppressed patients. Severe occlusive retinal vasculitis develops, followed by retinal necrosis and detachment. Type 1 antigens have been found in all layers of the retina, pigment epithelium, and choroid. Intravenous acyclovir prevents spread of the disease, and prophylactic retinal buckling may be useful.

Varicella-zoster virus is usually implicated in **acute retinal necrosis syndrome,** which produces a similar clinical picture but affects healthy individuals. However, herpes simplex types 1 and 2 and cytomegalovirus, albeit rarely, are now also associated with this condition. A 3-month course of oral acyclovir reduces the chances of involvement of the second eye.

VARICELLA-ZOSTER
(Chickenpox & Herpes Zoster)

First infection with varicella-zoster virus causes chickenpox (varicella). Swollen lids, conjunctivitis, vesicular conjunctival lesions, and (rarely) uveitis and optic neuritis may occur.

Herpes zoster is the response to the same virus in a partially immune person, ie, someone who has previously had chickenpox. It is usually confined to a single dermatome on one side and presents with malaise, headache, and fever followed by burning, itching, and pain in the affected area. The commonest ophthalmic manifestation is herpes zoster ophthalmicus, and the ocular complications are caused by ischemia, viral spread, or a granulomatous reaction. The acute stage is characterized by a virulent rash, conjunctivitis, keratitis, episcleritis, and uveitis when the nasociliary nerve is involved.

Treatment in the acute stages with high doses of oral acyclovir; 800 mg five times a day for 10 days, started within 72 hours after eruption of the rash, reduces ocular complications including postherpetic neuralgia. Anterior uveitis requires topical steroids and cycloplegics.

The acute retinal necrosis syndrome has been described following chickenpox and herpes zoster (see above). In immunocompromised individuals, both herpes zoster, which may become disseminated, and varicella are likely to be severe and may be fatal.

CYTOMEGALIC INCLUSION DISEASE

Infection with cytomegalovirus, also a member of the herpesvirus group, may range from a subclinical infection to classic manifestations of cytomegalic inclusion disease. The virus most frequently affects newborn infants and compromised hosts, and the disease can be acquired or congenital. The ocular findings in the newborn include focal necrotizing retinitis and choroiditis with perivascular infiltrates and retinal hemorrhages. Other reported ocular findings include microphthalmia, cataract, optic atrophy, and optic disk malformation.

Histopathologic examination of the retinal and choroidal lesion shows large inclusion-bearing cells characteristic of cytomegalovirus infections. There is disruption of the normal architecture of the retina and choroid, with evidence of necrosis and mononuclear and perivascular infiltration. Calcifications in the retina may be observed.

The differential diagnosis in the congenital disease should include toxoplasmosis, rubella, herpes simplex infection, and syphilis.

Ganciclovir is the drug of choice for cytomegalic inclusion retinitis. It halts the progression of the disease without eradicating the virus. (See section on AIDS, below.)

POLIOMYELITIS

Bulbar poliomyelitis severe enough to cause lesions of the third, fourth, or sixth cranial nerve is usually fatal. In survivors, any type of internal or external ophthalmoplegia may result. Supranuclear abnormalities ("gaze" palsies, paralysis of convergence or divergence) are rare residual defects. Optic neuritis is uncommon. Treatment is purely symptomatic, though occasionally a residual extraocular muscle imbalance can be greatly improved by strabismus surgery.

GERMAN MEASLES
(Rubella)

Maternal rubella during the first trimester of pregnancy causes serious congenital anomalies. The most common eye complication is cataract, which is bilateral in 75% of cases. Other congenital ocular anomalies are frequently associated with the cataracts, eg, uveal colobomas, nystagmus, microphthalmos, strabismus, retinopathy, and infantile glaucoma. Congenital cataract, especially if bilateral, may require surgical removal, but the prognosis is always guarded.

MEASLES
(Rubeola)

Acute conjunctivitis is common early in the course of measles. Koplik's spots may be seen on the conjunctiva, and epithelial keratitis occurs frequently.

The treatment of the eye complications of measles is symptomatic unless there is secondary infection, in which case local antibiotic ointment is used.

MUMPS

The most common ocular complication of mumps is dacryoadenitis. A diffuse keratitis with corneal edema resembling the disciform keratitis of herpes simplex occurs rarely.

INFECTIOUS MONONUCLEOSIS

The disease process can affect the eye directly, causing nongranulomatous uveitis, scleritis, conjunctivitis, retinitis, choroiditis, or optic neuritis. Complete recovery is usual, but residual visual loss can result.

FUNGAL DISEASE

CANDIDIASIS

Ocular involvement accompanies systemic *Candida* infection and candidemia in approximately two-thirds of cases. The initial *Candida* lesion is a focal necrotizing granulomatous retinitis with or without choroiditis, characterized by fluffy white exudative lesions associ-

ated with cells in the vitreous overlying the lesion. Such lesions may spread to involve the optic nerve and macula. Endophthalmitis, Roth's spots, and exudative retinal detachment may occur. Spread into the vitreous cavity may result in the formation of a vitreous abscess, sometimes described as "a string of pearls." Anterior uveitis occurs, and a hypopyon may form.

Treatment consists of systemic administration of amphotericin B, flucytosine, and ketoconazole. Early vitrectomy may prevent macular damage.

MUCORMYCOSIS

Mucormycosis is a rare, often fatal infection occurring in debilitated patients, particularly poorly controlled diabetics. The fungi (*Rhizopus, Mucor,* and *Absidia*) attack through the upper respiratory tract and invade the arterioles, producing necrotic tissue. Clinical features are the pathognomonic black hemipalate, proptosis, and an ischemic globe with blindness due to ophthalmic artery occlusion. Death occurs from cerebral abscess.

Treatment includes removal of the affected tissue, intravenous amphotericin B (preferably liposomal), and management of the underlying medical condition.

ACQUIRED IMMUNODEFICIENCY SYNDROME (AIDS)

AIDS is caused by human immunodeficiency virus (HIV), a retrovirus. The virus infects mature T helper cells and leads to immunosuppression, the severity of which depends on the balance between the rates of destruction and replacement of T cells. The persistent immunodeficiency gives rise to opportunistic infections. The virus has been recovered from various body fluids, including blood, semen, saliva, tears, and cerebrospinal fluid.

Transmission & Prevention of AIDS
Transmission of HIV is primarily by exchange of bodily fluids during sexual contact or through the use of contaminated needles by intravenous drug abuse. Transmission may also occur when contaminated blood products are transfused. The virus is not transmitted by casual contact, but because it is found in tears, conjunctival cells, and blood, health care workers must take reasonable precautions when handling infectious waste or when at risk of contact with body fluids.

Clinical Findings
The spectrum of clinical disease is wide, presumably due to the degree of immunologic damage and the frequency and nature of opportunistic infections. Typically, an acute flu-like illness occurs a few weeks after infection, followed months later by weight loss, fever, diarrhea, lymphadenopathy, and encephalopathy. The commonest ocular findings are retinal mi-

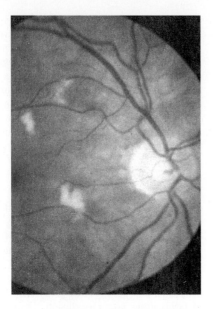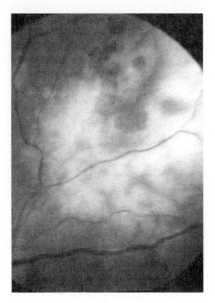

Figure 15–30. Retinal changes in AIDS. Multiple cotton-wool spots *(left)* and retinal necrosis with hemorrhage *(right)* due to opportunistic infection. (Courtesy of R Marsh.)

crovasculopathy with cotton-wool spots (Figure 15–30) and hemorrhages and conjunctival vasculopathy characterized by comma vessels, sludging of the blood, and linear hemorrhages. The cause of these findings is unknown, but they are sometimes associated with increased plasma viscosity and may represent immune complex deposition.

The hallmark of AIDS is the high incidence of infections, which are frequently multiple, opportunistic, and severe. The eye is involved in 30% of cases, and both the anterior segment and the retina may be affected. Viral opportunistic infections of the retina are most common, particularly cytomegalovirus. Typically there is a hemorrhagic necrotic retinopathy spreading from vascular arcades and associated with arteriolar occlusions. The vitreous is quiet; retinal detachment may occur. Involvement of the optic nerve results in gross optic disk edema and severe sudden and irreversible visual loss. Diagnosis is usually based on circumstantial evidence of positive antibody titers in blood, urine, or cerebrospinal fluid. Ocular fluids and retinal specimens are rarely examined. Treatment is with either ganciclovir or foscarnet. Both are virostatic drugs that stop progression of disease but do not eradicate the virus from the eye. Neutropenia is the most important side effect of ganciclovir, and renal damage of foscarnet. Local administration of both drugs is effective in controlling ocular infection but not systemic spread. A standard regimen is a 2-week induction course of intravenous therapy followed by maintenance oral therapy. Alternatively, intravitreal implant or repeated intravitreal injections may be supplemented by oral treatment. Cidofovir may also be used, but ocular complications include uveitis, ocular hypotension, and ciliary body necrosis.

Treatment of the HIV infection is complicated and involves combinations ("triple therapy") of protease inhibitors and reverse transcriptase inhibitors, usually given in 3-month cycles. These regimens may result in a dramatic drop in the HIV viral load, increase in CD4 counts, and improved well-being for the patient. It may be possible to stop anti-CMV therapy when the CD4 count has risen above 200/μL for 3 months.

Herpes simplex retinitis begins in the peripheral retina, advances to involve the entire fundus, and is associated with arteriolar occlusion. The retinitis almost always occurs concurrently with herpes simplex encephalitis, and this serves to distinguish herpes simplex from cytomegalovirus retinitis, which is rarely complicated by encephalitis. Treatment is with acyclovir, but maintenance therapy is required. A virulent form of retinitis, progressive outer retinal necrosis, is attributed to herpes zoster.

Toxoplasma chorioretinitis is usually bilateral, acquired (congenital infections are rarely reactivated in AIDS), and associated with substantial vitreous reaction; candidal endophthalmitis is rarely seen except in drug addicts. Less common organisms that typically involve the choroid are *Pneumocystis carinii, Cryptococcus,* and *Mycobacterium avium-intracellulare.* Choroidal infection is blood-borne and portends imminent demise.

Herpes zoster ophthalmicus is a rare presenting feature of HIV infection and may be very severe, with anterior segment necrosis and ophthalmoplegia. Similarly, syphilis in association with HIV infection produces a severe blinding uveitis. Herpes simplex, molluscum contagiosum, and Kaposi's sarcoma frequently affect the eyelids and surrounding tissues. The combination of rifabutin and clarithromycin or cidofovir may precipitate symptomatic uveitis.

Neuro-ophthalmologic problems are divided into those related directly to HIV infection of the brain, such as optic neuropathy and intranuclear ophthalmoplegia, and those caused by cerebral abscesses or encephalitis, commonly due to *Cryptococcus,* lymphoma, or toxoplasmosis.

MULTISYSTEM AUTOIMMUNE DISEASES

SYSTEMIC LUPUS ERYTHEMATOSUS

Systemic or disseminated lupus erythematosus is a multisystem disease manifested by facial "butterfly skin lesions," pericarditis, Raynaud's phenomenon, renal involvement, arthritis, anemia, and central nervous system signs. Ocular findings include episcleritis and scleritis and keratoconjunctivitis sicca (in 25% of cases). Uveitis rarely occurs, and retinal involvement produces signs of arteriolar occlusion as a result of immune complex deposition with associated choroidal vasculitis. The fundus picture may be complicated by a hypertensive retinopathy, which in severe cases can cause capillary occlusion or even proliferative retinopathy.

Pathogenesis & Diagnosis

The disease is an immunologic disorder marked by the presence of circulating immune complexes. Diagnostic tests include anti-DNA antibodies and mitochondrial type V antibodies. Active disease is associated with raised circulating immune complexes and reduced fractions of complement.

Treatment

Systemic steroids and pulsed intravenous cyclophosphamide are most effective. Hydroxychloroquine, methotrexate, and azathioprine may be useful.

ANTI-PHOSPHOLIPID ANTIBODY SYNDROME

This diagnosis should be considered in patients with recurrent thromboembolism, recurrent fetal loss, livedo reticularis, thrombocytopenia, and neurologic disease. Visual loss may be due to retinal vein or arterial occlusion or ischemic optic neuropathy. Choroidal infarcts may also occur (Figure 15–3). The diagnosis is confirmed by the presence of lupus anti-coagulant and high-titer IgG and IgM anticardiolipin antibodies.

DERMATOMYOSITIS

In this rare disease, there is characteristically a degenerative subacute inflammation of the muscles, sometimes including the extraocular muscles. The lids are commonly a part of the generalized dermal involvement and may show marked swelling and erythema. Retinopathy with cotton-wool spots and hemorrhages may occur. High doses of systemic corticosteroids will frequently effect a remission that continues even after cessation of therapy. The ultimate prognosis is poor, however.

SCLERODERMA

This rare chronic disease is characterized by widespread alterations in the collagenous tissues of the mucosa, bones, muscles, skin, and internal organs. Individuals of both sexes between 15 and 45 years of age are affected. The skin in local areas becomes tense and leathery, and the process may spread to involve large areas of the limbs, rendering them virtually immobile. The skin of the eyelids is often involved. Iritis and cataract occur less frequently. Retinopathy similar to that which occurs in lupus erythematosus and dermatomyositis may be present. Systemic corticosteroid treatment improves the prognosis.

POLYARTERITIS NODOSA

This collagen disease affects the medium-sized arteries, most commonly in men. There is intense inflammation of all the muscle layers of the arteries, with fibrinoid necrosis and a peripheral eosinophilia. The main clinical features include nephritis, hypertension, asthma, peripheral neuropathy, muscle pain with wasting, and peripheral eosinophilia. Cardiac involvement is common, though death is usually caused by renal dysfunction.

Ocular changes are seen in 20% of cases and consist of episcleritis and scleritis, which is often painless (see Chapter 7). When the limbal vessels are involved, guttering of the peripheral cornea may occur. A retinal microvasculopathy is common. Sudden dramatic visual loss may be due to ischemic optic neuropathy reflecting the severity of the vasculitis in the ciliary vessels or to a central retinal artery occlusion. Ophthalmoplegia may result from arteritis of the vasa nervorum (Figure 15–31). Systemic corticosteroids and cyclophosphamide are of some value. A few patients have a monophasic disease that resolves completely, but in the remainder the long-term prognosis is uniformly bad.

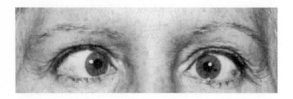

Figure 15–31. Polyarteritis nodosa. Bilateral sixth nerve palsies.

WEGENER'S GRANULOMATOSIS

This granulomatous process shares certain clinical features with polyarteritis nodosa. The three diagnostic criteria are (1) necrotizing granulomatous lesions of the respiratory tract, (2) generalized necrotizing arteritis, and (3) renal involvement with necrotizing glomerulitis.

Ocular complications occur in 50% of cases, and proptosis resulting from orbital granulomatous formation occurs with associated ocular muscle or optic nerve involvement (Figure 15–32). If the vasculitis affects the eye, conjunctivitis, peripheral corneal ulceration, episcleritis, scleritis, uveitis, and retinal vasculitis may occur. Nasolacrimal duct obstruction is a rare complication.

Antineutrophil cytoplasmic antibodies are present in most cases and have both diagnostic and prognostic value. Combined corticosteroids and immunosuppressives (particularly cyclophosphamide) often produce a satisfactory response.

RHEUMATOID ARTHRITIS

Rheumatoid arthritis, a disease that is more common in women than in men, rarely presents with uveitis, but scleritis and episcleritis are comparatively common.

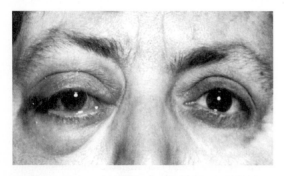

Figure 15–32. Classic Wegener's granulomatosis with proptosis, ptosis, and ophthalmoplegia. The condition has remained static for 10 years with use of corticosteroids and cyclophosphamide.

The scleritis may herald exacerbation of the systemic disease, tends to occur with widespread vasculitis and may lead to scleromalacia perforans (see Chapter 7).

Corticosteroid drops are helpful in episcleritis or anterior uveitis, but systemic treatment (nonsteroidal anti-inflammatory agents and corticosteroids) is necessary for scleritis. Keratoconjunctivitis sicca is present in 15% of cases (see Chapter 4). Peripheral corneal melting may occur in more severe cases.

JUVENILE RHEUMATOID ARTHRITIS (Still's Disease)

Ocular complications of Still's disease occur three times more frequently in girls with pauciarticular disease. The systemic disease appears to be disproportionately mild in children with severe visual loss, and diagnosis and treatment may therefore be delayed. Ocular involvement may occur before joint involvement. A chronic insidious uveitis with a high incidence of anterior segment complications develops (eg, posterior synechiae, cataract, secondary glaucoma, band-shaped keratopathy). Antinuclear antibodies are positive in 88% of patients with juvenile rheumatoid arthritis who develop uveitis, whereas they are positive in only 30% of the group as a whole.

SJöGREN'S SYNDROME

Sjögren's syndrome is a systemic disorder with diverse features. The disease is characterized by the clinical triad of keratoconjunctivitis sicca, xerostomia (dryness of the mouth), and a connective tissue disease, usually rheumatoid arthritis. It is more common in females. The onset of ocular symptoms occurs most frequently during the fourth, fifth, and sixth decades. Lymphoid proliferation is a prominent feature of Sjögren's syndrome and may involve the kidneys, the lungs, or the liver, causing renal tubular acidosis, pulmonary fibrosis, or cirrhosis. Lymphoreticular malignant disease such as reticulum cell sarcoma may complicate the benign course of Sjögren's syndrome many years after its onset.

The histopathologic changes in the lacrimal gland consist of infiltration of lymphocytes, histiocytes, and occasional plasma cells leading to atrophy and destruction of the glandular structures. These changes are part of the generalized polyglandular involvement in Sjögren's syndrome, which results in dryness of the eyes, mouth, skin, and mucous membranes.

Because of the relative inaccessibility of the lacrimal gland, the labial salivary gland biopsy serves as an important diagnostic procedure in patients with suspected Sjögren's syndrome.

Tear lysozyme and lactoferrin levels are absent or reduced in over 90% of patients, and very high titers of nuclear antibodies are present.

GIANT CELL ARTERITIS
(Including Temporal
or Cranial Arteritis)

This is a disease of elderly patients (mostly women over age 60). Medium-sized arteries are involved, particularly the intima of the vessels. Branches of the external carotid system are frequently involved, though pathologic studies have shown more diffuse arterial involvement. Polymyalgia rheumatica may precede or accompany the disease. Patients feel ill and have excruciating pain over the temporal or occipital arteries. Visual loss due to an ischemic optic neuropathy is frequent, and a few cases have a central retinal artery occlusion. Visual loss may also be due to cortical blindness. Other central nervous system signs include cranial nerve palsies and signs referable to brain stem lesions. The diagnosis is confirmed by a high erythrocyte sedimentation rate (ESR) and a positive temporal artery biopsy. In early stages of the disease, the ESR may be normal, but usually it is 80–100 mm in the first hour. It is important to make the diagnosis early, because immediate systemic corticosteroid administration produces dramatic relief of pain and prevents further ischemic episodes. The disease activity is monitored by the erythrocyte sedimentation rate and the clinical state. The corticosteroid dose may have to be maintained for several years and should be kept below 5 mg prednisolone daily if possible, since with higher doses toxic effects develop.

IDIOPATHIC ARTERITIS
OF TAKAYASU
(Pulseless Disease)

This disease, found most frequently in young women and occasionally in children, is a polyarteritis of unknown cause with increased predilection for the aorta and its branches. Manifestations may include evidence of cerebrovascular insufficiency, syncope, absence of pulsations in the upper extremities, and ophthalmologic changes compatible with chronic hypoxia of the ocular structures. Ophthalmodynamometry may be of value by demonstrating decreased carotid blood flow on one or both sides.

Thromboendarterectomy, prosthetic graft, and systemic corticosteroid therapy have been reported to be successful.

ANKYLOSING SPONDYLITIS

Ankylosing spondylitis occurs mainly in males 16–40 years of age. In most cases, an intermittent anterior uveitis is seen, but in a minority anterior and posterior uveitis exists with glaucoma and cataracts developing in the long term. In a few cases, aortic valve disease is also seen (see Chapter 7). There is a strong association with HLA-B27. Antigenic cross-reactivity is present between HLA-B27 and *Klebsiella pneumoniae,* but the etiology remains poorly understood.

REITER'S DISEASE

The diagnosis of Reiter's disease is based on a triad of signs that includes urethritis, conjunctivitis, and arthritis (see Chapter 16). Scleritis, keratitis, and uveitis may also be seen in addition to conjunctivitis.

BEHÇET'S DISEASE

Behçet's disease consists of the clinical triad of relapsing uveitis and aphthous and genital ulceration (Figure 15–33). Ocular signs occur in 75% of cases; the uveitis is severe, occasionally associated with hypopyon. Visual loss is due to inflammatory changes in the retinal vessels and retina, and there is a propensity to microvascular venous occlusions and retinal infiltrates. Treatment often involves multiple immunosuppression (eg, steroids, cyclosporine, azathioprine), but despite manipulation with these drugs the visual outcome is bad in 25% of cases. Ocular involvement is associated with the HLA-B5 haplotype.

HERITABLE CONNECTIVE
TISSUE DISEASES

MARFAN'S SYNDROME
(Arachnodactyly)
(Figure 15–34)

The most striking feature of this rare syndrome is increased length of the long bones, particularly of the fingers and toes. Other characteristics include scanty subcutaneous fat, relaxed ligaments, and, less commonly, other associated developmental anomalies, including congenital heart disease and deformities of the spine and joints. Ocular complications are often seen—in particular, dislocation of the lenses, usually superiorly and nasally. Less common ocular anomalies include severe refractive errors, megalocornea, cataract, uveal colobomas, and secondary glaucoma. There is a high infant mortality rate. Removal of a dislocated lens may be necessary. The disease is genetically determined, nearly always autosomal dominant, often with incomplete expression, so that mild, incomplete forms of the syndrome are seen. Several reports have correlated cytogenetic changes with Marfan's syndrome.

OSTEOGENESIS IMPERFECTA
(Brittle Bones
& Blue Scleras)

This rare autosomal dominant syndrome is characterized by multiple fractures, blue scleras, and, less commonly, deafness. The disease is usually manifest soon after birth. The long bones are very fragile, fracturing easily and often healing with fibrous bony union. The bones become more fragile with age. The very thin sclera allows the blue color imparted by the underlying uveal tract to show through. There is usually no visual impairment. Occasionally, abnormalities such as keratoconus, megalocornea, and corneal or lenticular opacities are also present.

Ophthalmologic treatment is seldom necessary.

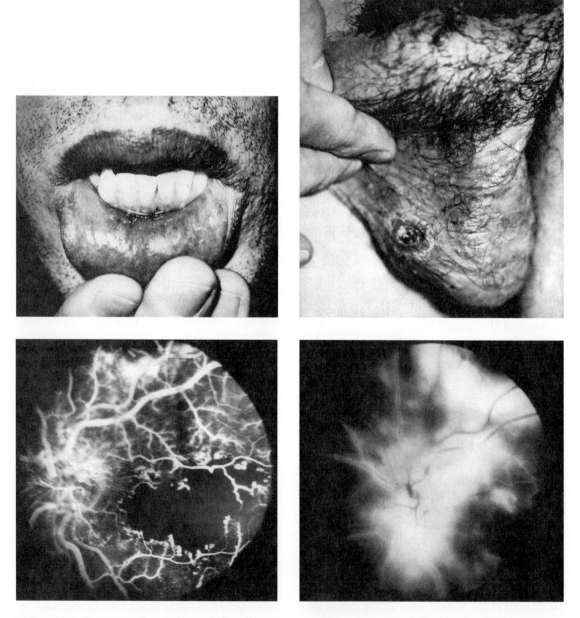

Figure 15–33. Behçet's disease. Clinical features include oral and genital ulcers. Ocular features include increased capillary permeability and areas of retinal ischemia and infiltration. Marked leakage of capillaries is seen in the late stages of fluorescein angiography (bottom right).

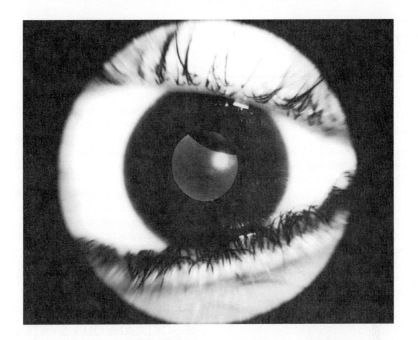

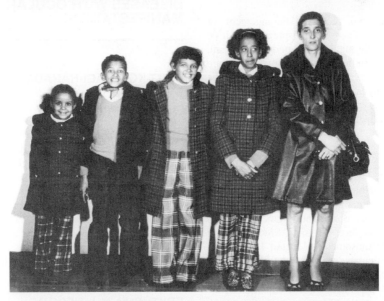

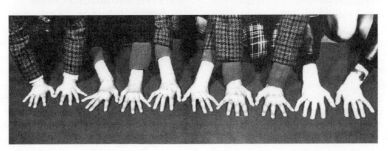

Figure 15–34. Marfan's syndrome. Familial expression of arachnodactyly and upward dislocation of the lens.

HEREDITARY METABOLIC DISORDERS

HEPATOLENTICULAR DEGENERATION (Wilson's Disease)

This rare autosomal recessive disease of young adults—characterized by abnormal copper metabolism—causes changes in the basal nuclei, cirrhosis of the liver, and a pathognomonic corneal pigmentation called the Kayser-Fleischer ring. The ring appears as a green or brown band peripherally and deep in the stroma near Descemet's membrane and may only be visible with a slitlamp. The disease is progressive and often results in death by age 40. Treatment with penicillamine has resulted in sustained clinical improvement in some cases.

CYSTINOSIS

This rare autosomal recessive derangement of amino acid metabolism causes widespread deposition of cystine crystals throughout the body. Dwarfism, nephropathy, and death in childhood from renal failure are the rule. Cystine crystals can be readily seen in the conjunctiva and cornea, where fine particles are seen predominantly in the outer third of the corneal stroma.

There is no treatment.

ALBINISM

Oculocutaneous albinism consists of a heterogeneous group of conditions characterized by generalized reduction in or absence of melanin pigmentation and inherited as autosomal recessive traits. Mutations have been found on chromosomes 9, 11, and 15. At birth there is little or no cutaneous pigmentation, such that the skin and hair, including the eyebrows and eyelashes, are white or paler than expected. In severely affected cases this situation persists throughout life, whereas in less affected individuals some pigmentation and tanning with sun exposure can develop during childhood. The ocular manifestations are reduced visual acuity (generally 20/200), nystagmus, pale irides that transilluminate, hypopigmented fundi, and hypoplastic foveas. Photophobia is a prominent symptom. Ocular albinism, an X-linked recessive trait, has the same ocular features as oculocutaneous albinism but generally without cutaneous manifestations, though the skin may be paler than that of first-degree relatives. It is an important cause of congenital nystagmus. Female carriers may be identified by the presence of iris transillumination and retinal abnormalities. In all types of albinism there is a characteristic increase in the propor-

tion of decussating axons in the optic chiasm, which can be identified by electrodiagnostic testing.

GALACTOSEMIA

Galactosemia is a rare autosomal recessive disorder of carbohydrate metabolism clinically manifested soon after birth by feeding problems, vomiting, diarrhea, abdominal distention, hepatomegaly, jaundice, ascites, cataracts, mental retardation, and elevated blood and urine galactose levels. Dietary exclusion of milk and all foods containing galactose and lactose for the first 3 years of life will prevent the clinical manifestations and will result in improvement of existing abnormalities. Even the cataract changes, which are characterized by vacuoles of the cortex, are reversible in the early stage.

Identification of the carrier state is possible by finding a 50% reduction of galactose 6-phosphatase.

MISCELLANEOUS SYSTEMIC DISEASES WITH OCULAR MANIFESTATIONS

VOGT-KOYANAGI-HARADA SYNDROME (Figure 15–35)

Bilateral uveitis associated with alopecia, poliosis, vitiligo, and hearing defects, usually in young adults, has been termed Vogt-Koyanagi disease. When the choroiditis is more exudative, serous retinal detachment occurs, and the complex is known as Harada's syndrome. There is a tendency toward recovery of visual function, but this is not always complete. Initial treatment is with local steroids and mydriatics, but systemic steroids in high doses are frequently required to prevent permanent visual loss.

ERYTHEMA MULTIFORME (Stevens-Johnson Syndrome)

Erythema multiforme is a serious mucocutaneous disease that occurs as a hypersensitivity reaction to drugs or food. Children are most susceptible. The manifestations consist of generalized maculopapular rash, severe stomatitis, and purulent conjunctivitis, sometimes leading to symblepharon and occlusion of the lacrimal gland ducts (dry eye syndrome). In severe cases, corneal ulcers, perforations, and panophthalmitis can destroy all visual function. Systemic corticosteroid treatment often favorably influences the course of the disease and usually preserves useful visual function. Secondary infection with *Staphylococcus aureus* is

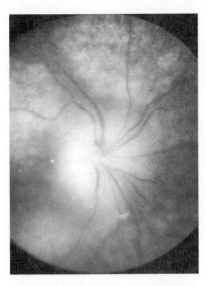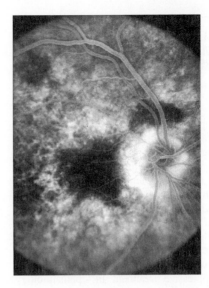

Figure 15–35. Vogt-Koyanagi-Harada syndrome. Acute pigment epithelial disease with disk swelling and cells in the vitreous *(left)*. Three months later, disk swelling has subsided and pigment epithelial damage is seen *(right)*.

common and must be vigorously treated with local antibiotics instilled into the conjunctival sac. Frequently there is marked reduction of tear formation that can be helped by instillation of artificial tears.

LAURENCE-MOON-BIEDL SYNDROME

Obesity, mental deficiency, polydactyly, hypogonadism, and retinitis pigmentosa form the complete syndrome. The retinal changes are not always typical of retinitis pigmentosa and may be present soon after birth or develop during adolescence. This rare syndrome is genetically determined and follows an autosomal recessive pattern with a high rate of consanguinity. The heterozygous state may be identified by mild incomplete evidence of the disease. It is interesting that a single abnormal gene can account for such a multiplicity of clinical findings.

ROSACEA (Acne Rosacea)

This disease of unknown cause is primarily dermatologic, beginning as hyperemia of the face associated with acneiform lesions and eventually causing hypertrophy of tissues (such as rhinophyma). Chronic blepharitis due to staphylococcal infection or seborrhea is often present. Rosacea keratitis develops in about 5% of cases. Episcleritis, scleritis, and nongranulomatous iridocyclitis are rare ocular complications.

Careful attention to lid hygiene is essential. Topical corticosteroids help in controlling keratitis or iridocyclitis. Long-term systemic tetracycline therapy is often beneficial.

LYME DISEASE

Lyme disease is a vector-mediated multisystem illness caused by the spirochete *Borrelia burgdorferi.* The usual vectors are small ixodid ticks that have a complex three-host life cycle involving multiple mammalian and avian species.

The disease has three major stages. Initially, in the area of the tick bite, there develops the characteristic skin lesion of erythema chronicum migrans, often accompanied by regional lymphadenopathy, malaise, fever, headache, myalgia, and arthralgia. Several weeks to months later there is a period of neurologic and cardiac abnormalities. After a few more weeks or even years, rheumatologic abnormalities develop—initially, migratory musculoskeletal discomfort, but later a frank arthritis that may recur over several years.

Conjunctivitis is a frequent finding in the first stage. Cranial nerve palsies—particularly of the seventh but also of the third, fourth, or sixth cranial nerves—often occur in the neurologic phase. Other ophthalmologic abnormalities that have been reported include uveitis, ischemic optic neuropathy, optic disk edema, bilateral keratitis, and choroiditis with exudative retinal detachments.

Laboratory diagnosis is by demonstration of specific IgM and IgG antibodies in serum or cerebrospinal fluid. The spirochetes may also be isolated from these sources.

Doxycycline and ampicillin are effective in curing the initial infection but unfortunately may not prevent late complications.

IMMUNOSUPPRESSIVE AGENTS USED IN MANAGEMENT OF EYE DISEASE

Immunosuppressive agents are used to suppress inflammatory reactions within the eye, particularly those affecting the uveal tract but also the sclera, retina, and optic nerve. Frequently, the cause of inflammation is not known, and the use of these drugs is therefore empirical. All patients must have a full medical examination before treatment is started. Special consideration must be given to patients with infections and blood diseases, and regular blood counts must be performed during the course of treatment.

Corticosteroids (eg, prednisolone) are the mainstay of immunosuppressive treatment in ophthalmology. High doses (eg, 60 mg of prednisolone daily) may be required to control inflammation, and there is a high incidence of side effects. Weight gain, acne, and hirsutism are common; peptic ulceration, myopathy, osteoporosis, and avascular necrosis are less frequently encountered. Alternate-day regimens produce fewer side effects in some patients. Azathioprine may be added as a corticosteroid-sparing drug; 2.5 mg/kg daily is an effective dose, and the total course should not last longer than 18 months. Intravenous methylprednisolone (1 g/d given over 3 hours in dextrose saline for 3 days) is an effective method of controlling exacerbations in patients already taking high doses of corticosteroids.

Cyclosporine is an immunosuppressive agent isolated from the fermentation products of a fungus that was recovered from Norwegian soil. It has an effective immunomodulating action and causes suppression of T helper cells. It is a useful alternative drug for refractory sight-threatening noninfectious inflammatory eye disease in patients who have not responded to corticosteroids or in whom the optimal therapeutic dose of corticosteroids is associated with intolerable side effects. The recommended dose is 5 mg/kg orally daily. The most important side effect is renal toxicity, but liver toxicity may also occur. Close surveillance and monitoring of kidney and liver function are mandatory on every patient receiving cyclosporine therapy. The drug should not be given to hypertensive patients. Reduction of the daily dose may be associated with troublesome rebound of the ocular inflammation.

Fortunately, **cytotoxic agents** are rarely indicated in the management of inflammatory eye disease except in severe cases of Behçet's syndrome and Wegener's granulomatosis. These drugs and their important side effects are listed in Table 15–3. Cytotoxic agents are sometimes used in the treatment of myasthenia gravis (see Figure 15–36).

OCULAR COMPLICATIONS OF CERTAIN SYSTEMICALLY ADMINISTERED DRUGS (See Also Chapter 3.)

AMIODARONE

Amiodarone is a benzofuran derivative used to treat cardiac dysrhythmias, particularly Wolff-Parkinson-White syndrome, and angina pectoris. Most patients develop small punctate deposits with a vortex pattern

Table 15–3. Cytotoxic agents used in the management of inflammatory eye disease.

Drug	Dose	Maximum Length of Treatment[1]	Side Effects
Azathioprine	2.5–3 mg/kg/d	1.5 years	Bone marrow depression (usually leukopenia, but may be anemia, thrombocytopenia, and bleeding) (irreversible in elderly patients). Skin rashes, drug fever, nausea and vomiting, sometimes diarrhea. Hepatic dysfunction (raised liver enzymes, mild jaundice). Lymphoma.
Chlorambucil	0.05–0.2 mg/kg/d	2.5 years (4 g)	Moderate depression of peripheral blood count. Excessive doses produce severe bone marrow depression with leukopenia, thrombocytopenia, and bleeding. Lymphoma. Prevent cystitis with adequate hydration. Chlorambucil: Leukemia may occur. Large doses near puberty may cause infertility. Cyclophosphamide: Nausea and vomiting acutely. Alopecia and hemorrhagic cystitis occasionally. Infertility may occur.
Cyclophosphamide	1.25–2.5 mg/kg/d	3 years	
Colchiciine	0.01–0.03 mg/kg/d	5 years	Occasionally nausea, vomiting, abdominal pain, diarrhea. Rarely, hair loss, bone marrow depression, peripheral neuritis, myopathy.
Methotrexate	7.5–15 mg/kg/wk	2.5 years (1.5 g)	Bone marrow depression. Skin rashes. Anorexia, nausea. Hepatic dysfunction with fibrosis, particularly in patients with excess alcohol consumption, obesity, and diabetes mellitus.

[1] Numbers in parentheses are maximum cumulative doses.

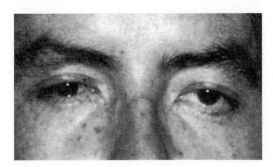 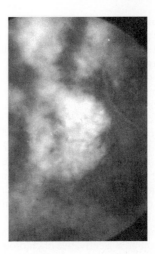

Figure 15–36. Retinitis in an immunosuppressed patient. ***Left:*** This patient with myasthenia gravis underwent thymectomy and received long-term immunosuppression with cytotoxic agents. ***Right:*** He developed retinal necrosis and Ramsay Hunt syndrome following infection with herpes zoster.

in the basal cell layer of the corneal epithelium (Figure 15–37). The severity of keratopathy is related to the total daily dose and is mild at a dose of less than 200 mg daily. The deposits rarely interfere with vision, and although they progress with continued treatment, even in low dosage, they always resolve completely when treatment is stopped. A small percentage of patients develop thyroid ophthalmopathy, though the mechanism is not fully understood.

ANTICHOLINERGICS (Atropine & Related Synthetic Drugs)

All of these drugs, when given preoperatively or for gastrointestinal disorders, may cause blurred vision in presbyopic patients because of a direct action on ac-

commodation. They also tend to dilate the pupils, so that in patients with narrow anterior chamber angles there is the added threat of angle-closure glaucoma. This is the cause of angle-closure glaucoma (frequently attributed to "nervousness") occasionally seen in patients hospitalized for general surgery.

ANTIDEPRESSANTS

Tricyclic antidepressants and monoamine oxidase inhibitors have an anticholinergic effect and theoretically may exacerbate open-angle glaucoma or provoke an attack of angle-closure glaucoma. However, these side effects are rare in clinical practice.

CHLORAMPHENICOL

Chloramphenicol, in addition to the possibility of causing severe blood dyscrasias, hepatic and renal disease, and gastrointestinal disturbances, can sometimes cause optic neuritis. This is especially true in children. Bilateral blurred vision with central scotomas occurs. Stopping the drug does not always restore vision.

Despite the possibility of toxic optic neuropathy, chloramphenicol may still be required for the treatment of bacterial endophthalmitis. The drug is generally not administered for more than 1 week.

CHLOROQUINE

Chloroquine is an effective antimalarial drug. With high dosage—often 250–750 mg daily administered for months or years—serious ocular toxicity has oc-

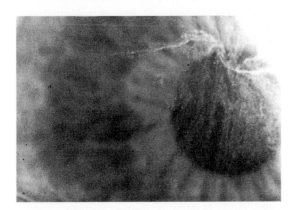

Figure 15–37. Amiodarone keratopathy. (Courtesy of DJ Spalton.)

curred. Corneal changes were described first and consisted of diffuse haziness of the epithelium and subepithelial area, occasionally sufficient to simulate an epithelial dystrophy. These changes cause only mild blurring of vision and are reversible upon drug withdrawal. Similar changes have been described in patients receiving quinacrine. Minimal corneal involvement is not necessarily an indication for discontinuance of chloroquine therapy.

A less common but more serious ocular complication of long-term chloroquine therapy is retinal damage, causing loss of central vision as well as constriction of peripheral visual fields. Pigmentary changes and edema of the macula, marked alteration of the retinal vessels, and in some cases peripheral pigmentary changes can be seen ophthalmoscopically. Hydroxychloroquine is a derivative of chloroquine that is regularly used in the treatment of collagen diseases (especially systemic lupus erythematosus), rheumatoid arthritis, and chronic skin disease, including discoid lupus and sarcoidosis. The range of ocular complications is the same as with chloroquine, but both their incidence and their severity are greatly reduced. If renal function is normal, routine ophthalmologic screening is probably required only if the daily dose of chloroquine exceeds 6.5 mg/kg or the total duration of treatment exceeds 6 years.

CHLOROTHIAZIDE

Xanthopsia (yellow vision) has been reported in patients taking this oral diuretic.

CONTRACEPTIVES, ORAL

Although numerous reports suggest that in predisposed individuals oral contraceptives can provoke or precipitate ophthalmic vascular occlusive disease or optic nerve damage, it is difficult to establish a definite cause and effect relationship. Optic neuritis, retinal arterial or venous thrombosis, and pseudotumor cerebri have been described in patients taking oral contraceptives. Since there is some uncertainty regarding the possibility of such ocular complications, oral contraceptives should be used only by healthy women with no history of vascular, neurologic, or ocular disease.

CORTICOSTEROIDS

It has been clearly demonstrated that long-term systemic corticosteroid therapy can cause chronic open-angle glaucoma and cataracts and can provoke and worsen attacks of herpes simplex keratitis. Locally administered corticosteroids are much more potent in this respect and have the added disadvantage of causing fungal overgrowth if the corneal epithelium is not intact. Steroid-induced subcapsular lens opacities cause some impairment of visual function but usually

do not progress to advanced cataract. Cessation of therapy will arrest progression of the lenticular opacities, but the changes are irreversible. Serous retinal detachments have been associated with systemic corticosteroids, particularly when these agents are used to treat the systemic vasculitides.

OXYGEN

Premature infants who are given any concentration of oxygen in excess of that in the air may develop retinopathy of prematurity (retrolental fibroplasia). These infants should receive only the amount of oxygen necessary for survival. The incidence of the condition was considerably reduced in the 1960s with rigid restriction of oxygen, but despite continued restriction, the incidence has recently risen again. This may be due to prematurity itself (with advanced medical techniques, smaller infants are surviving); the condition is found in 40–77% of infants weighing less than 1 kg.

In adults, administration of hyperbaric oxygen (3 atm) can cause constriction of the retinal arterioles.

PHENOBARBITAL & PHENYTOIN

Ocular complications relate to oculomotor involvement, producing nystagmus and weakness of convergence and accommodation. The nystagmus may persist for many months after cessation of the drug, and the degree of oculomotor abnormality is related to drug dosage. Early abnormalities include disturbance of smooth pursuit.

PHENOTHIAZINES

The phenothiazines usually exert an atropine-like effect on the eye so that the pupils may be dilated, especially with large doses. Of greater clinical significance, however, are the pigmentary ocular changes, which include pigmentary retinopathy and pigment deposits on the corneal endothelium and anterior lens capsule. The corneal and lens pigmentation may cause blurring of vision, but the pigment deposits usually disappear several months after the drug is discontinued. In pigmentary retinopathy, there is a diminution of central vision, night blindness, diffuse narrowing of the retinal arteries, and occasionally severe blindness.

The piperidine group (eg, thioridazine) has a higher risk of causing pigmentary retinopathy, and the maximum daily dose should not exceed 600 mg. The retinal changes are partly reversible under normal circumstances, but in some patients more severe irreversible changes occur at the "safe" dosage level.

The dimethylamine group (eg, chlorpromazine) rarely produces retinal pigmentary changes.

The piperazine group (eg, trifluoperazine) does not produce these retinal complications.

All of these drugs can produce an extrapyramidal syndrome that may involve eye movements. Large doses can provoke profound hypotension, which may produce ischemic optic neuropathy.

Patients receiving large doses or prolonged treatment with phenothiazines should be questioned regarding visual disturbances and should have periodic ophthalmoscopic examinations.

QUININE & QUINACRINE

Quinine and quinacrine, when used in the treatment of malaria, may cause bilateral blurred vision, sometimes following a single dose. There is constriction of the visual field and, rarely, total blindness. The tendency is toward partial recovery, though usually there are permanent peripheral field defects. The ganglion cells of the retina are affected first, presumably as a result of vasoconstriction of the retinal arterioles. Varying degrees of retinal edema occur early. Optic atrophy is a late finding.

SEDATIVE TRANQUILIZERS

When taken regularly, the so-called minor tranquilizers can decrease tear production by the lacrimal gland, thus resulting in ocular irritation because of dry eyes. Tear production returns to normal when the tranquilizers are discontinued.

The principal drugs in this group are meprobamate, chlordiazepoxide, and diazepam.

TAMOXIFEN

Asymptomatic intraretinal crystals are observed in 1–5% of patients who take 20 mg of tamoxifen twice daily. Corneal crystals and optic neuropathy have been reported in patients receiving 80–120 mg daily.

RADIATION

Both optic neuropathy and retinopathy may occur months or years after radiation treatment to the head and neck, particularly to the sinuses or the chiasm. The retinal endothelial cells are damaged, and ischemic retinopathy develops with cotton-wool spots, hemorrhages, and capillary closure. Patients with optic neuropathy present with arcuate field defects, and gadolinium-enhanced MRI reveals characteristic sharply demarcated lesions in the optic nerve. Both conditions progress slowly, and although there is no treatment, anticoagulation or aspirin may halt the process.

FETAL EFFECTS OF DRUGS

The visual pathways of the fetus are occasionally affected by drugs taken by the mother during pregnancy.

Phenytoin may cause optic nerve hypoplasia.

Pigmentary retinopathy has been reported in a child of a mother taking **busulfan** for acute myeloid leukemia.

Warfarin is teratogenic and may produce a hypoplastic nose, stippled epiphyses, and skeletal abnormalities. Affected children may present with recurrent sticky eyes from obstruction of the nasolacrimal duct secondary to malformation of the nose. Other ocular abnormalities include optic atrophy, microphthalmia, and lens opacities.

REFERENCES

Acheson JF, Green WT, Sanders MD: Optic nerve sheath decompression for the treatment of visual failure in chronic raised intracranial pressure. J Neurol Neurosurg Psychiatry 1994;57:1426.

Acheson JF, Sanders MD: Coagulation abnormalities in ischaemic optic neuropathy. Eye 1994;8:89.

Aiello LM, Cavallerano J: Diabetic retinopathy. Curr Ther Endocrinol Metab 1997;6:475.

Akduman L, Kaplan HJ, Tyschen L: Prevalence of uveitis in an outpatient juvenile arthritis clinic: Onset of uveitis more than a decade after onset of arthritis. J Pediatr Ophthalmol Strabismus 1997;34:101.

Akova YA, Jabbur NR, Foster CS: Ocular presentation of polyarteritis nodosa. Ophthalmology 1993;100:1775.

Akpek EK et al: Ocular rosacea: Patient characteristics and follow-up. Ophthalmology 1997; 104:1863.

Balcer LJ, Winterkorn JMS, Galetta SL: Neuro-ophthalmic manifestations of Lyme disease. J Neuroophthalmol 1997;17:108.

Barile GR, Flynn TE: Syphilis exposure in patients with uveitis. Ophthalmology 1997;104:1605.

Bartley GB et al: Long-term follow-up of Graves ophthalmopathy in an incidence cohort. Ophthalmology 1996;103:958.

Burgett RA, Purvin VA, Kawasaki A: Lumboperitoneal shunting for pseudotumor cerebri. Neurology 1997;49:734.

Carden SM et al: Albinism: Modern molecular diagnosis. Br J Ophthalmol 1998;82:189.

Central Retinal Vein Occlusion Study Group: Natural history and clinical management of central retinal vein occlusion. Arch Ophthalmol 1997; 115:486.

Chew EY: Diabetic retinopathy and lipid abnormalities. Curr Opin Ophthalmol 1997;8:59.

Clarkson JG for the Central Vein Occlusion Study Group: A randomized clinical trial of early panretinal photocoagulation for ischemic central vein occlusion: The Central Vein Occlusion Study Group N Report. Ophthalmology 1995;102:1434.

Dana M-R et al: Prognosticators for visual outcome in sarcoid uveitis. Ophthalmology 1996;103:1846.

de Boer JH et al: Detection of intraocular antibody production to herpesviruses in acute retinal necrosis syndrome. Am J Ophthalmol 1994;117:201.

Demiroglu H, Barista 1, Dündar S: Risk factor assessment and prognosis of eye involvement in Behçet's disease in Turkey. Ophthalmology 1997;104:701.

Dodson PM et al: Hypertensive retinopathy: A review of existing classification systems and a suggestion for a simplified grading system. J Hum Hypertens 1996;10:93.

Eggenberger ER, Miller NF, Vitale S: Lumboperitoneal shunt for the treatment of pseudotumor cerebri. Neurology 1996;46:1524.

El Sheikh M, McGregor AM: Graves' ophthalmopathy: Medical management. Curr Ther Endocrinol Metab 1997;6:90.

Fekrat S, Finkelstein D: Current concepts in the management of central retinal vein occlusion. Curr Opin Ophthalmol 1997;18:50.

Fong ACO, Schatz H: Central retinal vein occlusion in young adults. Surv Ophthalmol 1993;37:393.

Fox RI et al: Criteria for diagnosis of Sjögren's syndrome. Rheum Dis Clin North Am 1994;20:391.

Fraunfelder FT: *Drug-Induced Ocular Side-Effects and Drug Interactions.* Lea & Febiger, 1976.

Gass JDM, Olson CL: Sarcoidosis with optic nerve and retinal involvement. Arch Ophthalmol 1976;94:945.

Ghanchi FD, Dutton GD: Current concepts in giant cell (temporal) arteritis. Surv Ophthalmol 1997;42:99.

Glacet-Bernard A et al: Prognostic factors for retinal vein occlusion. Ophthalmology 1996;103:551.

Gold DH, Weingeist TA (editors): *The Eye in Systemic Disease.* Lippincott, 1990.

Hayreh SS: Anterior ischemic optic neuropathy. Clin Neurosci 1997;4:251.

Hayreh SS et al: Giant cell arteritis: Validity and reliability of various diagnostic criteria. Am J Ophthalmol 1997;123:285.

Henricsson M et al: The effect of glycaemic control and the introduction of insulin therapy on retinopathy in non-insulin-dependent diabetes mellitus. Diabet Med 1997;14:123.

Hutchinson BM, Kyle PM: Long-term visual outcome following orbital decompression for dysthyroid eye disease. Eye 1995;9:578.

Ischemic Optic Decompression Trial Research Group: Optic nerve decompression surgery for nonarteritic anterior ischemic optic neuropathy (NAION) is not effective and may be harmful. JAMA 1995;273:625.

Jabs DA et al: Rhegmatogenous retinal detachment in patients with cytomegalovirus retinitis: The Foscarnet-Ganciclovir Cytomegalovirus Retinitis Trial. Am J Ophthalmol 1997;124:61.

Jabs DA, Bartlett JG: AIDS and ophthalmology: A period of transition. Am J Ophthalmol 1997;124:61.

Jacobson DNL, Vierkant RA, Belongia EA: Nonarteritic anterior ischemic optic neuropathy. Arch Ophthalmol 1997;115:1403.

Jacobson MA: Treatment of cytomegalovirus retinitis in patients with the acquired immunodeficiency syndrome. N Engl J Med 1997;337:105.

Jennette JC, Falk RJ: Small-vessel vasculitis. N Engl J Med 1997;337 21:1512.

Kahn M et al: Immunocytologic findings in a case of Vogt-Koyanagi-Harada syndrome. Ophthalmology 1993;100:1191.

Kruize AA et al: Long-term followup of patients with Sjögren's syndrome. Arthritis Rheum 1996;39:297.

Levy GD et al: Incidence of hydroxychloroquine retinopathy in 1,207 patients in a large multicenter outpatient practice. Arthritis Rheum 1997;40:1482.

Lewis RA et al: Foscarnet-Ganciclovir Cytomegalovirus Retinitis Trial 5. Clinical features of cytomegalovirus retinitis at diagnosis. Am J Ophthalmol 1997;124:141.

Marsh RJ, Cooper M: Ophthalmic herpes zoster. Eye 1993;7:350.

Mavrikakis M et al: Retinal toxicity in long term hydroxychloroquine treatment. Ann Rheumat Dis 1996;55:187.

Mets MB et al: Eye manifestations of congenital toxoplasmosis. Am J Ophthalmol 1996;122:309.

Mizener JB, Podhajsky P, Hayreh SS: Ocular ischemic syndrome. Ophthalmology 1997;104:859.

Moorthy RS et al: Management of varicella zoster virus retinitis in AIDS. Br J Ophthalmol 1997;81:189.

Musch DC et al: Treatment of cytomegalovirus retinitis with a sustained-release ganciclovir implant. N Engl J Med 1997;337:83.

Nussenblatt RB: Uveitis in Behçet's disease. Int Rev Immunol 1997;14:67.

Nussenblatt RD, Palestine AG: *Uveitis: Fundamental and Clinical Practice.* Year Book, 1989.

Perry SR, Rootman J, White VA: The clinical and pathologic constellation of Wegener granulomatosis of the orbit. Ophthalmology 1997; 104:685.

Quaterman MJ et al: Ocular rosacea: Signs, symptoms, and tear studies before and after treatment with doxycycline. Arch Dermatol 1997;133:49.

Reed JB et al: Regression of cytomegalovirus retinitis associated with protease-inhibitor treatment in patients with AIDS. Am J Ophthalmol 1997;124:199.

Shalaby IA et al: Syphilitic uveitis in human immunodeficiency virus-infected patients. Arch Ophthalmol 1997;115:469.

Shields CL et al: Survey of 520 eyes with uveal metastases. Ophthalmology 1997; 104:1265.

Sjolie AK et al: Retinopathy and vision loss in insulin-dependent diabetes in Europe. The EURODIAB IDDM Complications Study. Ophthalmology 1997;104:252.

Spector SA: Current therapeutic challenges in the treatment of cytomegalovirus retinitis. J Acquir Immune Defic Syndr Hum Retrovirol 1997;14:S32.

Studies of Ocular Complications of AIDS Research Group in collaboration with the AIDS Clinical Trials Group. Parenteral cidofovir for cytomegalovirus retinitis in AIDS: The HPMPC Peripheral Cytomegalovirus Retinitis Trial. A randomized, controlled trial. Ann Intern Med 1997;126:264.

Wall M, George D: Idiopathic intracranial hypertension: A prospective study of 50 cases. Brain 1991;114:155.

Walsh JB: Hypertensive retinopathy: Description, classification, and prognosis. Ophthalmology 1982;89:1127.

Watson PG, Hazleman BL (editors): *The Sclera and Systemic Disorders.* Saunders, 1976.

Weinberg DV, Murphy R, Naughton K: Combined daily therapy with intravenous ganciclovir and foscarnet for patients with recurrent cytomegalovirus retinitis. Am J Ophthalmol 1994;117:776.

Weisman RA, Osguthorpe JD: Orbital decompression in Graves' disease. Arch Otolaryngol Head Neck Surg 1994;120:831.

Whitcup SM, Nussenblatt RB: Immunologic mechanisms of uveitis: New targets for immunomodulation. Arch Ophthalmol 1997;115:520.

Yohai RA et al: Survival factors in rhino-orbital-cerebral mucormycosis. Surv Ophthalmol 1994;39:3.

Immunologic Diseases of the Eye

16

William G. Hodge, MD, MPH, FRCS(C)

Ocular manifestations are a common feature of immunologic diseases even though, paradoxically, the eye is also a site of immune privilege. The propensity for immunologic disease to affect the eye derives from a number of factors, including the highly vascular nature of the uvea, the tendency for immune complexes to be deposited in various ocular tissues, and the exposure of the mucous membrane of the conjunctiva to environmental allergens. Inflammatory eye disorders are more obvious (and often more painful) than those of other organs such as the thyroid or the kidney.

Immunologic diseases of the eye can be grossly divided into two major categories: antibody-mediated and cell-mediated diseases. As is the case in other organs, there is ample opportunity for the interaction of these two systems in the eye.

ANTIBODY-DEPENDENT & ANTIBODY-MEDIATED DISEASES

Before it can be concluded that a disease of the eye is antibody-dependent, the following criteria must be satisfied:

(1) There must be evidence of specific antibody in the patient's serum or plasma cells.

(2) The antigen must be identified and, if feasible, characterized.

(3) The same antigen must be shown to produce an immunologic response in the eye of an experimental animal, and the pathologic changes produced in the experimental animal must be similar to those observed in the human disease.

(4) It must be possible to produce similar lesions in animals passively sensitized with serum from an affected animal upon challenge with the specific antigen.

Unless all of the above criteria are satisfied, the disease may be thought of as *possibly* antibody-dependent. In such circumstances, the disease can be regarded as antibody-mediated if only one of the following criteria is met:

(1) If antibody to an antigen is present in higher quantities in the ocular fluids than in the serum (after adjustments have been made for the total amounts of immunoglobulins in each fluid).

(2) If abnormal accumulations of plasma cells are present in the ocular lesion.

(3) If abnormal accumulations of immunoglobulins are present at the site of the disease.

(4) If complement is fixed by immunoglobulins at the site of the disease.

(5) If an accumulation of eosinophils is present at the site of the disease.

(6) If the ocular disease is associated with an inflammatory disease elsewhere in the body for which antibody dependency has been proved or strongly suggested.

HAY FEVER CONJUNCTIVITIS
(See Also Chapter 5.)

This disease is characterized by edema and hyperemia of the conjunctiva and lids (Figure 16–1) and by itching, which is always present, and watering of the eyes. There is often an associated itching sensa-

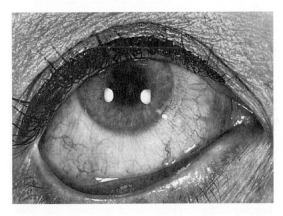

Figure 16–1. Hay fever conjunctivitis. Note edema and hyperemia of the conjunctiva. (Courtesy of M Allansmith and B McClellan.)

tion in the nose as well as rhinorrhea. The conjunctiva appears pale and boggy because of the intense edema, which is often rapid in onset. There is a distinct seasonal incidence, some patients being able to establish the onset of their symptoms at precisely the same time each year. These times usually correspond to the release of pollens by specific grasses, trees, or weeds.

Immunologic Pathogenesis

Hay fever conjunctivitis is one of the few inflammatory eye disorders for which antibody dependence has been definitely established. It is recognized as a form of atopic disease with an implied hereditary susceptibility. IgE (reaginic antibody) is attached to mast cells lying beneath the conjunctival epithelium. Contact of the offending antigen with IgE triggers the release of vasoactive substances, principally leukotrienes and histamine, in this area, and this in turn results in vasodilation and chemosis.

The role of circulating antibody to ragweed pollen in the pathogenesis of hay fever conjunctivitis has been demonstrated by passively transferring serum from a hypersensitive person to a nonsensitive one. When exposed to the offending pollen, the previously nonsensitive individual reacted with the typical signs of hay fever conjunctivitis.

Immunologic Diagnosis

Victims of hay fever conjunctivitis show many eosinophils in Giemsa-stained scrapings of conjunctival epithelium, and this is the test most commonly used to confirm the diagnosis. They show the immediate type of response, with wheal and flare, when tested by scratch tests of the skin with extracts of pollen or other offending antigens. Biopsies of the skin test sites have occasionally shown the full-blown picture of an Arthus reaction, with deposition of immune complexes in the walls of the dermal vessels. Passive cutaneous anaphylaxis can also be used to demonstrate the presence of circulating antibody.

Immunologic Treatment

Immunotherapy with gradually increasing doses of subcutaneously injected pollen extracts or other suspected allergens appears to reduce the severity of the disease in some individuals if started well in advance of the season. The mechanism is presumed to be production of blocking antibodies in response to the injection of small, graded doses of the antigen. This procedure cannot be recommended routinely, however, in view of the generally good results and relatively few complications of antihistamine therapy. Acute anaphylactoid reactions have occasionally resulted from overzealous immunotherapy. Topical antihistamines are the mainstay of treatment, and occasionally mast cell stabilizers and mild nonpenetrating corticosteroids.

Other forms of treatment are discussed in Chapter 5.

VERNAL CONJUNCTIVITIS & ATOPIC KERATOCONJUNCTIVITIS (See Also Chapter 5.)

These two diseases also belong to the group of atopic disorders. Both are characterized by itching and lacrimation of the eyes but are more chronic than hay fever conjunctivitis. Furthermore, both ultimately result in structural modifications of the lids and conjunctiva, especially atopic keratoconjunctivitis.

Vernal conjunctivitis characteristically affects children and adolescents; the incidence decreases sharply after the second decade of life. Like hay fever conjunctivitis, vernal conjunctivitis occurs only in the warm months of the year. Most of its victims live in hot, dry climates. The disease characteristically produces giant ("cobblestone") papillae of the tarsal conjunctiva (Figure 16–2). The keratinized epithelium from these papillae may abrade the underlying cornea, giving rise to complaints of foreign body sensation or even producing frank epithelial loss ("shield ulcer").

Atopic keratoconjunctivitis affects individuals of all ages and has no specific seasonal incidence. The skin of the lids has a characteristic dry, scaly appearance. The conjunctiva is pale and boggy. Both the conjunctiva and the cornea may develop scarring in the later stages of the disease. Atopic cataract has also been described. Staphylococcal blepharitis, manifested by scales and crusts on the lids, commonly complicates this disease. These patients are also more prone to herpes simplex ocular infections.

Although vernal and atopic disease may lie along a disease spectrum, often the two disorders can be differentiated. Atopic disease tends to occur in older patients, and there is little or no seasonal exacerbation. The papil-

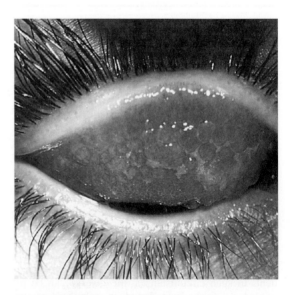

Figure 16–2. Giant papillae ("cobblestones") in the tarsal conjunctiva of a patient with vernal conjunctivitis.

lae in atopic disease are smaller than in vernal disease and are as often found on the lower palpebral conjunctiva as the upper. Furthermore, corneal vascularization and conjunctival scarring are much more common in atopic disease. Finally, in atopic disease eosinophils on smears are less numerous and less often degranulated.

Immunologic Pathogenesis

Reaginic antibody (IgE) is fixed to subepithelial mast cells in both of these conditions. Contact between the offending antigen and IgE is thought to trigger degranulation of the mast cell, which in turn allows for the release of vasoactive amines in the tissues. It is unlikely, however, that antibody action alone is responsible, since—at least in the case of papillae of vernal conjunctivitis—there is heavy papillary infiltration by mononuclear cells. Hay fever and asthma occur much more frequently in patients with vernal conjunctivitis and atopic keratoconjunctivitis than in the general population. Of the criteria outlined above for demonstration of *possibly* antibody-dependent diseases, (2), (5), and (6) have been met by atopic keratoconjunctivitis.

Immunologic Diagnosis

Patients with atopic keratoconjunctivitis and vernal conjunctivitis generally show large numbers of eosinophils in conjunctival scrapings. Skin testing with food extracts, pollens, and various other antigens reveals a wheal-and-flare type of reaction within 1 hour after testing, but the significance of these reactions is not established. Furthermore, the exact identification of the inciting antigens in these cases is usually unknown.

Immunologic Treatment

Avoidance of allergens (if known) is helpful; such objects as duck feathers, animal danders, and certain food proteins (egg albumin and others) are possible offenders. Specific allergens have been especially difficult to demonstrate in the case of vernal disease, though some workers feel that such substances as rye grass pollens may play a causative role. Installation of air conditioning in the home or relocation to a cool, moist climate is useful in vernal conjunctivitis.

Other treatments are discussed in Chapter 5.

JOINT DISEASES AFFECTING THE EYE

The diseases in this category vary greatly in their clinical manifestations depending upon the specific disease entity and the age of the patient. **Uveitis** and **scleritis** (Chapter 7) are the principal ocular manifestations associated with joint diseases. **Juvenile rheumatoid arthritis** affects females more frequently than males and is commonly accompanied by iridocyclitis of one or both eyes (see Chapter 17).

Ankylosing spondylitis affects males more frequently than females, and the onset is in the second to sixth decades. It may be accompanied by iridocyclitis of acute onset, often with fibrin in the anterior chamber (Figure 16–3).

Reiter's disease affects men more frequently than women. The first attack of ocular inflammation usually consists of a self-limited papillary conjunctivitis. It follows, at a highly variable interval, the onset of nonspecific urethritis and the appearance of inflammation in one or more of the weight-bearing joints. Subsequent attacks of ocular inflammation may consist of acute iridocyclitis of one or both eyes, occasionally with hypopyon (Figure 16–4). **Rheumatoid arthritis** of adult onset may be accompanied by acute scleritis or episcleritis but very rarely by uveitis (Figure 16–5). (See also Chapter 7.)

Immunologic Pathogenesis

Rheumatoid factor, an IgM autoantibody directed against the patient's own IgG, may play a major role in the pathogenesis of rheumatoid arthritis. The union of IgM antibody with IgG is followed by fixation of complement at the tissue site and the attraction of leukocytes and platelets to this area. An occlusive vasculitis, resulting from this chain of events, is thought to be the cause of rheumatoid nodule formation in the sclera as well as elsewhere in the body. The occlusion of vessels supplying nutrients to the sclera is thought to be responsible for the "melting away" of the scleral collagen that is so characteristic of rheumatoid arthritis (Figure 16–6).

While this explanation may suffice for rheumatoid arthritis, patients with the ocular complications of juvenile rheumatoid arthritis, ankylosing spondylitis, and Reiter's syndrome usually have negative tests for rheumatoid factor, so other explanations must be sought.

Outside the eyeball itself, the lacrimal gland has been shown to be under attack by circulating antibodies. Destruction of acinar cells within the gland and invasion of the lacrimal gland (as well as the salivary glands) by

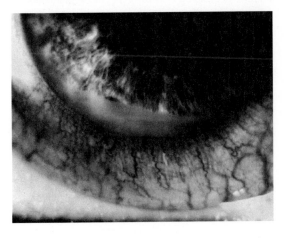

Figure 16–3. Acute iridocyclitis in a patient with ankylosing spondylitis. Note fibrin clot in anterior chamber.

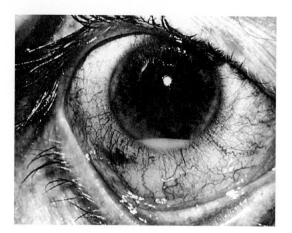

Figure 16–4. Acute iridocyclitis with hypopyon in a patient with Reiter's disease.

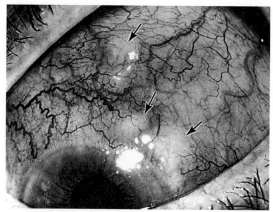

Figure 16–5. Scleral nodules in a patient with rheumatoid arthritis. (Courtesy of S Kimura.)

mononuclear cells result in decreased tear secretion. The combination of dry eyes (keratoconjunctivitis sicca), dry mouth (xerostomia), and rheumatoid arthritis is known as Sjögren's syndrome (see Chapter 15).

A growing body of evidence indicates that the immunogenetic background of certain patients accounts for the expression of their ocular inflammatory disease in specific ways. Analysis of the HLA antigen system shows that the incidence of HLA-B27 is significantly greater in patients with ankylosing spondylitis and Reiter's syndrome than could be expected by chance alone. It is not known how this antigen controls specific inflammatory responses. Other well-established HLA disease associations include HLA-A11 in sympathetic ophthalmia, HLA-A29 in birdshot choroidopathy, HLA-B51 in Behçet's syndrome, and HLA-B7 in macular histoplasmosis.

Immunologic Diagnosis

Rheumatoid factor can be detected in the serum by a number of standard tests involving the agglutination of IgG-coated erythrocytes or latex particles. Unfortunately, the test for rheumatoid factor is not positive in the majority of isolated rheumatoid afflictions of the eye.

The HLA types of individuals suspected of having ankylosing spondylitis and related diseases can be determined. HLA-B27 is associated with ankylosing spondylitis and Reiter's syndrome. X-ray of the sacroiliac area is a valuable screening procedure that may show evidence of spondylitis prior to the onset of low back pain in patients with the characteristic form of iridocyclitis.

OTHER ANTIBODY-MEDIATED EYE DISEASES
(See Also Chapter 15.)

The following antibody-mediated diseases are infrequently encountered by the practicing ophthalmologist.

Systemic lupus erythematosus, associated with the presence of circulating antibodies to DNA, produces an occlusive vasculitis of the nerve fiber layer of the retina. Such infarcts result in retinal cotton-wool spots (Figure 16–7).

Pemphigus vulgaris produces painful intraepithelial bullae of the conjunctiva. It is associated with the presence of circulating antibodies to an intercellular antigen located between the deeper cells of the conjunctival epithelium.

Cicatricial pemphigoid is characterized by subepithelial bullae of the conjunctiva. In the chronic stages of this disease, cicatricial contraction of the conjunctiva may result in severe scarring of the cornea, dryness of the eyes, and ultimate blindness. Pemphigoid is associated with local deposits of tissue antibodies directed against one or more antigens located in the basement membrane of the epithelium. Immunosuppressive treatment is often needed in the progressive stages of this disease.

Lens-induced uveitis is a rare condition that may be associated with circulating antibodies to lens proteins. It

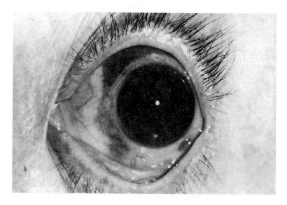

Figure 16–6. Scleral thinning in a patient with rheumatoid arthritis. Note dark color of the underlying uvea.

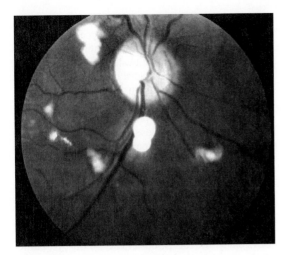

Figure 16–7. Cotton-wool spots in the retina of a patient with systemic lupus erythematosus.

is seen in individuals whose lens capsules have become permeable to these proteins as a result of trauma or other disease (see Chapter 7). Interest in this field dates back to Uhlenhuth (1903), who first demonstrated the organ-specific nature of antibodies to the lens. Witmer showed in 1962 that antibody to lens tissue may be produced by lymphoid cells of the ciliary body.

CELL-MEDIATED DISEASES

This group of diseases appears to be associated with cell-mediated immunity or delayed hypersensitivity. Various structures of the eye are invaded by mononuclear cells, principally lymphocytes and macrophages, in response to one or more chronic antigenic stimuli. In the case of chronic infections such as tuberculosis, leprosy, toxoplasmosis, and herpes simplex, the antigenic stimulus has clearly been identified as an infectious agent in the ocular tissue. Such infections are often associated with delayed skin test reactivity following the intradermal injection of an extract of the organism.

More intriguing but less well understood are the granulomatous diseases of the eye for which no infectious cause has been found. Such diseases are thought to represent cell-mediated, possibly autoimmune processes, but their origin remains obscure.

OCULAR SARCOIDOSIS

Ocular sarcoidosis is characterized by a panuveitis with occasional inflammatory involvement of the optic nerve and retinal blood vessels (see Chapter 7).

Immunologic Pathogenesis

Although many infectious or allergic causes of sarcoidosis have been suggested, none has been confirmed. Noncaseating granulomas are seen in the uvea, optic nerve, and adnexal structures of the eye as well as elsewhere in the body. The presence of macrophages and giant cells suggests that particulate matter is being phagocytosed, but this material has not been identified.

Patients with sarcoidosis are usually anergic to extracts of the common microbial antigens such as those of mumps, *Trichophyton, Candida,* and *Mycobacterium tuberculosis.* As in other lymphoproliferative disorders such as Hodgkin's disease and chronic lymphocytic leukemia, this may represent suppression of T cell activity such that the normal delayed hypersensitivity responses to common antigens cannot take place. Meanwhile, circulating immunoglobulins are usually detectable in the serum at higher than normal levels.

Immunologic Diagnosis

The diagnosis is largely inferential. Negative skin tests to a battery of antigens to which the patient is known to have been exposed are highly suggestive, and the same is true of the elevation of serum immunoglobulins. Biopsy of a conjunctival nodule or scalene lymph node may provide positive histologic evidence of the disease. X-rays of the chest reveal hilar adenopathy in many cases. Elevated levels of serum lysozyme, serum angiotensin-converting enzyme, or serum calcium may be detected.

Treatment

See Chapter 15.

SYMPATHETIC OPHTHALMIA & VOGT-KOYANAGI-HARADA SYNDROME

These two disorders are discussed together because they have certain common clinical features. Both are thought to represent autoimmune phenomena affecting pigmented structures of the eye and skin, and both may give rise to meningeal symptoms.

Clinical Features

Sympathetic ophthalmia is an inflammation in the second eye after the other has been damaged by penetrating injury. In most cases, some portion of the uvea of the injured eye has been exposed to the atmosphere for at least 1 hour. The uninjured or "sympathizing" eye develops minor signs of anterior uveitis after a period ranging from 2 weeks to many years. However, the vast majority of cases occur within 1 year. Floating spots and loss of the power of accommodation are among the earliest symptoms. The disease may progress to severe iridocyclitis with pain and photophobia. Usually, however, the eye remains relatively quiet and painless while the inflammatory disease spreads around the entire uvea. Despite the presence of panuveitis, the retina usually remains uninvolved except for perivascular cuffing of the retinal vessels with inflammatory cells. Optic nerve swelling and secondary glaucoma may occur. The disease may be accompanied by vitiligo (patchy depigmentation of the skin) and poliosis (whitening) of the eyelashes. For unknown reasons, the incidence of this disease has decreased markedly over the last several decades.

Vogt-Koyanagi-Harada syndrome consists of inflammation of the uvea of one or both eyes characterized by acute iridocyclitis, patchy choroiditis, and serous detachment of the retina (see Chapter 15). It usually begins with an acute febrile episode with headache, dysacusis, and occasionally vertigo. Patchy loss or whitening of scalp hair is described in the first few months of the disease. Vitiligo and poliosis are commonly present but are not essential for the diagnosis. Although the initial iridocyclitis may subside quickly, the course of the posterior disease is often indolent, with long-standing serous detachment of the retina and significant visual impairment.

Immunologic Pathogenesis

In both sympathetic ophthalmia and Vogt-Koyanagi-Harada syndrome, delayed hypersensitivity to melanin-containing structures is thought to occur. Although a viral cause has been suggested for both of these disorders, there is no convincing evidence of an infectious origin. It is postulated that some insult, infectious or otherwise, alters the pigmented structures of the eye, skin, and hair in such a way as to provoke delayed hypersensitivity responses to them. Soluble materials from the outer segments of the photoreceptor layer of the retina (retinal S-antigens) have been incriminated as possible autoantigens. Patients with Vogt-Koyanagi-Harada syndrome are usually Orientals, which suggests an immunogenetic predisposition to the disease.

Histologic sections of the traumatized eye from a patient with sympathetic ophthalmia may show uniform infiltration of most of the uvea by lymphocytes, epithelioid cells, and giant cells. The overlying retina is characteristically intact, but nests of epithelioid cells may protrude through the pigment epithelium of the retina, giving rise to **Dalen-Fuchs nodules.** The inflammation may destroy the architecture of the entire uvea, leaving an atrophic, shrunken globe.

Immunologic Diagnosis

Skin tests with soluble extracts of human or bovine uveal tissue are said to elicit delayed hypersensitivity responses in these patients. Several investigators have shown that cultured lymphocytes from patients with these two diseases undergo transformation to lymphoblasts in vitro when extracts of uvea or rod outer segments are added to the culture medium. Circulating antibodies to uveal antigens have been found in patients with these diseases, but such antibodies are to be found in any patient with long-standing uveitis, including those suffering from several infectious entities. The spinal fluid of patients with Vogt-Koyanagi-Harada syndrome may show increased numbers of mononuclear cells and elevated protein in the early stages. Treatment of both conditions requires at least systemic steroids and often oral immunosuppressive therapy.

OTHER DISEASES OF CELL-MEDIATED IMMUNITY

Giant cell arteritis (temporal arteritis) (see Chapter 15) may have disastrous effects on the eye, particularly in elderly individuals. The condition is manifested by temporal arteritis and polymyalgia rheumatica. Ocular complications include anterior ischemic optic neuropathy and central retinal artery occlusion. Such patients have an elevated sedimentation rate. Biopsy of the temporal artery reveals extensive infiltration of the vessel wall with giant cells and mononuclear cells.

Polyarteritis nodosa (see Chapter 15) is a vasculitis which predominantly affects small to medium-sized vessels. It can affect both the anterior and posterior segments of the eye. The corneas of such patients may show peripheral thinning and cellular infiltration. The retinal vessels reveal extensive necrotizing inflammation characterized by eosinophil, plasma cell, and lymphocyte infiltration.

Behçet's disease (see Chapter 15) has an uncertain place in the classification of immunologic disorders. It is characterized by recurrent iridocyclitis with hypopyon and occlusive vasculitis of the retinal vessels. Although it has many of the features of a delayed hypersensitivity disease, dramatic alterations of serum complement levels at the very beginning of an attack suggest an immune complex disorder. Furthermore, high levels of circulating immune complexes have recently been detected in patients with this disease. Most patients with eye symptoms are positive for HLA-B51, a subtype of HLA-B5.

Contact dermatitis of the eyelids represents a significant though minor disease caused by delayed hypersensitivity. Atropine, perfumed cosmetics, materials contained in plastic spectacle frames, and other locally applied agents may act as the sensitizing hapten. The lower lid is more extensively involved than the upper lid when the sensitizing agent is applied in drop form. Periorbital involvement with erythematous, vesicular, pruritic lesions of the skin is characteristic.

Phlyctenular keratoconjunctivitis (Figure 16–8) represents a delayed hypersensitivity response to certain microbial antigens, principally those of *M tuberculosis* and *Staphylococcus aureus* (see Chapters 5 and 6).

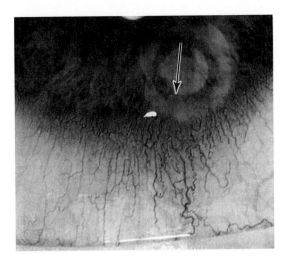

Figure 16–8. Phlyctenule (arrow) at the margin of the cornea. (Courtesy of P Thygeson.)

CORNEAL GRAFT REACTIONS
(Figure 16–9)

Blindness due to opacity or distortion of the central portion of the cornea is a remediable disease. If all other structures of the eye are intact, a patient whose vision is impaired solely by corneal opacity can expect great improvement from a graft of clear cornea into the diseased area (see Chapter 6). Trauma, including chemical burns, is one of the most common causes of central corneal opacity. Others include scars from herpetic keratitis, endothelial cell dysfunction with chronic corneal edema (including pseudophakic bullous keratopathy and Fuchs's dystrophy), keratoconus, and opacities from previous graft failures. All of these conditions represent indications for penetrating corneal grafts, provided the patient's eye is no longer inflamed and the opacity has been allowed maximal time to undergo spontaneous resolution (usually 6–12 months). It is estimated that approximately 10,000 corneal grafts are performed in the USA annually. Of these, about 90% can be expected to produce a beneficial result.

The cornea was one of the first human tissues to be successfully grafted. The fact that recipients of corneal grafts generally tolerate them well can be attributed to (1) the absence of blood vessels or lymphatics in the normal cornea, (2) the lack of presensitization to tissue-specific antigens in most recipients, and (3) anterior chamber acquired immune deviation (ACAID). This is a series of unique immunologic properties of the anterior chamber, conferring on the graft area the status of immune privilege. Reactions to corneal grafts do occur, however, particularly in indi-

viduals whose own corneas have been damaged by previous inflammatory disease. Such corneas may have developed both lymphatics and blood vessels, providing afferent and efferent channels for immunologic reactions in the engrafted cornea.

Although attempts have been made to transplant corneas from other species into human eyes (xenografts), particularly in countries where human material is not available for religious reasons, most corneal grafts have been taken from human eyes (allografts). Except in the case of identical twins, such grafts always represent the implantation of foreign tissue into a donor site; thus, the chance for a graft rejection due to an immune response to foreign antigens is virtually always present.

The cornea is a three-layered structure composed of a surface epithelium, an oligocellular collagenous stroma, and a single-layered endothelium. Although the surface epithelium may be sloughed and later replaced by the recipient's epithelium, certain elements of the stroma and all of the donor's endothelium remain in place for the rest of the patient's life. This has been firmly established by sex chromosome markers in corneal cells when donor and recipient were of opposite sexes. The endothelium must remain healthy in order for the cornea to remain transparent, and an energy-dependent pump mechanism is required to keep the cornea from swelling with water. Since the recipient's endothelium is in most cases diseased, the central corneal endothelium must be replaced by healthy donor tissue.

A number of foreign elements exist in corneal grafts that might stimulate the immune system of the host to reject this tissue. In addition to those mentioned above, the corneal stroma is regularly perfused

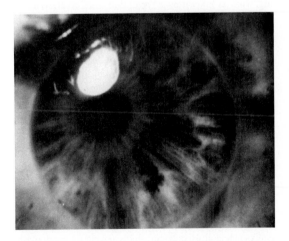

Figure 16–9. A cornea severely scarred by chronic atopic keratoconjunctivitis into which a central graft of clear cornea has been placed. Note how distinctly the iris landmarks are seen through the transparent graft. (Reproduced, with permission, from Stites DP, Terr AI [editors]: *Basic & Clinical Immunology,* 7th ed. Appleton & Lange, 1991.)

with IgG and serum albumin from the donor, although none of the other blood proteins are present—or only small amounts. While these serum proteins of donor origin rapidly diffuse into the recipient stroma and are thus removed from the graft site, they are theoretically immunogenic.

HLA incompatibility between donor and recipient has been shown by several authors to be significant in determining graft survival, particularly when the corneal bed is vascularized. It is known that most cells of the body possess these HLA antigens, including the endothelial cells of the corneal graft as well as certain stromal cells (keratocytes). The epithelium has been shown to possess a non-HLA antigen that diffuses into the anterior third of the stroma. Thus, while much foreign antigen may be eliminated by purposeful removal of the epithelium at the time of grafting, that amount of antigen which has already diffused into the stroma is automatically carried over into the recipient.

Despite numerous analytic studies supporting the role of HLA incompatibility in corneal graft rejection, a recent multicenter clinical trial found no use in HLA typing high risk grafts. In this study, ABO blood typing did provide a slight protective effect in high-risk cases. These surprising findings are leading many investigators to restudy the role of major and minor antigens in corneal graft rejection.

Both humoral and cellular mechanisms have been implicated in corneal graft reactions. It is likely that early graft rejections (2–4 weeks from surgery) are cell-mediated reactions. Cytotoxic lymphocytes have been found in the limbal area and stroma of affected individuals, and phase microscopy in vivo has revealed an actual attack on the grafted endothelial cells by these lymphocytes. Such lymphocytes generally move inward from the periphery of the cornea, making what is known as a "rejection line" as they move centrally. The donor cornea becomes edematous as the endothelium becomes compromised by an accumulation of lymphoid cells.

Late rejection of a corneal graft may occur several weeks to many months after implantation of donor tissue into the recipient eye. Such reactions may be antibody-mediated, since cytotoxic antibodies have been isolated from the serum of patients with a history of multiple graft reactions in vascularized corneal beds. These antibody reactions are complement-dependent and attract polymorphonuclear leukocytes, which may form dense rings in the cornea at the sites of maximum deposition of immune complexes. In experimental animals, similar reactions have been produced by corneal xenografts, but the intensity of the reaction can be markedly reduced either by decomplementing the animal or by reducing its leukocyte population through mechlorethamine therapy.

Treatment

The mainstay of the treatment of corneal graft reactions is corticosteroid therapy. This medication is generally given in the form of frequently applied eye drops (eg, 1% prednisolone acetate every hour) until the clinical signs abate. These clinical signs consist of conjunctival hyperemia in the perilimbal region, a cloudy cornea, cells and protein in the anterior chamber, and keratic precipitates on the corneal endothelium. The earlier treatment is applied, the more effective it is likely to be. Some cases may require systemic or periocular corticosteroids in addition to local eye drop therapy. High-dose intravenous steroids may also be efficacious if used sooner than 8 days after onset of the rejection period. Occasionally, vascularization and opacification of the cornea occur so rapidly as to make corticosteroid therapy useless, but even the most hopeless-appearing graft reactions have occasionally been reversed by corticosteroid therapy. Oral cyclosporine has been used successfully in the treatment of corneal graft rejection, and some benefit may be derived from cyclosporine eye drops.

Patients known to have rejected many previous corneal grafts are managed somewhat differently, particularly if disease affects their only remaining eye. Some surgeons may choose to find a close HLA match between donor and recipient, but conflicting analytic studies make doing so of questionable use. Pretreatment of the recipient with immunosuppressive agents such as azathioprine has also been resorted to in some cases.

REFERENCES

Bernauer W et al: The conjunctiva in acute and chronic mucous membrane pemphigoid: An immunohistochemical analysis. Ophthalmology 1993;100:339.

Boisjoly HM et al: Risk factors of corneal graft failure. Ophthalmology 1993;100:1728.

Foulks GN et al: Histocompatibility testing for keratoplasty in high-risk patients. Ophthalmology 1993;90:239.

Friedlaender MH, O'Connor GR: *Eye diseases.* In: *Medical Immunology,* 9th ed. Stites DP, Terr AI, Parslow TG (editors). Appleton & Lange, 1997.

Froebel KS et al: An investigation of the general immune status and specific immune responsiveness to retinal-(S)-antigen in patients with chronic posterior uveitis. Eye 1989;3:263.

Hylkema HA et al: Circulating immune complexes in uveitis patients. Int Ophthalmol 1989;13:253.

Jakobiec FA, Lefkowitch J, Knowles DM II: B- and T-lymphocytes in ocular disease. Ophthalmology 1984;91:635.

Kahn M et al: Immunocytologic findings in a case of Vogt-Koyanagi-Harada syndrome. Ophthalmology 1993;100:1191.

Kamp M et al: Patient-reported symptoms associated with graft reactions in high-risk patients in the collaborative corneal transplantation studies. Collaborative Corneal

Transplantation Studies Research Group. Cornea 1995;14:43.

Kaplan HJ, Waldrep JC: Immunologic insights into uveitis and retinitis: The immunoregulatory circuit. Ophthalmology 1984;91:655.

Klok AM et al: Antibodies against ocular and oral antigens in Behçet's disease associated with uveitis. Curr Eye Res 1989;8:957.

Larkin DFP: Corneal allograft rejection. Br J Ophthalmol 1994;78:649.

Mizuno K, Clark AF, Streilein JW: Anterior chamber-associated immune deviation induced by soluble antigens. Invest Ophthalmol Vis Sci 1989;30:1112.

Montan PG, van Hage-Hamsten M: Eosinophil cationic protein in tears in allergic conjunctivitis. Br J Ophthalmol 1996;80:556.

Nussenblatt RB: Immunoregulation of uveitis. Int Ophthalmol 1990;14:13.

Nussenblatt RB, Palestine AG: *Uveitis: Fundamentals and Clinical Practice.* Year Book, 1989.

Pepose JS, Holland GN, Wilhelmus KR (editors): *Ocular Infection and Immunity.* Mosby-Year Book, 1996.

Power WJ et al: Increasing the diagnostic yield of conjunctival biopsy in patients with suspected ocular cicatricial pemphigoid. Ophthalmology 1995;102:1158.

Rosenbaum JT: An algorithm for the systemic evaluation of patients with uveitis: Guidelines for the consultant. Semin Arthritis Rheum 1990;19:248.

Uusitalo RJ et al: Systemic cyclosporin treatment for high-risk corneal transplantation. Ocular Immunol Inflammation 1996;4:15.

17

Special Subjects of Pediatric Interest

Douglas R. Fredrick, MD

Pediatric ophthalmology offers particular challenges to the ophthalmologist, pediatrician, and family physician. Symptoms are often nonspecific, and the usual examination techniques require modification. Development of the visual system is still occurring during the first decade of life, with the potential for amblyopia even in response to relatively mild ocular disease. Because the development of the eye often reflects organ and tissue development of the body as a whole, many congenital somatic defects are mirrored in the eye. Collaboration with pediatricians, neurologists, and other health workers is essential in managing these conditions. Similar collaboration is required in assessing the educational needs of any child with poor vision.

Details of the embryology and the normal postnatal growth and development of the eye are discussed in Chapter 1.

NEONATAL OCULAR EXAMINATION

A careful eye examination soon after birth may reveal congenital abnormalities that suggest the presence of abnormalities elsewhere in the body and the need for further investigations. Recent demonstration of the value of retinal cryotherapy in the treatment of retinopathy of prematurity has highlighted the need for careful retinal examination of at-risk preterm babies.

The instruments required for the ocular examination of the newborn are a good hand light, direct and indirect ophthalmoscopes, a loupe for magnification, and occasionally a portable slitlamp. Phenylephrine 2.5% and cyclopentolate 1% or tropicamide 1% are generally safe for pupillary dilation in full-term neonates, though even these concentrations may have adverse effects on blood pressure and gastrointestinal function. The combination of cyclopentolate 0.2% and phenylephrine 1% (Cyclomydril) should be used to dilate the pupils of low-weight neonates.

Subjective response testing is limited to observing the following response to a visual target, of which the most effective is a human face—particularly the mother's face. Visual fixation and following move-

---

PEDIATRIC EYE EXAMINATION SCHEDULE
Neonatal Examination

External eye examination and ophthalmoscopic examination through dilated pupils as outlined in the text. Two drops of sterile 2.5% phenylephrine and 1% cyclopentolate or 1% tropicamide in each eye are instilled 1 hour prior to examination. (Cyclopentolate 0.2% and phenylephrine 1% combination [Cyclomydril] may be sufficient in babies with lightly pigmented eyes and low-weight neonates.) Special emphasis should be placed on the optic disks and maculas; detailed examination of the peripheral retinas is not necessary unless the baby is at risk for retinopathy of prematurity.

Age 6 Months

Test ocular fixation and ocular movement. Look for strabismus.

Age 4 years

Test visual acuity with illiterate "E" chart or HOTV matching optotypes, and stereopsis by the random dot "E" test or Titmus stereo test. Visual acuity should be normal 20/20 - 20/30.

Age 5–16 years

Test visual acuity at age 5. If normal, test visual acuity with the Snellen chart every 2 years until age 16. Color vision should be tested at ages 8–12. No other routine eye examination (eg, ophthalmoscopy) is necessary if visual acuity is normal and the eyes

---

ments can be demonstrated in most newborn babies. Following movements in this age group are usually coarse and jerky and should not be expected to resemble the smooth pursuit movements of older children and adults. The characteristics of the nystagmus induced by whole body rotation can be quite valuable in assessment of both the visual pathways and the control of eye movements in neonates, but their evaluation is complex.

External Inspection

The eyelids are inspected for growths, deformities, lid notches, and symmetric movement with opening and closing of the eyes. The absolute and relative size of the eyeballs is noted, as well as position and alignment. The size and luster of the corneas are noted, and the anterior chambers are examined for clarity and iris configuration. The size, position, and light reaction of the pupils are also noted. The pupils are normally relatively dilated until 29 weeks of gestation, at which time the pupillary light response first becomes apparent. The light response is not a reliable test until 32 weeks of gestation. Anisocoria of 0.5 mm can be seen in as many as 20% of neonates.

Ophthalmoscopic Examination

With undilated pupils, some information can be obtained by use of the ophthalmoscope in a dimly lighted room. Ideally, however, all newborns should be examined with an ophthalmoscope through dilated pupils. Ophthalmoscopic examination will demonstrate any corneal, lens, or vitreous opacities as well as abnormalities in the fundus. In premature infants, remnants of the tunica vasculosa lentis are frequently visible, either in front of the lens, behind the lens, or in both positions. The remnants are usually absorbed by the time the infant has reached term, but rarely they remain permanently and appear as a complete or partial "cobweb" in the pupil. At other times, remnants of the primitive hyaloid system fail to absorb completely, leaving either a cone on the optic disk that projects into the vitreous—Bergmeister's papilla—or a gliotic tuft on the posterior lens capsule called Mittendorf's dot.

Physiologic cupping of the disk is usually not seen in premature infants and is rarely seen at term; if seen then, it is usually very slight. In such cases the optic disk will appear gray, resembling optic nerve atrophy. This relative pallor, however, gradually changes to the normal adult pink color at about 2 years of age. Preretinal and intraretinal hemorrhages have been reported in 30–45% of newborns, usually clearing completely within a few weeks and leaving no permanent visual dysfunction.

OCULAR EXAMINATION OF INFANTS & YOUNG CHILDREN

Tests for Visual Acuity

In the early years, visual acuity should be appraised as part of each general "well child" examination. It is best not to wait until the child is old enough to respond to visual charts, since these may not furnish accurate information until school age.

During the first 3–4 years, estimations of vision rely greatly on observation and reports about the child's behavior both at play and during interactions with parents and with other children. Unfortunately, at this age seemingly normal visual performance is possible with relatively poor vision, and obviously abnormal performance probably reflects extremely poor acuity. The influence of visual impairment on motor and social development must always be borne in mind. The pupillary responses to light are a gross test of visual function and are reliable only for ruling out complete dysfunction of the anterior visual or efferent pupillary pathways. The ability to fixate and follow a target is much more informative. The target must be appropriate to the age of the child. Binocular following and converging reflexes are best examined first to establish the child's cooperation. Each eye should then be tested separately, preferably with occlusion of the fellow eye by an adhesive patch. Comparison of the performance of the two eyes will give useful information about their relative acuities. Resistance to occlusion of one eye strongly suggests it is the preferred eye and therefore that the fellow eye must have comparatively poor vision. In cases of latent nystagmus—nystagmus increasing with occlusion of one eye—the child is likely to resent occlusion of each eye because of the effect such nystagmus has on visual acuity. Manifest nystagmus may be indicative of an anterior visual pathway disorder or other central nervous system disease until these have been excluded. (Further discussion of the assessment of nystagmus is given in Chapter 14).

After 3 months of age, the presence of strabismus, detected by examining the relative position of the corneal light reflections, must also be regarded as indicative of poor vision in the deviated eye, particularly if this eye does not take up or is slow to take up fixation of a light upon occlusion of the fellow eye. (Further discussion of the assessment of strabismus is given in Chapter 12.)

These inferences about the status of the developing sensory systems can now be augmented by the quantitative techniques of optokinetic nystagmus, forced-choice preferential looking methods, and visually evoked responses (see Chapter 2). Although visually evoked potentials have suggested that normal adult visual acuity is attained before 2 years of age, this is probably an overestimate and it is likely that 3–4 years of age is a more accurate estimate (Table 17–1).

Table 17–1. Development of visual acuity (approximate).

Age	Visual Acuity
2 months	20/400
6 months	20/100
1 year	20/50
3 years	20/20

Forced-choice preferential looking methods have gained increasing popularity as a reliable and relatively easy assessment of visual acuity in preverbal children, even in the very young. This technique does, however, have a tendency to overestimate visual acuity in amblyopes.

From about age 4 on, it becomes possible to elicit subjective responses by use of the illiterate "E" chart, child recognition figures, Lea figures, or HOTV cards. Usually, at the first- or second-grade level, the regular Snellen chart may be employed. Stereoacuity can be shown to develop in most infants beginning at 3 months of age, but clinical testing is not generally possible until 3–4 years of age. Absence of stereopsis, as judged with the random dot "E" test or the Titmus stereo test, is suggestive of strabismus or amblyopia and the need for further investigation.

Refraction

Objective refraction is an important part of the pediatric ophthalmic examination, especially if there is any suggestion of poor vision or strabismus. In young children, this should be performed under cycloplegia in order to overcome the child's tendency to accommodate. In many circumstances, 1% cyclopentolate drops applied twice—separated by an interval of 5 minutes—30 minutes prior to examination will provide sufficient cycloplegia, but atropine is recommended if convergent strabismus is present or the eyes are heavily pigmented. Because atropine drops are commonly associated with systemic side effects, 1% atropine ointment applied once daily for 2 or 3 days prior to examination is the recommended regimen. The parents should be warned of the symptoms of atropine toxicity—fever, flushed face, and rapid pulse—and the necessity for discontinuing treatment, cooling the child with sponge bathing, and, in severe cases, seeking urgent medical assistance. Cycloplegic refraction provides the additional advantage of good mydriasis to facilitate fundal examination.

About 80% of children between the ages of 2 and 6 years are hyperopic, 5% are myopic, and 15% are emmetropic. About 10% have refractive errors that require correction before age 7 or 8. Hyperopia remains relatively static or gradually diminishes until 19 or 20 years of age. Myopia often develops between ages 6 and 9 and increases throughout adolescence, with the greatest change at the time of puberty. Astigmatism is relatively common in babies but decreases in prevalence during the first few years of life. Thereafter, it remains relatively constant in prevalence and degree throughout life.

Anterior & Posterior Segment Examination

Further examination needs to be tailored to each child's age and ability to cooperate. Anterior segment examination in the young child relies mainly upon the use of a hand light and magnifying loupe, but slitlamp examination is often possible in babies with the coop-

eration of the mother—and in young children with appropriate encouragement. Measurement of intraocular pressure and gonioscopy are more of a problem and frequently necessitate examination under anesthetic. Fundal examination relies upon good mydriasis. It is generally easier in neonates and babies than in young children because they can be restrained easily by being wrapped in a blanket.

The foveal light reflection is absent in infants. Instead, the macula has a bright "mother-of-pearl" appearance with a suggestion of elevation. This is more pronounced in black infants. At 3–4 months of age, the macula becomes slightly concave and the foveal light reflection appears.

The peripheral fundus in the infant is gray, in contrast to the orange-red fundus of the adult. In white infants, the pigmentation is more pronounced near the posterior pole and gradually fades to almost white at the periphery. In black infants, there is more pigment in the fundus, and a gray-blue sheen is seen throughout the periphery. In white infants, a white periphery is normal and should not be confused with retinoblastoma. During the next several months, pigment continues to be deposited in the retina, and usually at about 2 years of age the adult color is evident.

CONGENITAL OCULAR ABNORMALITIES

Congenital defects of the ocular structures fall into two main categories: (1) developmental anomalies, of which genetic defects are an important cause; and (2) tissue reactions to intrauterine insults (infections, drugs, etc).

Congenital Abnormalities of the Globe

Failure of formation of the optic vesicle results in **anophthalmos.** Failure of invagination leads to a **congenital cystic eye.** Failure of closure produces **colobomas of the iris, retina, and choroid. Cryptophthalmos** occurs when the eyelids fail to separate.

Abnormally small eyes can be divided into **nanophthalmos,** in which function is normal, and **microphthalmos,** in which function is abnormal and there may be other ocular abnormalities such as cataract, coloboma, or congenital cyst.

Lid Abnormalities

Congenital ptosis is commonly due to dystrophy of the levator muscle of the upper lid. Other causes are congenital Horner's syndrome and congenital third nerve palsy.

Palpebral coloboma is a cleft of usually the upper lid, due to incomplete fusion of fetal maxillary processes. Large defects require early repair to avoid corneal ulceration due to exposure. Congenital eyelid colobomas are commonly seen in association with craniofacial disorders such as Goldenhar's syndrome.

Corneal Defects

There may be partial or complete opacity of the corneas such as is found in congenital glaucoma, forceps injuries at birth, faulty development of the corneal endothelium, developmental anterior segment abnormalities with persistent corneal-lens attachments, intrauterine inflammation, interstitial keratitis, and mucopolysaccharide depositions of the cornea as in Hurler's syndrome. The most frequent cause of opaque corneas in infants and young children is congenital glaucoma, in which the eye is often larger than normal (buphthalmos). Forceps injuries at birth may cause extensive corneal opacities with edema as a result of rupture of Descemet's membrane. These usually clear spontaneously but frequently induce anisometropic amblyopia.

Megalocornea is an enlarged cornea with normal clarity and function, usually transmitted as an X-linked recessive trait. It must be differentiated from congenital glaucoma. There are usually no associated defects.

Iris & Pupillary Defects

Misplaced or ectopic pupils (corectopia) are frequently observed. The usual displacement is upward and laterally (temporally) from the center of the cornea. Such displacement is occasionally associated with ectopic lens, congenital glaucoma, or microcornea. Multiple pupils are known as **polycoria.** **Coloboma of the iris** indicates incomplete closure of the fetal ocular cleft and usually occurs inferiorly and nasally. It may be associated with coloboma of the lens, choroid, and optic nerve. **Aniridia** (absence of the iris) is a rare abnormality, frequently associated with secondary glaucoma and usually due to an autosomal dominant hereditary pattern. There is a significant association between sporadic aniridia and Wilms' tumor. Frequent abdominal examinations with periodic renal ultrasonography should be performed to detect Wilms' tumor at an early treatable stage.

The color of the iris is determined largely by heredity. Abnormalities in color include **albinism,** due to the absence of normal pigmentation of the ocular structures and frequently associated with poor visual acuity and nystagmus; and **heterochromia,** which is a difference in color in the two eyes that may be a primary developmental defect with no functional loss, due to congenital Horner's syndrome or secondary to an inflammatory process.

Lens Abnormalities

The lens abnormalities most frequently noted are cataracts, though there may be faulty development, forming colobomas, or subluxation, as seen in Marfan's syndrome.

Any lens opacity that is present at birth is a congenital cataract, regardless of whether or not it interferes with visual acuity. Congenital cataracts are often associated with other conditions. Maternal rubella during the first trimester of pregnancy is a common cause of congenital cataract. Other congenital cataracts have a hereditary background.

Congenital opacities may occur at any time during formation of the lens, and the stage during which the opacity started to develop is often measurable by the depth of the opacity. The innermost fetal nucleus of the lens forms early in embryonic life and is surrounded by the embryonic nucleus. During adult life, further growth in the lens is peripheral and subcapsular.

If the opacity is small enough so that it does not occlude the pupil, adequate visual acuity is attained by focusing around the opacity. If the pupillary opening is entirely occluded, however, normal sight does not develop, and the poor fixation may lead to nystagmus and profound amblyopia. Good visual results have been reported with both unilateral and bilateral cataracts treated by early surgery. Aphakic correction is then achieved usually with extended-wear contact lenses that need to be changed frequently to maintain optimal correction.

A major management problem in congenital cataracts is the associated amblyopia. Whether this can be dealt with adequately is a major determinant in deciding whether early surgery for monocular congenital cataract is justified. In the case of bilateral congenital cataracts, the time interval between operating on the two eyes must be as short as possible if amblyopia in the second eye is to be avoided. If early surgery is to be undertaken for congenital cataracts, it is best done within the first few weeks of life, and early referral to an ophthalmologist thus is essential. Surgery for congenital cataracts is discussed in Chapter 8.

Developmental Anomalies of the Anterior Segment

Failure of migration or subsequent development of neural crest cells produces abnormalities involving the anterior chamber angle, iris, cornea, and lens. Axenfeld's syndrome, Rieger's syndrome, and Peter's anomaly are examples. Glaucoma is a major clinical problem. The associated extraocular abnormalities are probably also manifestations of abnormal neural crest development.

Vitreous Abnormalities

Remnants of the hyaloid artery may be seen on the posterior surface of the lens (Mittendorf's dot) or on the optic disk (Bergmeister's papilla).

Persistent hyperplastic primary vitreous is an important cause of leukocoria that must be differentiated from retinoblastoma, congenital cataract, and retinopathy of prematurity.

Choroid & Retina

Gross defects of the choroid and retina are visible with the ophthalmoscope. The choroidal structures may show congenital colobomas, usually in the lower nasal region, which may also include the iris and all or part of the optic nerve. Choroidal colobomas are often associated with syndromes such as CHARGE association, Aicardi's syndrome, and Goldenhar's syndrome. Posterior polar chorioretinal scarring is a pigmentary disturbance often caused by intrauterine toxoplasmosis.

Optic Nerve

Congenital anomalies of the optic nerve are relatively common. They are usually benign, such as minor abnormalities of the retinal vessels at the nerve head and tilted disks due to an oblique entrance of the nerve into the globe, but they may be associated with severe visual loss in the case of optic nerve hypoplasia or the rare central coloboma of the disk (morning glory syndrome).

Optic nerve hypoplasia is a nonprogressive congenital abnormality of one or both optic nerves in which the number of axons in the involved nerve is reduced. Previously regarded as rare, it is now understood to be a major cause of visual loss in children. The degree of visual impairment varies from normal acuity with a wide variety of visual field defects to no perception of light. Clinical diagnosis is hampered by the difficulties of examining young children and the subtlety of the clinical signs. In more marked cases, the optic disk is obviously small and the circumpapillary halo of the normal-sized scleral canal produces the characteristic "double ring sign." In other cases, the hypoplasia may be only segmental and much more difficult to detect.

Optic nerve hypoplasia is frequently associated with midline deformities, including absence of the septum pellucidum, agenesis of the corpus callosum, dysplasia of the third ventricle, pituitary and hypothalamic dysfunction, and midline facial abnormalities. Jaundice and hypoglycemia in the neonatal period and growth retardation, hypothyroidism, and diabetes insipidus during childhood are important clinical effects of the resultant endocrine disturbances. More severe intracranial abnormalities such as anencephaly and porencephaly also occur. Endocrine and neuroradiographic investigations should be undertaken in all patients with optic nerve hypoplasia except perhaps those with unilateral segmental hypoplasia who are developing normally and have no other clinically evident congenital abnormalities.

Visual performance in children with optic nerve hypoplasia may be improved by occlusion therapy. Conversely, optic nerve hypoplasia is an important cause of poor vision that does not normalize with occlusion therapy in children with or without strabismus. A number of patients with optic nerve hypoplasia are not diagnosed until adult life because of the subtlety of the optic nerve abnormality.

Extraocular Dermoids

Congenital rests of surface ectodermal tissues may lead to formation of dermoids that occur frequently in the extraocular structures. These dermoids occur most commonly superolaterally, arising from the frontozygomatic suture.

Congenital Nasolacrimal Duct Obstruction

Canalization of the distal nasolacrimal duct normally occurs before birth or during the first month of life. As many as 30% of babies will have epiphora during this time. Approximately 6% have more prolonged symptoms, of which the majority will also resolve aided by lacrimal sac massage and treatment of episodes of conjunctivitis with topical antibiotics. Nasolacrimal probing is usually curative in the remainder and is best left until about 1 year of age. In the event of acute dacryocystitis, earlier probing is often indicated. The possibility of more extensive congenital nasolacrimal anomalies should be born in mind in patients with craniofacial anomalies. Epiphora may also be due to inflammatory anterior segment disease, lid abnormalities, and congenital glaucoma.

Orbital Abnormalities

Craniofacial dysostosis (Crouzon's disease) is a rare hereditary deformity due to an autosomal dominant gene, characterized by exophthalmos, hypoplasia of the maxilla, enlargement of the nasal bones, abnormal increase in the space between the eyes (ocular hypertelorism), optic atrophy, and bony abnormalities of the region of the perilongitudinal sinus. The palpebral fissures slant downward (in contrast to the upward slant of Down's syndrome). Strabismus is also present. The strabismus is secondary to both structural anomalies of the muscles and orbital angle anomalies.

Various congenital abnormalities of skull development—due to premature closure of the skull sutures—are associated with deformities of the orbits and ocular complications resembling those associated with Crouzon's disease. Examples are oxycephaly and acrobrachycephaly.

INVESTIGATION OF THE BLIND BABY WITH NORMAL OCULAR & NEUROLOGIC EXAMINATION

An important part of pediatric ophthalmology is the investigation of babies with poor visual performance for which clinical examination reveals no ocular or neurologic cause. This presumes that defects such as optic nerve hypoplasia, albinism, and high refractive errors have been excluded. The important conditions to be considered are Leber's congenital amaurosis, cortical blindness, cone dystrophy, oculomotor apraxia, and delayed visual maturation.

Leber's congenital amaurosis—as distinct from Leber's hereditary optic neuropathy—and cone dystrophy are congenital retinal dystrophies detectable by electroretinography. Visual evoked responses and neuroimaging studies are used to diagnose cortical blindness. In oculomotor apraxia, a defect in initiation of horizontal saccades gives the impression of visual unresponsiveness, though the visual pathways are normal. Affected children develop characteristic compensatory head movements to overcome the eye movement disorder. Delayed visual maturation is a rare condition in which vision does not develop until after 3 months of age. In some cases, there may be associated ocular and neurologic abnormalities that limit final visual performance, but normal vision is attained in those in which it is an isolated condition.

POSTNATAL PROBLEMS

The most common ocular disorders of children are external infections of the conjunctiva and eyelids (bacterial conjunctivitis, hordeola, blepharitis), strabismus, ocular foreign bodies, allergic reactions of the conjunctiva and eyelids, refractive errors, and congenital defects. Since it is more difficult to elicit an accurate history of causative factors and subjective complaints in children, it is not uncommon to overlook significant ocular disorders (especially in very young children). Aside from the altered frequency of occurrence of the types of ocular disorders, the causes, manifestations, and treatment of eye disorders are about the same for children as for adults. Certain special problems encountered more frequently in infants and children are discussed below.

Ophthalmia Neonatorum (Conjunctivitis of the Newborn)

Conjunctivitis of the newborn may be of chemical, bacterial, chlamydial, or viral origin. Differentiation is sometimes possible according to the timing of presentation, but appropriate smears and cultures are essential. Antenatal diagnosis and treatment of maternal genital infections should prevent many cases of neonatal conjunctivitis. The presence of active maternal genital herpes at the time of delivery is an indication for elective cesarean section.

A. Conjunctivitis Due to Chlamydial Infection: *Chlamydia* is now the commonest identifiable infectious cause of neonatal conjunctivitis in the USA. Inclusion blennorrhea due to chlamydial infection has its onset between the fifth and fourteenth days; the presence of typical inclusion bodies in the epithelial cells of a conjunctival smear confirms this diagnosis. Direct immunofluorescent antibody staining of conjunctival scrapings is a highly sensitive and specific diagnostic test. Systemic therapy with erythromycin is more effective than topical therapy and aids in the eradication of concurrent nasopharyngeal carriage, which may predispose to the development of pneumonitis.

B. Conjunctivitis Due to Chemical Trauma: Chemical conjunctivitis caused by the silver nitrate drops instilled into the conjunctival sac at birth is most apparent during the first or second day of life. Silver nitrate conjunctivitis is usually self-limited. Silver nitrate solution (1%) should be contained in sealed single-use disposable containers. Because of the possibility of chemical conjunctivitis, some authorities advocate use of topical erythromycin or tetracycline instead for prophylaxis. Instillation of silver nitrate or an antibiotic is still required by statute in most states in the USA.

C. Conjunctivitis Due to Bacterial Infection: Bacterial conjunctivitis, usually due to *Staphylococcus aureus, Haemophilus* species, *Streptococcus pneumoniae, Streptococcus faecalis, Neisseria gonorrhoeae,* or *Pseudomonas* species (the last two being the most serious because of potential corneal damage), presents between the second and fifth days after birth. Provisional identification of the causative organism may be made from conjunctival smears. Gonococcal conjunctivitis necessitates parenteral therapy with aqueous penicillin G procaine given intravenously for penicillin-sensitive strains and ceftriaxone given intravenously with topical erythromycin for penicillinase-producing strains. In all cases due to chlamydial or gonococcal infection, both parents should also be given systemic treatment. Other types of bacterial conjunctivitis require topical instillation of antibacterial agents, such as sodium sulfacetamide, bacitracin, or tetracycline, as soon as results of smears are known.

D. Conjunctivitis Due to Viral Infection: Herpes simplex virus produces characteristic giant cells and viral inclusions on cytologic examination. Herpetic keratoconjunctivitis usually resolves spontaneously but may require antiviral therapy, particularly when associated with disseminated infection that occurs chiefly in atopic individuals.

Uveitis in Childhood

Inflammatory eye disease is relatively uncommon in children, but there are a number of important syndromes. The conditions that are seen in the same form as in adults are acute nongranulomatous anterior uveitis associated with the HLA-B27 spondylarthritides, intermediate uveitis, Fuchs' heterochromic cyclitis, and idiopathic anterior uveitis. These are treated in the same way as in adults but with care in the use of systemic steroids because of their effects on growth. Uveitis in association with juvenile rheumatoid arthritis is generally asymptomatic in its early stages and often remains undetected until severe loss of vision due to glaucoma, cataract, or band keratopathy, has already occurred. Regular ophthalmic screening of children with juvenile rheumatoid arthritis is essential. Girls with a pauciarticular onset of juvenile rheumatoid arthritis, especially if they have circulating antinuclear antibody, are at particularly high risk for developing uveitis. Long-term use of topical steroids and mydriatics is effective in controlling the uveitis associated with juvenile rheumatoid arthritis. (Further discussion of uveitis in children is included in Chapter 7.)

Retinopathy of Prematurity

Retinopathy of prematurity, previously called retrolental fibroplasia, has been estimated to result in 550 new cases of infant blindness each year in the United States. Improved neonatal care may reduce the percentage of babies affected but has also greatly increased the total number at risk. Retinal cryotherapy is now recommended treatment for babies with severe active disease.

Retinal vascularization proceeds centrifugally from the optic nerve, beginning at the fourth month of gestation. Retinal vessels normally reach the nasal ora serrata at 8 months and the temporal ora serrata at 9 months. Retinopathy of prematurity develops if this process is disturbed. It is usually bilateral but often asymmetric. The active phase involves changes at the junction of vascularized and avascular retina, initially as an obvious demarcation line (stage 1), followed by formation of a distinct ridge (stage 2), then extraretinal fibrovascular proliferation (stage 3). Even among patients with stage 3 disease, there is a very high incidence of spontaneous regression. Consideration is also given to the location of the changes with respect to distance from the optic disk, the extent of the disease in clock hours, and the presence of venous dilation and arterial tortuosity in the posterior segment ("plus" disease). The cicatricial phase (stages 4 and 5) is manifested by increasingly severe retinal detachment.

The major risk factors for retinopathy of prematurity are decreasing gestational age and decreasing birth weight. Although recognition of the causative role of supplemental oxygen and its restriction seems to have reduced the incidence of retinopathy of prematurity, other factors must also be important. Associated risk factors include acidosis, apnea, patent ductus arteriosus, septicemia, blood transfusions, and intraventricular hemorrhage.

It is recommended that all babies with a birth weight of 1500 g or less and those that receive prolonged supplemental oxygen therapy should undergo repeated screening for retinopathy of prematurity. As many as 60% of such babies will develop the disease, even if only in its early stages. Screening should begin at 2–4 weeks after birth and continue until the retina is fully vascularized, until the changes of retinopathy of prematurity have undergone spontaneous resolution, or until appropriate treatment has been given. Pupillary dilation is achieved with Cyclomydril (cyclopentolate 0.2% and phenylephrine 1%). In eyes with five contiguous or eight cumulative clock hours of stage 3 "plus" disease, it is recommended that retinal cryotherapy or laser photocoagulation be applied to the entire avascular retina anterior to the ridge in order to reduce the risk of subsequent cicatricial disease. Whether treatment should be given to both eyes if they both fulfill the criteria has not been determined. Such treatment should be carried out with the assistance of an experienced neonatologist and under careful monitoring because of the risks of serious systemic complications including respiratory and cardiorespiratory arrest.

Vitrectomy and lensectomy may be beneficial in cicatricial disease but probably should be reserved for babies with severe disease in both eyes.

See also Chapter 10 and discussion of oxygen toxicity in Chapter 15.

Congenital Glaucoma

Congenital glaucoma (see Chapter 11) may occur alone or in association with many other congenital lesions. Early recognition is essential to prevent permanent blindness. Involvement is often bilateral. The most striking symptom is extreme photophobia. Early signs are corneal haze or opacity, increased corneal diameter, and increased intraocular pressure. Since the outer coats of the eyeball are not as rigid in the child, the increased intraocular pressure expands the corneal and scleral tissues, producing an eye that is larger than normal (buphthalmos). The major differential diagnoses are forceps injuries at birth, developmental anomalies of the cornea or anterior segment, and mucopolysaccharidoses such as Hurler's syndrome. All of these cause corneal clouding but none produce enlargement of the globe. Useful vision may be preserved by early diagnosis and medical and surgical treatment by an ophthalmologist.

Leukocoria
(White Pupil)

Parents will occasionally see a white spot through the infant's pupil (leukocoria). Although retinoblastoma must be ruled out, the opacity is more often due to cataract, retinopathy of prematurity, or persistent hyperplastic primary vitreous.

Retinoblastoma

This rare malignant tumor of childhood is fatal if untreated. In 90% of cases, the diagnosis is made before the end of the third year. In about 30% of cases, retinoblastoma is bilateral. Development of the tumor is thought to occur because of the loss—from both members of the chromosome pair—of the normally protective dominant allele at a single locus within chromosomal band 13q14 (see Chapter 18). This gene is normally responsible for production of a nuclear phosphoprotein with DNA binding activity. Loss of the allele is caused by mutations, either in the somatic retinal cells alone (nonheritable retinoblastoma) or in the germ line cells as well (heritable retinoblastoma). In heritable retinoblastoma, the genetic predisposition is inherited as an autosomal dominant trait; children of survivors have a nearly 50% chance of having the disease; and the tumor is more apt to be bilateral and multifocal. Parents who have produced one child with retinoblastoma run a 4–7% risk of having a subsequent child with the disease. Recent sequencing of the retinoblastoma gene locus now allows more specific genetic counseling and identification of individuals carrying the mutation. In sporadic cases, the tumor is usually not discovered until it has advanced far enough to produce an opaque pupil. Infants and children with presenting symptoms of strabismus should be examined carefully to rule out retinoblastoma, since a deviating eye may be the first sign of the tumor. In children of families affected by familial retinoblastoma, regular screening is important in the early detection of tumors.

Enucleation is the treatment of choice in nearly all extensive unilateral cases of retinoblastoma. In bilateral cases, conservative therapy with radiotherapy, either with episcleral plaques or external beam, and photocoagulation techniques are used increasingly to preserve the less severely affected eye. A collaborative study has been initiated to investigate the efficacy of chemotherapy in the treatment of advanced retinoblastoma.

Strabismus

Strabismus is present in about 2% of children. Its early recognition is often the responsibility of the pediatrician or the family physician. Occasionally, childhood strabismus has neurologic significance. The idea that a child may outgrow crossed eyes should be discouraged. Any child with evidence of strabismus after 3 months of age must be referred as soon as possible for ophthalmologic assessment. Neglect in the treatment of strabismus may lead to undesirable cosmetic effects, psychic trauma, and amblyopia (see below) in the deviating eye. Strabismus is covered in Chapter 12.

Amblyopia

Amblyopia is decreased visual acuity of one eye (uncorrectable with lenses) in the absence of organic eye disease. Organic eye disease may be present but insufficient to explain the level of vision.

Normal development of the physiologic mechanisms of the retina and visual cortex is determined by postnatal visual experience. Visual deprivation due to any cause, congenital or acquired, during the critical period of development (probably lasting up to age 8 in humans) prevents the establishment of normal vision in the involved eye. Reversal of this effect becomes increasingly difficult with increasing age of the child. Early suspicion and prompt referral for treatment of the underlying condition are important in preventing amblyopia.

The most common causes of amblyopia are strabismus, in which the image from the deviated eye is suppressed to prevent diplopia, and anisometropia, in which an inability to focus the eyes simultaneously causes suppression of the image of one eye

and high hypermetropia, in which both eyes may become amblyopic because of failure to form a focused image in either eye. All of these conditions are treatable.

Since poor visual function in a young child may go unnoticed, routine screening is advocated to detect amblyogenic factors (eg, by photorefraction of babies for refractive errors and strabismus) or established amblyopia (by testing visual acuity at age 4).

Child Abuse
(Shaken Baby Syndrome)

Child abuse is an increasingly recognized cause of childhood trauma. Making the diagnosis is essential if affected children are to be given the protection they must have, but wrong diagnosis must also be avoided if families are not to be unjustly treated.

In the shaken baby syndrome, external signs of head injury are absent, but intraretinal, preretinal, and vitreous hemorrhages are common. They are often accompanied by intracranial hemorrhage and may be indicative of the presence of subdural hemorrhage even if a CT scan is normal. Unexplained retinal hemorrhages in children less than 3 years of age without external evidence of head injury is strongly suggestive of child abuse.

Blunt trauma to the head and eyes is a more readily recognized form of child abuse. Ocular manifestations include subconjunctival hemorrhage, hyphema, cataract, lens subluxation, glaucoma; retinal, vitreous, intrascleral, and optic nerve hemorrhages; and papilledema.

Victims of child abuse may present initially to ophthalmologists, and the diagnosis must be kept in mind. Ophthalmologists may also provide evidence of injuries to the head and eyes in children presenting with unexplained injuries to other parts of the body.

Learning Disabilities & Dyslexia

Ophthalmologists are often asked to evaluate children with suspected learning disabilities in order to rule out ocular disorders. Dyslexia is the most common type of learning disability and is characterized by the inability to develop good reading and writing skills. Affected children are usually of normal intelligence and have no associated physical or visual abnormalities. Parents and educators sometimes attribute learning disabilities to visual perceptual abnormalities, but most of these affected children have no visual or ocular impairment. It is believed that dyslexia is caused by a specific defect of information processing in the central nervous system. The diagnosis of learning disabilities can be readily made by education specialists, and treatment is often effective in ameliorating this condition. When asked to evaluate a child with a learning disorder, the ophthalmologist should perform a complete examination and treat any refractive, strabismic, or amblyopic conditions identified. It is important to advise the parents that ocular or visual abnormalities generally do not lead to learning disabilities, and special educational programs may be necessary to treat these children. "Vision training," "visual therapy," and "perceptual training" programs have not been evaluated in a scientifically controlled, randomized, or prospective fashion, and thus their efficacy has not been proved. Ophthalmologists should provide indicated care of ocular problems and refer patients to appropriate educational programs for diagnosis and treatment of learning disabilities.

REFERENCES

Abrahamsson M, Sjöstrand J: Natural history of infantile anisometropia. Br J Ophthalmol 1996;80:860.

Akduman L, Kaplan HJ, Tyschen L: Prevalence of uveitis in an outpatient juvenile arthritis clinic: Onset of uveitis more than a decade after onset of arthritis. J Pediatr Ophthalmol Strabismus 1997;34:101.

Atkinson J et al: Two infant vision screening programmes: Prediction and prevention of strabismus and amblyopia from photo- and videorefractive screening. Eye 1996;10:189.

Awner S et al: Unilateral pseudophakia in children under 4 years. J Pediatr Ophthalmol Strabismus 1996;33:230.

Basti S, Ravishankar U, Gupta S: Results of a prospective evaluation of three methods of management of pediatric cataracts. Ophthalmology 1996;103;713.

Birch EE, Stager DR: The critical period for surgical treatment of dense congenital unilateral cataract. Invest Ophthalmol Vis Sci 1996;37:1532.

Bradford GM, Keech KV, Scott WE: Factors affecting visual outcome after surgery for bilateral congenital cataracts. Am J Ophthalmol 1994;117:58.

Brown GC et al: Systemic complications associated with retinal cryoablation for retinopathy of prematurity. Ophthalmology 1990;97:855.

Cryotherapy for Retinopathy of Prematurity Cooperative Group: Multicenter trial of cryotherapy for retinopathy of prematurity: Snellen visual acuity and structural outcome at 5 years after randomization. Arch Ophthalmol 1996;114:417.

Eden GF et al: Abnormal processing of visual motion in dyslexia revealed by functional brain imaging. Nature 1996;382:66.

Elner SG et al: Ocular and associated systemic findings in suspected child abuse: A necropsy study. Arch Ophthalmol 1990;108:1094.

Friendly DS, Jaafar MS, Morillo DL: A comparative study of grating and recognition visual acuity testing in children with anisometropic amblyopia without strabismus. Am J Ophthalmol 1990;110:293.

Fries PD, Katowitz JA: Congenital craniofacial anomalies of ophthalmic importance. Surv Ophthalmol 1990;35:87.

Good WV et al: Cortical visual impairment in children. Surv Ophthalmol 1994;38:351.

Harris CM et al: Intermittent horizontal saccade failure (ocular motor apraxia) in children. Br J Ophthalmol 1996;80:151.

Hungerford JL et al: External beam radiotherapy for retinoblastoma: I. Whole eye technique. Br J Ophthalmol 1995;79:109.

Johnson L et al: Severe retinopathy of prematurity in infants with birth weights less than 1250 grams: Incidence and outcome of treatment with pharmacologic serum levels of vitamin E in addition to cryotherapy from 1985 to 1991. J Pediatr 1995;127:632.

Kingston JE et al: Results of combined chemotherapy and radiotherapy for advanced intraocular retinoblastoma. Arch Ophthalmol 1996;114:1339.

Knight-Nanan DM et al: Advanced cicatricial retinopathy of prematurity: Outcome and complications. Br J Ophthalmol 1996;80:343.

Knight-Nanan DM, O'Keefe M: Refractive outcome in eyes with retinopathy of prematurity treated with cryotherapy or diode laser: 3 year follow-up. Br J Ophthalmol 1996;80:998.

Lambert SR, Taylor D, Kriss A: The infant with nystagmus, normal appearing fundi, but an abnormal ERG. Surv Ophthalmol 1989;34:173.

Lewis TL, Maurer D, Brent HP: Development of grating acuity in children treated for unilateral or bilateral congenital cataract. Invest Ophthalmol Vis Sci 1995; 36:2080.

Mercuri E et al: Visual function and perinatal focal cerebral infarction. Arch Dis Child 1996;75:F76.

Mets MB: Drops, drops, drops in pediatric ophthalmology. In: *Year Book of Ophthalmology 1988.* Deutsch E (editor). Year Book, 1988.

Nelson LB (editor): *Harley's Pediatric Ophthalmology,* 4th ed. Saunders, 1998.

Newman DK et al: Preschool vision screening: Outcome of children referred to the hospital eye service. Br J Ophthalmol 1996;80:1077.

Noorani HZ et al: Cost comparison of molecular versus conventional screening of relatives at risk for retinoblastoma. Am J Hum Genet 1996;59:301.

Quinn GE et al: Visual acuity of eyes after vitrectomy for retinopathy of prematurity: Follow-up at 5 years. Ophthalmology 1996;103;595.

Saunders KJ: Early refractive development in humans. Surv Ophthalmol 1995;40:207.

Schnall BM, Christian CJ: Conservative treatment of congenital dacryocele. J Pediatr Ophthalmol Strabismus 1996;33:219.

Shields CL et al: Treatment of retinoblastoma with indirect ophthalmoscope laser photocoagulation. J Pediatr Ophthalmol Strabismus 1995;32:317.

Strömland K, Miller M, Cook C: Ocular teratology. Surv Ophthalmol 1991;35:429.

Taylor D: *Pediatric Ophthalmology,* 2nd ed. Blackwell Science, 1997.

Toma NMG et al: External beam radiotherapy for retinoblastoma: II. Lens sparing technique. Br J Ophthalmol 1995;79:112.

Wilkins B: Head injury: Abuse or accident. Arch Dis Child 1997;76:393.

Young JDH, MacEwen CJ, Ogston SA: Congenital nasolacrimal duct obstruction in the second year of life: A multicentre trial of management. Eye 1996;10:485.

Genetic Aspects of Ocular Disorders

18

Paul Riordan-Eva, FRCS, FRCOphth, & Taylor Asbury, MD

Genetic influences are being described in an increasing number of diseases, and a primary causative role for genetic defects is being more clearly defined in many instances. Thus, it becomes increasingly important to understand the principles of genetic transmission. Much of the background work in clinical genetics has been done in ophthalmology. The eye seems to be unusually prone to genetically determined disease, and an accurate diagnosis of ocular disease can usually be arrived at on the basis of careful clinical examination.

Clinicians can estimate the risk of occurrence of many genetically determined diseases (usually the rare but severe ones), but the familial incidence of many other diseases also known to be genetically determined still cannot be accurately predicted.

Mechanisms of Inheritance

An individual's genetic identity (**genotype**) is carried in the DNA found in the cell nucleus and mitochondria. The DNA in the nucleus of the normal human somatic cell is organized into 23 pairs of **chromosomes.** Twenty-two of these pairs are somewhat similar (homologous) and are therefore termed **autosomal.** The twenty-third pair is composed of the **sex chromosomes** (X and Y). In the female, this pair is homologous (XX), whereas in the male it is heterologous (XY). A number of agents (quinacrine mustard, trypsin, Giemsa's stain) produce morphologic banding of human chromosomes that permits their identification and classification into a number of groups. Mitochondrial DNA is a double-stranded circular molecule of which each mitochondrion has several copies.

The genotype is composed of many small functional units termed **genes,** which are situated at specific sites (**loci**) along the length of the DNA. Genes are thus also arranged in pairs. The alternate forms of a gene at a locus controlling a particular characteristic are known as **alleles.** There are commonly two alternate forms, but there may be more. When the alleles at a particular locus are the same, the individual is said to be homozygous, and when they are different, heterozygous.

Genes exert their effects by controlling the production of proteins within the cell. Complementary copies of the DNA constituting specific genes are formed with RNA, and these are used to direct protein synthesis. The mechanisms regulating gene expression are complex.

DNA recombinant technology using isolated human DNA fragments inserted into bacterial cells has led to the identification of the DNA sequences and protein products of specific genes. Linkage studies and DNA probes have identified the position of specific gene loci and carriers for certain mutant genes.

The **gametes** (spermatozoon and ovum) are produced by a special type of cell division called **reduction-division meiosis,** in which the 23 pairs of chromosomes dissociate, each daughter cell receiving one chromosome of each pair. One of each pair passes into each daughter cell as a random occurrence. Exchange of chromosomal material (**translocation**) between the members of each pair also occurs. At fertilization, each chromosome of the spermatozoon joins its corresponding chromosome of the ovum to produce a cell with 46 chromosomes of unique genetic constitution. Mitochondrial DNA is derived entirely from the ovum. All cell divisions after fertilization (**mitosis**) involve duplication and separation of all the chromosomes to produce cells with the constant number of 46 chromosomes and identical genetic constitution.

The expression of the genotype in physical characteristics is known as the **phenotype.** The inheritance of certain characteristics of the human phenotype, such as eye color, can be explained on the basis of interaction between the two alleles at a single chromosomal locus. Each allele determines the development of one form of the particular characteristic. In the homozygous individual, this form is correspondingly expressed. In the heterozygous individual, one allele is said to be **dominant** because it determines the phenotype, while the other is **recessive** (not expressed). This is the basis of **mendelian inheritance,** from which are derived many of the terms used to describe patterns of inheritance. The inheritance of many phenotypic characteristics, however, cannot easily be classified in this way. This has led to modifications of the original mendelian concepts, including variable expression and variable penetration of genes. Recent improvements in the understanding of gene regulation and expression, as well as recognition of the role of environmental factors, have demonstrated why this model breaks down. Nevertheless, the framework of mendelian inheritance is still of immense value in clinical genetics as a means of describing modes of inheritance and estimating the risk of transmission of certain genetically determined abnormalities. The major alternative patterns of inheritance are those due to chromosomal abnormalities, maternal inheritance due to defects of mitochondrial DNA, and those described as multifactorial, involving multiple genes or major environmental influences.

MENDELIAN INHERITANCE

Mendelian inheritance can be divided into three main patterns: autosomal dominant, autosomal recessive, and X-linked recessive.

Autosomal Dominant Inheritance

An abnormal dominant gene produces its specific abnormality even though its paired gene (allele) is normal. Males and females are affected alike and—being heterozygous—have a theoretic 50% chance of passing along the affected gene (and therefore the abnormality) to each of their offspring even when mated to genotypically normal individuals (Figure 18–1).

Given a particular group of pedigrees, autosomal dominant inheritance is established if the following conditions are met: (1) Males and females are equally affected. (2) Direct transmission has occurred over two or more generations. (3) About 50% of individuals in the pedigrees are affected.

Quite a large number of uncommon but serious diseases with ocular manifestations are transmitted in this way: forms of juvenile glaucoma, Marfan's syndrome, congenital stationary night blindness (Figure 18–2), osteogenesis imperfecta, neurofibromatosis 1 and 2, Lindau-Von Hippel disease, and tuberous sclerosis. The process of natural selection tends to keep most of these serious diseases at a low incidence since many of these persons do not or cannot reproduce. By contrast, autosomal dominant optic atrophy, now known to have a genetic locus on chromosome 3, is in general a less serious disorder affecting many large families.

Dominant disease may be more or less severe from generation to generation depending upon its **expression;** a disease with "variable expression" is one that can occur in a mild or severe form. An example is neurofibromatosis 1, in which genotypically affected individuals may have merely café au lait spots or may have many serious manifestations. One cannot predict if or when the disease will be more serious (with central nervous system tumors or optic nerve gliomas) in a succeeding generation. In other autosomal dominant conditions, severity of expression increases with each successive generation. This phenomenon, known as **anticipation,** has been demonstrated in a number of neurologic conditions, such as Huntington's disease, to be due to increasing numbers of mutated copies of the same triplet of base pairs, from which DNA is made. Severity of expression may also depend upon whether the mutation is inherited from the father or the mother. If the genetic pattern is present but there is no evidence of the disease, one says that its **penetrance** is reduced. It may be quite difficult to differentiate dominant inheritance with reduced penetrance from recessive inheritance (see below).

In certain diseases such as hemoglobin S disease, there is a clearly defined intermediate phenotype that corresponds to the heterozygous individual. This is known as **codominant inheritance.**

Autosomal Recessive Inheritance

Abnormal recessive genes must lie in pairs (duplex state) to produce manifest abnormality. Thus, each parent must contribute one recessive abnormal gene. Each parent is clinically unaffected (genotypically affected but phenotypically normal), since a normal dominant gene makes the abnormal gene recessive (Figure 18–3).

It is difficult to establish that a given disease results from autosomal recessive inheritance. Some of the criteria used to establish recessive inheritance are the following:

(1) Occurrence of the same disease in collateral branches of the family.

(2) History of consanguinity. The higher the rate of consanguinity in the pedigrees of a given disease, the more likely the disease is to be recessive. Consanguinity creates greater opportunities for the genes to lie in the duplex state, inasmuch as an individual with two related parents can receive the same affected gene

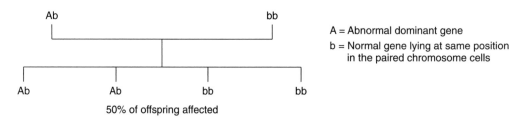

Figure 18–1. Autosomal dominant inheritance.

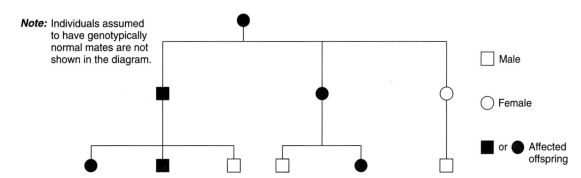

Note: Individuals assumed to have genotypically normal mates are not shown in the diagram.

☐ Male

◯ Female

■ or ● Affected offspring

Figure 18–2. Pedigree of congenital stationary night blindness (abnormal dominant gene).

from each, a common ancestor having originally passed on the affected gene.

(3) The occurrence of the disease in about 25% of siblings. This only holds for groups of pedigrees. There is a 25% chance that the two abnormal genes will be passed on to one individual. There is a 50% chance that a normal gene will modify the affected gene. In this case, the individual is a carrier of the disease (just like the parents) but is not affected with the disease (ie, genotypically affected but phenotypically normal). In the remaining 25% of siblings, two normal genes lie together and the abnormal gene is completely lost (ie, the individual is genotypically normal). Although a number of pedigrees are required to definitely establish recessive inheritance, even a single pedigree is suggestive if more than one sibling is similarly affected without an antecedent history.

Many disease processes have been definitely established as resulting from autosomal recessive inheritance, and many others are suspected of having such a genetic background. Included among the definite cases are Laurence-Moon-Biedl syndrome and inborn errors of metabolism such as oculocutaneous albinism (Figure 18–4), galactokinase deficiency, and Tay-Sachs disease.

X-Linked (Sex-Linked) Recessive Inheritance

Many of the genes of the X chromosome are unopposed by a gene of the Y chromosome. Abnormalities of these genes cause disease in the male, whereas in the female an abnormal recessive gene of the sex chromosome is masked by its normal allele. There-

fore, nearly all of the X-linked diseases are manifested in males, whereas the disease is passed through the female. A male and his maternal grandfather are affected, and the intervening female is the carrier.

The criteria for X-linked inheritance are (1) that only males are affected, (2) that the disease is transmitted through carrier females to half of the sons, and (3) that there is no father-to-son transmission.

Among the important eye diseases with an X-linked genetic pattern are color blindness (Figure 18–5), ocular albinism, and one type of retinitis pigmentosa.

Females have a mosaic of somatic cells consisting of cell groups with one X chromosome functioning and cell groups with the other X chromosome functioning (Lyon hypothesis). When the female is a carrier of an X-linked disease, this mosaicism is occasionally detectable. Such is the case in female carriers of ocular albinism, in whom groups of pigmented and albino retinal pigment epithelial cells are visible ophthalmoscopically.

MATERNAL INHERITANCE

Maternal inheritance, in which a condition is inherited only from the mother, does not obey the accepted rules of any form of mendelian inheritance. It has particular relevance to ophthalmology because its existence was recognized through the study of inheritance patterns in Leber's hereditary optic neuropathy, which causes severe bilateral optic neuropathy in young adults. The explanation for maternal inheritance is a

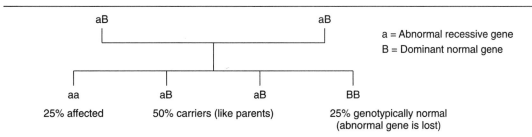

aB

aB

a = Abnormal recessive gene
B = Dominant normal gene

aa
25% affected

aB

aB

50% carriers (like parents)

BB
25% genotypically normal
(abnormal gene is lost)

Figure 18–3. Autosomal recessive inheritance. Mating of two carriers.

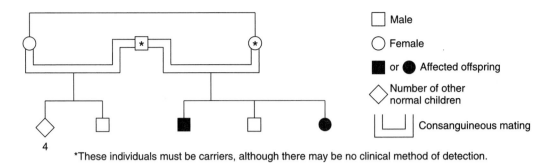

*These individuals must be carriers, although there may be no clinical method of detection.

Figure 18–4. Pedigree of oculocutaneous albinism (autosomal recessive gene). In this case a man married successively two sisters, his first cousins.

defect in mitochondrial DNA, which is derived entirely from the individual's mother.

Maternal inheritance should produce a genetic abnormality that is transmitted only through the female line and then potentially to all offspring, that is never found in the offspring of an affected male, and that is detectable in every generation, with males and females being equally affected.

In almost all families affected by Leber's hereditary optic neuropathy, a mitochondrial DNA point mutation involving a gene responsible for the production of a protein involved in oxidative phosphorylation can be identified. The most frequent mutation, known as the Wallace mutation, is at base pair 11778 (see Chapter 14). The inheritance pattern of Leber's hereditary optic neuropathy does not in fact fulfill all the features outlined above, which suggests the presence of other influences. The significant anomaly is a marked male gender bias in clinical expression of the disease.

CHROMOSOMAL ABNORMALITIES

When mitosis is interrupted in metaphase, the chromosomes can be spread on a slide, counted, and photographed. These cytogenetic studies have made pos-

sible the classification of chromosomes into seven groups based upon characteristics such as size and the position of the centromere. The study of cytogenetics has also established that some clinical states can be correlated with an abnormal number of chromosomes, most frequently one more (trisomy) or occasionally one less (monosomy) than the normal number of 46. A few of the more common syndromes are summarized briefly below. Since the addition or subtraction of an entire gene is obviously a major genetic abnormality, these syndromes are characterized by many and extensive deformities. Many such abnormal fertilizations result in early abortions and stillbirths.

1. SYNDROMES ASSOCIATED WITH AN ABNORMAL NUMBER OF CHROMOSOMES

Trisomy 13 (Patau's Syndrome)

Anophthalmos, microphthalmos, retinal dysplasia, optic atrophy, coloboma of the uvea, and cataracts are the major eye anomalies; cerebral defects, cleft palate, heart lesions, polydactyly, and hemangiomas are the

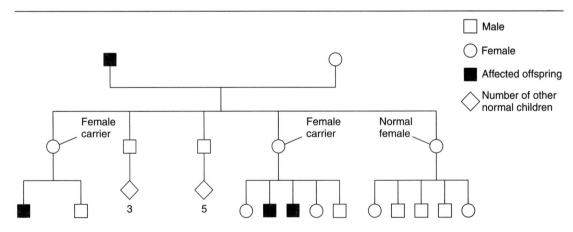

Figure 18–5. Pedigree of red-green color blindness (X-linked recessive inheritance).

more severe nonophthalmic changes. Death by age 6 months is the rule.

Trisomy 18
(Edwards' Syndrome)

The main features of this rare syndrome are mental and physical retardation, congenital heart defects, and renal abnormalities. Corneal and lenticular opacities, unilateral ptosis, and optic atrophy have been described.

Trisomy 21
(Down's Syndrome)

Although Down's syndrome is a fairly common and well-known entity, the hereditary pattern was long ill-defined. Waardenburg originally suggested that Down's syndrome was a chromosomal problem in 1932. Cytogenetic studies in 1958 revealed an extra chromosome indistinguishable from chromosome 21. The principal manifestations are small stature, a flattened, round, mongoloid facies, saddle nose, thick lower lip, large tongue, soft, seborrheic skin, smooth hair, obesity, small genitalia, short fingers, a simian fold, congenital heart anomalies, mental retardation, and frequent psychic disturbances. The ocular signs include hyperplasia of the iris, narrow palpebral fissures with Oriental slant, strabismus, epicanthus, cataract, high myopia (33%), keratoconus, and Brushfield (silver-gray) spots on the iris.

The incidence of Down's syndrome is significantly increased in children born to older women, particularly those past age 35.

2. ABNORMALITIES INVOLVING SEX CHROMOSOMES

Turner's syndrome is a monosomy (45 chromosomes). For some reason, the affected female receives only one X chromosome. Clinically, growth retardation, rudimentary ovaries and female genitalia, amenorrhea, pterygium colli, epicanthus, cubitus valgus, and ptosis occur. Of particular ophthalmic interest is the high incidence of color blindness (8%). This is the same frequency as for males (the female incidence is 0.4%) and is readily explained by the fact that the normally recessive gene is unopposed and is expressed just as in the male.

Klinefelter's syndrome is a trisomy involving the X chromosomes. These phenotypical males have 47 chromosomes: the normal 44 autosomes and three sex chromosomes, XXY. These individuals are sterile, with small testes, a eunuchoid physique, and frequently gynecomastia. The ocular finding of interest is the very rare occurrence of color blindness, since the recessive X chromosome is masked by a normal dominant (as in the normal female).

OTHER GENETIC CONSIDERATIONS

Genetic Counseling

Valuable advice can often be given to families concerned with the percentage risk of transmitting serious disease to future generations. This entails a working knowledge of basic genetic principles and sensitive counseling skills. A careful history of the pedigree in question is very important, since a single disease may have more than one mode of transmission (eg, retinitis pigmentosa has three or more basic patterns, and within each of these there is a wide variation in severity of disease between families). On the other hand, careful inquiries about maternal health during pregnancy may suggest that the anomaly—eg, congenital cataracts—is developmental and therefore unrelated to the genes.

Consanguineous mating increases the prevalence of autosomal recessive traits, and the most likely explanation for two individuals' having the same recessive gene is the fact that they are related.

Prenatal Diagnosis

In some cases it is possible to offer families at risk for a specific hereditary disease the option of prenatal diagnosis. This may involve searching for chromosomal abnormalities or specific structural protein defects such as enzyme deficiencies. Currently, techniques are being devised to identify abnormalities at the gene level using DNA linkage studies (eg, in X-linked retinitis pigmentosa) or DNA probes. Prenatal diagnosis by testing amniotic fluid cells obtained by amniocentesis at 14–16 gestational weeks has become a safe and practical procedure. The list of hereditary diseases that can be diagnosed with this method is rapidly increasing. There is, however, a 3-week delay before results of cytogenetic analysis become available. Chorionic villus sampling has certain advantages: It can be undertaken at 8–12 gestational weeks, and results are known within 24 hours. Its overall safety is still being determined.

Genetic Carrier State

Recognition of the genetic carrier state makes possible more accurate prediction of possible disease transmission and helps to establish the genetic nature of a disease by providing an occasion for examination of relatives of affected individuals. Detection is possible in many diseases. There are three types:

(1) Autosomal dominant diseases in which the disease appears in a mild or subclinical form (low expression). Because the offspring of such individuals still have the theoretic 50% chance of passing on the disease process, the recognition of this carrier state is important in genetic counseling.

(2) Autosomal recessive diseases with heterozygous manifestations. Affected genes that are normally balanced by a normal allele may cause minor subclinical abnormalities that disclose the presence of the abnormal gene. One can predict the 25% possibility of occurrence of some autosomal recessive diseases if the carrier state can be recognized in both potential mates.

(3) Female carrier in X-linked recessive disease. Subclinical evidence of the disease in daughters of af-

fected fathers differentiates carriers from noncarriers in a number of X-linked recessive diseases (often quite obvious in tapetoretinal degenerative conditions).

Mutation

Mutation occurs when a gene undergoes alteration in the germ cell as a result of spontaneous chemical change within the gene and the change is manifested by a new characteristic. The causes of the change are not well understood, but such extrinsic environmental factors as heat, x-rays, and exposure to radioactive materials may induce it. Most often, the new characteristic is unfavorable (ie, disease-producing), but some mutations are favorable and account for the evolution of species (Darwin).

Certain mutations occur repeatedly in specific genes and cause specific disease. Hemophilia, which follows an X-linked pattern, and retinoblastoma, in which a single locus on chromosome 13 is involved, are examples of disease occurring as a result of mutation. Very few individuals with severe abnormalities reproduce, so that the incidence of such diseases is dependent very highly upon mutation. Mutations causing less severe diseases are inherited as dominant, recessive, or X-linked traits depending upon the type of mutated gene. Research into the genetics of retinitis pigmentosa has demonstrated that clinically identical patterns of disease may be caused by many different mutations.

Retinoblastoma

Recent advances in our understanding of the genetic basis of retinoblastoma illustrate many of the points discussed above. Retinoblastoma is a malignant tumor of retinal photoreceptors seen in childhood. Most cases are sporadic, without transmission to subsequent generations, but a significant proportion are familial. The "two-hit" hypothesis of oncogenesis for this and other hereditary cancers proposes that tumor development is a recessive trait at the cellular level and that two separate mutations are necessary to produce the required homozygous state. In retinoblastoma, the relevant mutation is deletion at the chromosomal locus 13q14. In sporadic cases, both mutations occur in the somatic cells of the retina, and for that reason the disease is not genetically transmissible. In familial cases, the first mutation is present in the germ cells, and the second develops in retinal cells.

In familial cases, predisposition for tumor development is inherited as an autosomal dominant trait, being present in 50% of children of retinoblastoma patients. Nine out of ten individuals who inherit the germ cell mutation develop the tumor. Familial cases tend to be bilateral and multifocal and to have onset at an early age, whereas sporadic cases are unilateral, unifocal, and appear later. Individuals who inherit the germ cell mutation are also known to have a greatly increased risk for development of independent second primary tumors—particularly osteosarcoma—in later life.

Present practice consists of regular screening of all siblings and children of retinoblastoma patients for the development of retinoblastoma. This necessitates frequent general anesthesia for ophthalmoscopy. It would be advantageous to be able to restrict the screening procedure to individuals truly at risk, ie, those who have inherited the germ cell mutation.

All bilateral cases and those with a family history can be assumed to be familial; unilateral cases may be familial or sporadic. Cases without a family history may be sporadic or may be the first of a series of familial cases following de novo mutation in the germ line. However, these features are not sufficient to reliably identify only those with the germ line mutation.

Fortunately, the necessary process of gene tracking is now becoming possible both by gene linkage studies, using the esterase-D protein, which has a gene locus close to that of the retinoblastoma gene; and by DNA probes for the esterase-D and retinoblastoma genes. These techniques are also applicable to prenatal diagnosis, using chorionic villus sampling. Consequently, it is theoretically possible to identify exactly which retinoblastoma cases are familial and to determine even before birth which siblings or children also possess the germ cell mutation, thus allowing termination of the pregnancy or a much more specific childhood screening program.

GLOSSARY OF GENETIC TERMS*

Abiotrophic disease: Genetically determined disease which is not evident at birth but which becomes manifest later in life.

Acquired: Contracted after birth or in utero.

Alleles: Alternative forms of an individual gene.

Anticipation: Progressive increase in severity of autosomal dominant disease in successive generations.

Autosomes: The chromosomes (22 pairs of autosomes in humans) other than the sex chromosomes.

Chromosome: A small thread-like or rod-like structure into which the nuclear chromatin separates during mitosis. The number of chromosomes is constant for any given species (23 pairs in humans: 22 pairs of autosomes and one pair of sex chromosomes).

Codominant inheritance: Inheritance pattern in which the individuals heterozygous for the abnormality have a phenotype distinguishable from that of the homozygote.

* Modified from Krupp MA et al: *Physician's Handbook,* 21st ed. Lange, 1985.

Congenital: Existing at or before birth; not necessarily hereditary.

DNA probes: DNA fragments used to locate specific gene sequences to which they are complementary.

Dominant: Designating a gene whose phenotypic effect largely or entirely obscures that of its allele.

Expressivity: Variability of phenotype amongst genotypically identical individuals.

Familial: Pertaining to traits, either hereditary or acquired, which tend to occur in families.

Gamete (germ cell): A cell that is capable of uniting with another cell in sexual reproduction (ie, the ovum and spermatozoon).

Gene: A unit of heredity which occupies a specific locus in the chromosome which, either alone or in combination, produces a single characteristic. It is usually a single unit that is capable of self-duplication or mutation.

Genetic carrier state: A condition wherein a given hereditary characteristic is not manifest in one individual but may be genetically transmitted to the offspring of that individual.

Genotype: The hereditary constitution, or combination of genes, that characterizes a given individual or a group of genetically identical organisms.

Germ cell: See Gamete, above.

Hereditary: Transmitted from ancestor to offspring through the germ plasm.

Heterozygous: Having two members of a given hereditary factor pair that are dissimilar, ie, the two genes of an allelic pair are not the same.

Homozygous: Having two members of a given hereditary factor pair that are similar, ie, the two genes of an allelic pair are identical.

Linkage studies: Statistical analysis of frequency of association of genetic abnormalities to estimate the proximity of the gene loci.

Lyon hypothesis: Inactivation of one X chromosome in each somatic cell of the female, the inactivated chromosome forming the sex chromatin (Barr) body.

Meiosis: A special type of cell division occurring during the maturation of sex cells, by which the normal diploid set of chromosomes is reduced to a single (haploid) set, two successive nuclear divisions occurring, while the chromosomes divide only once.

Mitosis: Cell division in which daughter nuclei receive identical components of the number of chromosomes characteristic of the species.

Monosomy: The existence of one chromosome of one variety, rather than the normal pair of chromosomes.

Mosaicism: The presence of cells of functionally different genetic constitution within the same individual. Normally present in the female in respect of the X chromosome (Lyon hypothesis).

Mutation: A transformation of a gene, often sudden and dramatic, with or without known cause, into a different gene occupying the same locus as the original gene on a particular chromosome; the new gene is allelic to the normal gene from which it has arisen.

Penetrance: The likelihood or probability that a gene will become morphologically (phenotypically) expressed. The degree of penetrance may depend upon acquired as well as genetic factors.

Phenotype: The visible characteristics of an individual or those which are common to a group of apparently identical individuals.

Recessive: Designating a gene whose phenotypic effect is largely or entirely obscured by the effect of its allele.

Sex chromosome: The chromosome or pair of chromosomes that determines the sex of the individual. (In the human female, the sex chromosome pair is homologous, XX; in the male, heterologous, XY.)

Sex linkage: See X linkage, below.

Somatic cells: Cells incapable of reproducing the organism.

Translocation: Exchange of DNA fragments between chromosomes at the time of meiosis.

Trisomy: The existence of three chromosomes of one variety, rather than the normal pair of chromosomes.

X linkage: The pattern of inheritance of genes located on the X chromosome.

Zygote: The cell formed by the union of two gametes in sexual reproduction.

REFERENCES

Bird AC: Retinal photoreceptor dystrophies. Am J Ophthalmol 1995;119:543.

Charles SJ et al: Genetic counselling in X-linked ocular albinism: Clinical features of the carrier state. Eye 1992;6:75.

Damji KF, Allingham RR: Molecular genetics is revolutionizing our understanding of ophthalmic disease. Am J Ophthalmol 1997;124:530.

Della NG: Molecular biology in ophthalmology: A review of principles and recent advances. Arch Ophthalmol 1996;114:457.

Dryja TP: Doyne Lecture: Rhodpsin and autosomal dominant retinitis pigmentosa. Eye 1992;6:1.

Harper PS: *Practical Genetic Counselling,* 3rd ed. Wright, 1988.

Jay B: New light on visual pigment genes. Br J Ophthalmol 1990;74:238.

Jones KL: *Smith's Recognizable Patterns of Human Malformation,* 4th ed. Saunders, 1988.

Lichter PR: Genetic clues to glaucoma's secrets. Am J Ophthalmol 1994;117:706.

MacDonald IM, Sasi R: Molecular genetics of inherited eye disorders. Clin Invest Med 1994;17:454.

McKusick VA: The defect in Marfan syndrome. Nature 1991;352:279.

McKusick VA: *Mendelian Inheritance in Man,* 8th ed. Johns Hopkins Univ Press, 1988.

Moore AT, Evans K: Molecular genetics of central retinal dystrophies. Aust N Z J Ophthalmol 1996;24:189.

Musarella MA: Gene mapping of ocular diseases. Surv Ophthalmol 1992;36:285.

Newman NJ: Mitochondrial disease and the eye. Ophthalmol Clin North Am 1992;5:405.

Noorani HZ et al: Cost comparison of molecular versus conventional screening of relatives at risk for retinoblastoma. Am J Hum Genet 1996;59:301.

Pagon RA: Retinitis pigmentosa. Surv Ophthalmol 1988; 33:137.

Pyeritz RE: Medical genetics. In: *Current Medical Diagnosis & Treatment 1998.* Tierney LM Jr, McPhee SJ, Papadakis MA (editors). Appleton & Lange, 1998.

Ragge NK: Clinical and genetic patterns of neurofibromatosis 1 and 2. Br J Ophthalmol 1993;77:662.

Rennie WA (editor): *Goldberg's Genetic and Metabolic Eye Diseases,* 2nd ed. Little, Brown, 1986.

Wiggs JL: *Molecular Genetics of Ocular Disease.* Wiley-Liss, 1995.

Ocular & Orbital Trauma

19

Taylor Asbury, MD, & James J. Sanitato, MD

Ocular trauma is a common cause of unilateral blindness in children and young adults; persons in these age groups sustain the majority of severe ocular injuries. Young adults—especially men—are the most likely victims of penetrating ocular injuries. Domestic accidents, violent assaults, exploding batteries, sports-related injuries, and motor vehicle accidents are the most common circumstances in which ocular trauma occurs. Increasingly, ocular injuries are the result of paintball air gun mishaps and air bag deployment in automobile accidents.

INITIAL EXAMINATION OF OCULAR TRAUMA

The history should include an estimate of visual acuity prior to and immediately following the injury. It should be noted whether any visual loss was slowly progressive or sudden in onset. An intraocular foreign body must be suspected if there is a history of hammering, grinding, or explosions. Injuries in a child with a history that is not appropriate for the injury sustained should raise a suspicion of child abuse (see Chapter 17).

Physical examination begins with the measurement and documentation of visual acuity. If visual loss is severe, check for light projection, two-point discrimination, and the presence of an afferent pupillary defect. Test ocular motility and periorbital skin sensation, and palpate for defects in the bony orbital rim. At the bedside, the presence of enophthalmos can be determined by viewing the profiles of the corneas from over the brow. If a slitlamp is not available in the emergency room, a penlight, loupe, or direct ophthalmoscope set on +10 (black numbers) can be used to examine the tarsal surfaces of the lids and the anterior segment for injury.

The corneal surface is examined for foreign bodies, wounds, and abrasions. The bulbar conjunctiva is inspected for hemorrhage, foreign material, or lacerations. The depth and clarity of the anterior chamber are noted. The size, shape, and light reaction of the pupil should be compared with the other eye to ascertain if an afferent pupillary defect is present in the injured eye. If the eyeball is undamaged, the lids, palpebral conjunctiva, and fornices can be more thoroughly examined, including inspection after eversion of the upper lid. The direct and indirect ophthalmoscopes are used to view the lens, vitreous, optic disk, and retina. Photographic documentation is useful for medicolegal purposes in all cases of external trauma. In all cases of ocular trauma, the apparently uninjured eye should also be carefully examined.

Immediate Management of Ocular Trauma

If there is obvious rupture of the globe, one should avoid further manipulation until the patient has been given general anesthesia. No cycloplegic agents or topical antibiotics should be applied prior to surgery because of potential toxicity to exposed intraocular tissues. A Fox shield (or the bottom third of a paper cup) is taped over the eye, and parenteral broad-spectrum antibiotics are started. Analgesics, antiemetics, and tetanus antitoxin are given as needed, with restriction of food and fluids. Induction of general anesthesia should not include the use of depolarizing neuromuscular blocking agents, because these transiently increase pressure on the globe and thus increase any tendency to herniation of intraocular contents. Small children may also be better examined initially with the aid of a short-acting general anesthetic.

In severe injuries, it is important for the nonophthalmologist to bear in mind the possibility of causing further damage by unnecessary manipulation while attempting to do a complete ocular examination.

Caution: Topical anesthetics, dyes, and other medications placed in an injured eye *must be sterile.* Both tetracaine and fluorescein are available in sterile, individual dose units.

ABRASIONS & LACERATIONS OF THE LIDS

Particulate matter should be removed from abrasions of the lids to reduce skin tattooing. The wound is then irrigated with saline and covered with an antibiotic ointment and sterile dressing. Avulsed tissue is cleaned and reattached. Because of the excellent vascularity of the lids, there is a good chance that ischemic necrosis will not occur.

Partial-thickness lacerations of the lids not involving the lid margin may be surgically repaired in the same way as other skin lacerations. Full-thickness lid lacerations involving the lid margin, however, must be repaired carefully to prevent marginal lid notching and trichiasis (Figure 19–1).

Correct lid repair requires precise approximation of the lacerated lid margin, tarsal plate, and skin (Figure 19–1A). This is initiated by placing a double-armed 6-0 silk or nylon suture in mattress fashion through the edge of the tarsal plate. The needle is first passed through corresponding edges of the tarsal plate before exiting the meibomian gland orifice on the opposing side. The other needle with 6-0 silk is then passed similarly with a 3–4 mm spacing (Figure 19–1B). A second 6-0 silk suture is preplaced through lash follicles 2 mm equidistant on either side of the laceration. These sutures are not tied until the tarsus has been repaired with interrupted absorbable 5-0 sutures (Figure 19–1C). Finally, the skin is closed with interrupted 6-0 nylon sutures (Figure 19–1D). Antibiotic ointment is then applied to the repaired lid tissue.

If primary repair is not effected within 24 hours, edema may necessitate delayed closure. The wound should be cleaned thoroughly and antibiotics administered. After swelling has subsided, repair may be performed. Debridement should be minimized, especially if the skin is not lax.

Lacerations near the inner canthus frequently involve the canaliculi. Early repair is desirable, since the tissue becomes more difficult to identify and repair when swollen. The value of direct repair of canalicular lacerations is debated. Simple apposition of the cut ends is often sufficient. Stenting or intubation may exacerbate the degree of canalicular damage and thus the risk of stenosis and may even result in damage to other parts of the canalicular system during surgical manipulation. Nevertheless, sharp lacerations through the distal canaliculus may benefit from repair with a Veirs rod or other form of stent. Similarly, avulsions or proximal canalicular lacerations may require silicone nasocanalicular intubation with Quickert probes. Various methods of intubating a single canaliculus have been described that serve to avoid the risky and traumatic use of pigtail probes, which are particularly likely to damage other parts of the canalicular system.

FOREIGN BODIES ON THE SURFACE OF THE EYE & CORNEAL ABRASIONS

Corneal foreign bodies and abrasion cause pain and irritation that can be felt during eye and lid movement, and corneal epithelial defects may cause a similar sensation. Fluorescein will stain the exposed basement membrane of an epithelial defect and can highlight aqueous leakage from penetrating wounds

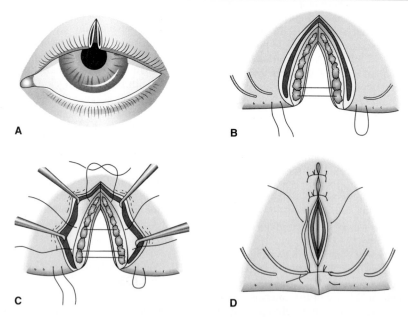

Figure 19–1. Repair of full-thickness lid laceration. **A:** The defect shown. **B:** Initial vertical mattress suture through tarsal plate. **C:** Interrupted suture closure of tarsal plate. **D:** Interrupted suture closure of skin. (Reproduced, with permission, from Phelps C: *Manual of Common Ophthalmic Surgical Procedures.* Churchill Livingstone, 1986.)

(positive Seidel test). A pattern of vertical scratch marks on the cornea indicates foreign bodies embedded on the tarsal conjunctival surface of the upper lid. Contact lens overwear produces corneal edema.

Simple corneal epithelial defects are treated with antibiotic ointment and a pressure patch to immobilize the lids. For removal of foreign matter, a topical anesthetic can be given and a spud or fine-gauge needle used to remove the material during slitlamp examination. A cotton-tipped applicator should not be used because it rubs off a large area of epithelium, often without removing the foreign body. Metallic rings surrounding copper or iron fragments (Figure 19–2) can be removed with a battery-operated drill with a burr tip. Deeply embedded inert materials (eg, glass, carbon) may be allowed to remain in the cornea. If removal of deeply embedded fragments is necessary or if there is an aqueous leak requiring sutures or cyanoacrylate glue, the procedure should be undertaken by microsurgical technique in an operating room, where the anterior chamber can be re-formed, if necessary, with or without viscoelastics under sterile conditions.

Following removal of a foreign body, antibiotic ointment should be instilled and the eye patched. The wound should be examined daily for evidence of infection until it is completely healed.

Never give a topical anesthetic solution to the patient for repeated use after a corneal injury, as this delays healing, masks further damage, and can lead to permanent corneal scarring. In addition, chronic anesthetic use can cause corneal infiltrates and ulceration which clinically can mimic the appearance of an infectious ulcer. Steroids should be avoided while an epithelial defect exists. Because corneal abrasions are a frequent complication of general anesthesia, care should be taken to avoid this injury during induction and throughout the procedure by taping the lids closed or instilling a lubricating ophthalmic ointment in the conjunctival fornices. Recurrent epithelial erosions sometimes follow corneal injuries and are treated with patching or a bandage contact lens.

PENETRATING INJURIES & CONTUSIONS OF THE EYEBALL

Rupture of the eyeball can occur as a result of sharp penetrating injury or blunt contusive force. Blunt trauma produces a rise in orbital and intraocular pressure, with deformation of the globe. Rapid decompression occurs when the eye wall ruptures or the orbital contents herniate into adjacent sinuses (blowout fracture; see below). The superonasal limbus is the most common site of globe rupture (contrecoup effect—the lower temporal quadrant being most exposed to trauma). Generally, blunt traumatic injuries have a worse prognosis than penetrating injuries because of the increased incidence of retinal detachment and intraocular tissue avulsion and herniation.

While most penetrating injuries cause a marked loss of vision, injuries due to small high-velocity particles generated by grinding or hammering might present with only mild pain and blurring. Other signs include hemorrhagic chemosis, conjunctival laceration, a shallow anterior chamber with or without an eccentrically placed pupil, hyphema, or vitreous hemorrhage. The intraocular pressure can be low, normal, or, rarely, slightly elevated.

In addition to rupture of the scleral wall, contusive forces to the eyeball can result in motility disorders, subconjunctival hemorrhage, corneal edema, iritis, hyphema, angle-recession glaucoma, traumatic mydriasis, rupture of the iris sphincter, iridodialysis, paralysis of accommodation, lens dislocation, and cataract. Injuries sustained by posterior structures include vitreal and retinal hemorrhages, retinal edema (commotio retinae, or Berlin's edema), retinal holes, vitreous base avulsions, retinal detachment, choroidal rupture, and optic nerve contusion or avulsion (Figures 19–3 and 19–4).

Many of these injuries cannot be seen upon external examination. Some, such as cataract, may not develop until days or weeks after the injury. The use of ultrasonic biomicroscopy has recently aided in diagnosing angle recession, iridodialysis, lens subluxation, and intraocular foreign bodies when visualization is limited by media opacities.

Treatment

Except for injuries involving rupture of the eyeball itself, most of the effects of contusion of the eye do not require immediate surgical treatment. However, any injury severe enough to cause intraocular hemorrhage increases the risk of delayed secondary hemorrhage and possible intractable glaucoma and permanent damage to the eyeball. The further management of these cases is described in the section below on hyphema.

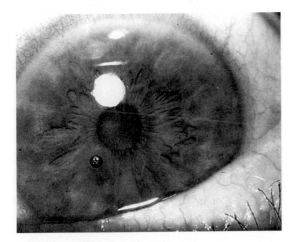

Figure 19–2. Metallic corneal foreign body. (Courtesy of A Rosenberg.)

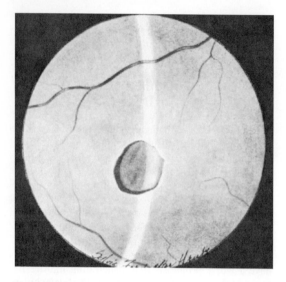

Figure 19–3. Hole in retina, macular area, posttraumatic.

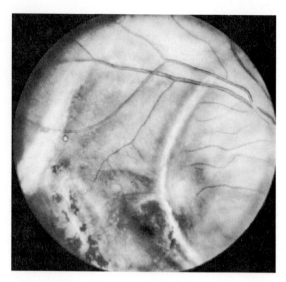

Figure 19–4. Choroidal ruptures. (Photo by Diane Beeston.)

In the closure of anterior segment wounds, microsurgical techniques should be used. Corneal lacerations are repaired with 10-0 nylon sutures to form a watertight closure. An incarcerated iris or ciliary body exposed for less than 24 hours can be reposited in the globe with viscoelastics or by introducing a cyclodialysis spatula through a limbal stab incision and sweeping the tissue out of the wound. If this cannot be achieved, if the tissue has been exposed for more than 24 hours, or if it is ischemic and severely damaged, then the prolapsing tissue should be excised at the level of the wound lip. Any excised tissue should be sent for pathologic examination. Cultures are taken for investigation of possible bacterial or fungal infection. Lens remnants and blood are removed with mechanical irrigation and aspiration or vitrectomy equipment. Anterior chamber reformation during repair is achieved with viscoelastics, air, or physiologic intraocular fluids.

Scleral wounds are closed with interrupted 8-0 or 9-0 nonabsorbable sutures. The rectus muscles may be temporarily disinserted to provide better exposure. Posterior scleral exit wounds in a double penetrating injury are self-sealing, and generally no attempt is made at closure.

The prognosis for traumatic retinal detachments is poor because of macular injury, giant retinal tears, and formation of intravitreal fibrovascular membranes that occur with penetrating injury. Such intravitreal membranes generate sufficient contractile force to detach the retina. Vitrectomy is effective in their treatment, but the timing of this procedure remains controversial. Early vitrectomy with intravitreal antibiotics is indicated for endophthalmitis. In noninfected cases, delaying surgery for 10–14 days may decrease the risk of intraoperative hemorrhage and per-

mit a posterior vitreous detachment to develop, making surgery technically easier.

Vitreoretinal surgery in the presence of large corneal wounds can be done through a temporary Landers-Foulks keratoprosthesis prior to corneal grafting. Primary enucleation or evisceration should only be considered when the globe is completely disorganized. The fellow eye is susceptible to sympathetic ophthalmia whenever penetrating ocular trauma occurs, particularly if there has been damage to the uveal tissues; fortunately, this complication occurs very rarely.

INTRAOCULAR FOREIGN BODIES
(Figure 19–5)

A complaint of discomfort or blurred vision in an eye with a history of striking metal upon metal, ex-

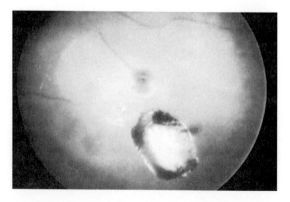

Figure 19–5. Ophthalmoscopic view of intraocular metallic (iron) foreign body in vitreous.

plosion, or high-velocity projectile injury should arouse a strong suspicion of intraocular foreign body. The anterior portion of the eye should be inspected with a loupe or slitlamp in an attempt to localize the wound of entry. Direct and indirect ophthalmoscopic visualization of an intraocular foreign body should be attempted. An orbital soft tissue x-ray or CT scan must be taken to verify the presence of a radiopaque foreign body as well as for medicolegal reasons. MRI is absolutely contraindicated in the identification and localization of intraocular foreign bodies because of the risk of movement of a metallic foreign body in the magnetic field.

Foreign bodies that have been identified and localized within the eye must be removed whenever possible. Particles of iron or copper must be removed to prevent later disorganization of ocular tissues from toxic degenerative changes (siderosis from iron and chalcosis from copper). Some of the newer alloys are more inert and may be tolerated. Other kinds of particles, such as glass or porcelain, may be tolerated indefinitely and are usually better left alone.

Localization of intraocular foreign bodies includes the geometric method of Sweet, the Comberg contact lens (containing a post and ring), ultrasonography, and coronal CT scan of the orbits. MRI is contraindicated in localizing intraocular metallic foreign bodies because the magnetic field produced during scanning can cause the foreign bodies to become high-velocity intraocular projectiles with catastrophic ocular effects.

Treatment

If the foreign body is anterior to the lens zonules, it should be removed through a limbal incision from the anterior chamber. If it is located behind the lens and anterior to the equator, it should be removed through the area of pars plana that is nearest to the foreign body because less retinal damage is caused in that manner. If the foreign body is posterior to the equator, it is best removed via the pars plana by vitrectomy and intraocular forceps, thus avoiding major choroidal hemorrhages from incisions of the posterior wall of the eyeball. This method is used for both magnetic and nonmagnetic foreign bodies. Special forceps are available for grasping spherical pellets.

Any damaged area of the retina must be treated with diathermy, photocoagulation, or endolaser coagulation to prevent retinal detachment.

HYPHEMA

Contusive forces will frequently tear the iris vessels and damage the anterior chamber angle. Blood in the aqueous may settle out in a visible layer (hyphema). Acute glaucoma occurs if the trabecular meshwork is blocked by fibrin and cells or if clot formation produces pupillary block.

Treatment

Patients with visible hyphema filling more than 5% of the anterior chamber should be placed at bed rest, and steroid drops should be instilled in the affected eye for 5 days. Pupillary dilation may increase the risk of rebleeding and thus is often deferred until the hyphema has resolved. Initial assessment for posterior segment damage may thus require ultrasound examination. The eye should be examined frequently for secondary bleeding, glaucoma, or corneal blood staining from iron pigment. Rebleeding occurs in 16–20% of cases within 2–3 days. This complication carries a high risk of glaucoma and corneal staining. Several studies indicate that the use of oral aminocaproic acid to stabilize clot formation reduces the risk of rebleeding. A dose of 100 mg/kg every 4 hours up to a maximum of 30 g/d for 5 days is a good regimen. If glaucoma occurs, management includes the use of ocular timolol 0.25% or 0.5.% applied twice a day; acetazolamide, 250 mg orally four times a day; and hyperosmotic agents (mannitol, glycerol, and sorbitol). Other ocular antihypertensives that may be used with timolol are dorzolamide applied three times a day and apraclonidine applied twice a day.

The hyphema must be surgically evacuated if the intraocular pressure remains elevated (> 35 mm Hg for 7 days or 50 mm Hg for 5 days) to avoid optic nerve damage and corneal staining. If the patient has a hemoglobinopathy, glaucomatous optic atrophy is likely to develop much more readily, and surgical evacuation of the clot should be considered much earlier. Vitrectomy instruments are used to remove the central clot and lavage the anterior chamber. The mechanized probe and irrigation port are introduced anterior to the limbus through clear cornea to avoid damage to the iris and lens. No attempt is made to extract the clot from the anterior chamber angle or from iris tissue. A peripheral iridectomy is then performed. Another means of clearing the anterior chamber is by viscoelastic evacuation. A small limbal incision is made to inject the viscoelastic, and a larger incision 180 degrees away allows the hyphema to be pushed out.

Late-onset glaucoma may follow months to years later as a result of angle recession. With rare exceptions, corneal blood staining clears slowly over a period of up to 1 year.

BURNS OF THE EYE

Chemical Burns

All chemical burns must be treated as ophthalmic emergencies. Immediate tap-water lavage should be started at the site of injury before the patient is transported. Any obvious foreign bodies should also be irrigated away if possible. In the emergency room, a brief history and examination precedes copious irrigation of the ocular surfaces, including the conjunctival fornices. Sterile isotonic saline (several liters per injured eye) is instilled with standard intravenous tubing. A lid speculum and local anesthetic infiltration of the lids may be necessary to overcome blepharospasm. Analgesics and topical anesthetic and cycloplegic agents are nearly always indicated. Use a moistened cotton-tipped applicator and jeweler's forceps to remove particulate matter from the fornices. Watch for respiratory distress due to soft tissue swelling of the upper airways. The pH of the ocular surface is checked by placing a strip of indicator paper in the fornix; resume irrigation if the pH is not between 7.3 and 7.7. After lavage, apply an antibiotic ointment and a pressure dressing.

Since alkali rapidly penetrates through ocular tissues and will continue to cause damage long after the injury is sustained, prolonged lavage and repeated pH checks are needed. Acids form a barrier of precipitated necrotic tissue that tends to limit further penetration and damage. Alkali burns cause an immediate rise in intraocular pressure owing to contraction of the sclera and trabecular meshwork damage. A secondary pressure rise occurs 2–4 hours later from the release of prostaglandins, which potentiate an intense uveitis. This is difficult to monitor through the opaque cornea. Treatment is with topical steroids, antiglaucoma agents, and cycloplegics during the first 2 weeks. Beyond 2 weeks, steroids must be used with caution because they inhibit reepithelialization. Corneal melting and possible perforation from continued collagenase activity can then occur. Ascorbate (vitamin C) and citrate drops are minimally effective for preventing corneal melting in patients with severe burns or persistent corneal epithelial defects. A trial with collagenase inhibitors (acetylcysteine) may prove beneficial. Corneal exposure and persistent epithelial defects are treated with artificial lubricants, tarsorrhaphy, or a bandage contact lens.

Long-term complications of chemical burns include angle-closure glaucoma, corneal scarring, symblepharon, entropion, and keratitis sicca. Competency of the conjunctival and scleral vasculature has been shown to be of prognostic value. A greater loss of perilimbal epithelium and conjunctival and scleral vasculature indicates a poorer prognosis.

Thermal Burns

Thermal burns of the lids are treated with topical antibiotics and sterile dressings. If corneal damage is sustained, the extensive lid swelling initially makes pressure patching unnecessary. After 2–3 days, ectropion and lid retraction begin. Tarsorrhaphies and moisture chambers fashioned from plastic wrap then protect the cornea. Full-thickness skin grafts are delayed until skin contraction is no longer progressing.

Ultraviolet irradiation, even in moderate doses, often produces a painful superficial keratitis. Pain often begins 6–12 hours after exposure. This keratitis follows exposure to an electric welding arc without the protection of a filter, short circuits in high-voltage

lines, or exposure to the reflections from snow without protective sunglasses ("snow blindness").

In severe cases of "flash burn," instillation of a sterile topical anesthetic may be necessary for examination. Treatment consists of pressure patching with an antibiotic ointment. A mydriatic is instilled if there is iritis.

Infrared exposure rarely produces an ocular reaction. ("Glassblower's cataract" is rare today but once was common among workers who were required to watch the color changes in molten glass in furnaces without proper filters.) Radiant energy from viewing the sun or an eclipse of the sun without an adequate filter, however, may produce a serious burn of the macula, resulting in permanent impairment of vision.

Excessive exposure to radiation (x-ray) produces cataractous changes that may not appear for many months after the exposure. The same risk is inherent with exposure to nuclear radiation.

INJURIES INVOLVING THE ORBIT & ITS CONTENTS

Orbital Fractures
(Figure 19–6)

Orbital fractures commonly occur with facial trauma. Fractures of the maxilla are classified by the Le Fort system: type I is below the orbital floor; type II passes through the nasal and lacrimal bones in addition to the maxilla forming the medial orbital floor; and type III involves the medial and lateral walls and the orbital floor in the presence of separation of the facial skeleton from the cranium. Orbital roof fractures are rare and are generally caused by penetrating injuries. If visual loss is progressing in the presence of an optic canal fracture, steroids and surgical decompression may be necessary. When visual loss is sudden and complete, however, recovery is less likely. Carotid-cavernous sinus fistulas are associated with

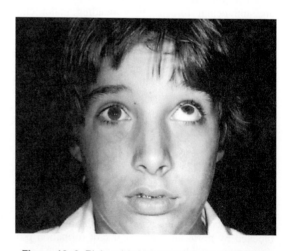

Figure 19–6. Right orbital blowout fracture in upgaze.

orbital apex fractures, and the orbit should therefore be auscultated for bruits.

Tripod fractures of the zygoma involve the orbital floor but in the absence of dislocation may not need surgical repair. Zygomatic arch fractures do not involve the orbit. Telescoping fractures of the frontal process of the maxilla and the lacrimal and ethmoid bones produce a saddle-nose deformity with telecanthus and lacrimal system obstruction.

When the orbital entrance receives a blow, the compressive forces can fracture the thin medial and inferior walls, with prolapse and possible entrapment of soft tissues. There may be associated intraocular injury, including hyphema, angle recession, and retinal detachment. If the blowout is large, enophthalmos of the globe may develop immediately. Enophthalmos can occur later after the swelling subsides and atrophy or scarring of the soft tissues develops.

Diplopia can be caused by direct neuromuscular damage or swelling of orbital contents. This must be differentiated from entrapment of the inferior rectus and oblique muscle or adjacent tissue within the fracture. When entrapment is present, passive movement of the eye with forceps (forced ductions test) is restricted. Sufficient time should pass to allow for spontaneous improvement in eye movements with the resolution of swelling. Sensation is tested in the distribution of the infraorbital nerve. Hypesthesia is present with orbital floor fractures. CT scanning with axial and coronal views provides the best assessment of orbital trauma. Plain x-rays may be helpful in the initial identification of bony injury.

The indications for surgical repair of the blowout fracture are (1) persistent diplopia within 30 degrees of the primary position of gaze in the presence of entrapment; (2) enophthalmos of 2 mm or more; or (3) a large fracture (half the orbital floor), which is likely to cause late enophthalmos. Delaying surgery for 1–2 weeks helps the surgeon to assess whether the diplopia will resolve without intervention. Longer delays decrease the likelihood of successful repair of enophthalmos and strabismus because of progressive scarring.

Surgical repair is usually accomplished via an infraciliary or transconjunctival route, though transantral and infraorbital approaches are also done. The periorbita is incised and elevated to expose the fracture site in the floor and medial walls. Herniated tissue is pulled back into the orbit, and the defect is covered by an alloplastic implant, with care being taken not to damage the infraorbital neurovascular bundle. Complications include blindness, diplopia, extrusion of the implant, or migration of the implant to press against the lacrimal sac, causing obstruction and dacryocystitis. Other complications include hemorrhage, infection, lower eyelid retraction, and infraorbital anesthesia. Subsequent procedures for strabismus and ptosis may be needed.

Penetrating Injury of the Orbit

Penetrating injuries of the orbital tissue may be produced by high-velocity projectiles or sharp instruments. Radiopaque foreign bodies can be localized by methods similar to those used in locating intraocular foreign bodies within the eye.

Contusions of the Orbit

Contusion injuries to the orbital contents may result in hemorrhage or subsequent atrophy of the tissue, with enophthalmos. Traumatic paresis of the extraocular muscles occasionally occurs but is usually transient.

Pulsating Exophthalmos Following Orbital Injury

Pulsating exophthalmos occasionally follows a penetrating or contusion injury to the orbital contents due to the formation of an arteriovenous shunt. A common site of involvement is a bone fracture into the cavernous sinus. Spontaneous resolution is uncommon, and closure of the shunt, usually by embolization, is often required.

PREVENTION OF INJURIES TO THE EYE (See Also Chapter 21.)

Persons engaging in industrial or athletic activities while wearing prescription lenses made of glass or plastic are at increased risk from shattered lens fragments. The eyewear most effective in preventing injuries consists of polycarbonate lenses in polyamide frames with a posterior retention rim. Solid wraparound frames should be used (rather than hinged frames) because they better withstand lateral blows. In athletic or high-risk recreational activities (eg, air or paint-pellet gun "war games"), guards without lenses do not always protect the eye adequately. Proper eye protection is particularly indicated for those playing racquetball, handball, and squash. The sight of many eyes has been lost in these sports, particularly from ocular contusion trauma in the absence of adequate eye protection.

REFERENCES

Aiello LP, Iwamoto M, Guyer DR: Penetrating ocular fishhook injuries. Surgical management and long-term visual outcome. Ophthalmology 1992;99:862.

Beare JD: Eye injuries from assault with chemicals. Br J Ophthalmol 1990;74:514.

Berinstein DM et al: Ultrasound biomicroscopy in anterior ocular trauma. Ophthalmic Surg Lasers 1997;28:201.

Brackup AB et al: Long-term follow-up of severely injured eyes following globe rupture. Ophthal Plast Reconstr Surg 1991;7:194.

Cooney MJ, Pieramici DJ: Eye injuries caused by bungee cords. Ophthalmology 1997;104:1644.

Dannenberg AL et al: Penetration eye injuries in the workplace. The National Eye Trauma System Registry. Arch Ophthalmol 1992;110:843.

Dannenberg AL, Parver LM, Fowler CJ: Penetrating eye injuries related to assault. The National Eye Trauma System Registry. Arch Ophthalmol 1992;110:849.

DeBustros S, Michels RG, Glaser BM: Evolving concepts in the management of posterior segment penetrating ocular injuries. Retina 1990;10(Suppl):S72.

Dhir SP et al: Ocular fireworks injuries in children. J Pediatr Ophthalmol Strabismus 1991;28:354.

Enger C, Schein OD, Tielsch JM: Risk factors for ocular injuries caused by air guns. Arch Ophthalmol 1996;114:469.

Farber MD, Fiscella R, Goldberg MF: Aminocaproic acid versus prednisone for the treatment of traumatic hyphema: A randomized clinical trial. Ophthalmology 1991;98:279.

Fuller DG, Hutton WL: Prediction of postoperative vision in eyes with severe trauma. Retina 1990;10(Suppl 1):20.

Green MA et al: Ocular and cerebral trauma in non-accidental injury in infancy: Underlying mechanisms and implications for paediatric practice. Br J Ophthalmol 1996;80:282.

Groessl S, Nanda SK, Mieler WF: Assault-related penetrating ocular injury. Am J Ophthalmol 1993;116:26.

Harris GJ, Fuerste FH: Lacrimal intubation in the primary repair of midfacial fractures. Ophthalmology 1987;94:242.

Jain BK, Talbot EM: Bungee jumping and intraocular haemorrhage. Br J Ophthalmol 1994;78:236.

Kearns P: Traumatic hyphaema: A retrospective study of 314 cases. Br J Ophthalmol 1991;75:137.

Klopfer J et al: Ocular trauma in the United States. Eye injuries resulting in hospitalization, 1984 through 1987. Arch Ophthalmol 1992;110:838.

Macewen CJ: Eye injuries: A prospective survey of 5671 cases. Br J Ophthalmol 1989;73:888.

Macken PL et al: Intralenticular foreign bodies: Case reports and surgical review. Ophthalmic Surg 1995;26:250.

Mamalis N et al: Blunt ocular trauma secondary to "war games." Ann Ophthalmol 1990;22:416.

Manchee FF, Goldberg RA, Mondino BJ: Air bag-related ocular injuries. Ophthalmic Surg Lasers 1997;28:246.

Meredith TA, Gordon PA: Pars plana vitrectomy for severe penetrating injury with posterior segment involvement. Am J Ophthalmol 1987;103:549.

Meyer DR et al: Management of canalicular injury associated with eyelid burns. Arch Ophthalmol 1995;113;900.

Mitchell GC et al: A two-year prospective study of penetrating ocular trauma at the Wilmer Ophthalmological Institute. Ann Ophthalmol 1987;19:104.

Napier SM et al: Eye injuries in athletes and recreation. Surv Ophthalmol 1996;41:229.

Ng CS et al: Factors related to the incidence of secondary haemorrhage in 462 patients with traumatic hyphema. Eye 1992;6:308.

Punnonen E, Laatikainen L: Prognosis of perforating eye injuries with intraocular foreign bodies. Acta Ophthalmol 1989;67:483.

Sharif KW, McGhee CN, Tomlinson RC: Ocular trauma caused by air-gun pellets: A ten year survey. Eye 1990;4:855.

Spaulding SC, Sternberg P Jr: Controversies in the management of posterior segment ocular trauma. Retina 1990;10(Suppl 1):S76.

Steinsapir KD, Goldberg RA: Traumatic optic neuropathy. Surv Ophthalmol 1994;38:487.

Strahlman E et al: Causes of pediatric eye injuries. A population-based study. Arch Ophthalmol 1990;108:603.

Teboul BK et al: Clinical evaluation of aminocaproic acid for managing traumatic hyphema in children. Ophthalmology 1995;102:1646.

Thompson JT et al: Infectious endophthalmitis after penetrating injuries with retained intraocular foreign bodies. Ophthalmology 1993;100:1468.

Verma L et al: Retinopathy after solar eclipse, 1995. Natl Med J India 1996;9:266.

Wagoner MD: Chemical injuries of the eye. Current concepts in pathophysiology and therapy. Surv Ophthalmol 1997;41:275.

Williams C et al: Outpatient management of small traumatic hyphaemas: Is it safe? Eye 1993;7:155.

Wilson TW, Jeffers JB, Nelson LB: Aminocaproic acid prophylaxis in traumatic hyphema. Ophthalmic Surg 1990;21:807.

Wilson WB et al: Magnetic resonance imaging of nonmetallic orbital foreign bodies. Am J Ophthalmol 1988;105:612.

Zachariades N, Papavassiliou D, Christopoulos P: Blindness after facial trauma. Oral Surg Oral Med Oral Pathol Oral Radiol Endod 1996;81:34.

Optics & Refraction

20

Paul Riordan-Eva, FRCS, FRCOphth

The correct interpretation of visual information depends on the eye's ability to focus incoming rays of light on the retina. An understanding of this process and how it is influenced by normal variations or ocular disease is essential to the successful use of any optical aid, eg, glasses, contact lenses, intraocular lenses, or low-vision aids. To achieve this understanding, it is necessary to master the concepts of geometric optics, which define the effect on light rays as they pass through different surfaces and media.

GEOMETRIC OPTICS

Speed, Frequency, & Wavelength of Light

Speed, frequency, and wavelength of light are related by the following expression:

$$\text{Frequency} = \frac{\text{Speed}}{\text{Wavelength}}$$

In different optical media, speed and wavelength of light change, but frequency is constant. Color depends on frequency, so that the color of a ray of light is not altered as it passes through optical media except by selective nontransmittance or fluorescence. The optical characteristics of a substance can only be defined with respect to clearly specified frequencies of light. A substance to be used for lenses to refract visible light is usually tested with the yellow sodium light (D line) and the blue (F line) and the red (C line) of a rarefied hydrogen discharge tube.

In a vacuum, the speed of all frequencies of light is the same, ie, 299,792.46 kilometers per second (186,282.40 statute miles per second). Since the frequency of the yellow D line is approximately 5.085×10^{14} Hz, the wavelength of this line in a vacuum is 0.5896 μm. Similarly, the wavelengths in a vacuum of the blue F and red C lines are 0.4861 μm and 0.6563 μm, respectively.

Index of Refraction

If the speed of a light ray is altered by a change in the optical medium, refraction of the ray will also occur (Figure 20–1). The effect of an optical substance on the speed of light is expressed as its index of re-

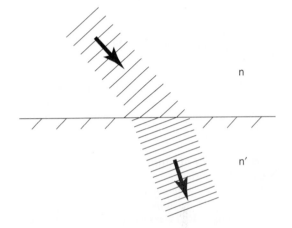

Figure 20–1. Refraction of light as it enters a transparent medium of higher refractive index n′.

fraction, n. The higher the index, the slower the speed and the greater the effect on refraction.

In a vacuum, n has the value of 1.00000. The **absolute index of refraction** of a substance is the ratio of the speed of light in a vacuum to the speed of light in the substance. The **relative index of refraction** of a substance is calculated with reference to the speed of light in air. The absolute index of refraction of air varies with the temperature, pressure, and humidity of the air and the frequency of the light, but it is about 1.00032. In optics, n is assumed to be relative to air unless specified as absolute.

Thermal Coefficient of Index of Refraction

The index of refraction changes with the temperature of the medium—it is higher when the substance is colder. This lability of n to temperature is different for different substances. The change in n per degree Celsius for the following substances (all to be multiplied by 10^{-7}) is as follows: glass, 1; fluorite, 10; plastic, 140; water, aqueous, and vitreous, 185. This makes plastic undesirable for precision optical devices. (Plastic also has eight times the thermal expansion of glass.) Water lenses date back to antiquity but are not practical, because of problems with thermal instability, evaporation, freezing, and susceptibility to contamination. It is interesting that in the eye, these objections all but disappear, making the fluid lenses of the eye acceptable.

Dispersion of Light

In a vacuum, the speed of all frequencies of light is the same; thus, the index of refraction is also the same for all colors (1.00000). In all substances, n is different for each color or frequency, being larger at the blue end and smaller at the red end of the spectrum. This difference can be quantified as the dispersion value, V:

$$V = \frac{n_D - 1}{n_F - n_C}$$

where n_D, n_F, and n_C are the indices of refraction for the yellow sodium line and the blue and the red hydrogen lines.

The higher the value of V, the less the dispersion of colors. Table 20–1 gives the indices of refraction and some dispersion values for substances of ophthalmologic interest.

Transmittance of Light

Optical materials vary in their transmittance or transparency to different frequencies. Some "transparent" materials such as glass are almost opaque to ultraviolet light. Red glass would be almost opaque to

the green frequency. Optical media must be selected according to the specific wavelength of light with which they are to be used.

Laws of Reflection & Refraction

The laws of reflection and refraction were formulated in 1621 by the Dutch astronomer and mathematician Willebrod Snell at the University of Leyden. These laws, together with Fermat's principle, form the basis of applied geometric optics. They can all be stated as follows (Figure 20–2).

(1) Incident, reflected, and refracted rays all reside in a plane known as the plane of incidence, which is normal (at a right angle) to the interface.

(2) The angle of incidence equals the angle of reflection but has the opposite sign: $I = -I'$.

(3) The product of the index of refraction of the medium of the incident ray and the sine of the angle of incidence of the incident ray is equal to the product of the same terms of the refracted ray. The refracted ray is designated by a prime: $n \sin I = n' \sin I'$ (**Snell's law**).

(4) A ray of light passing from one point to another follows the path that takes the least time to negotiate (**Fermat's principle**). Optical path length is the index of refraction times the actual path length.

Critical Angle & Total Reflection

In Figure 20–2, consider the ray in the more dense medium as the arriving ray. We see that it is refracted into the less dense medium away from the normal. If we gradually increase the angle of incidence (Figure 20–3) in the denser medium until we reach the critical angle, a startling event takes place: None of the light escapes, but all is suddenly, totally, and perfectly reflected (total internal reflection). This angle is reached as the sine of the incident ray in the denser medium reaches the value $-n'/n$. This is one method used to

Table 20–1. Indices of refraction and dispersion values of some substances of ophthalmologic interest.

Substance (20 °C unless noted)	Indices of Refraction (n_D)	Dispersion Values (V)
Water	1.33299	
Water 37 °C	1.33093	55.6
Sea water	1.344	
Sea water, 11,000 meters' depth	1.361	
Polymethylmethacrylate	1.49166	57.37
Polymethylmethacrylate 37 °C	1.48928	
Acrylonitrile styrene copolymer	1.56735	34.87
Polystyrene	1.59027	30.92
Fluorite	1.4338	95.2
Spectacle crown glass	1.523	58.8
Flint glass	1.617	36.6
Aqueous and vitreous 37 °C	1.3337	55.6
Hydroxyethylmethacrylate (HEMA)	1.43	
Cellulose acetate butyrate (CAB)	1.47	
Silicone	1.439	

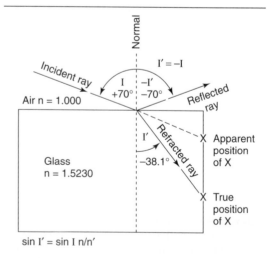

sin I' = sin I n/n'

Figure 20–2. Example of the laws of reflection and refraction.

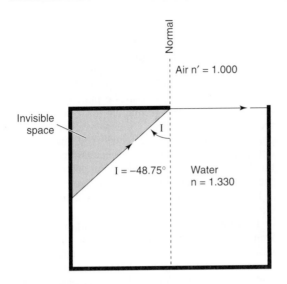

Figure 20–3. Example of the critical angle.

determine the index of refraction. For water, with an index of refraction of 1.330, the critical angle has the sine of –1/1.330, or –48.75 degrees.

Total reflection obeys the laws of regular reflection, ie, $I = -I'$. This allows perfect reflection without coatings and is used extensively in prisms and fiberoptics.

In Figure 20–3, the shaded area is not visible from the surface. This is why the angle of the eye cannot be inspected except with the gonioscopic lens (see Chapter 2). The index of refraction of the *aqueous*—and not the index of refraction of the tears or cornea, as is frequently stated—is the determining factor in this context.

CALCULATIONS USED IN OPTICS

There are two approaches to the application of the principles of geometric optics to single lenses or to compound lens systems. **Trigonometric ray tracing** is the more valid and exact approach, as it makes no assumptions other than those already determined by the laws of refraction. The **algebraic method** is a system based on a number of assumptions that greatly simplify calculation of the effects of various lens systems but also limit accuracy to an ever-increasing extent as the lens systems become more complex. The algebraic method cannot be relied on for accurate results, particularly in the assessment of the optical effects of contact lenses, intraocular lenses, and keratorefractive procedures—all of which are becoming more frequently used in the practice of ophthalmology.

Certain considerations are universal to optical calculations whatever method is used. For any optical system, the object and its image are said to lie in **conjugate planes.** If the object were to be placed in the plane of its own image, the optical system would produce its new image in the original object plane. Thus, the effects of any optical system will be the same for whichever direction light travels through the system. Each optical system has an infinite number of pairs of conjugate planes. Corresponding points on conjugate planes are known as **conjugate points.**

Trigonometric Ray Tracing

The trigonometric method of ray tracing consists of mathematically plotting the course of certain specified rays through the lens systems. The three rays most frequently traced are shown in Figure 20–4. They are named according to their positions relative to the first refracting surface. The marginal ray enters at the margin of the lens, the paraxial ray very near the optical axis (center of the lens), and the zonal ray in the portion of the lens where the average luminous flux of light passes through the lens. At each refracting surface, the change in direction of each of these rays is calculated according to the principles of Snell's law. This requires knowledge of the radius of curvature of the surface, the index of refraction of the medium on each side of the refracting surface, and the distance to the next surface. Elementary trigonometry is the only mathematical skill necessary for such calculations, though a programmable calculator greatly assists with the number of such calculations that have to be carried out.

Trigonometric ray tracing provides an exact determination of the point of focus and information on the quality of the image formed by a lens system. The difference between the back focal lengths (distance along the optical axis from the last refracting surface to the point of focus) of the marginal and paraxial rays is a measure of the "spread of focus," thus indicating the degree of **spherical aberration** (see below). Similarly, if rays of different color (frequency), with their different indices of refraction in each medium, are traced through the system, the degree of **chromatic aberration** (see below) will be determined. The optical pathway is the sum of the actual distance a ray

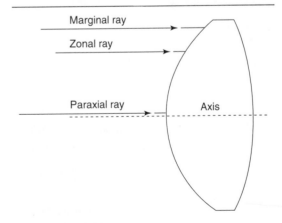

Figure 20–4. Illustration of three rays traced in trigonometric ray tracing.

passes through the substances multiplied by the index of refraction in the various substances through which it passes. How closely the optical pathways of the marginal and paraxial rays match determines the brightness and contrast of the final image.

Trigonometric ray tracing permits determination of the performance of each refracting surface relative to the contribution to the final image. For example, it is easily shown that a planoconvex intraocular lens gives a better image with the convex surface forward and the flat surface closer to the retina. The point of focus often requires—and is easily adjusted by—postoperative refraction. *However, the distorted image caused by selecting an intraocular lens of improper shape cannot be repaired by refraction. Suitability in this respect must be achieved by proper preoperative lens design, and this can only be achieved by calculation using the trigonometric method of ray tracing.*

Graphic ray tracing is a system comparable to trigonometric ray tracing that uses drawings to determine the optical properties of lens systems; it should not be confused with the method of "ray tracing" described in several books, in which tracings of an image are based on nodal points and focal planes (a derivation of the algebraic method of optical calculations discussed below).

Algebraic Method

Karl Friedrich Gauss (1777–1855) is responsible for refining a method of optical calculations that dispensed with the sines and cosines of the trigonometric method. This assumed that the lenses are "infinitely thin," placed close together, and of small diameter, such that any angle will be so small that the size of the angle measured in radians will have the same value as the sine of the angle and that the sine and the tangent of the angle can be assumed to be the same. The results are the **thin lens equations** used by opticians to calculate curves for lenses. "Fudge factors" derived from experience are then necessary to correct for the inaccuracies of these equations.

Use of the algebraic method depends on certain definitions. The position of the lens, reduced to a single line, is the **principal plane,** which intersects the optical axis at the **nodal point** (optical center). The **primary focal point (F)** is that point along the optical axis where an object must be placed to form an image at infinity. The **secondary focal point (F′)** is that point along the optical axis where parallel incident rays are brought to a focus. If the medium on either side of the lens is of the same refractive index, the distance between the nodal point and each of the focal points, the **focal length,** is the same.

Figure 20–5 shows some of the important thin lens equations.

The **diopter (D)** is a measure of lens power derived from the algebraic method of optical calculations. It is defined as the reciprocal of the focal length of a lens in air measured in meters. Diopters are additive, but only for low-power lenses. The result of combining lenses of high power varies greatly with their thickness and the separation distance. High-power lenses must be described by three values: (1) radii of curvature, (2) index of refraction, and (3) thickness.

In Gaussian optics, a thick lens is treated as if there are two nodal points and two principal planes (n and n′ and H and H′ in Figure 20–6). The nodal points lie on the principal planes only if the refractive medium is the same on either side of the lens. The true focal lengths are measured from the principal planes to the focal points, but the front and back focal lengths—essential to the prescription of corrective lenses—are measured from the respective surfaces of the lens to the focal points. The reciprocal of the back focal length corresponds to the back vertex power as measured with a lensometer.

For making high plus contact lenses or thick spectacle lenses, the equation for dioptric power according to the algebraic method is as follows:

$$\text{Dio} \cong \frac{1}{F} \cong (n-1)\left[\frac{1}{r_1} - \frac{1}{r_2} - \frac{(n-1)d}{n r_1 r_2}\right]$$

$$\text{Diopters} \cong \frac{1}{\text{Focal length}} \cong \frac{1}{\text{Distance of image}} - \frac{1}{\text{Distance of object}}$$

$$\text{Diopters} \cong (n-1)\frac{1}{\text{Radius}_1} - \frac{1}{\text{Radius}_2}$$

$$\frac{\text{Size of image}}{\text{Distance of image}} \cong \frac{\text{Size of object}}{\text{Distance of object}}$$

$$\text{Magnification} = \frac{\text{Size of image}}{\text{Size of object}} \cong \frac{\text{Distance of image}}{\text{Distance of object}}$$

Power for Several Lenses Combined
Diopters total $\cong$ Dio$_1$ + Dio$_2$ + Dio$_3$, etc

Figure 20–5. Algebraic thin lens approximations. All lengths in meters.

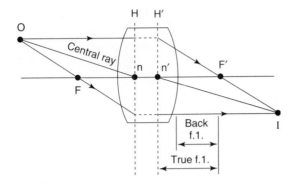

Figure 20–6. Description of a thick lens in Gaussian optics.

Magnification

Linear magnification is the ratio of the height of the image to the height of the object. For an infinitely thin lens in air—as assumed by the algebraic method of optical calculation—this ratio is equal to the ratio of the distance of the image to the distance of the object. For real lens systems, such as those of the eye, a more complex equation including the index of refraction of the initial and final media must be used. Trigonometric ray tracing quickly provides other information necessary for the calculation.

Change of Vertex Distance

If the vertex distance (the distance from the eye) of a lens of given power is altered, the effective power of the lens will also change. To calculate a new lens that will have the same effect at the new distance, a derivation of the thin lens equations can be used:

where F = focal length, r = radius, and d = thickness of lens, all measured in meters, and n = refractive index.

For contact lenses, a derivation of the thin lens equations is presently used to relate dioptric power to radius of curvature:

$$Dio \approx \frac{(n-1)}{r} \approx \frac{1.3375-1}{r} \approx \frac{337.5}{rmm} \text{ and } rmm \approx \frac{337.5}{Dio}$$

n of "cornea" is for this purpose assumed to be 1.3375. rmm = radius in millimeters. These equations are only approximations.

The ray tracing method commonly described in ophthalmic optics texts is a graphic representation of the algebraic system of optical calculations—in comparison to true graphic ray tracing, which is a graphic representation of the trigonometric system. Rays are traced through the optical system to connect conjugate points. The positions of the conjugate planes are derived mathematically from the thin lens equations. The size and orientation of the object are then determined by tracing the central ray, which passes straight through the tip of the image, the nodal point of the lens (without being refracted), and the tip of the object. The rays that traverse the focal points of the lens are derived by extrapolation (Figure 20–7).

For multiple lens systems, the conjugate planes and the path of the central ray are determined for each lens in succession, producing an image that becomes the object for the next lens until the size and orientation of the final image is located. In the case of a thick lens, refraction occurs at the principal planes of the lens, the position of rays being translated from one principal plane to another without any change in their vertical separation from the optical axis (Figure 20–6). The central ray passes from the tip of the object to the first nodal point and then emerges from the second nodal point parallel to its original direction to reach the tip of the image. When the media on either side of the lens have different refractive indices, the nodal points do not coincide with the principal planes.

(Dio = Power in diopters)

$$Dio_2 \approx \frac{1}{\frac{1}{Dio_1} - (Dist_1 - Dist_2)}$$

Example 1: A + 13 diopter lens at 11mm (0.011 m) is to be replaced by a lens at 9mm (0.009 m)

$$Dio_2 \cong \frac{1}{\frac{1}{13} - (0.011 - 0.009)} \cong 13.347 \text{ diopters}$$

Example 2: Same lens to be replaced by a contact lens

$$Dist_2 = 0$$

$$Dio_2 \cong \frac{1}{\frac{1}{13} - (0.011)} \cong 15.169 \text{ diopters}$$

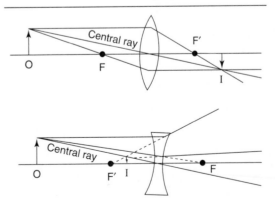

Figure 20–7. Ray tracing through plus and minus lenses.

This vertex equation is also an approximation and should not be used for intraocular lens calculations, but it is useful for conversion from spectacle to contact lens powers.

Aberrations of Spherical Lenses

Spherical lenses are subject to a number of aberrations that reduce the quality of image produced. The variation of refractive index with frequency of light (dispersion) results in greater refraction of blue than red light **(chromatic aberration)** (Figure 20–8). Marginal rays are refracted more than paraxial rays, producing **spherical aberration** (Figure 20–9). **Coma,** a characteristic comet-shaped blur, is the result of spherical aberration of light originating away from the optical axis of the lens. When light traverses a spherical lens obliquely, there is an additional cylindrical lens effect—**astigmatism of oblique incidence. Curvature of field** is the production of a curved image from a flat object. Prismatic effects of the lens periphery also cause image distortion. Achromatic lenses may be made by cementing together plus and minus lenses of different refractive indices. The nonchromatic aberrations are overcome by combining or shaping lenses to reduce the power of the lens periphery, by restricting the area of the lens used to the paraxial zones, and by use of meniscus lenses.

Cylindrical Lenses

A **planocylindrical lens** (Figure 20–10) has one flat surface and one cylindrical surface, producing a lens with no optical power in the meridian of its axis and maximum power in the meridian 90 degrees away from the axis meridian. The total effect is the formation of a line image, parallel to the axis of the lens, from a point object. The orientation of a planocylindrical lens is specified by the meridian of its axis. The ophthalmic convention for specifying the orientation of the axis of a cylindrical lens is shown in Figure 20–11. Zero begins nasally in the right lens and temporally in the left lens and proceeds in a counterclockwise direction to 180 degrees.

In a **spherocylindrical lens,** the cylindrical surface is curved in two meridians but not to the same extent. In ophthalmic lenses, these principal meridians are at 90 degrees to each other. The effect of a spherocylindrical lens on a point object is to produce a geometric figure known as the **conoid of Sturm** (Figure 20–12), consisting of two focal lines separated by the interval of Sturm. The position of the focal lines relative to the lens is determined by the power of the two meridians and their orientation by the angle between the meridians. Cross-sections through the conoid of Sturm reveal lines at the focal lines and generally ellipses elsewhere. In one position, the cross-section will be a circle that represents the **circle of least confusion.**

A spherocylindrical lens can be thought of as a combination of a spherical lens and a planocylindrical lens. It can then be specified by the orientation of principal meridians and the power acting in each (Figure 20–13). In a cross diagram, the arms are drawn parallel to the principal meridians and labeled with the relevant power. In longhand notation, the cylinder is specified by the orientation of its axis, which is 90 degrees away from the meridian of maximum power.

Writing prescriptions for spherocylindrical lenses uses longhand notation, and the lens can be specified

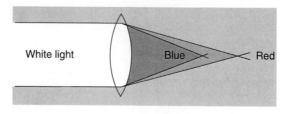

Figure 20–8. Chromatic aberration of lenses.

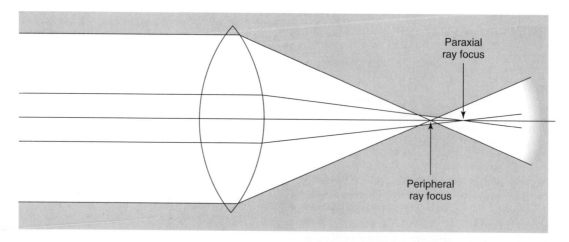

Figure 20–9. Spherical aberration of a biconvex lens.

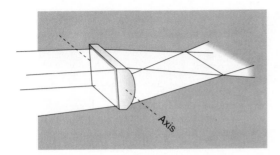

Figure 20–10. A planocylindrical lens with axis in the horizontal meridian.

in either plus or minus cylinder form (Figure 20–13). The procedure for transposing between these forms is as follows: (1) algebraically sum the original sphere and cylinder; (2) reverse the sign of the cylinder; and (3) change the axis of the cylinder by 90 degrees.

If their principal meridians correspond, combinations of spherocylindrical lenses can be summed mathematically. Otherwise, trigonometric formulas are required. Alternatively, the power of such combinations can be determined by placing them together in a lensometer. The principal meridians of any such combination will be 90 degrees apart.

Prisms

A prism consists of a transparent material with nonparallel flat surfaces. In cross-section, it has an apex and a base. The prism is specified by its power and the orientation of its base.

A prism refracts light toward its base, whereas an object seen through a prism appears deviated toward the apex of the prism. The amount of deviation varies according to the tilt of the prism, ie, the angle of incidence of the light. For glass prisms, calibration is performed in the **Prentice position,** in which the incident light is perpendicular to the face of the prism (Figure 20–14). For plastic prisms and in general optics, a prism is calibrated in the **position of minimum deviation,** in which the amount of refraction at the two surfaces of the prisms is equal (Figure 20–14). When prisms are used in clinical practice, these orientations must be adhered to for accurate results.

For a glass prism in the Prentice position, the incident ray is not refracted at the first surface because the surfaces are perpendicular to one another (Figure 20–15). At the second surface, the angle of incidence is the same as the apex angle of the prism (A). If I' is the angle of the final refracted ray, from Snell's law, sin I' = (n/n') sin A, n being the refractive index of the prism and n' the refractive index of the surrounding medium. For example, if the prism is of glass with

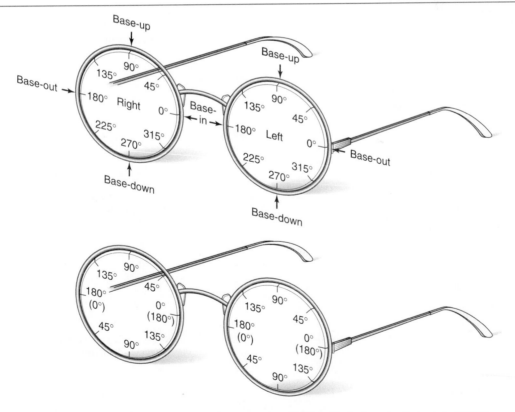

Figure 20–11. ***Top:*** Illustration of prism base notation. ***Bottom:*** Illustration of cylinder axis notation.

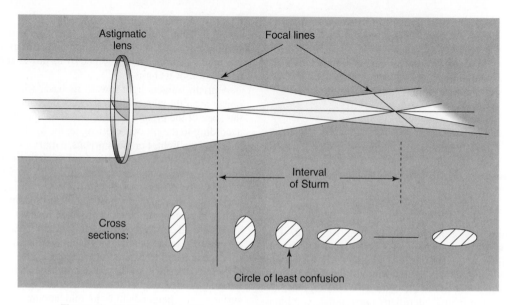

Figure 20–12. The conoid of Sturm, formed by light refracted by an astigmatic lens.

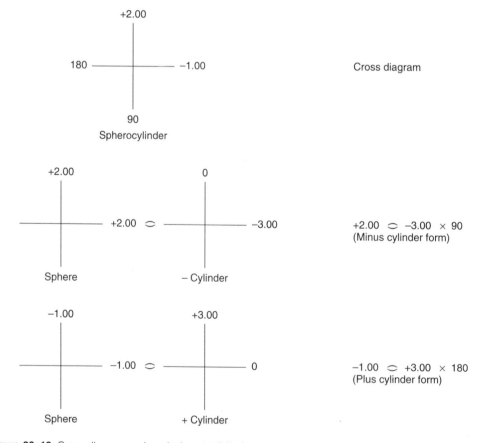

Figure 20–13. Cross diagram and equivalent combinations, including longhand notations, for a spherocylindrical lens.

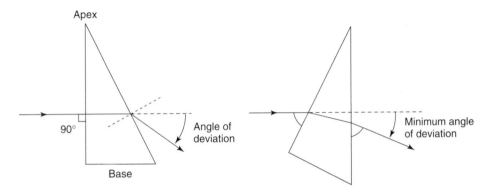

Figure 20–14. Calibration of prisms. Glass prisms and spectacle prisms are calibrated according to the Prentice position, whereas plastic prisms are calibrated according to the position of minimum deviation.

n = 1.523 and A = 30 degrees, then sin I′ is 1.523 × 0.5, or 0.7615. I′ is 49.6 degrees. The angle of deviation is I′ − A, or 19.6 degrees.

The power of a prism is measured in prism diopters (Δ). One prism diopter deviates an image 1 cm at 1 m (Figure 20–16). The arc tangent of 1/100 is 0.57 degrees. So 1$^\Delta$ produces an angle of deviation of almost one-half degree. The "rule of thumb" is that a prism of 2$^\Delta$ produces an angle of deviation of 1 degree, but this cannot be applied to prisms of more than 100$^\Delta$.

Prisms are used in ophthalmology both to measure and to treat heterotropia and heterophoria. The orientation of a prism's base is indicated by its direction, usually descriptively, ie, "base-up right eye," "base-down left eye," "base-in" or "base-out," or occasionally by a mathematical system (Figure 20–11).

Fresnel prisms are lightweight plastic prisms consisting of narrow, parallel strips of prism with the same apex angle as the desired single prism (Figure 20–17). They are available as press-on prisms for at-tachment to the back of spectacle lenses, providing an easily adjusted temporary prismatic correction that is less heavy than conventional glass prisms. Their disadvantages are the image degradation due to light scatter and dirt within the grooves.

Prismatic Effect of Spherical Lenses

Spherical lenses have increasing prismatic power as the light path moves away from the optical center of the lens. The amount of prism power can be calculated from Prentice's rule, which states that the prism power in prism diopters is equal to the dioptric power of the lens in diopters multiplied by the displacement from the optical center in centimeters. For example, at 0.5 cm away from the optical center of a 6$^\Delta$ lens, the prismatic power is 3$^\Delta$. Plus lenses produce prism power with the base oriented toward the optical center of the lens, and minus lenses produce prism power with the base oriented away from their optical center.

The prismatic effect of spherical lenses is an important consideration in the correction of anisometropia. Appropriate spectacle lenses may produce significant vertical prismatic deviation when the peripheral portions of the lenses are used. This occurs mainly when the patient attempts to read. The prismatic effect can be overcome by adopting a chin-down position, thus using the optical centers of the lenses once again, by grinding of a compensatory prism into the reading segment of the glasses (**slab-off prism**), or by changing to contact lenses.

If a prism needs to be incorporated into a patient's spectacle correction, such as in the control of hyper-

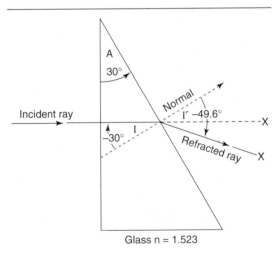

Figure 20–15. Example of the prism as used in ophthalmology.

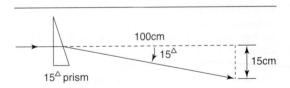

Figure 20–16. Power of a prism in prism diopters.

Fresnel prism

Apex 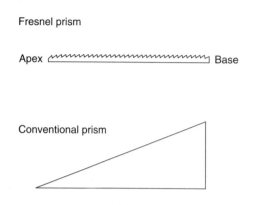 Base

Conventional prism

Figure 20–17. The Fresnel prism.

Power = +60 D

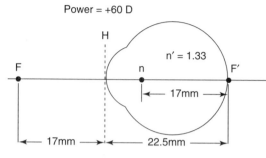

Figure 20–18. The reduced schematic eye.

tropia, it may be achieved by decentration of the spherical lens rather than by addition of a prism to the spherical component.

Rapid Detection of Lens Characteristics

The nature of a spherical lens may be rapidly detected by looking through it 0.5 m (19 inches) or so from the eye and moving the lens at right angles to the visual axis. The image seen through a minus (concave) lens will tend to move *with* the lens. The same test with a plus (convex) lens causes the image to tend to move *away from* the direction of motion. This effect is due to the prismatic effect of the periphery of the lens. The power of the lens can be approximated by neutralization of these movements by lenses of known power. A cylindrical lens shows changing distortion of the image when the lens is rotated about the visual axis. (Spherical lenses do not.) The orientations of the lens in which the image is clearest indicate the principal meridians. The power in each of the principal meridians can then be determined by the method described above for spherical lenses. A prism is recognized by deviation of the image as the static lens is viewed through its center.

OPTICS & THE EYE

Many attempts have been made to simplify the optical system of the human eye, particularly using the thick lens equations of the algebraic method of optical calculations. Much has been made of the concept that the image on the retina is formed by two lens elements, the cornea contributing about 43 D and the lens the remaining 19 D, but this is a gross oversimplification. The **schematic eye of Gullstrand** and its reduced form (Figure 20–18) are models from which mathematical values for the optical characteristics of the eye were derived. For instance, in the reduced schematic eye, the cornea is assumed to be the only refracting surface, the principal plane (H) being placed at its apex and a single nodal point (n) at its center of curvature. The globe has an axial length of 22.5 mm, and the refractive index of the eye is said to

be 1.33. Unfortunately, these numbers have become accepted by many as true physiologic values rather than as the convenient mathematically derived values they really are. The refractive index of aqueous is about 1.3337 (for the sodium D line at 37 °C).

Trigonometric ray tracing demonstrates that the optical system of the human eye is more accurately conceptualized as a three-lens system: the aqueous lens, the lens lens, and the vitreous lens (Figure 20–19). Contrary to popular belief, the cornea itself has almost no power of refraction in the optical system but is important only in shaping the anterior curve of the aqueous lens. The crystalline lens is an interesting optical component because its index of refraction varies throughout its thickness rather than being constant, as assumed in most optical calculations. The vitreous lens is particularly important because of its major effect on magnification.

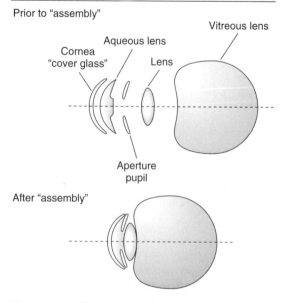

Figure 20–19. The optical system of the eye, illustrating the three-lens concept.

Reassessment of models for the optical system of the human eye is essential now that much of ophthalmic surgery, whether it be cataract surgery, keratorefractive procedures, or vitreous surgery, produces profound effects on individual components of the system. Gullstrand's models, in which the system is assumed to function as an integrated unit, cannot be applied under such circumstances.

Accommodation

The eye changes refractive power to focus on near objects by a process called accommodation. Study of Purkinje images, which are reflections from various optical surfaces in the eye, has shown that accommodation results from changes in the crystalline lens. Contraction of the ciliary muscle results in thickening and increased curvature of the lens, probably due to relaxation of the lens capsule.

Visual Acuity

Assessment of visual acuity with the Snellen chart is described in Chapter 2. The average resolving power of the normal human eye is 1 minute of arc. Since the Snellen letters are made from squares of 5×5 units (Figure 20–20), the 20/20 size letter has a visual angle of 5 minutes of arc at 20 feet. This is equivalent to 8.7 mm (0.35 inch) width and height. The eye minifies an image at 20 feet by about 350 times. Therefore, the size of the 20/20 letter on the retina is 0.025 mm high and wide. This is equivalent to a resolution capacity of 100 lines per millimeter. For a 6-mm pupil and light of wavelength 0.56 μm (in air), the absolute theoretic limit would be 345 lines per millimeter.

REFRACTIVE ERRORS

Emmetropia is absence of refractive error and **ametropia** is the presence of refractive error.

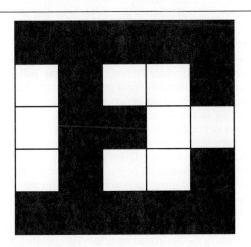

Figure 20–20. Snellen block E.

Table 20–2. Table of accommodation.

Age (Years)	Mean Accommodation (Diopters)
8	13.8
25	9.9
35	7.3
40	5.8
45	3.6
50	1.9
55	1.3

Presbyopia

The loss of accommodation that comes with aging to all people is called presbyopia (Table 20–2). A person with emmetropic eyes (no refractive error) will begin to notice inability to read small print or discriminate fine close objects at about age 44–46. This is worse in dim light and usually worse early in the morning or when the subject is fatigued. Many people complain of a feeling of sleepiness when reading. These symptoms increase until about age 55, when they stabilize but persist.

Presbyopia is corrected by use of a plus lens to make up for the lost automatic focusing power of the lens. The plus lens may be used in several ways. Reading glasses have the near correction in the entire aperture of the glasses, making them fine for reading but blurred for distant objects. Half-glasses can be worn to abate this nuisance by leaving the top open and uncorrected for distance vision. Bifocals do the same but allow correction of other refractive errors. Trifocals correct for distance vision by the top segment, the middle distance by the middle section, and the near distance by the lower segment. Progressive power lenses similarly correct for far, middle, and near distances but by progressive change in lens power rather than stepped changes.

Myopia

When the image of distant objects focuses in front of the retina in the unaccommodated eye, the eye is myopic, or nearsighted (Figure 20–21). If the eye is longer than average, the error is called axial myopia. (For each additional millimeter of axial length, the eye is approximately 3 diopters more myopic.) If the refractive elements are more refractive than average, the error is called curvature myopia or refractive myopia. As the object is brought closer than 6 meters, the image moves closer to the retina and comes into sharper focus. The point reached where the image is most sharply focused on the retina is called the "far point." One may estimate the extent of myopia by calculating the reciprocal of the far point. Thus, a far point of 0.25 m would suggest a 4-diopter minus lens correction for

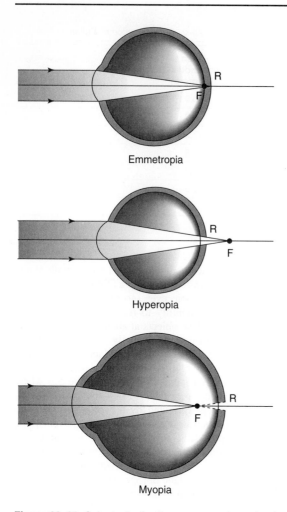

Figure 20–21. Spherical refractive errors as determined by the position of the secondary focal point with respect to the retina.

distance. The myopic person has the advantage of being able to read at the far point without glasses even at the age of presbyopia. A high degree of myopia results in greater susceptibility to degenerative retinal changes, including retinal detachment.

Concave spherical (minus) lenses are used to correct the image in myopia. These lenses move the image back to the retina.

Hyperopia

Hyperopia (hypermetropia, farsightedness) is the state in which the unaccommodated eye would focus the image behind the retina (Figure 20–21). It may be due to reduced axial length (axial hyperopia), as occurs in certain congenital disorders, or reduced refractive error (refractive hyperopia), as exemplified by aphakia.

Hyperopia is a more difficult concept to explain than myopia. The term "farsighted" contributes to the difficulty, as does the prevalent misconception among laymen that presbyopia is farsightedness and that one who sees well far away is farsighted. If hyperopia is not too great, a young person may obtain a sharp distant image by accommodating, as a normal eye would to read. The young hyperopic person may also make a sharp near image by accommodating more—or much more than one without hyperopia. This extra effort may result in eye fatigue that is more severe for near work. The degree of hyperopia a person may have without symptoms is—like most clinical conditions—variable. However, the amount decreases with age as presbyopia (decrease in ability to accommodate) increases. Three diopters of hyperopia might be tolerated in a teenager but will require glasses later, even though the hyperopia has not increased. If the hyperopia is too high, the eye may be unable to correct the image by accommodation. The hyperopia that cannot be corrected by accommodation is termed manifest hyperopia. This is one of the causes of deprivation amblyopia in children and can be bilateral. There is a reflex correlation between accommodation and convergence of the two eyes. Hyperopia is therefore a frequent cause of esotropia (crossed eyes) and monocular amblyopia (see Chapter 12).

Latent Hyperopia

As explained above, a prepresbyopic person with hyperopia may obtain a clear retinal image by accommodation. The degree of hyperopia overcome by accommodation is known as latent hyperopia. It is detected by refraction after instillation of cycloplegic drops, which determines the sum of both manifest and latent hyperopia. Refraction with a cycloplegic is very important in young patients who complain of eyestrain when reading and is vital in esotropia, where full correction of hyperopia may achieve a cure.

Remember that a moderately "farsighted" person may see well for near or far when young. However, as presbyopia comes on, the hyperope first has trouble with close work—and at an earlier age than the non-hyperope. Finally, the hyperope has blurred vision for near *and far* and requires glasses for both near and far.

Astigmatism

In astigmatism, the eye produces an image with multiple focal points or lines. In **regular astigmatism,** there are two principal meridians, with constant power and orientation across the pupillary aperture, resulting in two focal lines. The astigmatism is then further defined according to the position of these focal lines with respect to the retina (Figure 20–22). When the principal meridians are at right angles and their axes lie within 20 degrees of the horizontal and vertical, the astigmatism is subdivided into **astigmatism with the rule,** in which the greater refractive power is in the vertical meridian; and **astigmatism against the rule,** in which the greater refractive power is in the horizontal meridian. Astigmatism with the rule is more commonly found in younger patients

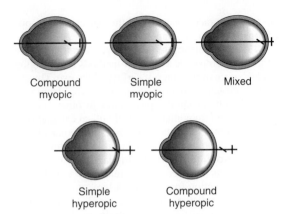

Figure 20–22. Types of regular astigmatism as determined by the positions of the two focal lines with respect to the retina.

and astigmatism against the rule more commonly in older patients (Figure 20–23). **Oblique astigmatism** is regular astigmatism in which the principal meridians do not lie within 20 degrees of the horizontal and vertical. In **irregular astigmatism,** the power or orientation of the principal meridians changes across the pupillary aperture.

The usual cause of astigmatism is abnormalities of corneal shape. The crystalline lens may also contribute. In contact lens terminology, lenticular astigmatism is called residual astigmatism because it is not corrected by a spherical hard contact lens, which does correct corneal astigmatism.

Astigmatic errors can be corrected with cylindrical lenses, frequently in combination with spherical lenses. Because the brain is capable of adapting to the visual distortion of an uncorrected astigmatic error, new glasses that do correct the error may cause temporary disorientation, particularly an apparent slanting of images.

Natural History of Refractive Errors

Most babies are slightly hyperopic at birth. The hyperopia slowly decreases, with a slight acceleration in the teens, to approach emmetropia. The corneal curvature is much steeper (6.59 mm radius) at birth and flattens to nearly the adult curvature (7.71 mm) by about 1 year. The lens is much more spherical at birth and reaches adult conformation at about 6 years. The axial length is short at birth (17.3 mm), lengthens rapidly in the first 2 or 3 years (to 24.1 mm), then moderately (0.4 mm per year) until age 6, and then slowly (about 1 mm total) to stability at about 10 or 15 years. Presbyopia becomes manifest in the fifth decade.

Refractive errors are inherited. The mode of inheritance is complex, as it involves so many variables. Refractive error, though inherited, need not be present at birth any more than tallness, which is also inherited, need be present at birth. For example, a child who reaches emmetropia at age 10 years will probably soon become myopic. Myopia usually increases during the teens. This should be expected, just as the need for larger shoes is expected, and not looked on with alarm by the patient and parents. In a similar way, hyperopia usually decreases slightly during the teens. Myopia does not generally decrease with age, as is popularly believed, nor does farsightedness come with aging.

Anisometropia

Anisometropia is a difference in refractive error between the two eyes. It is a major cause of amblyopia because the eyes cannot accommodate independently and the more hyperopic eye is chronically blurred. Refractive correction of anisometropia is complicated by differences in size of the retinal images (**aniseikonia**) and oculomotor imbalance due to the different degree of prismatic power of the periphery of the two corrective lenses. Aniseikonia is predominantly a problem of monocular aphakia. Spectacle correction produces a difference in retinal image size of approx-

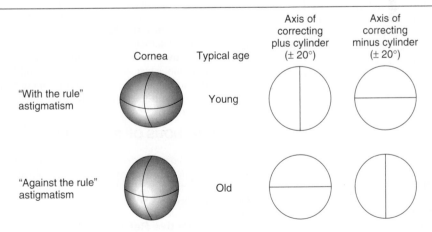

Figure 20–23. Types of astigmatism as determined by the orientation of the principal meridians and the orientation of the correcting cylinder axis.

imately 25%, which is rarely tolerable. Contact lens correction reduces the difference in image size to approximately 6%, which can be tolerated. Intraocular lenses produce a difference of less than 1%.

Correction of Refractive Errors

A. Spectacle Lenses: Spectacles continue to be the safest method of refractive correction. To reduce nonchromatic aberrations, the lenses are made in meniscus form (corrected curves) and tilted forward (pantascopic tilt).

B. Contact Lenses: The first contact lenses were glass fluid-filled scleral lenses. These were difficult to wear for extended periods and caused corneal edema and much ocular discomfort. Hard corneal lenses, made of polymethylmethacrylate, were the first really successful contact lenses and gained wide acceptance for cosmetic replacement of glasses. Subsequent developments include gas-permeable rigid lenses, made of cellulose acetate butyrate, silicone, or various silicone and plastic polymers, and soft contact lenses, made of various hydrogel plastics, all of which provide increased comfort but greater risk of serious complications.

Hard and gas-permeable lenses correct refractive errors by changing the curvature of the anterior surface of the eye. The total refractive power consists of the power induced by the back curvature of the lens, the base curve, together with the actual power of the lens due to the difference between its front and back curvatures. Only the second is dependent on the refractive index of the contact lens material. Hard and gas-permeable lenses overcome corneal astigmatism by modifying the anterior surface of the eye into a truly spherical shape.

Soft contact lenses, particularly the more flexible forms, adopt the shape of the patient's cornea. Thus, their refractive power resides only in the difference between their front and back curvature, and they correct little corneal astigmatism unless a cylindrical correction is incorporated to make a toric lens.

Contact lens base curves are selected according to corneal curvature, as determined by keratometry or trial fittings. The front curvature is then calculated from the results of overrefraction with a trial contact lens, or from the patient's spectacle refraction as corrected for the corneal plane.

Hard contact lenses are specifically indicated for the correction of irregular astigmatism, such as in keratoconus. Soft contact lenses are used for the treatment of corneal surface disorders, but for control of symptoms rather than for refractive reasons. All forms of contact lenses are used in the refractive correction of aphakia, particularly in overcoming the aniseikonia of monocular aphakia, and the correction of high myopia, in which they produce a much better visual image than spectacles. But the vast majority of contact lenses worn are for cosmetic correction of low refractive errors. This has important implications for the risks that can be reasonably accepted in the use of contact lenses. (Further discussion of therapeutic and cosmetic contact lens use, and the associated complications, is given in Chapter 6.)

C. Keratorefractive Surgery: Keratorefractive surgery encompasses a range of methods for changing the curvature of the anterior surface of the eye. The expected refractive effect is generally derived from empirical results of similar procedures in other patients and not based upon mathematical optical calculations. Further discussion of the methods and outcome of keratorefractive procedures is included in Chapter 6.

D. Intraocular Lenses: Implantation of an intraocular lens has become the preferred method of refractive correction for aphakia. A large number of designs are available, including rigid lenses, most commonly consisting of an optic made of polymethylmethacrylate and loops (haptics) made of the same material or polypropylene; and foldable lenses, made of silicone or hydrogel plastics, which can be inserted into the eye through a much smaller incision. The safest position for an intraocular lens is within an intact capsular bag following extracapsular surgery.

The most popular method of determining the necessary intraocular lens power is the empirical regression method of analyzing experience with lenses of one style in many patients, from which is derived a mathematical formula based on a constant for the particular lens *(A)*, average keratometer readings *(K)*, and axial length in millimeters *(L)*. An example is the **SRK (Sanders-Retzlaff-Kraff) equation:**

$$\text{Power IOL} = A - 2.5\ L - 0.9\ K$$

This formula gives clinically satisfactory results in most cases. When the eye is not of average dimensions, such as in high myopia, the results are less good, and various modifications have been derived.

Certain theoretic formulas are also available, also utilizing a lens constant, keratometer readings, and axial length, together with estimated anterior chamber depth following surgery. Unfortunately, none of these formulas are based on trigonometric ray tracing methods, which do accurately predict the correct power of intraocular lens for an individual patient.

E. Clear Lens Extraction for Myopia: Extraction of noncataractous lenses has been advocated for the refractive correction of myopia. For the process to have any success, the eye must be highly myopic, and the surgery is then sufficiently likely to have an adverse result that it is rarely justifiable.

METHODS OF REFRACTION

Determination of a patient's refractive correction can be achieved by objective or subjective means and is best accomplished by a combination of the two methods where possible.

Objective Refraction

Objective refraction is performed by retinoscopy, in which a streak of light, known as the **intercept,** is pro-

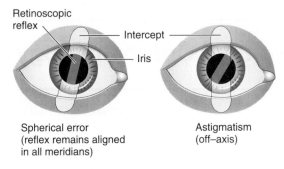

Figure 20–24. The retinoscopic reflex.

jected into the patient's eye to produce a similarly shaped reflex, the **retinoscopic reflex,** in the pupil (Figure 20–24). Parallel alignment of the intercept and the retinoscopic reflex indicates the presence of only a spherical error, or an additional cylindrical error in which the intercept coincides with one of the principal meridians. Rotation of the projected streak will determine which of these applies and the location of the other principal meridian in the case of a cylindrical error.

The intercept is then swept across the patient's pupil, and the effect on the retinoscopic reflex is noted (Figure 20–25). If it moves in the same direction **(with movement),** plus lenses are placed before the patient's eye; and if it moves in the opposite direction **(against movement),** minus lenses are added—until the pupillary reflex fills the whole pupillary aperture and no movement is detected **(point of neutralization).** When the point of neutralization has been reached, the patient's refractive error has been corrected with an additional correction related to the distance between the patient and examiner **(working distance).** Spherical power equal to the reciprocal of the working distance (measured in meters) is subtracted to compensate for this additional correction and obtain the patient's refractive correction. The working

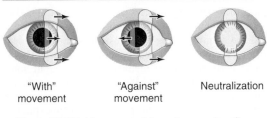

"With" movement   "Against" movement   Neutralization

Figure 20–25. Movement of the retinoscopic reflex.

distance is usually $2/3$ m, and the correction to be subtracted for the working distance thus is usually 1.5 D.

Automated refractors are available to rapidly determine the objective refraction, but they are not useful in young children or in adults with significant anterior segment disease.

Subjective Refraction

In cooperative patients, subjective refraction produces more accurate results than objective refraction. It relies on the patient's response to alterations in lens power and orientation, using objective refraction or the patient's current refractive correction as the starting point.

The spherical correction is checked by small changes, initially increasing the plus power so as to overcome any accommodative effort, until the clearest image is obtained. The duochrome test of black letters on red and green backgrounds uses the normal chromatic aberration of the eye to refine spherical correction. When the black letters of the two halves of the chart are equally clear, the end point has been reached.

A **cross cylinder** consists of two planocylindrical lenses of equal power but opposite sign superimposed such that their axes of refractive power lie at right angles to one another. This is equivalent to a spherocylindrical lens in which the power of the cylinder is twice the power of the sphere and of the opposite sign. The cross cylinder allows rapid small changes in the axis and power of a cylindrical correction.

Cycloplegic Refraction

In the determination of full hyperopic refractive correction, either in the management of childhood esotropia or the assessment of eyestrain in adult hyperopes, it is necessary to overcome accommodation. This can usually be achieved in adults by fogging techniques in which plus lenses are used to overcome accommodative effort. But otherwise—and always in children—accommodation has to be relaxed by cycloplegic drugs. Cyclopentolate 1%, 1 drop instilled twice 30 minutes prior to refraction, may be sufficient, but atropine 0.5% or 1% ointment, applied twice a day for 3 days, may be necessary in children with dark irides and in the initial assessment of accommmodative esotropia. Parents should be warned of the symptoms of atropine toxicity (fever, flushed face, and rapid pulse) and the necessity for discontinuing treatment, cooling the child with sponge bathing, and—in severe cases—seeking urgent medical assistance.

21

Preventive Ophthalmology

John P. Whitcher, MD, MPH

Preventive medicine is increasingly important in attempts to fulfill society's expectations of modern medicine with the resources available. Although prevention is a logical approach to the solution of many problems in all branches of medicine, in practice there are a number of hurdles to be overcome. For any particular condition, it is essential that individuals at risk be easily identified. If their identification requires population screening, the screening process should be easy to perform, accurate, and reliable. Preventive measures must be both effective and acceptable to the target population. Unwarranted interference with the at-risk individual's lifestyle only leads to poor compliance. Legislation may be required for certain measures but may engender resentment when it is felt to infringe on personal liberty. For preventive medicine to be successful, there must be cooperation among all segments of society—not just the medical community—in identifying problem areas, establishing workable solutions, and disseminating information. The successes that have been achieved in occupational health are an example of what can be accomplished if a consensus of opinion is established.

In ophthalmology, the major avenues for preventive medicine are ocular injuries and infections, genetic and systemic diseases with ocular involvement, and ocular diseases in which the early treatable stages are often unrecognized or ignored.

PREVENTION OF OCULAR INJURIES

Approximately 1 million Americans have visual loss due to trauma, of which 75% are blind in one eye, and approximately 50,000 suffer serious sight-threatening injuries each year. Young men and children are particularly prone to suffer major ocular trauma. Simple measures are available for preventing many injuries to the eye.

Occupational Injuries

Many manufacturing processes pose a particular threat to the eye. Grinding or drilling commonly propels small fragments of metal into the environment at high velocity, and these missiles can easily lodge on the cornea or penetrate the globe through the cornea

or sclera. Tools with sharp ends, such as screwdrivers, are also commonly involved in producing penetrating ocular injuries. Welding arcs produce ultraviolet radiation that may cause epithelial keratitis ("arc eye"). Industrial chemicals—particularly those containing high concentrations of alkali or acid—can rapidly produce severe ocular damage that is often bilateral and associated with a poor visual outcome.

Workers must be properly trained in the use of tools, machinery, and chemicals. Safety guards must be fitted to all machinery, and safety goggles must be worn whenever the worker is doing hazardous work or is in the workplace area where such hazards exist. It is surprising how many workers assume that they are no longer at risk of injury when they are not themselves performing hazardous tasks even though they are in the vicinity of work being performed by others.

The growing interest in "do-it-yourself" projects in the home exposes many more individuals to the risks of ocular injury from machinery, tools, and chemicals. Education of the public about these matters is particularly important, since the risks involved may not be obvious to the ordinary householder or hobbyist.

Early recognition and urgent expert ophthalmologic assessment of any injuries sustained is essential. In the case of chemical injuries, immediate copious lavage of the eyes with sterile water, saline if available, or tap water for at least 5 minutes is the most important method of limiting the damage incurred. Neglect of penetrating injuries or corneal foreign bodies markedly increases the potential for long-term morbidity. Obtaining an accurate history is crucial in identifying the possibility of a penetrating injury. This is particularly true when medical help is sought some time after the injury and the patient may not realize the importance of a seemingly minor episode of trauma. Any worker who presents with unexplained visual loss or intraocular inflammation must be carefully questioned about the possibility of recent ocular injuries and the possibility of an occult intraocular foreign body borne in mind.

Chronic exposure to some industrial processes may lead to ocular damage. For example, improperly screened nuclear materials can lead to early and rapid cataract formation in exposed workers.

Nonoccupational Injuries

The marked reduction in the incidence of severe ocular and facial damage associated with car windshield injuries as a result of legislation requiring the wearing of seat belts is a testament to the effectiveness of such legislation. Similar attempts to reduce the incidence of injuries from fireworks by limiting their availability have not yet been as successful.

Various sports are notorious for the high incidence of severe injuries to the eye, eg, blunt injuries such as in racquetball or penetrating injuries such as in ice hockey. The availability of toughened plastic protective glasses—which can be fitted with refractive correction if required—is a major advance in preventing such injuries.

A large number of ocular injuries are suffered in the home. Corks from bottles of champagne or other sparkling wines can produce severe blunt injuries, and explosion of any bottle containing carbonated beverages may lead to penetrating eye injuries from glass fragments. Unless adequately supervised, children using pencils, scissors, or airguns may sustain or cause serious penetrating injuries.

Unfortunately, a significant proportion of serious ocular trauma results from violent assaults, notably those involving firearms. Prevention requires a reduction in the frequency of such incidents.

Acute keratitis from **ultraviolet irradiation** as seen after exposure to a welding arc may also occur during skiing if protective goggles are not worn. The role of long-term exposure to ultraviolet light in the etiology of cataract and age-related macular degeneration is still debated. Since the cornea and crystalline lens are effective barriers to the transmission of ultraviolet light—becoming even more effective with age in the case of the crystalline lens—it is hardly surprising that the development of age-related macular degeneration in phakic individuals has not been shown to be related to ultraviolet exposure and thus is not preventable by the use of sunglasses. The effect of ultraviolet light on the maculas of the increasing numbers of aphakic and pseudophakic individuals has yet to be fully assessed. Largely on empirical grounds, ultraviolet filters have been incorporated into many of the intraocular lenses implanted. And individuals without such filters in their intraocular lenses or who are aphakic have been encouraged to incorporate ultraviolet filters in their spectacle lenses or wear appropriate sunglasses whenever possible. There is substantial evidence linking ultraviolet exposure to the development of cataract. But since ultraviolet exposure occurs from the time of birth, advocating the regular use of ultraviolet filters in spectacle lenses or sunglasses as a preventive measure is unlikely to be workable or effective. The role of ultraviolet light exposure in the etiology of certain corneal disorders—particularly pterygium—and of basal cell carcinoma and melanoma of the eyelids is much more widely accepted. Education of the public about the dangers of skin cancer following prolonged sun exposure is very important. Ultraviolet-blocking skin creams should not be used around the eyes, and for that reason reliance must be placed on avoiding unnecessary exposure to the sun or the use of sunglasses. In patients with xeroderma pigmentosum, the eyelids and bulbar conjunctiva frequently develop carcinomas and melanomas, and their development can be minimized, if not prevented entirely, by protective lenses.

Solar retinitis (eclipse retinopathy) is a specific type of radiation injury that usually occurs after solar eclipses as a result of direct observation of the sun without an adequate filter. Under normal circumstances, sun-gazing is difficult because of the glare, but cases have been reported in young people who have suffered self-inflicted macular damage by deliberate sun-gazing, perhaps while under the influence of drugs.

The optical system of the eye behaves as a strong magnifying lens, focusing the light onto a small spot on the macula, usually in one eye only, and producing a thermal burn. The resulting edema of the retinal tissue may clear with minimal loss of function, or it may cause significant atrophy of the tissue and produce a defect that is visible ophthalmoscopically as a macular hole. In the latter event, a permanent central scotoma results. Eclipse retinopathy can easily be prevented by the use of adequate filters when observing eclipses, but the surest way to prevent it is to watch the eclipse on television.

Similar to eclipse retinopathy is the iatrogenic retinal damage that may occur from use of the operating microscope and indirect ophthalmoscope (photic retinopathy). The risk of damage from the operating microscope can be reduced by the use of filters to block both ultraviolet light and the blue portion of the visible spectrum, light barriers such as an opaque disk placed on the cornea, or air injected into the anterior chamber.

PREVENTION OF ACQUIRED OCULAR INFECTION

Infections are a major cause of preventable ocular morbidity. Preventive measures are based on maintenance of the integrity of the normal barriers to infection and the avoidance of inoculation with pathogenic organisms. The pathogenicity of various organisms and the size of the inoculum required to establish infection vary enormously according to the state of the eye. A compromised eye is highly susceptible to infection.

The major barrier to exogenous ocular infection is the epithelium of the cornea and conjunctiva. This can be damaged directly by trauma, including surgical trauma and contact lens wear, or by the secondary effects of other abnormalities of the outer eye, such as lid abnormalities or tear deficiency. In all such situations, particular care must be taken to avoid or recognize secondary infection in its earliest stages.

In the presence of a corneal or conjunctival epithelial defect, particularly when there is an associated full-thickness wound of the cornea or sclera—eg, following penetrating trauma or intraocular surgery—it is essential to use prophylactic antibiotic therapy and most importantly to make certain that any drops or ointments are sterile. Accidental epithelial injury should be avoided whenever possible, particularly in compromised eyes, eg, dry eyes, eyes with corneal exposure due to exophthalmos or abnormal eyelid function such as produced by facial nerve paralysis or ectropion, and eyes with reduced corneal sensation. The classic situation is the combination of fifth and seventh nerve dysfunction such as occurs with cerebellopontine angle tumors, producing a dry, anesthetic eye with poor eyelid closure. Any comatose patient is also at risk of corneal exposure, and prophylactic eyelid taping should be undertaken.

Any unnecessary exposure of the eye to pathogenic organisms should be avoided, but it becomes critical in certain situations. During intraocular surgery, the normal barriers to infection are circumvented, and meticulous attention must be paid to avoiding contamination of the eye with organisms. The ocular environment must be assessed preoperatively to identify and treat any sources of pathogenic organisms. These include colonization or infection of the lacrimal sac, the lid margins, the conjunctiva, and the cornea. In emergency situations, it may only be possible to identify such sources and use prophylactic antibiotic therapy to reduce the chances of subsequent infection, whereas for elective surgery more definitive therapy to eradicate or minimize the pathogenic organisms should be possible. There is much debate about the value of preoperative and perioperative prophylactic antibiotics in patients with no identifiable external ocular disease. It is important to recognize that one of the major causes of endophthalmitis after cataract surgery is *Staphylococcus epidermidis,* which frequently colonizes normal eyelids. Considerations may need to be given to other sites of bacterial colonization or infection such as the bladder, throat, nose, and skin. Sterility must be ensured of the operative field, instruments, intraocular and topical medications, and other fluids introduced into the eye. During the postoperative period, sterile medications must be used and contact with other patients with established ocular infections avoided.

Contact lens wear is strongly associated with suppurative keratitis due to the combination of an abnormal load of pathogenic organisms and probable recurrent minor trauma to the corneal epithelium. The incidence of suppurative keratitis is particularly high with soft lenses, especially with extended wear. It is apparent that many people wearing contact lenses for cosmetic reasons are not aware of the risks involved. Whereas it may be reasonable to face the risks of infection with extended-wear soft lenses in elderly aphakes who are dependent on contact lenses for refractive correction and cannot cope with daily-wear lenses—or in patients with highly compromised eyes that are symptomatic from bullous keratopathy—the arguments in favor of extended-wear soft lenses for refractive correction in patients with low refractive errors are less strong. A number of patients in this latter group start off their contact lens career using extended-wear disposable lenses, which is of course an attractive arrangement because it dispenses with the need for lens cleaning and the associated paraphernalia, but this practice is likely to require an unwelcome sacrifice of safety for convenience. Contact lens wear exposes the eye to an abnormal load of pathogenic organisms, which have been shown to adhere with particular tenacity to soft lenses, unless the user is absolutely meticulous about contact lens hygiene. The development of toxic reactions to preservatives within the contact lens solutions with the necessary dependence on preservative-free solutions increases the chances of suppurative keratitis from organisms capable of surviving in such solutions, eg, *Pseudomonas* and *Acanthamoeba.*

All contact lens wearers must be apprised of the relative risk of suppurative keratitis and the need for meticulous contact lens hygiene. They should be advised to keep a pair of spectacles available so that contact lens wear be discontinued immediately whenever an eye becomes uncomfortable or inflamed. If ocular discomfort or inflammation persists, the wearer should seek ophthalmologic advice without delay.

Neonatal conjunctivitis (see Chapter 17) is a good example of exposure to a heavy load of pathogenic organisms with the added inherent susceptibility of the poorly developed immune mechanisms of the neonatal eye. The major organisms that may produce neonatal conjunctivitis are *Neisseria gonorrhoeae,* chlamydiae, herpes simplex, *Staphylococcus aureus, Haemophilus* species, and *Streptococcus pneumoniae.* Exposure to these organisms occurs during passage down the birth canal. It should be possible to prevent neonatal conjunctivitis by treating mothers harboring these organisms prior to delivery, and this has been achieved for the bacteria, including *Chlamydia.* The alternative approach is the routine ocular prophylaxis of neonates. This started with the silver nitrate prophylaxis of Credé and has been superseded in a number of centers by topical erythromycin in view of the predominance of chlamydial neonatal conjunctivitis.

Shedding of herpes simplex virus by the expectant mother is not necessarily associated with clinically obvious lesions, and shedding may occur in mothers who do not have any history of such lesions. Identification of mothers likely to infect their babies would require routine viral cultures from all women prior to delivery, and even then it would not be possible to identify specifically those actually shedding virus at the time of delivery. In the presence of frank clinical lesions at the time of delivery, elective cesarean section may be advisable.

PREVENTION OF IATROGENIC OCULAR INFECTION

Ophthalmologists have been clearly implicated in the transmission of infectious eye disease. Outbreaks of **epidemic keratoconjunctivitis** have been traced to contamination in the ophthalmologist's office. The adenovirus is transmitted via the ophthalmologist's hands, a tonometer, or solutions contaminated by droppers accidentally rubbed against the infected conjunctiva or lid margin of a patient. Contaminated ophthalmic solutions have also been the source of infection in bacterial corneal ulcers and endophthalmitis following intraocular surgery. *Pseudomonas aeruginosa* used to be a common contaminant of ophthalmic solutions, particularly fluorescein. Instillation of contaminated fluorescein solution to delineate corneal epithelial defects (eg, after removal of a corneal foreign body) may result in severe pseudomonal keratitis and, frequently, loss of the eye.

Other infections can be similarly spread, but their occurrence is not generally recognized. The ophthalmologist should be alert to the possibility that if ophthalmic instruments are improperly sterilized (as by cold sterilization), they may be contaminated with hepatitis B virus. Identification of the AIDS virus in tears has suggested a small possibility of transmission by ophthalmologists. To date, no such incident has occurred.

There is good experimental evidence that applanation tonometer tips can be adequately sterilized, particularly with respect to human immunodeficiency virus type 1, herpes simplex virus, and adenovirus, by wiping with 70% isopropyl alcohol swabs and then allowing the instrument to evaporate dry. It is imperative that the tonometer tip be completely dry before use on the next patient or corneal epithelial damage will result. This method of sterilization is more practical than immersion in alcohol, hypochlorite, or hydrogen peroxide and less likely to damage the tonometer tip, though immersion in such disinfectant solutions at the end of each working day and after examination of high-risk patients is probably advisable. In this case, the tonometer tip should be rinsed in tap water and dried before use. Goldmann three-mirror and similar contact lenses used for patient examination are also susceptible to damage from immersion in disinfectants and should be treated in a similar manner to tonometer tips. The Schiotz tonometer needs to be immersed in disinfectant, autoclaved, or exposed to ethylene oxide for effective sterilization. The noncontact tonometer is recommended for reducing the risks of disease transmission, but it may generate an aerosol spray that endangers the individual operating the tonometer.

Ophthalmologists and their staffs must maintain the highest level of personal hygiene at all times and must use standard sterile technique when appropriate, keeping in mind the possibility of contamination of any solution brought into contact with the eye.

Hands play a major role in the transmission of infection. They should be washed or disinfected (eg, with isopropyl alcohol) before and after the examination of every patient, especially if an ocular infection is thought to be present.

PREVENTION OF OCULAR DAMAGE DUE TO CONGENITAL INFECTIONS

Viral disease of the mother with resultant embryopathy may lead to such ocular anomalies in the offspring as retinopathy, infantile glaucoma, cataract, uveal tract coloboma, etc, and prevention may in some cases be possible. Two viruses, rubella and cytomegalovirus, can be extremely damaging to the infant, and one of them—rubella virus—can be prevented by vaccination. Once a common childhood disease, rubella led to lifelong immunity, but vaccination is now indicated for susceptible young women approaching childbearing age. Susceptibility can be determined by assessing the antibody content of the young woman's blood. If a mother contracts rubella during early pregnancy, she should be informed of the likelihood of ocular and other abnormalities in her baby, and the arguments for and against abortion should be presented.

Unfortunately, cytomegalovirus (the other virus causing a high incidence of congenital anomalies) continues to be a serious and unsolved threat. No protective vaccine is currently available, though one is currently under study.

Toxoplasmosis is another important cause of congenital infection, leading to (1) chorioretinitis, which may be apparent at birth or may remain subclinical until reactivation occurs later in life; (2) cerebral or cerebellar calcification; (3) hydrocephalus; and occasionally (4) more severe central nervous system abnormalities. Unless the mother is immunocompromised, fetal infection occurs only if she acquires primary infection during pregnancy. This can be prevented by eating only meat that is well cooked, by washing vegetables and fruits, and by wearing gloves when disposing of cat litter or working in the garden so that contact with viable oocysts and tissue cysts is avoided. It has been shown that if acute maternal infection during pregnancy can be identified—such as with the serial serologic tests that are required by law in France and Austria—appropriate antibiotic treatment in those pregnancies allowed to proceed, with adjustments according to whether fetal infection is also present, reduces the incidence of congenital infection and improves the clinical outcome in fetuses that are infected.

PREVENTION OF GENETIC DISEASES WITH OCULAR INVOLVEMENT

Until recently, the prevention of genetic disorders received little attention. Now, however, there are genetic counseling centers in many medical centers, and the genetic nature of many disorders that affect the eye is recognized and their transmission better understood than formerly. In conference with internists and pediatricians, it is up to the ophthalmologist to recommend genetic counseling for patients contemplating marriage and children. Patients with histories of childhood diabetes, retinitis pigmentosa, consanguineous mating, retinoblastoma, neurofibromatosis, etc, need genetic counseling to prevent disaster for their offspring.

Some clinical conditions, eg, Down's syndrome (trisomy 21), are associated with an abnormal number of chromosomes or with abnormalities of the sex chromosomes. Prenatal diagnosis can now be made by testing amniotic fluid cells obtained by amniocentesis (a safe and practical procedure), and a positive diagnosis gives the patient the option of abortion.

EARLY DETECTION OF TREATABLE OCULAR DISEASE

A number of primary ocular diseases are treatable only during their early stages or are more effectively treated at that time. Detection of such diseases may be possible through the timely recognition of relevant symptoms or may require specific vigilance on the part of medical workers because of the absence of symptoms.

Age-Related Macular Degeneration

Age-related macular degeneration is the leading cause of permanent visual loss in the elderly in industrialized countries, and its incidence is increasing with each decade over age 50. There are two major forms of the disease: (1) atrophic ("dry") degeneration, in which there is progressive degeneration of the outer retina, retinal pigment epithelium, Bruch's membrane, and choriocapillaris; and (2) exudative ("wet") degeneration, in which there is a sudden onset of visual loss due to leakage of serous fluid or blood into the retina followed by new vessel formation under the retinal pigment epithelium (subretinal neovascular membrane).

Laser photocoagulation of subretinal neovascular membranes may delay the onset of central visual loss but only when the membrane is far enough away from the fovea to permit treatment. Elderly patients developing sudden visual loss due to macular disease—particularly paracentral distortion or scotoma, with preservation of central acuity—should undergo urgent ophthalmic assessment, including fluorescein angiography, to determine their suitability for laser treatment. There is no effective treatment for the atrophic form of macular degeneration except for the provision of low vision aids.

Primary Open-Angle Glaucoma

Primary open-angle glaucoma is a major cause of preventable blindness worldwide, particularly among individuals of African racial origin. About two million Americans have the disease, though half are undiagnosed. The prevalence of primary open-angle glaucoma increases from 0.1% for those aged 40–49 to 3% for those over age 70. Symptoms do not usually occur until there is advanced visual field loss. For treatment to be effective, the disease must be detected at a much earlier stage. Specific screening programs are hampered by the high prevalence of raised intraocular pressure in the absence of glaucomatous visual field loss (ocular hypertension), which is ten times more common than primary open-angle glaucoma, the high frequency of normal intraocular pressure on a single reading in untreated open-angle glaucoma, and the complexities of screening for optic disk or visual field abnormalities.

The best means of detecting primary open-angle glaucoma early is performance of tonometry and direct ophthalmoscopy of the optic disk on all adult patients every 3 years, with referral to ophthalmologists of all those with relevant abnormalities. In the case of patients at high risk of developing primary open-angle glaucoma, such as first degree relatives of affected individuals, formal ophthalmic assessment should take place every year.

PREVENTION OF AMBLYOPIA ("LAZY EYE")

Amblyopia can be defined for the purposes of this discussion as diminished visual acuity in one eye in the absence of organic eye disease. Central vision develops from birth to age 6 or 7; if vision has not developed by then, there is little or no chance that it will develop later. In the absence of eye disease, the two main abnormalities that will prevent a child from acquiring binocular vision are strabismus and anisometropia.

Strabismus

Esotropia or exotropia in a young child causes double vision. The child quickly learns to suppress the image in the deviating eye and learns to see normally with one eye. Unfortunately, vision does not develop in the unused eye; unless the good eye is patched, thus forcing the child to use the deviating eye, sight will never develop in that eye. The child will grow up with one perfectly normal eye that is essentially blind, since it has never developed a functional connection with the visual centers of the brain. This is more likely to occur with esotropia than with exotropia.

Anisometropia

Young children are more concerned with the perception of near objects than with those at a distance. If one eye is nearsighted (myopic) and the other farsighted (hyperopic), the child will favor the nearsighted eye. Thus, the farsighted eye will not be used even though it is straight. The result will be the same as in untreated strabismus, ie, monocular blindness due to failure of visual development in an unused eye. The incidence of anisometropia is about 0.75–1%.

Early Diagnosis

The best way to prevent amblyopia is to test the visual acuity of all preschool children. By the time a child reaches school, it is usually too late for occlusion therapy. The parents can perform the test at home with the illiterate "E" chart. This is sometimes known as the "Home Eye Test." Pediatricians and others responsible for the care of small children should test visual acuity no later than age 4.

Photorefraction is said to be useful in screening for anisometropia, ametropia, astigmatism, and strabismus in preschool children. Any child observed to have strabismus after the age of 3 months should be seen by an ophthalmologist.

PREVENTION OF OCULAR DAMAGE DUE TO SYSTEMIC DISEASES

It is important for nonophthalmologic practitioners, particularly internists, general practitioners, and pediatricians, to be aware of the systemic diseases that have an ophthalmic component which may produce asymptomatic ocular damage.

Diabetic retinopathy is the most common cause of blindness developing between ages 20 and 64. Treatment is available to prevent such blindness, but for best effect it must be administered before visual loss has occurred, ie, diabetics must undergo regular fundal examination and be referred whenever treatment is indicated. The major abnormalities that must be recognized are new vessel formation on the optic disk and exudates around the macula. Any diabetic developing visual loss should also be referred for ophthalmic assessment. (The management of diabetic retinopathy is discussed further in Chapters 10 and 15.)

Uveitis associated with juvenile rheumatoid arthritis is generally asymptomatic in its early stages and often remains undetected until severe loss of vision due to glaucoma, cataract, or band keratopathy has already occurred. Regular ophthalmic screening should take place, particularly of girls with a pauciarticular onset of the disease and circulating antinuclear antibody.

Even in the USA, where it should now be all but unknown, occasional cases of xerophthalmia still occur, and in the underdeveloped areas the world over, where nutrition is often poor, it is still common. Vitamin A deficiency disease, in which the eye changes (xerophthalmia and keratomalacia) are the most damaging and often cause blindness (see Chapter 23), is usually the result of a deficient diet associated with poverty. It should be borne in mind, however, that it may also be associated with chronic alcoholism, weight-reducing diets, dietary management of food allergy, or poor absorption from the gastrointestinal tract due to the use of mineral oil or gastrointestinal disease such as chronic diarrhea.

In vitamin A-deficient children, measles may result in severe corneal disease. Because of the eye signs (ie, night blindness, Bitot's spots, or a lackluster corneal epithelium), the ophthalmologist may be the first to recognize vitamin A deficiency. Early recognition and treatment can prevent loss of vision or blindness due to secondary infection and corneal perforation. Treatment of the acute condition may require large intramuscular doses of vitamin A followed by corrective diet and careful analysis of all possible causes.

PREVENTION OF VISUAL LOSS DUE TO DRUGS

All drugs can cause adverse reactions. It is the ophthalmologist's responsibility to prevent visual loss or major ocular disability from drugs used to treat eye diseases.

Ophthalmic drugs should be packaged and labeled so that mistakes are not made by elderly or poorly sighted patients. Atropine and other strong medications may call for color-labeling. On the first visit to a new ophthalmologist, the patient should be asked to bring along any previously prescribed medications in order to avoid duplication and possible overdosage.

Certain ophthalmic drugs have such frequently occurring and damaging side effects that their use requires special monitoring and special warnings to the patient. Atropine and scopolamine, used to dilate the pupil in iridocyclitis, may precipitate acute glaucoma in certain patients with narrow anterior chamber angles. After prolonged use, they can also lead to conjunctivitis and allergic eczema of the eyelids. Many antiglaucoma drugs can produce stenosis of the puncta and shrinkage of the conjunctiva. Topical anesthetics should never be prescribed or made available for long-term use because severe corneal ulceration and scarring may result.

Corticosteroids used locally in drop or ointment forms may depress the local defense mechanisms and precipitate corneal ulceration, often fungal. They may also worsen herpetic keratitis and other corneal infections and on prolonged use may lead to open-angle glaucoma and to posterior subcapsular cataract. Much of the severity of both herpes simplex virus and varicella-zoster virus corneal infections can be blamed on the unwise use of topical corticosteroids. In this situation, short-term improvement has been traded for long-term disaster.

Many drugs used **systemically** have serious ocular side effects, eg, keratopathy, retrobulbar neuritis, retinopathy, and Stevens-Johnson syndrome (erythema multiforme). For this reason, the ophthalmologist must take a careful history of the patient's use of drugs as part of the initial examination. Of special interest are the keratopathy and retinopathy that may follow the use of chloroquine in discoid lupus erythematosus. It is the function of the consulting ophthalmologist to detect any early ocular changes and to inform the dermatologist of them so that he can substitute another medication.

REFERENCES

Apt L et al: The effects of povidone-iodine solution applied at the conclusion of ophthalmic surgery. Am J Ophthalmol 1995;119:701.

Azar MJ et al: Possible consequence of shaking hands with your patients with epidemic keratoconjunctivitis. Am J Ophthalmol 1996;121:711.

Batisse D et al: Acute retinal necrosis in the course of AIDS: Study of 26 cases. AIDS 1996;10:55.

Bird AC et al: An international classification and grading system for age-related maculopathy and age-related macular degeneration. The International ARM Epidemiological Study Group. Surv Ophthalmol 1995;39:367.

Chen CJ et al: Managing diabetic retinopathy: The partnership between ophthalmologist and primary care physician. J Miss State Med Assoc 1995;36:201.

Cheung J et al: Microbial etiology and predisposing factors among patients hospitalized for corneal ulceration. Can J Ophthalmol 1995;30:251.

Chitkara DK et al: Risk factors, complications, and results in extracapsular cataract extraction. J Cat Refract Surg 1997;23:570.

Cumming RG et al: Use of inhaled corticosteroids and the risk of cataracts. N Engl J Med 1997;337:8.

Darzins P et al: Sun exposure and age-related macular degeneration. An Australian case-control study. Ophthalmology 1997;104:770.

De Respinis PA et al: Survey of severe eye injuries in children. Am J Dis Child 1989;143:711.

Duttner LR et al: Potential bacterial contamination in fluorescein-anesthetic solutions. Am J Ophthalmol 1990; 110:426.

Eaton RB et al: Multicenter evaluation of a fluorometric enzyme immunocapture assay to detect toxoplasmosis-specific immunoglobulin M in dried blood filter paper specimens from newborns. J Clin Microbiol 1996;34: 3147.

Givens KT et al: Congenital rubella syndrome and associated systemic disorders. Br J Ophthalmol 1993;77:358.

Gordon YJ et al: Prolonged recovery of desiccated adenoviral serotypes 5, 8 and 19 from plastic and metal surfaces in vitro. Ophthalmology 1993;100:1835.

Gottsh JD: Surveillance and control of epidemic keratoconjunctivitis. Trans Am Ophthalmol Soc 1996;94:539.

Haefliger IO et al: The logic of prevention of glaucomatous damage progression. Curr Opin Ophthalmol 1997;8:64.

Javitt JC: Universal coverage and preventable blindness. Arch Ophthalmol 1994;112:453.

Kristinsson JK et al: Active prevention in diabetic disease. A 4 year follow-up. Acta Ophthalmol Scand 1997;75: 249.

Larrison WI et al: Sports related ocular trauma. Ophthalmology 1990;97:1265.

Lee GA et al: Knowledge of sunlight effects on the eyes and protective behaviors in the general community. Ophthalmol Epidemiol 1994;1:67.

Liggett PE et al: Ocular trauma in an urban population. Review of 1132 cases. Ophthalmology 1990;97:581.

McCarthy CA et al: Recent developments in vision research: Light damage in cataracts. Invest Ophthalmol Vis Sci 1996;37:1720.

Mulvihill A et al: Uniocular childhood blindness: A prospective study. J Pediatr Ophthalmol Strabismus 1997;34:111.

Ng EW et al: Postoperative endophthalmitis: Risk factors and prophylaxis. Int Ophthalmol Clin 1996;36:109.

Ratelle S et al: Neonatal chlamydial infections in Massachusetts, 1992–1993. Am J Prev Med 1997;13:221.

Rosenwasser GOD et al: Topical anesthetic abuse. Ophthalmology 1990;97:962.

Silvestri G: Age-related macular degeneration: Genetics and implications for detection and treatment. Mol Med Today 1997;3:84.

Sjostrand J et al: Prevention of amblyopia and the concept of cure. Eur J Ophthalmol 1997;7:121.

Speaker MG et al: Role of external bacterial flora in the pathogenesis of acute postoperative endophthalmitis. Ophthalmology 1991;98:639.

Threlkeld AB et al: Efficacy of a disinfectant wipe method for the removal of adenovirus 8 from tonometer tips. Ophthalmology 1993;100:1841.

von Setten GB: The clinical use of contact lenses and collagen shields. Curr Opin Ophthalmol 1996;7:17.

Wagner PH et al: Mechanical ocular trauma. Curr Opin Ophthalmol 1996;7:57.

Low Vision

22

Eleanor E. Faye, MD, FACS

In every subspecialty of ophthalmology, the patient with impaired vision represents a challenge in management. Whether reduced vision is temporary or permanent, it is the consequence of an eye disorder and, as such, is the responsibility of the ophthalmologist and optometrist. If the outcome of optimal medical and surgical intervention is diminished functional vision, the patient needs vision rehabilitation. No person with low vision should have to search far and wide for low-vision care. Some level of care should be integrated into every ophthalmic practice whether it is on-site or referral to a low-vision center.

Low-vision patients typically have impaired visual performance, ie, visual acuity is not correctable with conventional glasses or contact lenses. They may have cloudy vision, constricted fields, or large scotomas. There may be additional functional complaints: glare sensitivity, abnormal color perception, difficulty with diminished contrast. Some patients have diplopia. A frequent complaint is confusion from overlapping but dissimilar images from each eye.

The term "low vision" covers a wide range. A person in the early stages of an eye disease may have near-normal vision. Others may have moderate to severe loss. All low-vision patients have some degree of useful vision even though they might have a profound loss. They should not be considered "blind" unless their level of function is near-blind. Performance varies with each individual

In the United States, over 6 million persons are visually impaired but not classified as legally blind.* Over 75% of patients seeking treatment are age 65 or older. Age-related macular degeneration accounts for an increasing number of cases. Other common causes of low vision are complicated cataract, corneal dystrophy, glaucoma, diabetic retinopathy, optic atrophy, stroke, degenerative myopia, and retinitis pigmentosa.

Effective low-vision intervention starts as soon as the patient experiences difficulty performing ordinary tasks. A treatment plan should consider the level of function, realistic goals for intervention, and the varieties of devices that could be helpful. Patients must face the fact that impaired vision is usually progressive. The sooner they adapt to low-vision devices, the sooner they can adjust to the new techniques of using their vision. Low-vision evaluation should never be delayed unless the person is undergoing active medical or surgical treatment.

Visual performance can be improved by the use of optical and nonoptical devices. The general term for corrective devices is "low-vision aids." In this chapter, the emphasis will be on assessment techniques, descriptions of useful devices, and a discussion of some of the functional aspects of common eye diseases.

MANAGEMENT OF THE PATIENT WITH LOW VISION

Comprehensive management includes (1) history of onset, and the effect of the eye condition on daily life; (2) examination for best corrected acuity, visual fields, contrast sensitivity, color perception, and glare sensitivity if it pertains to the patient's symptoms; (3) evaluation of near vision and reading skills; (4) selection and prescription (or lending) of aids that accomplish task objectives; (5) instruction in correct use and application of devices; and (6) follow-up to reinforce new patterns.

1. HISTORY TAKING

Specific features of the onset, treatments given, and current medications should be verified. Patients' responses indicate their understanding of their condition. Are there unrealistic or unreasonable attitudes? Does the person understand what can be achieved with low-vision rehabilitation? It is helpful to list a number of common daily activities the patient can no longer perform efficiently (Table 22–1). From this list it is possible to arrive at realistic objectives for that person.

2. EXAMINATION

The patient should not have pupillary dilation before a low-vision evaluation. Refractive status should be confirmed to rule out a significant change. A pa-

---

* Legal blindness—defined as best corrected visual acuity of 20/200 or less in the better eye or a visual field of 20 degrees or less—affects 1,000,000 individuals in the USA (see Chapter 23).

Table 22–1. Common activities that are adversely affected by visual impairment are listed with suggestions for low vision aids.

Activity	Optical Aids	Nonoptical Aids
Shopping	Hand magnifier	Lighting, color cues
Fixing a snack	Bifocals	Color cues, consistent storage plan
Eating out	Hand magnifier	Flashlight, portable lamp
Identifying money	Bifocal, hand magnifier	Arrange wallet in compartments
Reading print	High power spectacle, bifocal, hand magnifier, stand magnifier, closed circuit television	Lighting, high-contrast print, large print, reading slit
Writing	Intermediate add hand magnifier, focusable telescope, closed circuit television	Lighting, bold tip pen, black ink
Dialing a telephone	Hand magnifier	Large print dial, hand-printed directory
Crossing streets	Telescope	Cane, ask directions
Finding taxis and bus signs	Telescope	
Reading medication labels	Hand magnifier	Color codes, large print
Reading stove dials	Hand magnifier	Color codes
Thermostat adjustment	Hand magnifier	Enlarged print model
Using a computer	Intermediate add spectacles	High-contrast color, large print program
Reading signs	Spectacle	Move closer
Watching sporting event	Telescope	Sit in front rows

tient may have become myopic (cataract) or astigmatic (corneal or cataract surgery). The most accurate acuity test is the ETDRS chart (Figure 22–1), which has 14 five-letter lines of 0.1 log unit size difference and a convenient metric or Snellen conversion table. A 4 meter test distance is used when acuity is 20/20 to 20/200; a 2 meter distance for acuities less than 20/200 but 20/400 or better; and the 1 meter distance for acuities less than 20/400. The ETDRS chart makes obsolete the imprecise expression "finger counting only."

Projector charts are not recommended for testing subnormal vision because of low contrast and insufficient letter choice at low acuities. Any Snellen chart may be hand-held at 10 feet or less.

The dominant eye and preferred eye should be noted.

The Amsler grid is the traditional test for evaluating the central field. Although it is relatively insensitive, it can be used to advantage in low vision, particularly to identify the dominant eye. At the test distance of 33 cm, the patient should first look at the chart binocularly. ("Can you see the dot?") Observe for eye or head turn. If the dot is seen, the patient is using either a viable macular area or an eccentric viewing region. An eye turn or head tilt may confirm this. Ask the patient to report distortion or blank areas seen binocularly. Then check the grid monocularly and again ask the patient to report seeing the center fixation dot and any distortion or scotoma. If the grid is presented in this manner, the patient understands what is expected and the test can provide helpful data. For example, if

a large scotoma in the dominant eye overrides the better nondominant eye, the patient probably will require occlusion of the dominant eye. If the dominant eye "fills in" the defect of the poorer eye, the patient can benefit from binocular correction.

Tests of contrast express the functional level of retinal sensitivity more accurately than any other test, including acuity. Of the available tests for contrast sensitivity,* the test using sine wave gratings (Vistech) covers the greatest number of retinal receptor channels. The resulting curve measures the contrast levels attained in each of five channels covering low, middle, and high contrast. Contrast sensitivity is a predictor of the retina's response to magnification. Regardless of acuity, if contrast is subthreshold, the patient is unlikely to respond to optical magnification. The contrast curve is analogous to the curve produced in audiometry (pitch and volume).

Simple color identification tests are done if the patient's complaints include difficulty with color cues.

3. NEAR VISION

Near vision may be evaluated with a combination of single-letter tests (Figure 22–2) and graded text. Single letters and short words are presented first to establish near acuity. Graded text is presented after the

* Vistech Contrast Sensitivity Vision Test, Pelli-Robson, Lea Test System and Symbols available from The Lighthouse Low Vision Catalog, 111 East 59th Street, New York, NY 10022.

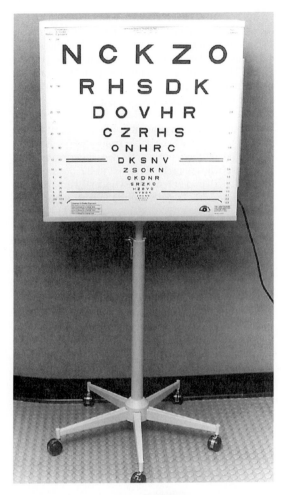

Figure 22–1. Lighthouse modification of the Ferris-Bailey ETDRS chart in a movable light box.

function tests to establish reading skills with the selected optical devices.

4. SELECTION OF DEVICES & PATIENT INSTRUCTION

The dioptric range is selected from the outcome of acuity tests, modified by the results of the Amsler grid and contrast sensitivity tests. A rule of thumb for the starting power is to calculate the reciprocal of a visual acuity—eg, an acuity of 20/160 (160/20) suggests a starting lens of 8 diopters. Keep in mind that visual acuity is not a particularly sensitive measure of function. Scotomas within the reading field and the contrast sensitivity of the paramacular retina have a greater influence on ability to read through an optical lens.

After the dioptric range has been agreed upon, the three major categories of devices are presented in sequence in the selected power.

5. INSTRUCTION

Part of effective management of every low-vision patient is skilled instruction in using a device. Attention should be paid to daily living activities, which can be complemented by low-vision lenses, but may also require referral to an agency for the visually impaired.

The patient uses the various devices under the supervision of an instructor until proficiency is achieved. During the instruction time, mechanics of the aids are reviewed, questions are answered, and goals reexamined. The patient is allowed ample time to learn correct techniques in one or more sessions, and possibly a loaner lens for home or job trial. Older patients usually need more adaptation time and reinforcement than younger or congenitally impaired persons.

Practitioners and staff benefit from training programs to learn how to manage a low-vision patient in the office. Basic setups for incorporating low vision into a practice are reviewed in a number of publications.

Instruction is the key to success in vision rehabilitation. Over 90% of patients succeed with instruction, whereas a 50% success rate (no better than chance) results from prescribing an aid without training.

6. FOLLOW-UP

In two to three weeks the patient's progress is reviewed, adjustments are made, and prescriptions are finalized. If minor problems arise within the first few days after the appointment they can usually be resolved by telephone.

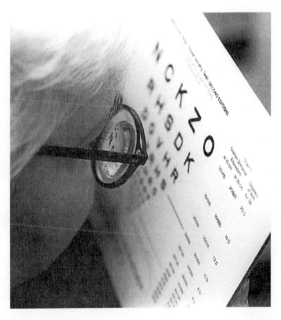

Figure 22–2. Low-vision spectacle aid. Patient demonstrates close reading distance (with lenticular spectacle) but with both hands free to hold reading material.

LOW-VISION AIDS

There are five types of low-vision aids: (1) convex lens aids such as spectacle, hand-held, and stand-mounted magnifiers; (2) telescopic systems, either spectacle-mounted or hand-held; (3) nonoptical (adaptive) devices such as large print, lighting, reading stands, marking devices, talking clocks, timers, and scales; (4) tints and filters, including antireflective lenses; and (5) electronic reading systems such as closed-circuit television reading machines, optical print scanners, computers with large print programs, and computers equipped with voice commands to access the programs.

1. CONVEX LENS AIDS

Spectacles and hand and stand magnifiers are prescribed for over 90% of patients. Various mountings have inherent advantages and disadvantages. If the patient uses spectacles, reading material must be held at the focal distance of the lens, eg, 10 cm for a 10-diopter lens. The stronger the lens, the shorter the reading distance, which tends to obstruct light (Figure 22–2) The advantage of spectacles is that both hands remain free to hold the reading material. Lamps with flexible arms can be adjusted for uniform lighting.

Patients who have binocular potential may use spectacles in the 4- to 14-diopter range with base-in prism to aid convergence. Above 14 diopters, a monocular sphere must be used for the better eye.

Hand magnifiers are convenient for shopping, reading dials and labels, identifying money, etc (Figure 22–3). They are often used by older people in conjunction with their reading glasses to enlarge print. The advantage of the hand-held lens is a greater working space between the eye and lens. Holding a lens, however, may be a disadvantage for a trembling hand or stiff joints. Hand magnifiers are available from 4 to 68 diopters.

Stand magnifiers are convex lenses mounted on a rigid base whose height is related to the power of the lens, eg, a 10 diopter lens is just under 10 cm from the page (Figure 22–4). Because the lens mounting may block light, a lens with a battery-powered light may be the best choice. Patients with corneal and lens pathology may not be able to tolerate the glare from an illuminated device.

2. TELESCOPIC SYSTEMS

Telescopic systems are the only devices that can be focused from infinity to near. For low vision, the simplest device is the hand-held monocular for short-term viewing, particularly of signs. For patients with vocational or hobby interests, Galilean or Keplerian telescopes (internal prism systems) in a spectacle frame are practical (Figure 22–5). A recent development is a monocular autofocus telescope. The practical limit of power for hand-held units is 2–8×. Spectacle tele-

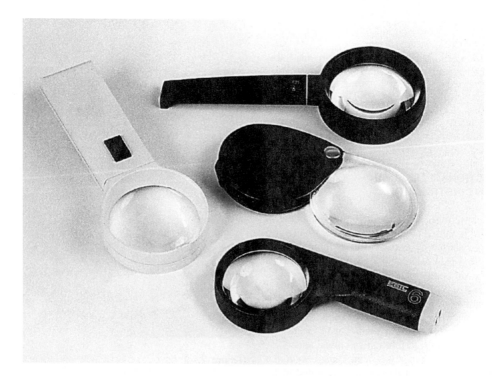

Figure 22–3. Hand magnifiers of varius types and strengths.

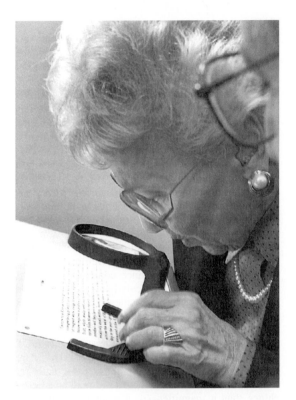

Figure 22–4. A woman with macular degeneration uses a fixed-focus stand magnifier. Her hand tremor prevented her from using a hand magnifier.

scopes are difficult to use above 6×. All telescopes share the disadvantage of a small field diameter and shallow depth of field.

3. NONOPTICAL (ADAPTIVE) DEVICES

There are many practical items that augment or replace visual aids. They are traditionally called "nonoptical devices," though "adaptive aids" is probably a better term. In daily life, difficulty reading is not the only frustrating experience for the low-vision person. Cooking, setting thermostats and stove dials, measuring, reading a scale, putting on makeup, selecting the correct illumination, identifying paper money, and playing cards are only a few things that sighted people take for granted. A catalog from The Lighthouse lists practical articles for every facet of daily life. Patients and family members appreciate it as a handout to review at home.

4. TINTS & COATINGS

Many low-vision patients complain of poor contrast and glare, which particularly hampers getting around by themselves. A basic approach is to consider the effect of short-wave light on cloudy media and to remember that contrast is also affected by time of day, weather, and textures and colors in the surroundings. As a rule, light or medium gray lenses are prescribed

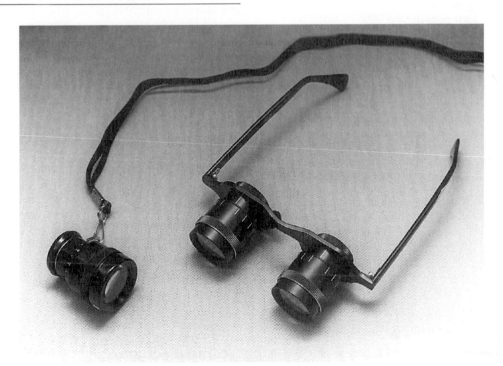

Figure 22–5. Low-vision telescopes. *A:* Hand-held monocular telescope. *B:* Spectacle-mounted Galilean focusable telescope.

to reduce light intensity. To improve contrast and reduce the effect of short-wave light rays, amber or yellow lenses are suggested. Companies such as Corning and NoIR design and manufacture lenses specifically for low-vision patients. An additional antireflective coating should be considered for patients who are mildly glare sensitive.

5. ELECTRONIC READING SYSTEMS

Electronic devices are the only ones that encourage a natural reading posture. A closed-circuit television reading machine (CCTV) consists of a high-resolution television monitor with a built-in camera with a zoom lens, an accessory lamp, and an X-Y reading platform. The patient sits comfortably in front of the screen, moving the print back and forth on the platform. Magnification from 1.5× to 45× is possible with adjustable font sizes, and the background can be reversed from white to dark gray. Some models have choices of print colors. Recent developments include a hand-held camera, the Mouse-Cam, that can be carried around and plugged into any TV; computers with voice output and scrolling of text; and optical scanners that can read text aloud. Standard personal computers can be easily modified for large print programs. Laptop computers have insufficient contrast and screen size for the average low-vision patient.

THE EFFECT OF THE EYE DISORDER

Treatment plans should take into account the effect of the eye disorder on both visual acuity and visual field. The type and strength of visual aid are influenced by the type and extent of the deficit.

Diseases resulting in low vision can be classified in four categories: (1) blurred or hazy vision throughout the visual field, characteristic of cloudy media (cornea, lens, lens capsule, vitreous); (2) impaired resolution without central scotoma with normal peripheral retina, characteristic of macular edema or albinism; (3) central scotomas, characteristic of degenerative, congenital, or inflammatory macular disorders, and the cecocentral scotoma of optic nerve disease; and (4) peripheral scotomas, typical of retinitis pigmentosa, advanced glaucoma, stroke, and any peripheral retinal disorder, including diabetic retinopathy.

1. BLURRED, HAZY VISION

Generalized blurring and haziness of vision is the rule in any abnormality of the optical media. Glare and photophobia may also be factors. Any corneal disease, cataracts, capsular opacification, or vitreous opacities interfere with refraction of light rays entering the eye.

Such random refraction causes reduced acuity, glare, and decreased contrast. Pupillary miosis further restricts the quantity of light reaching the retina. Patients have difficulty seeing stairs and steps and other low-contrast objects. Acuity varies with ambient light.

Useful tests of visual function include Snellen visual acuity, glare test, and contrast sensitivity. A potential acuity meter (PAM) used in conjunction with a glare test helps to differentiate retinal from media pathology.

Management

Refraction should always be carefully done, including multiple pinholes, stenopeic slit, and keratometry. Modification of illumination and attention to details of room and task lighting are most important. Antireflective lens coatings and neutral gray lenses reduce light intensity (and therefore glare). Yellow and amber lenses enhance contrast. Ultraviolet filters should be used particularly for pseudophakic patients. Large bold print provides the higher contrast the patient needs.

Magnification may or may not be effective depending on the patient's level of contrast sensitivity. A magnified image itself has low contrast. The glare from an illuminated stand magnifier may actually reduce reading acuity. Large bold print may be a better choice than a magnifier—or a reading slit of matte black plastic to reduce glare and outline the text. Contact lenses, keratoplasty, LASIK refractive surgery, posterior capsulotomy, and intraocular lens implants may also be considered in specific cases. The cataract surgeon may wish to discuss overcorrecting the power of the implant by a few diopters. The resulting myopia would allow the low-vision patient useful uncorrected vision in the intermediate range.

2. IMPAIRED RESOLUTION

Macular edema from a variety of disorders and congenital foveal aplasia of albinism affect only a few degrees of the fovea. As a rule, the acuity is in the higher range from 20/50 to 20/200.

Useful tests of visual function include Snellen visual acuity, Amsler grid, and contrast sensitivity.

Management

Careful refraction should be done to rule out astigmatic error. Patients usually accept reading adds of +4 to +10 D and are proficient readers. Bifocals or contact lenses should be considered for stable or congenital conditions. Albinos with nystagmus can wear toric contact lenses successfully.

3. CENTRAL SCOTOMAS

Central vision is essential for details, color vision, and daylight vision. The macula consists predominately of cones. The two commonest causes of macular disease are atrophic (dry) and exudative (wet) macular degeneration, both of which are more prevalent in today's aging society. Other causes are macular holes, myopic macular degeneration, optic nerve disease (cecocentral scotoma), and congenital macular disorders. Laser treatment near the fovea may result in a dense scotoma.

In the early stages of macular disease, patients most often report blurred or distorted central vision. Peripheral vision is unaffected unless there is a cataract to complicate the picture. The loss of central vision interferes with reading, seeing facial features, and other details. Dense scotomas are not present unless there is scarring following choroidal or subretinal hemorrhage (disciform disease). Contrast sensitivity decreases as the disease extends beyond the fovea. Macular degeneration generally does not hinder safe travel because the peripheral vision is effective for orientation purposes.

Tests of visual function include Snellen acuity, Amsler grid, and contrast sensitivity. Reduced contrast indicates the need for higher magnification, more contrast, and more illumination than predicted from the Snellen acuity.

Management

Patients often spontaneously adopt an eccentric head tilt or eye turn to move images from nonseeing retina to a viable parafoveal area. The ability to move the scotoma may be demonstrated to a patient during the Amsler grid test. Some patients respond to bilateral prisms in spectacles to relocate the image.

Magnifying lenses enlarge the retinal image beyond the scotoma. The power of the lens is related to the near acuity and contrast sensitivity, as well as location and density of the scotoma. Patients may use different types of devices for various tasks: spectacles for reading, hand magnifier for shopping, CCTV for writing and typing. Most people learn to use low-vision aids successfully, particularly after instruction sessions to reinforce correct usage. Older people may require more time and repetition. All patients need to be reassured about the remote possibility of blindness.

4. PERIPHERAL SCOTOMA

Scotomas in the peripheral field are characteristic of end stage glaucoma, retinitis pigmentosa, diabetic retinopathy treated with photocoagulation, and central nervous system diseases and disorders such as tumor, stroke, or trauma. The peripheral field is essential for orienting oneself in space, detecting motion, and for awareness of potential hazards in the environment. The predominantly rod vision is most sensitive in twilight and at night. A person with a constricted field may be able to read small print yet need a cane or guide dog to get around.

Management

Adequate task and ambient lighting is essential for persons who depend for vision principally on the macula. Photophobia often results from using high levels of light, which may be relieved by introducing amber to yellow filters that block ultraviolet and visible blue light below 527 nm.

If a cataract seems to interfere with optimal function, a combination of contrast sensitivity and glare tests may indicate the best timing for cataract surgery. The posterior chamber implant should contain an ultraviolet blocking agent.

When the central field diameter is less than 7 degrees, magnification may not be advantageous to the patient. Telescopes and spectacle magnifiers may enlarge the image beyond the useful field. Hand magnifiers and closed-circuit television or computers may be the equipment of choice because the size of the image can be adjusted to match the size of the field.

REFERENCES & RESOURCES

Faye EE (editor): *Clinical Low Vision,* 2nd ed. Little, Brown, 1984.

Faye EE: Low vision aids. In: *Clinical Ophthalmology.* vol 1: *Refraction.* Duane TD (editor). Harper & Row, 1990.

Faye EE: Pathology and visual function. In: *Functional Assessment of Low Vision.* Rosenthal BP, Cole RG (editors). Mosby, 1996.

Faye EE, Stuen CS: *The Aging Eye and Low Vision: A Study Guide.* The Lighthouse, 1995.

Freeman PB, Jose RT: *The Art and Practice of Low Vision.* Butterworth-Heinemann, 1997.

The Lighthouse Catalog. Consumer catalog featuring products for the visually impaired and blind. Phone: 800-346-9579

Lighthouse Continuing Education. Annual catalog of courses, seminars and symposia. Fax: 212-821-9705; e-mail: kseidman@lighthouse.org

Lighthouse Information and Resource Service: Information and pamphlets about eye conditions, visual impairment, and blindness. Phone: 212-821-9200, XT 798.

23

Blindness

John P. Whitcher, MD, MPH

In this chapter we shall discuss blindness as a worldwide health problem, summarizing information about its epidemiology, emphasizing the value of community-based methods to prevent or treat its causes, and outlining resources available in more developed countries for rehabilitation of the blind. All of the disorders that may cause blindness are discussed more fully in other parts of this book.

DEFINITION OF BLINDNESS

The World Health Organization defines visual impairment as shown in Table 23–1. WHO officials encourage investigators and reporting agencies in all countries to report blindness and near blindness according to the categories defined in this table.

In the USA, the most widely used definition of partial blindness is that used by the Internal Revenue Service for the purpose of determining who is eligible for tax deductions on that basis: *central visual acuity 20/200 or less in the better eye with best correction, or widest diameter of visual field subtending an angle of no greater than 20 degrees.* An alternative functional definition is *loss of vision sufficient to prevent one from being self-supporting in an occupation, making the individual dependent on other persons, agencies, or devices in order to live.*

"Industrial blindness" is said to be present when a worker can no longer pursue an occupation because of poor vision; "automobile blindness" when vision is so poor that the responsible licensing agency in that state will not issue a driver's license. The term color blindness is a misnomer since this genetically transmitted disorder is not blindness as that term is generally understood and is only a minor handicap to a few people. Loss of vision may affect only the central fields, only the peripheral fields, or only specific portions of the peripheral fields in one or both eyes. Total loss of vision in one eye is said to reduce visual capacity by only 10%, though it makes the other eye infinitely more valuable.

Table 23–1. Categories of visual impairment. (Adapted from the International Classification of Diseases, World Health Organization, 1977.)

Category of Visual Impairment	Visual Acuity (Best Corrected)
Low Vision 1	6/18 3/10 (0.3) 20/70
Low Vision 2	6/60 1/10 (0.1) 20/200
Blindness 3	3/60 (finger counting at 3m) 1/20 (0.05) 20/400
Blindness 4	1/60 (finger counting at 1m) 1/50 (0.02) 5/300
Blindness 5	No light perception

Visual Field

Patients with a visual field radius no greater than 10 degrees but greater than 5 degrees around central fixation should be placed in category 3 and patients with a field no greater than 5 degrees around central fixation in category 4—even if the central acuity is not impaired.

PREVALENCE OF BLINDNESS THROUGHOUT THE WORLD

WHO estimates that there are between 27 and 35 million blind people in the world today. This figure rises to at least 42 million if the criterion is extended to visual acuity of 20/200 or worse. Even where health statistics are most reliable, the methods of counting the blind are often crude and may be applied according to different criteria in different places and at different times within any extensive geographic area. Furthermore, extrapolations are often made from small sample studies to large populations. Ninety percent of the world's blind live in developing countries, mostly in Asia (approximately 20 million) and Africa (approximately 6 million), clustered largely in disadvantaged communities in rural areas and urban slums. The risk of blindness in many of these neglected communities is 10–40 times higher than in the industrially developed regions of Europe and America.

Table 23–2 lists some countries where fairly reliable data are available about the prevalence of blindness.

Table 23–2. Approximate prevalence of blindness (%)
(Estimates based on WHO surveys.)[1]

Chad	3.2–5	Malawi	1
Liberia	3.2	Brazil	0.3
Egypt	2.6	Mexico	0.3
Phillipines	2.1	Australia	0.2
Afghanistan	2	Japan	0.2
Bangladesh	2	USA	0.2
Pakistan	2	UK	0.18
Saudi Arabia	2	Canada	0.15
India	1.5	USSR	0.12
Indonesia	1.3	China	0.1
Chile	1	Germany	0.1

[1] Based on available data, 1969–1980. Some data were only rough estimates when obtained and may have changed markedly since then. In some cases, the survey criteria used did not correspond to WHO definitions. Data taken from Maitchouk IF: Data on blindness: Prevalence and causes throughout the world. In: Lim ASM, Jones BR (editors): World's major blinding conditions. *Vision* 1982;1:99. (International Agency for the Prevention of Blindness.)

CAUSES OF BLINDNESS & METHODS OF PREVENTION & TREATMENT

The relative importance of various causes of blindness differs according to the level of social development in the geographic area being studied. In developing countries, cataract is the leading cause, with trachoma, leprosy, onchocerciasis, and xerophthalmia also being important. In more developed countries, blindness is to a great extent related to the aging process. Cataract is still important despite the availability of facilities for its treatment, along with age-related macular degeneration and glaucoma. Other causes are diabetic retinopathy, herpes simplex keratitis, retinal detachment, and inherited retinal degenerative disorders.

In terms of the worldwide prevalence of blindness, the vastly greater number of people in the developing world and the greater likelihood of their being affected mean that the causes of blindness in those areas are numerically more important. Cataract is responsible for an estimated 17 million cases of blindness, trachoma between 6 and 9 million, leprosy at least 1 million, and onchocerciasis 1 million. Xerophthalmia is estimated to affect 5 million children each year; 500,000 develop active corneal involvement, and half of these go blind.

WHO estimates that up to 80% of cases of blindness in developing countries are avoidable, ie, preventable or treatable. The worldwide eradication of smallpox demonstrates what can be achieved in the area of infectious disease and the superiority of prevention over treatment. Similar efforts are being made to prevent the infectious diseases trachoma, leprosy, and onchocerciasis as well as the noninfectious xerophthalmia. The sheer numbers of individuals blinded by cataract continues to overwhelm the resources available. In all programs to reduce blindness

in the developing world, cooperation between governments and nongovernmental charitable organizations has proved to be essential. The WHO Prevention of Blindness Programme has established centers in about 60 developing countries to undertake collaborative studies, particularly generating epidemiologically sound information to form the basis for rational planning, implementation, and proper evaluation of programs for prevention of blindness.

In more developed countries, the causes of blindness are less amenable to prevention. In general, it is necessary to rely on recognition and treatment of the early stages of the disease. This depends on education of ophthalmologists, nonophthalmologic medical personnel, and lay people about the necessity for screening for glaucoma and diabetic retinopathy and about the importance of the early symptoms of retinal detachment, age-related macular degeneration, and herpes simplex keratitis. The inherited conditions are amenable to prevention by genetic counseling.

Cataract

Cataract accounts for at least 50% of cases of blindness worldwide. As life expectancy increases, there is a continuing rise in the total number of people affected. In many parts of the developing world, the facilities available for treating cataract are grossly inadequate, hardly sufficient to cope with the new cases arising and completely inadequate for dealing with the backlog of existing cases, which is conservatively estimated to be 10 million worldwide.

It is not clearly understood why the frequency of cataract in different geographic areas varies so greatly, though exposure to ultraviolet radiation and recurrent episodes of dehydration, such as occur in severe diarrheal diseases, are thought to be important. If medical means could be found to delay the development of cataract by 10 years, it is estimated that this would reduce the number of individuals requiring surgery by 45%.

Mobile eye camps have aided in management, but there are too few to control the disorder. Many more cataract surgeons are needed in countries such as India and Pakistan. In a number of blindness surveys, the problem of uncorrected aphakia is particularly apparent. It has been suggested that intraocular lens implantation at the time of surgery, though requiring greater expertise, may be a better solution than relying on the subsequent provision of spectacles.

Trachoma

Trachoma causes bilateral keratoconjunctivitis, generally in childhood, that leads in adulthood to corneal scarring, which, when severe, causes blindness. About 400 million people have trachoma, most of them in Africa, the Middle East, and Asia. Trachoma can be treated with sulfonamides or various antibiotics such as tetracyclines or erythromycin and related agents, and an estimated 60 million individuals currently require treatment. But prevention of spread of infection by provision of proper sanitary facilities, including clean water for drinking and washing, is more effective in eliminating the disease.

Leprosy

Leprosy (Hansen's disease) affects 15–16 million people in the world and has a higher percentage of ocular involvement than any other systemic disease. Up to 10% of leprosy patients are blind from the disease. The social stigma attached to leprosy has greatly hindered its treatment, but there are effective chemotherapeutic agents and the possibility of a vaccine.

Onchocerciasis

Onchocerciasis is transmitted by bites of the blackfly, which breeds in clear running streams (hence the name river blindness). It is endemic in the greater part of tropical Africa and Central and South America. The most heavily infested zone is the Volta River basin, which extends over parts of Dahomey, Ghana, Ivory Coast, Mali, Niger, Togo, and Upper Volta. Worldwide, 28 million people are affected by onchocerciasis, with 20% of individuals in endemic areas being blind from the disease.

The major ophthalmic manifestations of onchocerciasis are keratitis, uveitis, retinochoroiditis, and optic atrophy. The disease is prevented by insect eradication and personal protection by screening. Treatment is with ivermectin.

Xerophthalmia

Xerophthalmia is due to hypovitaminosis A. Clinically, there is xerosis of the conjunctiva with characteristic Bitot's spots and softening of the cornea (keratomalacia), which may lead to corneal perforation. Protein malnutrition exacerbates the condition and renders it refractory to treatment. Xerophthalmia is a common cause of blindness in infants, particularly in India, Bangladesh, Indonesia, and the Philippines. Affected infants often do not reach adulthood, dying from malnutrition, pneumonia, or diarrhea.

Xerophthalmia can be prevented by general dietary improvement or vitamin A supplementation. If the problems of distribution and administration were solved, the cost of a quantity of the vitamin sufficient to prevent blindness in 1000 infants would be only about $25.00.

Other Causes

Glaucoma, retinal detachment, diabetic retinopathy, and herpes simplex keratitis are discussed in greater detail elsewhere in this text. The incidence of blindness due to glaucoma has decreased in recent years as a result of earlier detection, improved medical and surgical treatment, and a greater awareness and understanding of the disorder by the lay population.

Diabetic retinopathy is an increasingly more common cause of blindness everywhere in the world. Recent advances in surgical treatment (vitrectomy, laser therapy) are of some help, but many patients still suffer from proliferative retinopathy, recurrent vitreous hemorrhages, and eventual bilateral blindness. A vast research effort directed at all aspects of diabetes is in progress, and there is justification for hoping that the next generation of diabetics will benefit greatly from what is being done now.

Hereditary conditions are important causes of blindness but should gradually decrease in incidence in response to the efforts of genetic counselors to increase public awareness of the preventable nature of these disorders.

As is true also in other countries where medical care and social services are widely available, blindness in the USA is to a great extent related to the aging process, and about half of the legally blind people in this country are over age 65. The leading causes of blindness in this age group are degenerative retinal disorders, glaucoma, diabetes, and vascular diseases.

COSTS OF AVOIDING BLINDNESS

Some examples of what can be achieved for modest outlays of scarce funds are as follows:

(1) To cure one person of trachoma in Saudi Arabia: $1.25.

(2) To restore vision to one person in India blinded by cataracts: $30.00.

(3) To prevent blindness due to xerophthalmia in one infant in Indonesia: 30 cents.

On the advice of WHO experts, the World Council for the Welfare of the Blind and several international professional ophthalmic societies and agencies agreed to take the initiative, which led to the establishment in 1974 of the International Agency for Prevention of Blindness (Vision International), with Sir John Wilson, a blind barrister, as president. The aim of this agency is to work with groups formed for the purpose of preventing blindness. Its theme, Foresight Prevents Blindness, was brought into prominent display when WHO celebrated the first World Health Day on April 7, 1976. Its goal was stated as follows: "In every donor country during 1976, every family should be asked—in thanksgiving for sight—to give $10.00 to save the sight of its fellow countrymen or of the millions in the third world."

REHABILITATION OF THE BLIND

Although no completely reliable statistics are available, the most widely used estimates place the legally blind population of the USA at 2.24 per thousand (ie, approximately 500,000). Approximately 50,000 become legally blind annually, and many others have enough visual loss to constitute a serious employment problem.

Blindness does not necessarily imply helplessness. Individual adjustment to marked visual impairment or total blindness varies with age at onset, temperament, education, economic resources, and many other factors. The older patient, for example, may accept blindness quite stoically, whereas for the younger patient the vocational or social impact of blindness is often catastrophic. Blindness is accepted more easily by persons who are born blind and by persons of any age who lose their vision gradually rather than suddenly.

The aim of rehabilitation is to enable the patient to lead as nearly normal a life as possible. Approximately 5000 blind persons in the USA are rehabilitated and obtain paid employment each year. An additional larger number of blind homemakers are able to perform their household duties without assistance or are able to live independently of others.

Rehabilitation must be individualized. Many special services (see Appendix III) and increasingly complex optical and nonoptical aids (see Chapter 22) are available, but they are not universally helpful. Different categories of the blind have different needs, and some blind people simply cannot benefit from a number of services or aids available. It has been said that over half of the blind people in the USA are over age 65. The elderly widowed housewife may need or want no more than mobility training in home care and a steady supply of Talking Books. A young person facing blindness in later life due to retinitis pigmentosa requires the full range of social services, including educational assessment, job rehabilitation, and psychologic counseling as well as a number of sophisticated aids.

The responsibility of the physician clearly does not end with the diagnosis, prevention, and treatment of ocular disorders that might result in blindness. The physician caring for the patient who is suddenly faced with actual or imminent blindness is in a position to be of great assistance. When blindness is a possibility but is not inevitable (eg, during acute ocular inflammation), optimism and reassurance are warranted. However, it is unwise to offer false hope or to delay "breaking the news" when blindness is inevitable. If it is certain that blindness will occur, it is important to extend to the distraught patient as well as to the patient's family the warmth, understanding, encouragement, and assistance so desperately needed. The physician should be alert to the severe depressive reactions that may occur.

It is especially important to assist the patient in making the adjustment to blindness while some vision is still present. Early referral to rehabilitation agencies is essential for recently blinded adults and those with irreversible progressive visual loss. Training programs or reeducation for the many changes involved in daily living and employment are greatly simplified if the patient has the partial support provided by even limited vision.

The physician should work actively with both the patient and the family and with other professional people concerned with rendering services to the blind. The physician must know what referral sources are available and how to use them skillfully. Medical social workers, public health nurses, and counseling services and agencies serving the blind and visually handicapped are common sources of reliable information. It may be valuable to have the patient talk with a blind person who has made a satisfactory adjustment to blindness.

Mobility Training & Guide Dogs

Mobility training is most important in rehabilitation of the blind. Many state commissions for the blind offer a wide variety of mobility training courses, either directly or in cooperation with private agencies. The courses are offered on an outpatient and residential basis and have varied objectives according to the special needs of the people who apply for help. The curriculum commonly includes self-care, home functions, and mobility within the community. Several universities* have undergraduate and postgraduate programs in mobility training for the blind.

The usefulness of guide dogs is limited by their daily care needs and the physical strength required to hold them in check. They are most useful for students and professional men and women in good health who lead fairly well organized lives. At this time, less than 2% of blind people in the USA use guide dogs. Sonar sensor canes may ultimately be a better answer to the mobility problem even for those who are now using a dog successfully.

Braille

This remarkably effective system of reading for the blind was introduced in 1825. The braille characters consist of raised dots arranged in two columns of three. The system is so simple that a blind child can quickly learn to read braille, and proficient readers can learn to read braille as fast as they can talk. The system has been adapted to musical notation and technical and scientific uses also. An international braille code was introduced in 1951.

Braille is used less commonly now than formerly, since many blind people prefer auditory aids both for informational and recreational purposes. But the recent availability of portable data storage systems with braille-encoded input and conventional or braille form printed output has brought about a resurgence of interest. Braille continues to be essential on tags attached to items in common personal use even for people who do not wish to use it for reading.

---

* Undergraduate level programs are at Cleveland State University in Ohio, Florida State University in Florida, and Stephen F. Austin University in Texas. Graduate programs are available at Boston University, California State University (Los Angeles), Northern Colorado University, San Francisco State University, University of Arkansas, University of Wisconsin, and Western Michigan State University.

All paper money in the Netherlands and Switzerland is braille-printed to show the denomination.

Electronic Devices

Optacon is an electronic device that converts visual images of letters into tactile forms. It is easily portable and can be used with almost any kind of reading matter. Auditory aids are becoming increasingly important (eg, talking calculators, clocks, paper money identifiers).

FINANCIAL ASSISTANCE PROGRAMS

It is unfortunate that over half of the blind people in the USA are essentially dependent upon Social Security and whatever local supplemental aid may be available to them. For the younger blind population, rehabilitation programs are commonly administered at the state level by a division of the department of education specifically set up to serve blind people in the state. Some of these programs are better than oth-ers, and all physicians should support efforts to increase the effectiveness of such programs in their geographic area of influence. The programs are of wide scope and offer preliminary counseling followed by academic or vocational training as the circumstances warrant. Once a realistic vocational objective has been established, full financial support is commonly available. This single resource is probably the most crucial referral available to the ophthalmologist, particularly in the case of young patients. Counseling services are available as early as the junior high school years to ensure compliance with a curriculum consistent with measured aptitudes and interests. In many states, such rehabilitation programs as mobility training are administered under state auspices but contracted to private agencies for operational purposes.

In many countries, the blind receive no financial or other support from their governments and are either cared for by their families or left to manage by themselves in any way they can.

Special services available to the blind in the USA are listed and discussed in Appendix III.

REFERENCES

Abiose A et al: Distribution and aetiology of blindness and visual impairment in mesoendemic onchocercal communities, Kaduna State, Nigeria. Br J Ophthalmol 1994;78:8.

Adeoye A: Survey of blindness in rural communities of South-Western Nigeria. Trop Med Int Health 1996;1:672.

Courtright P et al: Multidrug therapy and eye disease in leprosy: A cross-sectional study in the Peoples Republic of China. Int J Epidemiol 1994;23:835.

Dolin PJ et al: Reduction of trachoma in a sub-Saharan village in absence of a disease control programme. Lancet 1997;349:1511.

Evans JG et al: Cost effectiveness and cost utility of preventing trachomatous visual impairment: Lessons from 30 years of trachoma control in Burma. Br J Ophthalmol 1996;80:880.

Fielder AR et al: The management of visual impairment in childhood. Clin Develop Med 1993;128:1.

Foster A et al: Epidemiology of cataract in childhood: A global perspective. J Cataract Refract Surg 1997(23 Suppl)1:601.

Global scale of avoidable blindness. Lancet 1990;336:1038.

Gulliford MC et al: Counting the cost of diabetic hospital admissions from a multi-ethnic population in Trinidad. Diabet Med 1995;12:1077.

Lewallen S: Prevention of blindness in leprosy: An overview of the relevant clinical and programme-planning issues. Ann Trop Med Parasitol 1997;91:341.

Lim AS: Mass blindness has shifted from infection (onchocerciosis, trachoma, corneal ulcers) to cataract. [Letter.] Ophthalmologica 1997;211:270.

Lim ASM: Eye surgeons seize the opportunity. Am J Ophthalmol 1996;122:571.

Moll AC et al: Prevalence of blindness and low vision of people over 30 years in the Wenchi District, Ghana, in relation to eye care programmes. Br J Ophthalmol 1994;78:275.

Narita AS et al: Blindness in the tropics. Med J Aust 1993;159:416.

Pitakiripan S et al: An outbreak of post-operative endophthalmitis in Lampang Hospital. J Med Assoc Thai 1995;78(Suppl 2):S95.

The Prevention of Blindness: Report of WHO Study Group. World Health Organization Technical Report Series 518, 1973. [Entire issue.]

Rait JI: Seven million too many. Br J Ophthalmol 1996;80:385.

Randy MJ et al: Blindness from uveitis in a hospital population in Sierra Leone. Br J Ophthalmol 1994;78:690.

Robin AL et al: A long-term approach to eliminate cataract blindness. [Editorial.] Ophthalmology 1997;104:571.

Schwab L et al: The epidemiology of trachoma in rural Kenya: Variation in prevalence with lifestyle and environment. Study Survey Group. Ophthalmology 1995;102:475.

Sekhar GC et al: Ocular manifestations of Hansen's disease. Doc Ophthalmol 1994;87:211.

Smith AF et al: The economic burden of global blindness: A price too high! Br J Ophthalmol 1996;80:276.

Taylor HR et al: Increase in mortality associated with blindness in rural Africa. Bull WHO 1991;69:335.

Thylefors B et al: Developments for a global approach to trachoma control. Rev Int Trachom 1994;71:63.

Thylefors B et al: Global data on blindness. Bull WHO 1995;73:115.

Thylefors B: The role of international ophthalmology in blindness prevention. Am J Ophthalmol 1995;119:229.

Van Laethern Y et al: Treatment of onchocerciasis. Drugs 1996;52:861.

Whitcher JP et al: Corneal ulceration in the developing world: A silent epidemic. Br J Ophthalmol 1997; 81:622.

Zerihum N et al: Blindness and low vision in Jimma zone, Ethiopia: Results of a population-based survey. Ophthalmol Epidemiol 1997;4:19.

24

Lasers in Ophthamology

James Berry Wise, MD

Ophthalmology was the first medical specialty to utilize laser energy in patient treatment, and it still accounts for more laser operations than any other specialty. The transparency of the optical media allows laser light to be focused upon the intraocular structures without the need for endoscopy. Laser therapy has made the treatment of a number of serious ocular diseases much safer and more effective. Lasers are also used to alter the refractive state of the eye and to perform cosmetic surgery upon the eyelids. Low-energy scanning laser systems are useful for diagnostic imaging of ocular structures and for measuring blood flow by interferometry. Because laser surgery irreversibly changes tissue, ocular laser surgery should be performed only by ophthalmologists with laser experience.

OCULAR LASER SYSTEMS

A laser consists of a transparent crystal rod (solid-state laser) or a gas- or liquid-filled cavity (gas or fluid laser) constructed with a fully reflective mirror at one end and a partially reflective mirror at the other. Surrounding the rod or cavity is an optical or electrical source of energy that will raise the energy level of the atoms within the rod or cavity to a high and unstable level, a process known as population inversion. When the excited atoms spontaneously decay back to a lower energy level, their excess energy is released in the form of light. This light can be emitted in any direction. In a laser cavity, however, light emitted in the long axis of the cavity can bounce back and forth between the mirrors, setting up a standing wave that stimulates the remaining excited atoms to release their energy into the standing wave, producing an intense beam of light that exits the cavity through the partially reflective mirror. The light beam produced is all of the same wavelength (monochromatic), with all of the light waves in phase with each other (coherent). The light waves follow closely parallel courses with almost no tendency to spread out. These unique properties of laser light allow the beam to be focused down to extremely small spots with very high energy densities. The laser light energy can be emitted continuously or in pulses, which may have pulse durations of nanoseconds or less.

MECHANISMS OF LASER EFFECTS

Photocoagulation

The principal lasers used in ophthalmic therapy are the thermal lasers, in which tissue pigments absorb the light and convert it into heat, thus raising the target tissue temperature high enough to coagulate and denature the cellular components. These lasers are used for retinal photocoagulation, for treatment of diabetic retinopathy (Figure 24–1) and sealing of retinal holes, and for photocoagulation of the trabecular meshwork, iris, and ciliary body in the treatment of glaucoma. They can be used at higher energy levels to evaporate tissue, as in laser iridotomy. These laser photocoagulators operate in continuous mode or very rapidly pulsed (thermal) mode. The (blue)-green argon laser is the workhorse of this class. Others include the krypton red laser; the solid-state diode laser, producing a near infrared wavelength; the tunable dye laser, producing wavelengths from green to red; the frequency-doubled Nd:YAG laser, producing green light; and the thermal mode Nd:YAG laser, producing infrared light. Because laser light is monochromatic, selective absorption into specific tissues by specific wavelengths is possible, while adjacent tissues are spared. An example is the yellow wavelength of the tunable dye laser, which can be used to treat neovascularization near the macula because the yellow light

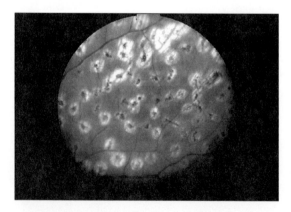

Figure 24–1. Argon laser burn scars in retina after panretinal photocoagulation for diabetic retinopathy.

is absorbed by hemoglobin but not by the yellow xanthophyll pigment of the macula. Absorption of laser light by specific tissues can be enhanced by intravenous injection of absorbing dyes such as fluorescein or indocyanine green.

Photodisruption

Photodisruption lasers release a giant pulse of energy with a pulse duration of a few nanoseconds. When this pulse is focused to a 15–25 μm spot, so that the nearly instantaneous light pulse exceeds a critical level of energy density, "optical breakdown" occurs in which the temperature rises so high (about 10,000 °K) that electrons are stripped from atoms, resulting in a physical state known as a plasma. This plasma expands with momentary pressures as high as 10 kilobars (150,000 psi), producing a cutting effect upon the ocular tissues. Because the initial plasma size is so small, it has little total energy and produces little effect away from the point of focus. Though a significant shock wave is produced, studies on polyethylene membranes indicate that direct contact with the plasma is required for cutting tissue. Photodisruptors are used principally for perforating cloudy posterior capsules after cataract extraction and for performing laser iridotomy. The principal laser of this class is the Q-switched neodymium:YAG laser.

Photo-evaporation

The prototype of this class is the carbon dioxide laser, which produces a long-wavelength infrared heat beam. The beam is absorbed by water and therefore will not enter the interior of the eye. This laser can evaporate away surface lesions such as lid tumors and can be used for bloodless incisions in skin or sclera. The carbon dioxide laser beam can also be delivered through probes for contact photo-incision and photocoagulation within the eye. Used in a rapidly pulsed mode, this laser produces a controlled superficial skin burn that can tighten the eyelid skin for cosmetic improvement. The erbium and holmium lasers produce similar effects.

Photodecomposition

Photodecomposition lasers produce very short wavelength ultraviolet light that interacts with the chemical bonds of biologic materials, breaking the bonds and converting biologic polymers into small molecules that diffuse away. These lasers collectively are called excimer ("excited dimer") lasers because the cavity contains two gases, such as argon and fluorine, that react into unstable molecules which then emit the laser light. They can precisely recontour the corneal surface by computer-controlled ablation of successive thin layers of the cornea, correcting refractive errors such as myopia, hyperopia, and astigmatism. Photodecomposition lasers can also remove shallow corneal opacities resulting from injuries or dystrophies.

THERAPEUTIC APPLICATION OF LASERS

DIABETIC RETINOPATHY

In nonproliferative diabetic retinopathy, vision may be impaired by macular edema and exudates resulting from breakdown of the inner blood-retinal barriers at the level of the retinal capillary endothelium. Many patients with long-term diabetes mellitus will gradually develop diffuse obliteration of the retinal microcirculation, especially of the capillaries, resulting in generalized retinal ischemia. This ischemic state leads to neovascularization of the retina and iris, at least partly mediated by diffusible vasoproliferative factors released from the ischemic retina into the ocular fluids. Untreated retinal neovascularization leads to vitreous hemorrhages and traction retinal detachment. Iris neovascularization produces neovascular glaucoma. (The clinical features of diabetic retinopathy are more fully discussed in Chapter 10.)

Diabetic macular edema is treated by focal or grid pattern laser photocoagulation, which principally acts by augmenting the function of the retinal pigment epithelium. Burns 50-100 μm in diameter are applied, avoiding the foveal avascular zone, which is approximately 300 μm in diameter. The areas of leakage to be treated can be identified by fluorescein angiography (areas of discrete or diffuse fluorescein leakage and areas of capillary nonperfusion associated with retinal thickening) or by clinical examination (zones of retinal thickening). The most effective treatment for retinal and iris neovascularization is panretinal photocoagulation (PRP), which usually consists of treating the entire retina—except for the area within the temporal vascular arcades—with 200-500 μm diameter burns placed one to two burn widths apart. PRP requires a total of at least 2000 and sometimes 6000 or more burns, usually delivered over two or more sessions spaced about 2 weeks apart. Retrobulbar or peribulbar anesthesia is sometimes required, particularly if areas of the retina need to be re-treated because of recalcitrant or recurrent neovascularization. Treatment is staged to reduce the incidence of uveitis, macular edema, exudative retinal detachment, and even shallowing of the anterior chamber with secondary angle closure. In the presence of significant macular edema, focal macular photocoagulation should be carried out prior to or together with the PRP to avoid increase in edema.

Adequate PRP is highly effective in producing regression of neovascularization. The exact mechanism of action has not been established, but reduction in the degree of retinal ischemia and production of diffusible vasostimulative substances are thought to be important. The type of laser used does not appear to influence the efficacy of PRP, but particular characteristics can be important in treatment, eg, the easier use of the diode infrared laser in the presence of vitreous hemorrhage. Direct treatment of retinal neovascularization is rarely necessary but can be performed if there are residual new vessels after extensive PRP, particularly if they are responsible for vitreous hemorrhage.

PRP does not cause regression of the fibrosis associated with retinal neovascularization, which is responsible for tractional retinal detachment. Furthermore, PRP can be precluded by vitreous hemorrhage. Thus, PRP should be undertaken as soon as high-risk clinical features have developed: optic disk neovascularization, retinal neovascularization at other sites associated with vitreous hemorrhage, and iris neovascularization. Retinal neovascularization away from the optic disk without vitreous hemorrhage may be treated either by scatter photocoagulation limited to the adjacent areas of retina or by PRP, particularly if there is advanced or rapidly proliferative disease in the other eye. Because timely PRP is so effective in preventing blindness in diabetes, any diabetic with retinopathy greater than scattered microaneurysms should be seen on a regular basis by an ophthalmologist.

CENTRAL RETINAL VEIN THROMBOSIS

Thrombosis involving the central retinal vein produces the classic fundus appearance of disk swelling, marked venous dilation, and almost confluent retinal hemorrhages (see Chapter 10). While these changes can progress to retinal neovascularization, vitreous hemorrhage, and fibrosis, a more common complication is the development of rubeosis iridis with neovascular glaucoma. If severe retinal ischemia is present on fluorescein angiography, there is a 60% chance of this complication. In neovascular glaucoma, substances produced by the ischemic retina diffuse forward and stimulate formation of a fibrovascular membrane that grows across the iris surface and covers the trabecular meshwork, resulting in glaucoma characterized by very high pressure, pain, and marked resistance to medical and surgical therapy, so that enucleation of the blind and painful eye may be required. PRP as described above for treatment of proliferative diabetic retinopathy—preferably with the krypton red or diode infrared laser to avoid preretinal fibrosis caused by heat absorption in the hemorrhages—can greatly reduce the incidence of neovascular glaucoma in ischemic central retinal vein thrombosis. It is most effectively applied when iris neovascularization is present but before neovascular glaucoma has developed. However, in clinical practice this timing can be difficult to achieve. Once neo-

vascular glaucoma is present, adequate panretinal photocoagulation will usually cause regression of the anterior segment neovascularization, allowing the glaucoma to be controlled medically or by filtering surgery. Unfortunately, established neovascular glaucoma is often associated with corneal edema, miosis, or hyphema so that PRP cannot be performed and only cyclophotocoagulation or enucleation can be used. For this reason, prophylactic PRP may be advisable in all cases of ischemic central retinal vein thrombosis. A relative afferent pupillary defect, vision of 20/200 or less, and multiple retinal cotton-wool spots are highly suggestive of ischemia severe enough to warrant prophylactic PRP. Electroretinography and fluorescein angiography provide further evidence when needed.

BRANCH RETINAL VEIN THROMBOSIS

This condition varies from localized areas of venous congestion and hemorrhage to hemiretinal involvement from thrombosis of the superior or inferior division of the central retinal vein. The principal complications are chronic macular edema (with or without exudates) and retinal neovascularization followed by vitreous hemorrhage and traction retinal detachment. When the area of ischemic retina is demonstrated by fluorescein angiography to exceed five disk diameters in extent, prophylactic scatter photocoagulation of the ischemic area can be performed to reduce the risk of retinal neovascularization, which usually develops in the region of the retinal vascular arcades. If retinal neovascularization does develop, laser treatment should be performed promptly, preferably before vitreous hemorrhage occurs. Focal and grid-pattern argon green laser photocoagulation is used to treat macular edema and exudates by obliteration of areas of retinal leakage as demonstrated by fluorescein angiography.

RETINAL TEARS

When a peripheral retinal tear occurs—usually due to senile vitreous degeneration causing vitreous traction—the patient often notices the sudden appearance of dot-like floaters. The tear can cause retinal detachment, but if detected prior to the accumulation of subretinal fluid it can be walled off by applying a double ring of laser burns around it to create an adhesion of the adjacent attached retina to the pigment epithelium. Once retinal detachment has occurred, surgery is required. Prompt retinal examination through a dilated pupil is therefore indicated in any eye with sudden onset of floaters, particularly dot-like floaters suggesting red blood cells.

MACULAR DEGENERATION & RELATED DISEASES

Bruch's membrane forms a barrier layer between the retinal pigment epithelium and the choriocapillaris, which is the capillary layer of the choroid. If Bruch's membrane deteriorates or is damaged, capillary nets can grow through the break beneath the pigment epithelium, first causing exudative pigment epithelial detachment with distortion and edema of the overlying retina and later causing hemorrhage and fibrosis with destruction of retinal function in that area. The macular retina is particularly likely to develop Bruch's membrane breaks and neovascularization, though these changes can occur anywhere in the fundus. The most frequent cause is age-related macular degeneration, which begins as asymptomatic yellowish deposits (drusen) in the macular area. As the years advance, pigment epithelial atrophy and clumping are seen, and finally Bruch's membrane breaks appear, leading to fluid leaks, neovascularization, fibrosis, and loss of central vision. This condition is the leading cause of legal blindness in the older population. Bruch's membrane breaks and neovascular nets can occur at sites of old chorioretinitis from childhood histoplasmosis, toxoplasmosis, and various other inflammatory disorders. They can develop from traumatic choroidal ruptures, even in children, and can occur in a host of hereditary diseases involving the retina. If sub-pigment epithelial neovascular nets are located away from the central foveal area, they can be destroyed by careful laser photocoagulation to preserve central vision. The yellow macular pigment (xanthophyll) strongly absorbs blue light, weakly absorbs green light, and does not absorb yellow, orange, or red light. Hemoglobin strongly absorbs blue, green, yellow, and orange light but very weakly absorbs red light. Melanin absorbs all visible wavelengths. Selective absorption of laser energy is therefore possible. If the neovascular net has melanin pigment in it or is bleeding, then krypton red laser light allows deep penetration to the choriocapillaris without hemoglobin or xanthophyll absorption. If the net does not have much melanin and has not bled, argon green or dye laser yellow or orange will be absorbed by hemoglobin to coagulate the net but the scattered light will not be absorbed by xanthophyll. The whole neovascular net must be heavily treated for control. Unfortunately, in many cases the net is already under the fovea at the time of diagnosis, or bleeding is already so extensive that laser treatment is not possible. Early diagnosis is therefore of utmost importance in this group of diseases, and patients at risk must diligently look for and report the small blurs and distortions of vision that are the first signs of neovascular growth. Fluorescein angiography can then be used to demonstrate the retinal circulation, including areas of neovascularization and abnormal vascular permeability. Direct laser treatment of subfoveal neovascular membranes produces an immediate permanent reduction in central acuity but may lead to a better long-term outcome than can be expected without treatment.

GLAUCOMA

Treatment of open-angle glaucoma, angle-closure glaucoma, and glaucoma resistant to surgery has been radically altered by availability of effective laser techniques.

Angle-Closure Glaucoma

In primary angle-closure glaucoma, aqueous flow through the pupil is blocked by contact of the lens with the posterior surface of the iris. The resulting pressure in the posterior chamber forces the peripheral iris forward into contact with the trabecular meshwork, blocking outflow and increasing intraocular pressure. While the classic, dramatic acute glaucoma attack is usually considered the prototype of angle-closure glaucoma, acute attacks are actually very rare. Creeping or subacute angle-closure glaucoma is far more common, especially in darkly pigmented eyes, and can occur with a normal central anterior chamber depth. Angle closure can be determined only by examining the angle, which is usually done by slitlamp gonioscopy through a gonioscopy contact lens containing a mirror. Because angle closure is the commonest type of glaucoma in Asian populations, it is probably the most common type of glaucoma worldwide. Surgical iridectomy was the standard treatment for angle-closure glaucoma for decades but carried the risks of hemorrhage, infection, anesthetic accidents, and even sympathetic ophthalmia. Studies of ruby laser iridotomy began in animals in 1964, but not until 1975 was an effective argon laser technique developed for human eyes. In 1979, laser iridotomy was made more effective by the Abraham contact lens, whose 66-diopter focusing button increased iris energy density. The more recent Wise iridotomy-sphincterotomy lens has a 103-diopter button that gives the highest energy density possible with a practical contact lens. With these high-energy densities, laser iridotomy (Figure 24–2) is nearly 100% successful with either the argon laser or the Q-switched Nd:YAG laser, failing only when the cornea is so cloudy that the laser cannot be focused upon the iris. With the argon laser, the beam is focused through the Wise lens upon the far peripheral iris fibers, which are cut in a line parallel to the limbus by multiple shots at 0.01-s or 0.02-s exposures and energy levels of 1–2 W. With the Nd:YAG laser, iridotomy can be done through the Wise lens by a high-power single-point method using about 8 mJ per shot in a single-shot or a two- or three-shot burst, or it can be done by cutting the far peripheral iris fibers in a line parallel to the limbus with multiple shots at

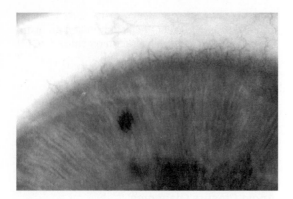

Figure 24–2. Laser iridotomy for angle-closure glaucoma.

1–1.5 mJ. The argon laser is preferable for dark brown, thick irides, which tend to bleed with the Nd:YAG laser, while light blue irides do not absorb argon laser energy well and are more easily perforated with the Nd:YAG laser. If both lasers are available, a very efficient method for thick brown irides is to cut the thick stroma with the argon laser and then remove strands and pigment with a few low-power Nd:YAG laser bursts. Because of its safety, laser iridotomy should be done not only for established angle-closure glaucoma but whenever progressive pupillary block is occurring, before irreversible damage from angle closure has occurred.

Primary Open-Angle Glaucoma

This is the most common type of glaucoma in Western countries and is characterized by painless gradual reduction in trabecular meshwork function with decreasing outflow, increasing intraocular pressure, progressive cupping of the optic nerve, and insidious loss of visual field, leading ultimately to blindness. Topical medical therapy is the standard approach. If medical therapy is not adequate, laser trabeculoplasty is usually the next therapy (Figure 24–3). This consists of spacing 100 or more nonperforating argon laser burns 360 degrees around the trabecular meshwork to shrink the collagen in the tissues of the trabecular ring, reducing the circumference and therefore the diameter of the trabecular ring, pulling the trabecular layers apart with reopening of the intertrabecular spaces and of Schlemm's canal. Growth of new trabecular cells may also occur. Trabeculoplasty increases outflow and has no influence upon aqueous secretion. Though in some eyes the abnormal meshwork can continue to deteriorate, with late failure requiring filtration surgery, 10-year control of glaucoma has been reported. Most eyes continue to require some medical therapy. The value of trabeculoplasty lies in reducing medical therapy and postponing or avoiding the risks of filtration surgery. The only significant side effects are a rise in pressure for 1–4 hours in about one-third of eyes (preventable by apraclonidine drops) and a rise in pressure for 1–3 weeks in about 2% of treated eyes. To reduce the severity of these pressure rises, many laser surgeons do trabeculoplasty with 50 laser burns in 180 degrees of the trabecular meshwork, reserving the other 180 degrees

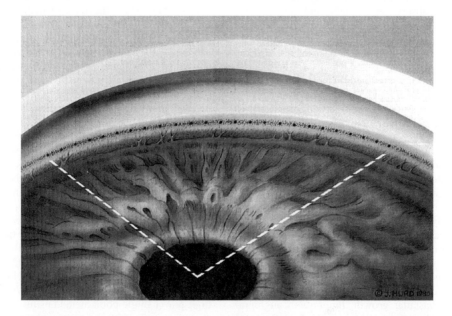

Figure 24–3. Laser trabeculoplasty. The laser is focused upon the trabecular meshwork to increase outflow. (Reproduced, with permission, from Schwartz A, et al: Argon laser trabecular surgery in uncontrolled phakic open-angle glaucoma. Ophthalmology 1981; 88: 205.)

for treatment later if necessary. Trabeculoplasty with other laser wavelengths, such as green, yellow, red, and infrared, is also effective. In a large randomized trial, primary argon laser trabeculoplasty gave better control of open-angle glaucoma than did primary medical therapy alone.

Cyclophotocoagulation

Glaucoma refractory to the usual operative procedures can often be controlled by direct destruction of the ciliary processes. This was first done by diathermy and later by cryosurgery. Cyclophotocoagulation through intact conjunctiva and sclera was originated by Beckman, using a high-energy ruby laser, but is currently performed by contact delivery through a fiberoptic probe with the thermal-mode Nd:YAG laser or the diode laser (Figure 24–4). Good control is usually obtained, but multiple treatments may be required. Side effects such as pain, inflammation, and reduction of vision are significantly less severe than with cryosurgery. Laser endocyclophotocoagulation can be performed using a fiberoptic probe passed through the pars plana during vitrectomy.

Laser Suture Lysis

Trabeculectomy is currently the procedure of choice for glaucoma drainage surgery (see Chapter 11) because the partial-thickness scleral flap reduces the incidence of complications caused by early postoperative hypotony. In order to increase the degree of drainage and perhaps achieve greater long-term reduction in intraocular pressure—similar to that obtained with the older full-thickness drainage procedures—laser lysis of the scleral flap sutures can be carried out 7–14 days after standard trabeculectomy and 3–8 weeks after trabeculectomy augmented by antifibrotic therapy with mitomycin. The black 10-0 nylon sutures

are cut by focusing short laser pulses upon them through the transparent conjunctiva, aided by compressing the overlying tissues with the Hoskins suture lens. The argon laser may be used, but if hemorrhage is present the krypton red or diode infrared laser is preferred to avoid flap perforation by hemoglobin absorption of argon blue-green laser wavelengths.

LASER PHOTOMYDRIASIS & LASER SPHINCTEROTOMY

For a variety of reasons, but most frequently because of long-term miotic therapy, the pupil can become fixed at a very small size, reducing vision and interfering with pupillary dilation for retinal examination or treatment. Multiple laser burns of 200 μm diameter placed on the iris in a ring outside the pupil will produce temporary enlargement, but marked uveitis and intraocular pressure rises can occur and the dilating effect disappears over time. A better method is argon laser sphincterotomy, in which one or more linear cuts across the iris sphincter are made by focusing the argon laser through the Wise iridotomy-sphincterotomy lens, using numerous shots at 0.01-s exposure and about 1 W energy. This produces permanent enlargement of the pupil with less irritation. Energy levels must be kept low to avoid lens burns. The Nd:YAG laser at very low energy levels can be used to cut persistent nonpigmented bridging strands.

POSTERIOR CAPSULOTOMY AFTER CATARACT SURGERY

Modern cataract surgery uses extracapsular extraction or phacoemulsification followed by posterior chamber intraocular lens (IOL) implantation (see Chapter 8). If the posterior capsule supporting the IOL later opacifies, vision can be restored by focusing Q-switched Nd:YAG laser pulses just posterior to the capsule to produce a central capsulotomy (thus avoiding further intraocular surgery). Careful focus through a condensing contact lens is necessary to avoid damage to the IOL. A small increase in the risk of retinal holes and retinal detachment is present after capsulotomy. Opacification of the capsule is not preventable at present, so that some eyes will require capsulotomy for useful vision. However, the risk of retinal detachment from delaying capsulotomy until vision is actually impaired is almost certainly less than the risk from primary capsulotomy during cataract surgery, which also carries the additional risks of IOL malposition and vitreous complications.

CUTTING VITREOUS BANDS & OPACITIES

Incomplete clearance of vitreous from the anterior chamber during the management of vitreous loss sec-

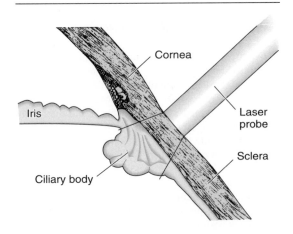

Figure 24–4. Laser cyclophotocoagulation. The laser light passes through the conjunctiva and sclera and is absorbed by the pigment in the ciliary body, producing thermal coagulation of secreting epithelium.

ondary to trauma or surgery may result in pupillary distortion, chronic uveitis, and cystoid macular edema. These bands can be cut with the Q-switched Nd:YAG laser, either directly through the cornea by focusing on the band through a condensing contact lens such as the Wise lens, or in the angle by focusing through the mirror of a condensing goniolens such as the Trokel lens or the Lasag CGA lens. Multiple shots at minimal optical breakdown levels should be used to minimize concussion to cornea and iris. Eyes with chronic cystoid macular edema have improved after cutting of vitreocorneal bands. Localized opacities and bands in the anterior vitreous can be cut with the Nd:YAG laser to clear the visual axis or reduce traction upon the retina. Much of the time, however, such vitreous abnormalities are widespread, and surgical vitrectomy is required.

VAPORIZATION OF LID TUMORS

The carbon dioxide laser has been used to bloodlessly remove both benign and malignant lid tumors. However, because of scarring, lack of a histologic specimen, and inability to assess margins, laser treatment for this purpose appears inferior to surgery in most cases.

REFRACTIVE SURGERY

The excimer lasers, particularly the 193-nm wavelength argon fluoride laser, can evaporate tissue very cleanly with almost no damage to cells adjacent to or under the cut. By using multiple pulses and progressively changing spot size to evaporate successive thin layers of the cornea, computer-controlled recontouring of the cornea (photorefractive keratectomy; PRK) can precisely and it would seem permanently correct moderate myopic and astigmatic refractive errors (Figure 24–5). Initial difficulties with superficial corneal haze appear to have been overcome. Hyperopic and highly myopic (over 6 diopters) errors do not respond as well to PRK. Many thousands of eyes have been successfully treated for myopia in Europe, Asia, and the USA. Where available, PRK has largely replaced surgical radial keratotomy, which is less predictable and which is associated with complications, such as deep scarring, ocular perforation, intraocular infection, and late hyperopic shift, that do not occur with the laser. PRK does remove Bowman's membrane, to which the corneal epithelium adheres, which can sometimes produce corneal haze. To preserve this membrane, an alternative procedure commonly known by the acronym LASIK (laser in situ keratomileusis) consists of cutting a hinged lamellar flap of cornea with a mechanical keratome, performing the refractive laser ablation in the corneal bed, and then replacing the flap. LASIK has not so far been compared with PRK in prospective controlled studies.

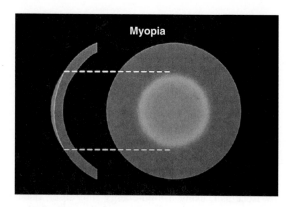

Figure 24–5. Excimer laser photorefractive keratectomy. The laser cleanly photodecomposes corneal tissue in a controlled pattern to reshape the corneal curvature. (Photo courtesy of T Clapham, VISX Inc.)

COSMETIC LASER EYELID SURGERY

Exposing wrinkled eyelid skin to repeated 1 ms pulses from the carbon dioxide laser, obtained by rapid pulsing of the laser tube or by computer-controlled rapid scanning of a continuous small laser beam, evaporates the epidermis and induces collagen contraction in the dermis. When the epithelium regenerates, the skin is tightened and small wrinkles and crow's-feet are removed. The technique is more precise than older methods such as dermabrasion or chemical peels, but it still can sometimes be complicated by keloid scarring, hyperpigmentation, and herpesvirus infection. Surgeon experience is very important in obtaining good results. The erbium:YAG laser can be used in the same manner.

LASER DIAGNOSTIC IMAGING

Confocal imaging is a video method that uses a rapidly scanning tiny laser spot whose reflected light is imaged through a pinhole upon a detector, thus suppressing all reflections except those from the focal plane. By scanning at multiple levels and then combining the images by computer processing, precise and reproducible three-dimensional images of ocular structures can be produced. The principal use of these instruments is to evaluate and follow glaucoma-induced changes in the optic nerve head, but other uses include macular, lens, and corneal imaging. Laser interferometry is used to measure blood flow in the ciliary body and retinal blood vessels. Ocular coherence tomography can produce very high resolution optical sections of the cornea and retina to allow evaluation of diseases such as corneal dystrophies and macular degeneration.

REFERENCES

Branch Vein Occlusion Study Group: Argon laser scatter photocoagulation for prevention of neovascularization and vitreous hemorrhage in branch vein occlusion: A randomized clinical trial. Arch Ophthalmol 1986;104:34.

Cioffi BA, Rovin AL, Eastman RD: Confocal laser scanning ophthalmoscope: Reproducibility of optic nerve head topographic measurements with the confocal scanning laser ophthalmoscope. Ophthalmology 1993;100:57.

Glaucoma Laser Trial Research Group: The glaucoma laser trial (GLT). 2. Results of argon laser trabeculoplasty versus topical medications. Ophthalmology 1990;97:1403.

Goldberg MF, Jampol LM: Knowledge of diabetic retinopathy before and 18 years after the Airlie House Symposium on Treatment of Diabetic Retinopathy. Ophthalmology 1988;94:741.

Klapper RM et al: Transscleral neodymium:YAG thermal cyclophotocoagulation in refractory glaucoma. Ophthalmology 1988;95:719.

Macular Photocoagulation Study Group: Argon laser photocoagulation for neovascular maculopathy: Five-year results from randomized clinical trials. Arch Ophthalmol 1991;109:1109.

Macular Photocoagulation Study Group: Laser photocoagulation of subfoveal neovascular lesions in age-related macular degeneration: Results of a randomized clinical trial. Arch Ophthalmol 1991;109:1220.

Patel A et al: Endolaser treatment of the ciliary body for uncontrolled glaucoma. Ophthalmology 1986;93:831.

Tengroth B et al: Excimer laser photorefractive keratectomy for myopia. Clinical results in sighted eyes. Ophthalmology 1993;100:739.

Wise JB: Iris sphincterotomy, iridotomy, and synechiotomy by linear incision with the argon laser. Ophthalmology 1985;92:641.

Wise JB: Low-energy linear-incision neodymium:YAG laser iridotomy versus linear-incision argon laser iridotomy. Ophthalmology 1987;94:1531.

Wise JB: Ten year results of laser trabeculoplasty. Does the laser avoid glaucoma surgery or merely defer it? Eye 1987;1:45.

Wise JB, Munnerlyn CR, Erickson PJ: A high-efficiency laser iridotomy-sphincterotomy lens. Am J Ophthalmol 1986;101:546.

Appendix I: Visual Standards

Eleanor E. Faye, MD, FACS

Standards for evaluating visual impairment have been provided for many years by the American Medical Association (AMA) in its *Guides to the Evaluation of Permanent Impairment,* also reproduced in the *Physicians' Desk Reference for Ophthalmology.* Standards are also set forth in the *International Classification of Diseases,* in sections relating to blindness and low vision.

ASSESSMENT OF VISUAL IMPAIRMENT

Three equally important criteria are used to assess visual impairment: visual acuity, visual field, and ocular motility. The percentage impairments of the three criteria are summed to produce an overall assessment of impairment of the visual system. This can then be converted to a percentage of whole-person impairment, to which 10% impairment can be added for cosmetic deformities of the eyes or orbits.

Visual Acuity

In line with improvements in test optotype design, the most acceptable charts for testing visual acuity for distance, such as the ETDRS chart (Figure 22–1), utilize the ten equally difficult block letters (D, K, R, H, V, C, N, Z, S, and O) developed by Louise L. Sloan. Also acceptable are Snellen test charts with block (sans serif) letters or numbers, illiterate E charts, or Landolt ring charts. Acceptable near vision charts have print similar to the Sloan optotypes, Revised Jaeger Standard print, or American point-type notation. Test distance is 35 cm (14 inches). Both distance and near acuity should be tested with best spectacle correction, or with contact lenses if the subject wishes.

The AMA Standards assign to acuities a percentage loss (Table 1). The percentage losses for distance and near vision are averaged to determine the overall loss of visual acuity. Allowance is also made for monocular pseudophakia or aphakia.

Visual Field

The traditional standard method of assessing visual field impairment uses kinetic perimetry, with the III4e

Table 1. AMA method of estimation of percentage loss of visual acuity.

Distance Visual Acuity	Percentage Loss	Revised Jaeger Near Visual Acuity
20/15, 20/20	0	1, 2
20/25	5	3
	7	4
20/30	10	5
20/40	15	
20/50	25	
20/60	35	
20/80	45	
20/100	50	6
	55	7
20/125	60	8
20/150	70	
20/200	80	9
20/300	85	10
20/400	90	12

stimulus of the Goldmann perimeter, to determine the full extent of the visual field of each eye. For each of eight principal meridians, the amount in degrees by which the visual field is reduced compared with a standard normal field is then calculated and an overall percentage loss is derived for each eye. The cumulative total of the maximum allowed extent of the standard normal visual field along the eight principal meridians is 500 degrees (Figure 1). Thus, the percentage visual field loss equals the total difference between the test and normal fields divided by 5. If the boundary of the visual field coincides with a principal meridian, the mean of the values of the ends of the boundary along the meridian is used. Furthermore, the extent of any scotoma lying across a meridian is deducted. Owing to the greater functional importance of inferior compared with superior field loss, the percentage field loss is further increased by 5% for inferior quadrantanopic and 10% for inferior hemianopic loss.

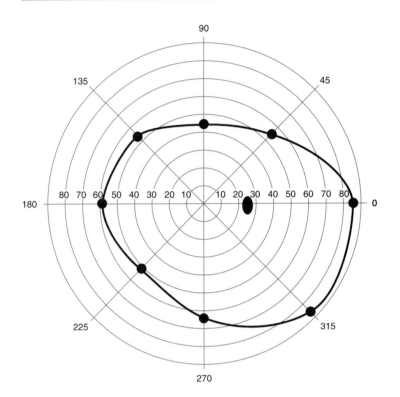

Normal Right Field	
Temporally	85°
Inferotemporally	85°
Inferiorly	65°
Inferonasally	50°
Nasally	60°
Superonasally	55°
Superiorly	45°
Superotemporally	55°
TOTAL	**500°**

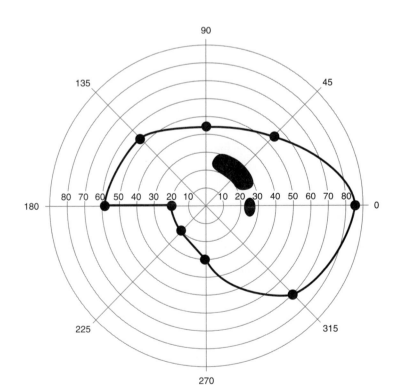

Abnormal Right Field[1]	
Temporally	85°
Inferotemporally	70°
Inferiorly	30°
Inferonasally	20°
Nasally	40°
Superonasally	55°
Superiorly	45°
Superotemporally	45°
TOTAL	**390°**

[1]Inferior nasal step and superior arcuate scotoma with 32% loss, including 10% for the inferior hemianopic field defect.

Figure 1. Quantification of monocular visual field determined by kinetic perimetry.

Ocular Motility

The extent of diplopia on ocular excursion up to 40 degrees—or, conversely, the field of binocular single vision within this area—is usually determined with a bowl (eg, Goldmann) or arc perimeter, using a III4e or equivalent target and with the subject viewing binocularly. A tangent screen can also be used. The presence or absence of diplopia at 10-degree intervals along the eight principal meridians is then determined and the meridian of maximum impairment is identified. Diplopia on excursion of less than 20 degrees is considered 100% impairment. Diplopia between 20 and 30 degrees looking upward—or upward and to either side—is 10% impairment; between 20 and 40 degrees looking laterally—or down and to either side—corresponds to 20% (20–30 degrees) or 10% (30–40 degrees) impairment. Diplopia on looking downward is functionally most disabling and thus corresponds to 50% impairment if between 20 and 30 degrees or 30% if between 30 and 40 degrees of ocular excursion.

ICD-9-DM STANDARDS

The *International Classification of Diseases* defines visual impairment as distinct from visual disability and visual handicap. **Visual impairment** is a functional limitation of the eye. **Disability** is the resulting limitation of the individual's ability to read or do close detailed work. A **visual handicap** is the impact on personal or socioeconomic independence (restricted mobility, unsuitable employment) and has been classified into various levels by the World Health Organization (Table 23–1), though definitions of blindness do still vary between countries.

VISUAL STANDARDS FOR DRIVERS' LICENCES, AIRCRAFT PILOTS, & THE ARMED SERVICES ACADEMIES

Visual standards for persons applying for drivers' licences vary between states, and some allow driving using telescopic low-vision aids. The visual standards for commercial drivers, for aircraft pilots, and for admission to service academies are listed in the *Physicians' Desk Reference for Ophthalmology*.

EDUCATION OF VISUALLY IMPAIRED CHILDREN

The education of visually impaired children has changed since passage of the Individuals with Disabilities Education Act of 1990 (IDEA—P.L. 101-476, amended by the IDEA Amendments of 1991, P.L. 102-119), which reads in part: "Each State and its public agencies must ensure that all children with specified disabilities have available to them a free appropriate public education." Because of the scattered nature of the provisions throughout the document for visually impaired children, the American Foundation for the Blind in 1993 prepared a summary of the pertinent sections. For example, subchapter II (Part B) covers special class settings and subchapter III (Part C) covers centers and services to meet unique needs.

Each child's needs must be evaluated before placement so that decisions can be made about whether to provide print or braille education, orientation and mobility, social interaction skills, career education, etc.

Placement options to be considered by a group "knowledgeable about the child" can be (1) in a regular classroom with needed support services by a special teacher in or outside of the classroom, (2) in a self-contained classroom in a regular school, or (3) in a special school with residential option.

Part B provides that a due process hearing may be initiated by the parents "when an agreement cannot be reached on important educational decisions."

REFERENCES

Guides to the Evaluation of Permanent Impairment, 4th ed. American Medical Association, 1993.

Individuals with Disabilities Act of 1990, Public Law 101-476. October 30, 1990), Title 20, U.S.C. 1400-1485: U.S. Statutes at Large, 104, 1103-1151. Washington, DC: U.S. Government Printing Office.

International Classification of Diseases (ICD-9-CM), 9th Revision, 3rd ed. Blindness and Low Vision, pp 84–85. (Order from Practice Management Information Corporation, 8330 West Third Street, Suite 200, Los Angeles, CA 90048.)

Physicians' Desk Reference for Ophthalmology, 26th ed. Medical Economics, 1998.

Appendix II: Practical Factors In Illumination

Eleanor E. Faye, MD, FACS

The physical aspects of illumination are of practical interest to the physician in evaluating the environmental setting of patients of all ages. Children in school, younger and older adults in the workplace, and the older person experience demands on their vision with little knowledge of correct illumination, often working under less than ideal circumstances.

Proper illumination increases the speed and efficiency of reading. It also encourages correct posture. Reflected glare, for example, may cause discomfort as the reader shifts position to avoid the reflection. With increasing age also comes increasing need for greater illumination to maintain reading proficiency. Corrective lenses are not the complete answer to seeing and reading at an acceptable level. Increasing the luminous intensity may be more effective than an increase in the prescription. Many eye conditions—macular degeneration, glaucoma, and diabetic retinopathy—are associated with reduced contrast sensitivity as well as acuity and may require not only magnification but increased illumination as well. Conditions that affect the optical media (corneal dystrophies, cataracts) may be worsened by increased lighting—indeed, in some cases the light source may become a glare source rather than a help.

The commonest sources of light are daylight, incandescent light (standard frosted, reflector, halogen), and fluorescent light. Daylight is composed of the entire spectrum of color; it is "white light." Incandescent light is formed by heating a tungsten filament and is the closest to the sun's spectrum. However, incandescent bulbs produce more heat than fluorescent tubes, which may become a safety issue particularly with halogen lamps. With high-efficacy fluorescent tubes coated with halophosphors (cool white), there are peaks particularly in the blue-violet range that may increase scatter and therefore glare unless the lamp is designed to reduce the blue and fill in with warmer red and yellow (warm white, yellow). The new compact bent or folded fluorescent lamps are coated with rare earth phosphors with greater efficacy and improved color rendering. A 15-watt compact lamp may produce as much as 75 watts of light energy.

DEFINITIONS RELATED TO ILLUMINATION

Color rendering: The effect of the light from the light source on the color of objects.

Color temperature: Indicates the hue of light (how white it looks). Incandescent lamps have low color temperature; sunlight has a high temperature.

Luminous efficacy: The luminous efficacy of a lamp is expressed in lumens per watt (lm/W). The fluorescent lamp is more efficient than the incandescent lamp.

Luminous intensity: The amount of light falling on a surface expressed in lux. For example, an 80 lux source for reading would be inefficient, whereas 500 lux would be efficient for reading and for desk or bench work.

Luminance: The light reflected from an area expressed in candelas per square meter (cd/m^2).

CHOOSING LAMPS

The basic requirement of any light source is that it be appropriate for the task. The wattage, color temperature, and luminous intensity are important considerations. The style of the luminaire (fixture), its placement, the shade, and the type of lamp (bulb) all have to be considered. Since intensity is inversely proportionate to the square of the distance from the light source, a reading luminaire should be flexible (gooseneck, spring arm) so that the source may be placed at the optimal distance from the task. The shade should be opaque for minimal lateral dispersion of light and maximum concentration on the area of the task. An incandescent flood bulb of 50 or 75 watts provides double the illumination of a standard incandescent bulb for the wattage; for example, a 50-watt reflector bulb provides 100 watts of energy. This lamp is therefore cooler than the nonreflector type.

There is a relationship between aging and light requirement. As long as accommodation is normal—up to the mid 40s—light intensity is not crucial to reading efficiency. After the onset of presbyopia, however, reading glasses must be augmented with stronger light. A rule of thumb is that a postpresbyope needs 1% more light each year.

CONTRAST

Contrast is another important factor in efficient reading. Highest contrast is achieved by black letters on a white background. Color contrast is also important in visibility of print. There are standards of color contrast that should be observed by all printers of pamphlets, brochures, and advertisements. One of the guidelines is to exaggerate differences between foreground and background colors. Another is to avoid using contrasting hues from adjacent colors of the hue spectrum—eg, a bad choice is orange against yellow rather than blue against yellow. As the normal eye ages, color discrimination is reduced, particularly if the lens has become yellow or amber, blocking some of the blue light rays: yellow may appear white or beige; blue may appear dark, almost black; and pale blue may appear aqua.

SOME FACTORS IN LIGHTING SELECTION

Younger children and young people in general do not specifically need bright light to read or perform tasks. The comfort factor, however, indicates that as a rule, incandescent lamps are best. Fluorescent light may cause glare unless it is modified with a warm white lamp or a tube with a higher proportion of red and yellow. An incandescent desk light can reduce the discomfort of fluorescent ceiling fixtures. In general, accent lighting should not be a glare source, and indirect lighting is best for ambient light. Halls and stairs should be well-lighted. And daylight is the best light, particularly when used in conjunction with artificial light sources.

REFERENCES

Arditi A, Knoblauch K: *Color Contrast and Partial Sight.* The Lighthouse, Inc,1997.
Florentine FA et al: Museum and Art Gallery Lighting: A Recommended Practice. Transaction of the Illuminating Engineering Society of America, 1996.
Lampi E: The sources of light and lighting at work. Presented at Ergophthalmology Symposium, Tempere, Finland, 1983. Acta Ophthalmologica 1984;191(Suppl):66.
Rosenberg R: (1984) Light, glare , and contrast in low vision care. In: *Clinical Low Vision,* 2nd ed. Faye EE (editor). Little, Brown, 1984.

Appendix III: Resources for Special Services for the Blind & Visually Impaired

Eleanor E. Faye, MD, FACS

Physicians and staff caring for blind and visually impaired individuals should be familiar with the many services and programs available from local, state, and national organizations. Video and computer technology has made an enormous difference in education of blind and low-vision students. The availability of information through websites has changed the way basic information is transmitted for everyone. Although braille is still useful for teaching blind children how the printed page is formatted and for personal tasks such as marking clothing, taking notes, and making checkbook entries, in competitive employment the voice output computer and scanner fill the gap in performance. Large print and low vision magnifying devices allow a person with useful residual vision to read.

The largest and most up-to-date database for information related to blindness and low vision is maintained by The Lighthouse at 111 East 59th Street, New York, NY 10022. The Lighthouse Information & Resource Service, which provides current names, addresses, and contact numbers from on-site files as well having the capacity to locate other information sources, can be reached at 1-800-334-5497, Fax: 212-821-9705, TTY: 212-821-9713, or website: www.lighthouse.org.

INFORMATION SOURCES AVAILABLE FROM THE LIGHTHOUSE

Fifty State Commissions for the Blind and Visually Impaired. Information can then be requested directly from the state for specific subjects such as state schools for the blind, libraries, special education programs, Americans with Disabilities Act (1990) information, low vision services, reader services, rehabilitation services, vocational services, social services, and funding.

Local agencies for the blind and visually impaired throughout the United States. Information can be obtained directly from the agency.

Location of low vision services and low vision specialists around the United States and abroad.

Information in the files on a variety of eye disorders and medically related conditions

Pamphlets on specific eye diseases, requests for resource information, individualized answers to questions about ocular and related conditions. Access to the major eye resource organizations such as the National Eye Institute (research, pamphlets), American Academy of Ophthalmology (informational material about eye conditions and treatment), American Academy of Optometry (informational pamphlets about many eye conditions).

Guide dog organizations around the United States.

Recordings for the Blind, including Choice, Library of Congress, Reader's Digest, and Recording for the Blind, Inc.

Printed and recorded material from American Printing House for the Blind, Howe Press of Perkins School for the Blind, Library of Congress, Reader's Digest, large print publications.

Home study courses, braille from The Hadley School for the Blind.

Information specifically for blind people from the American Foundation for the Blind as well as various sources for braille material, textbooks on low vision, mobility, education of visually impaired children, and rehabilitation of visually impaired persons.

Consumer catalogs for products for the blind and visually impaired.

Veterans Blind Rehabilitation Centers throughout the United States. Get information on available programs, funding, and transportation directly from the center.

Statistics on blindness and low vision.

Printouts and detailed information on the latest high-tech computer and closed-circuit television models.

SELECTED NATIONAL AGENCIES & ORGANIZATIONS

Administration on Aging. U.S. Department of Health and Human Services, 300 Independence Avenue S.W., Washington, DC 20201; 202-245-0724.

American Association of Retired Persons (AARP), 1909 K Street, N.W., Washington, DC 20049; 202-872-4700.

Association for Macular Diseases, 210 East 64th Street, New York, NY 10021; 212-605-3719.

Center for Independent Living (CIL) Publications and Audio Books for People Who Are Visually Impaired Home Page hftp://www.cilpubs.com.

Descriptive Video Service, WGBH-TV, 125 Western Avenue, Boston, MA 02134; 617-492-2777. (Monthly catalogue of programs that carry descriptions for the visually impaired.)

Library of Congress, National Library Service for the Blind and Physically Handicapped, 1291 Taylor Street, N.W., Washington, DC 20542; 800-424-9100 or 202-287-5100.

Glossary of Terms Relating to the Eye*

Accommodation: The adjustment of the eye for seeing at near distances, accomplished by changing the shape of the lens through action of the ciliary muscle, thus focusing a clear image on the retina.

Agnosia: Inability to recognize common objects despite an intact visual apparatus.

Albinism: A hereditary deficiency of melanin pigment in the retinal pigment epithelium, iris, and choroid.

Amaurosis fugax: Transient loss of vision.

Amblyopia: Reduced visual acuity (uncorrectable with lenses) in the absence of detectable anatomic defect in the eye or visual pathways.

Ametropia: See Refractive error.

Amsler grid: A chart with vertical and horizontal lines used for testing the central visual field.

Angiography: A diagnostic test in which the vascular system is examined. The ocular circulation can be highlighted by intravenous injection of either fluorescein, which particularly demonstrates the retinal circulation, or indocyanine green, to demonstrate the choroidal circulation.

Aniridia: Congenital absence of the iris.

Aniseikonia: A condition in which the image seen by one eye differs in size or shape from that seen by the other.

Anisocoria: Unequal pupillary size.

Anisometropia: Difference in refractive error of the eyes.

Anophthalmos: Absence of a true eyeball.

Anterior chamber: Space filled with aqueous bounded anteriorly by the cornea and posteriorly by the iris.

Aphakia: Absence of the crystalline lens.

Aqueous: Clear, watery fluid that fills the anterior and posterior chambers.

Asthenopia: Eye fatigue from muscular, environmental, or psychologic causes.

Astigmatism: Refractive error that prevents the light rays from coming to a point focus on the retina because of different degrees of refraction in the various meridians of the cornea or crystalline lens.

Axis: The meridian specifying the orientation of a cylindric lens.

Binocular vision: Ability of the eyes to focus on one object and then to fuse two images into one.

Biomicroscope: See Slitlamp.

Bitot's spots: Keratinization of the bulbar conjunctiva near the limbus, resulting in a raised spot—a feature of vitamin A deficiency.

Blepharitis: Inflammation of the eyelids.

Blepharoptosis: Drooping of the eyelid.

Blepharospasm: Involuntary spasm of the lids.

Blind spot: "Blank" area in the visual field, corresponding to the light rays that come to a focus on the optic nerve.

Blindness: In the USA, the usual definition of blindness is corrected visual acuity of 20/200 or less in the better eye, or a visual field of no more than 20 degrees in the better eye.

Botulinum toxin: Neurotoxin A of the bacterium *Clostridium botulinum* used in very small doses to produce temporary paralysis of the extraocular or facial muscles.

Buphthalmos: Large eyeball in infantile glaucoma.

Canal of Schlemm: A circular modified venous structure in the anterior chamber angle that drains aqueous to the aqueous veins.

Canaliculus: Small tear drainage tube in inner aspect of upper and lower lids leading from the punctum to the common canaliculus and then to the tear sac.

Canthotomy: Usually implies lateral canthotomy—cutting of the lateral canthal tendon for the purpose of widening the palpebral fissure.

Canthus: The angle at either end of the eyelid aperture; specified as outer and inner.

Cataract: An opacity of the crystalline lens.

Cataract extraction: Removal of a cataract, either by removal of the lens complete with its capsule (intracapsular cataract extraction), or by removal of the lens contents after opening the capsule (extracapsular cataract extraction).

Chalazion: Granulomatous inflammation of a meibomian gland.

Chemosis: Conjunctival edema.

Choroid: The vascular middle coat between the retina and sclera.

Ciliary body: Portion of the uveal tract between the iris and the choroid. It consists of ciliary processes and the ciliary muscle.

Coloboma: Congenital cleft due to the failure of some portion of the eye or ocular adnexa to complete growth.

Color blindness: Diminished ability to perceive differences in color.

Concave lens: Lens having the power to diverge rays of light; also known as diverging, reducing, negative, or minus lens, denoted by the sign (–), used to correct myopia.

---

* See also Definitions of Strabismus, Chapter 12, and Glossary of Genetic Terms, Chapter 18.

Cones and rods: Two kinds of retinal receptor cells. Cones are concerned with visual acuity and color discrimination; rods, with peripheral vision under decreased illumination.

Conjunctiva: Mucous membrane that lines the posterior aspect of the eyelids and covers the anterior sclera.

Convergence: The process of directing the visual axes of the eyes to a near point.

Convex lens: Lens having power to converge rays of light and to bring them to a focus; also known as converging, magnifying, or plus lens, denoted by the sign (+), used to correct hyperopia or presbyopia.

Cornea: Transparent portion of the outer coat of the eyeball forming the anterior wall of the anterior chamber.

Corneal contact lenses: Thin lenses that fit directly on the cornea.

Corneal graft (keratoplasty): Operation to restore vision by replacing a section of opaque cornea with transparent cornea, either involving the full thickness of the cornea (penetrating keratoplasty) or only a superficial layer (lamellar keratoplasty). The donor cornea may be from the same human (autograft), another human (homograft), or another species (heterograft).

Cover test A method of determining the presence and degree of phoria or tropia by covering one eye with an opaque object, thus eliminating fusion.

Cross cylinder: A specialized spherocylindrical lens used to measure astigmatism.

Crystalline lens: A transparent biconvex structure suspended in the eyeball between the aqueous and the vitreous. Its function is to bring rays of light to a focus on the retina. Accommodation is produced by variations in the magnitude of this effect. (Now usually called simply the lens.)

Cyclodestructive procedures: Surgical techniques to reduce aqueous production by destroying portions of the ciliary body in the treatment of intractable glaucoma, using cryotherapy (cyclocryotherapy), lasers (cyclophotocoagulation), or diathermy.

Cycloplegic: A drug that temporarily puts the ciliary muscle at rest, paralyzing accommodation.

Cylindrical lens: A segment of a cylinder the refractive power of which varies in different meridians, used to correct astigmatism.

Dacryocystitis: Infection of the lacrimal sac.

Dacryocystorhinostomy: A procedure by which a communication is made between the nasolacrimal duct and the nasal cavity to relieve an obstruction in the nasolacrimal duct, or sac.

Dark adaptation. The ability to adjust to decreased illumination.

Diopter: Unit of measurement of refractive power of lenses.

Diplopia: Seeing one object as two.

"E" test: A system of testing visual acuity in illiterates, particularly preschool children.

Ectropion: Turning out of the eyelid.

Emmetropia: Absence of refractive error.

Endolaser: Application of laser from a probe inserted into the globe.

Endophthalmitis: Extensive intraocular infection.

Enophthalmos: Abnormal retrodisplacement of the eyeball.

Entropion: A turning inward of the eyelid.

Enucleation: Complete surgical removal of the eyeball.

Epicanthus: Congenital skin fold that overlies the inner canthus.

Epiphora: Tearing.

Esophoria: A tendency of the eyes to be convergent.

Esotropia: A manifest inward deviation of one eye.

Evisceration: Removal of the contents of the eyeball.

Exenteration: Removal of the entire contents of the orbit, including the eyeball and lids.

Exophoria: A tendency of the eyes to be divergent.

Exophthalmos: Abnormal protrusion of the eyeball.

Exotropia: A manifest outward deviation of one eye.

Far point: The point at which the eye is focused when accommodation is completely relaxed.

Farsightedness: See Hyperopia.

Field of vision: The entire area that can be seen without shifting the gaze.

Floaters: Moving images in the visual field due to vitreous opacities.

Focus: A point to which rays of light are brought together to form an image; focal distance is the distance between a lens and its focal point.

Fornix: The junction of the palpebral and bulbar conjunctiva.

Fovea: Depression in the macula adapted for most acute vision.

Fundus: The posterior portion of the eye visible through an ophthalmoscope.

Fusion: Coordinating the images received by the two eyes into one image.

Glaucoma: Disease characterized by abnormally increased intraocular pressure, optic atrophy, and loss of visual field.

Gonioscopy: A technique of examining the anterior chamber angle, utilizing a corneal contact lens, magnifying device, and light source.

Hemianopia: Blindness in one-half of the field of vision of one or both eyes.

Heterophoria (phoria): A tendency of the eyes to be misaligned.

Heterotropia: See Strabismus.

Hippus: Exaggerated spontaneous rhythmic movements of the iris.

Hordeolum, external (sty): Infection of the glands of Moll or Zeis.

Hordeolum, internal: Meibomian gland infection.

Hyperopia, hypermetropia (farsightedness): A refractive error in which the focus of light rays from a distant object is behind the retina.

Hyperphoria: A tendency of one eye to deviate upward.

Hypertropia: A manifest upward deviation of one eye in relation to the other.

Hyphema: Blood in the anterior chamber.

Hypopyon: Pus in the anterior chamber.

Hypotony: Abnormally soft eye from any cause.

Injection: Congestion of blood vessels.

Iris: Colored, annular membrane, suspended behind the cornea and immediately in front of the lens.

Ishihara color plates: A test for color vision based on the ability to see patterns in a series of multicolored charts.

Isopter: An object for testing visual fields. Isopters can be of different colors and sizes so as to differentiate relative visual field defects from absolute defects.

Jaeger test: A test for near vision using lines of various sizes of type.

Keratic precipitate (KP): Accumulation of inflammatory cells on the posterior cornea in uveitis.

Keratitis: Inflammation of the cornea.

Keratoconus: Cone-shaped deformity of the cornea.

Keratomalacia: Corneal softening, usually associated with avitaminosis A.

Keratometer: An instrument for measuring the curvature of the cornea, used in fitting contact lenses.

Keratopathy, bullous: Swelling of the cornea with painful blisters in the epithelium due to excessive corneal hydration.

Keratoplasty: See Corneal graft.

Keratoprosthesis: Plastic implant surgically placed in an opaque cornea to achieve an area of optical clarity.

Keratotomy: An incision in the cornea. Radial keratotomy is a procedure in which radial incisions are made in the cornea to correct myopia.

Koeppe nodule: Accumulation of inflammatory cells on the iris in uveitis.

Lacrimal sac: The dilated area at the junction of the nasolacrimal duct and the canaliculi.

Lens: A refractive medium having one or both surfaces curved. (See also Crystalline lens.)

Limbus: Junction of the cornea and sclera.

Macula lutea: The small avascular area of the retina surrounding the fovea, containing yellow xanthophyll pigment.

Maddox rod: A red lens composed of parallel series of strong cylinders through which a point of light is viewed as a red line—used to measure phorias.

Magnification: The ratio of the size of an image to the size of its object.

Megalocornea: Abnormally large cornea (> 13 mm in diameter).

Metamorphopsia: Wavy distortion of vision.

Microphthalmos: Abnormally small eye with abnormal function (see Nanophthalmos).

Miotic: A drug causing pupillary constriction.

Mydriatic: A drug causing pupillary dilation.

Myopia (nearsightedness): A refractive error in which the focus for light rays from a distant object is anterior to the retina.

Nanophthalmos: Abnormally small eye with normal function (see Microphthalmos).

Near point: The point at which the eye is focused when accommodation is fully active.

Nearsightedness: See Myopia.

Nystagmus: An involuntary oscillation of the eyeball that may be horizontal, vertical, torsional, or mixed.

Ophthalmia neonatorum: Conjunctivitis in the newborn.

Ophthalmoscope: An instrument with a special illumination system for viewing the inner eye, particularly the retina and associated structures.

Optic atrophy: Optic nerve degeneration.

Optic disk: Ophthalmoscopically visible portion of the optic nerve.

Optic nerve: The nerve that carries visual impulses from the retina to the brain.

Orbital cellulitis: Inflammation of the tissues surrounding the eye.

Orthoptics: The study and treatment of defects of binocular visual function or of the muscles controlling movement of the eyeballs.

Oscillopsia: The subjective illusion of movement of objects that occurs with some types of nystagmus.

Palpebral: Pertaining to the eyelid.

Pannus: Infiltration of the cornea with blood vessels.

Panophthalmitis: Inflammation of the entire eyeball.

Papilledema: Swelling of the optic disk due to raised intracranial pressure.

Papillitis: Optic nerve head inflammation.

Partially seeing child: For educational purposes, a partially seeing child is one who has a corrected visual acuity of 20/70 or less in the better eye.

Perimeter: An instrument for measuring the field of vision.

Peripheral vision: Ability to perceive the presence, motion, or color of objects outside of the direct line of vision.

Phacoemulsification and phacofragmentation: Techniques of extracapsular cataract extraction in which the nucleus of the lens is disrupted into small fragments by ultrasonic vibrations, thus allowing aspiration of all the lens matter through a small wound.

Phakomatoses: A group of hereditary diseases characterized by the presence of spots, cysts, and tumors in various parts of the body—eg, neurofibromatosis, Von Hippel-Lindau disease, tuberous sclerosis.

Phlyctenule: Localized lymphocytic infiltration of the conjunctiva.

Phoria: See Heterophoria.

Photocoagulation: Thermal damage to tissues due to absorption of high levels of light (including laser) energy.

Photodecomposition: Tissue damage by direct separation of chemical bonds by absorption of very short wavelength ultraviolet light (eg, from excimer lasers).

Photodisruption: Tissue damage produced by the breakdown of "plasma," which is a state of ionization created by spot focusing a high-energy laser source (eg, neodymium:YAG).

Photophobia: Abnormal sensitivity to light.

Photopsia: Appearance of sparks or flashes within the eye due to retinal irritation.

Phthisis bulbi: Atrophy of the eyeball with blindness and decreased intraocular pressure, due to end-stage intraocular disease.

Placido's disk: A disk with concentric rings used to determine the regularity of the cornea by observing the ring's reflection on the corneal surface.

Poliosis: Depigmentation of the eyelashes.

Posterior chamber: Space filled with aqueous anterior to the lens and posterior to the iris.

Presbyopia ("old sight"): Physiologically blurred near vision, commonly evident soon after age 40, due to reduction in the power of accommodation.

Prism: A wedge of transparent material that deviates light rays without changing their focus.

Prism diopter: The unit of prism power.

Pseudoisochromatic charts: Charts with colored dots of various hues and shades forming numbers, letters, or patterns, used for testing color discrimination.

Pseudophakia: Presence of an artificial intraocular lens implant following cataract extraction.

Pterygium: A triangular growth of tissue that extends from the conjunctiva over the cornea.

Ptosis: Drooping of the eyelid.

Puncta: External orifices of the upper and lower canaliculi.

Pupil: The round hole in the center of the iris that corresponds to the lens aperture in a camera.

Refraction: (1) Deviation in the course of rays of light in passing from one transparent medium into another of different density. (2) Determination of refractive errors of the eye and correction by lenses.

Refractive error (ametropia): An optical defect that prevents light rays from being brought to a single focus on the retina.

Refractive index: The ratio of the speed of light in a vacuum to the speed of light in a given material.

Refractive keratoplasty: Surgery of the cornea to correct refractive errors.

Refractive media: The transparent parts of the eye having refractive power.

Retina: Innermost coat of the eye, consisting of the sensory retina, which is composed of light-sensitive neural elements connecting to other neural cells, and the retinal pigment epithelium.

Retinal detachment: A separation of the neurosensory retina from the pigment epithelium and choroid.

Retinitis pigmentosa: A hereditary degeneration of the retina.

Retinoscope: An instrument specially designed for refracting an eye objectively.

Rods: See Cones and rods.

Sclera: The white part of the eye—a tough covering that, with the cornea, forms the external protective coat of the eye.

Scleral spur: The protrusion of sclera into the anterior chamber angle.

Scotoma: A blind or partially blind area in the visual field.

Slitlamp: A combination light and microscope for examination of the eye.

Snellen chart: Used for testing central visual acuity. It consists of lines of letters or numbers, in graded sizes drawn to Snellen measurements.

Sphincterotomy: A surgical incision of the iris sphincter muscle.

Staphyloma: A thinned part of the coat of the eye, causing protrusion.

Strabismus (heterotropia, tropia): Misalignment of the eyes.

Sty: See Hordeolum, external.

Symblepharon: Adhesions between the bulbar and palpebral conjunctiva.

Sympathetic ophthalmia: Inflammation in both eyes following trauma.

Synechia: Adhesion of the iris to the cornea (anterior synechia) or lens (posterior synechia).

Syneresis: A degenerative process within a gel, involving a drawing together of particles of the dispersed medium, separation of the medium, and shrinkage of the gel. Specifically applied to the vitreous.

Tarsorrhaphy: A surgical procedure by which the upper and lower lid margins are united.

Tonometer: An instrument for measuring intraocular pressure.

Trabeculectomy: Surgical procedure for creating an additional aqueous drainage channel in the treatment of glaucoma.

Trabeculoplasty: Laser photocoagulation of the trabecular meshwork in the treatment of open-angle glaucoma.

Trachoma: A serious form of infectious keratoconjunctivitis.

Trichiasis: Inversion and rubbing of the eyelashes against the globe.

Tropia: See Strabismus.

Uvea (uveal tract): The iris, ciliary body, and choroid.

Uveitis: Inflammation of one or all portions of the uveal tract.

Visual acuity: Measure of the optical resolution of the eye.

Visual axis: An imaginary line that connects a point in space (point of fixation) with the fovea centralis.

Vitiligo: Localized patchy decrease or absence of pigment on the skin.

Vitreous: Transparent, colorless mass of soft, gelatinous material filling the eyeball behind the crystalline lens.

Xerosis: Drying of tissues lining the anterior surface of the eye.

Zonule: The numerous fine tissue strands that stretch from the ciliary processes to the crystalline lens equator (360 degrees) and hold the lens in place.

Zonulolysis: Lysis of the zonule, as with chymotrypsin, to facilitate removal of the lens in intracapsular cataract surgery.

INDEX